Atlas of Clinical
DERMATOLOGY

Atlas of Clinical
DERMATOLOGY

Anthony du Vivier MD, FRCP
Physician in Charge
The Skin Department
King's College Hospital
London, UK

Advisor on Pathology
Phillip H McKee MB BCh, BaO, MRCPath
Senior Lecturer and Honorary Consultant in Histopathology
St Thomas's Hospital Medical School
London, UK

Foreword by
Richard B Stoughton MD
Professor of Dermatology
University of California at San Diego
California, USA

W.B. Saunders Company   PHILADELPHIA • TORONTO

Gower Medical Publishing   LONDON • NEW YORK

Distributed in the USA and Canada by:
W.B. Saunders Company
West Washington Square
Philadelphia, PA 19105, USA

**Distributed in all countries except USA,
Canada & Japan by:**
Churchill Livingstone
Medical Division of Longman Group UK Limited
Robert Stevenson House
1-3 Baxter's Place
Leith Walk
Edinburgh EH1 3AF, UK

Distributed in Japan by:
Nishimura Company Ltd
1-754-39 Asahimachi-dori
Niigata-Shi 951, Japan

ISBN 0-906923-29-8 (Gower)
0-03-011443-8 (W.B. Saunders Company)

Library of Congress Catalog Card Number: 86-62028

Library of Congress Cataloging in Publication Data
is available

Project Editor: Fiona Lake

Design: Michael Laake
Mehmet Hussein

Printed in Hong Kong by South China Printing

Typeset by TNR Productions in Itek Bookface
and Helvetica Light

Foreword

This new splendid collection of colour plates of skin diseases is a welcome addition to our teaching resources in dermatology.

The only way one learns to recognize skin diseases is by seeing them. The old adage that a picture is worth a thousand words is not correct in dermatology because no quantity of words can substitute for a good colour picture of the disease.

This assemblage of 1552 colour photographs along with the informative text for each disease will be extremely useful not only for those who are in the early stages of learning the specialty of dermatology, but for trained dermatologists. Also it should be very helpful to those who are not dermatologists but want to identify the type of skin disease with which they are confronted.

The quality of the colour plates is excellent throughout and special diagrams add to the text by elucidating the nature of these skin diseases.

I was very fortunate in having Dr. du Vivier as my associate at the Scripps Clinic and Research Foundation in La Jolla, California for two years. During this time he conducted original clinical and laboratory investigations which led to the discovery of glucocorticoid tachyphylaxis in human skin and the development of useful animal models for the study of cellular proliferation in normal and diseased skin.

I am grateful to Dr. du Vivier for allowing me to present this brief foreword to his excellent book.

Richard B. Stoughton MD
Professor of Dermatology
University of California at San Diego

Preface

Skin diseases are mysterious to most non-dermatologists. This is mainly because they have not had the opportunity to learn how to interpret cutaneous physical signs and hence to make a dermatological diagnosis. Dermatology is a visual art depending largely on accurate observation and is a subject which lends itself *par excellence* to illustration. The object of this atlas is to aid the learning of the subject by providing illustrations of the common skin disorders and, where relevant, their differential diagnoses. An integrated text accompanies the photographs. This is not meant to be an exhaustive account of the skin diseases which are described but rather concentrates on their clinical aspects with the emphasis on how the diagnosis may be made.

Although common diseases are the focus of the atlas, certain rarer conditions are included where a therapeutic, diagnostic or mechanistic point needs to be made.

A. du V.
115a Harley Street,
London W1, 1986

Acknowledgements

The vast majority of the illustrations are, unless otherwise stated, of patients under the care of myself or members of the department of dermatology at King's College Hospital, London. The photographs have largely been taken by the medical illustration department of King's College Hospital or myself. The rest come from the photographic departments of the hospitals where I trained viz. St. Bartholomew's, St. Mary's and St. John's, London. I particularly wish to thank therefore Mr. E. Blewitt, Mr. D. Tredinnick, Dr. P. Cardew, Mr. B. Pike, Mr. E. Sparkes and Mr. S. Robertson and their departments for the help they have given me over the years.

I wish also to acknowledge with deep gratitude the physicians who have taught me dermatology and influenced me. They are Drs. Dowling Munro, Julian Verbov, Michael Feiwel, Richard Stoughton, Gerald Levene, Eugene van Scott, Peter Samman, Bob Marten, Professor Malcolm Greaves and the late Dr. Peter Borrie.

I am indebted to Dr. Phillip McKee for his help regarding the biology and pathology of diseases of the skin included in this atlas and to Drs. Andrew Pembroke and Jeremy Gilkes, my colleagues, for their advice and support.

I thank Mrs. Fiona Lake of Gower Medical Publishing for her great patience and editorial and creative assistance.

Finally the atlas is dedicated to my wife, Judith, who makes everything worthwhile.

All histopathology transparencies have been provided by Dr. Phillip McKee unless otherwise stated.

Contents

1 The Structure and Function of Normal Skin

Phillip H. McKee MB BCh, BaO, MRC Path

In addition to its obvious property of enveloping the body, the skin has a wide range of diverse functions including protection against injury, thermoregulation, waterproofing and fluid conservation. It is of considerable importance in the absorption of ultraviolet radiation and in the production of vitamin D; it acts as a barrier to pathogenic organisms and functions in the detection of sensory stimuli.

The .skin conveniently divides into two distinct layers, the epidermis and its appendages, derived from ectoderm, and the dermis with the underlying subcutaneous fat, derived from mesoderm. (The nerves and melanocytes are of neuroectodermal origin). The epidermis is a multilayered (stratified) squamous epithelium from which arises the pilosebaceous follicles, apocrine glands and eccrine sweat glands. The dermis consists of the ground substance plus a fibrous component (collagen and elastin).

There is considerable regional variation in skin structure and to some extent function (Figs. 1.1 & 1.2). Skin is divided into two types, glabrous and hairy. Glabrous skin (typified by a thick keratin layer) covers the surfaces of the palms and soles whilst hairy skin covers the rest of the body. Hair production is maximum about the head, the axillae and pubic regions, and on the face of males. Sebaceous glands are especially numerous about the face and nose whilst eccrine glands are most commonly found on the palms and soles. The surface of the skin is far from regular, being marked by a series of complex creases determined by the underlying epidermal ridge pattern. This is clearly demonstrated by the whorls, loops and arches that constitute fingerprints. Mucous membranes differ from skin by the absence of both granular and horny layers.

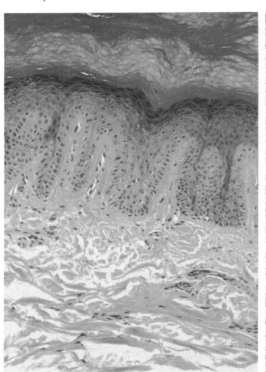
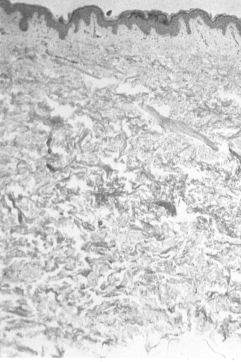

Fig. 1.1 Marked regional variations of normal skin structures as seen in sections from: (left) fingertip of young male and (right) abdomen of young female. Haematoxylin & eosin stains.

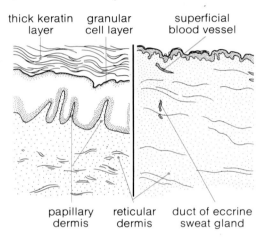

thick keratin layer — granular cell layer — superficial blood vessel

papillary dermis — reticular dermis — duct of eccrine sweat gland

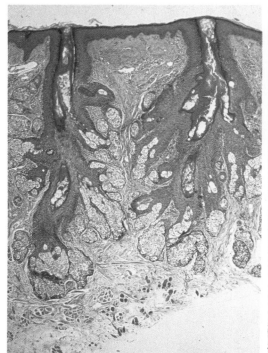
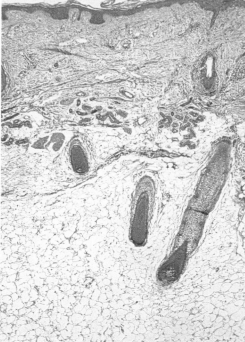

Fig. 1.2 Marked regional variations of normal skin structures as seen in sections from (left) nose of young female and (right) scalp of elderly female. H & E stains.

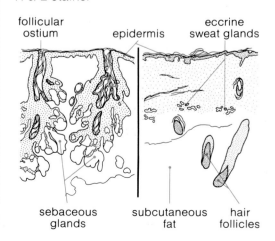

follicular ostium — epidermis — eccrine sweat glands

sebaceous glands — subcutaneous fat — hair follicles

EPIDERMIS

Histologically the epidermis consists of at least four cell types (keratinocytes, melanocytes, Merkel cells and Langerhans cells) and has four clearly defined layers, the basal cell, prickle cell, granular cell and keratin layers. A fifth layer may be interposed between the granular and keratin layers on the palms and soles. The basal cell layer is the germinative layer of the epidermis. With each division, approximately fifty percent of the daughter population contributes to the developing epidermis. It is thought that the epidermal transit time is approximately thirty days. Maturation consists of the conversion of columnar basal cells into the fully keratinized cells of the epidermal horn and involves a transformation of cellular polarity, basal cells being arranged at right angles to the basement membrane whilst the cellular residues of the keratin layer lie parallel.

These perpendicularly-orientated columnar cells have baso-philic cytoplasm and round to oval hyperchromatic nuclei and, when mature, acquire the polyhedral outline of the prickle cell layer. The acquisition of keratohyalin granules (Fig. 1.3) characterizes the granular cell layer. Further maturation leads to loss of nuclei and flattening of the cellular outline until the flattened plates of the keratin layer are fully formed. The keratinocytes are united at their free borders by intercellular bridges (desmosomes) best seen in the prickle cell layer. They are much more conspicuous in the disease states of the skin involving intercellular oedema (Fig. 1.4). The epidermis lies on a thin basement membrane, clearly visualized by periodic acid-Schiff staining (Fig. 1.5).

Under the electron microscope the basement membrane of the epidermis is no longer the homogeneous entity suggested by light microscopic examination but instead is seen to be quite a heterogeneous structure (Fig. 1.6).

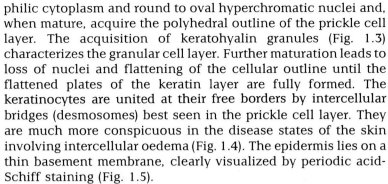

Fig. 1.3 Normal skin from the palm showing basophilic granular cell layer. H & E stain.

keratin

granular cell layer

prickle cell layer

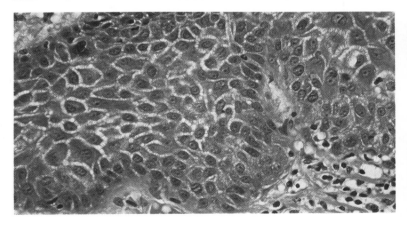

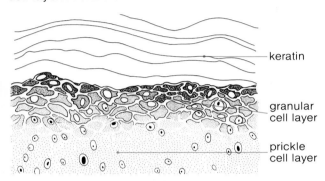

Fig. 1.4 Epidermis showing slight intercellular oedema, thus exaggerating the intercellular junctions (desmosomes). H & E stain.

Fig. 1.5 Normal skin showing purple-staining basement membrane. Periodic acid-Schiff stain.

Fig. 1.6 Basement membrane region of normal epidermis. Note conspicuous hemidesmosomes, lamina lucida and lamina densa. EM, x 20,200.

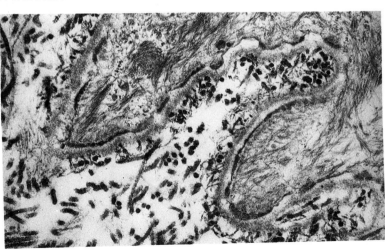

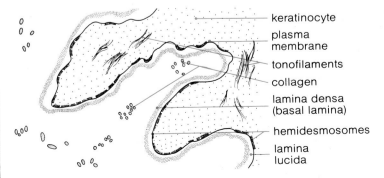

keratinocyte

plasma membrane

tonofilaments

collagen

lamina densa (basal lamina)

hemidesmosomes

lamina lucida

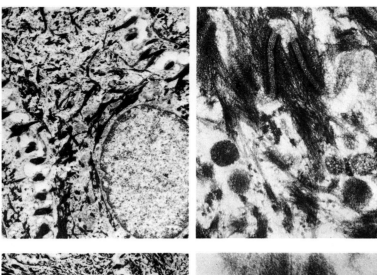

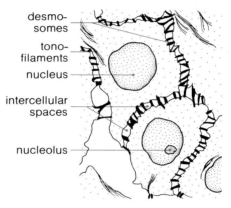

Fig. 1.7 Lower prickle cell layer of normal skin showing (left) tonofilaments and dilated intercellular spaces; (right) tonofilaments inserting into desmosomes. EMs, x 5200 (left), x 30,300 (right).

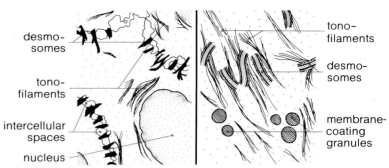

Fig. 1.8 Prickle cell layer showing conspicuous desmosomes (left); the multilayered nature of the desmosome (intercellular bridge) is clearly seen (right). EMs, x 2200 (left), x 71,000 (right).

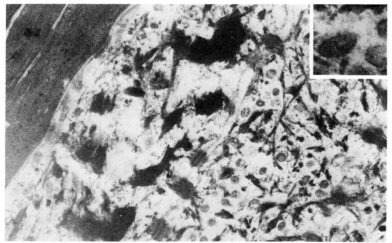

Fig. 1.9 Keratohyalin and membrane-coating granules are present in the granular cell layer; the lamellated structure of membrane-coating granules is seen (inset). EM, x 17,500, (inset) x 48,000.

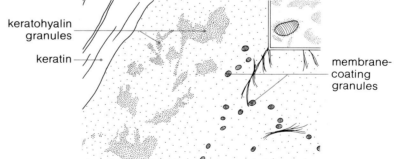

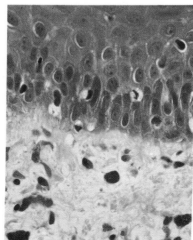
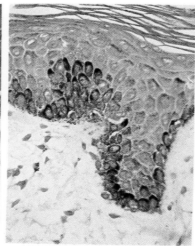

Fig. 1.10 Melanocytes appear as clear cells in the basal layer of the epidermis. Pigment is abundant in this section of skin from a black African (left). Positive staining of melanin pigment in a biopsy of simple lentigo from a young female (right). H & E (left), Masson-Fontanna (right) stains.

Hemidesmosomes are seen at intervals along the basal cell plasma membrane and, beneath this, a clear zone intervenes before the electron-dense lamina densa (basal lamina). Anchoring filaments adjoin the hemidesmosomes to the lamina densa and its fibrils may be seen spreading from the lamina densa into the papillary dermis. Basal cells contain tonofilaments loosely aggregated into bundles or tonofibrils while in the prickle cell layer the tonofibrils form an interlacing network occupying much of the cytoplasm (Fig. 1.7). The cytoplasmic membrane is infolded and shows numerous desmosomes (Fig. 1.8). The prickle cells also contain lamellated oval structures known as membrane-coating granules or Odland bodies, measuring 100-500nm in diameter. Covered by a double-layered membrane, they contain parallel lamellae about 20Å thick orientated along the short axis of the granule and are located particularly in the region of the plasma membrane (Fig. 1.9). In addition to the membrane-coating granules, the granular cells contain kerato-hyalin granules which are not membrane-bound and consist of closely packed amorphous particles (Fig. 1.9). The cells of the keratin layer contain tonofibrils embedded in an amorphous matrix and are characterized by a thickened cytoplasmic membrane. The intercellular spaces contain a material probably derived from the membrane-coating granules which functions as an intercellular cement.

Tonofilaments and keratohyalin granules are largely composed of protein whilst membrane-coating granules contain large amounts of lipids and hydrolytic enzymes (possibly involved in exocytosis of the granules).

Keratinization is the process of epidermal differentiation by which basal cells are converted into the protective membranous horny layer. Its exact mechanism is not fully understood but it depends on the development and interplay of the three intracellular organelles, namely tonofibrils, keratohyalin granules and membrane-coating granules.

Maturation of the epidermis involves an increase in the number of tonofibrils followed by their incorporation by the amorphous substance of the keratohyalin granules. There is some evidence suggesting that desmosomes play an important role in keratinization, possibly functioning as attachment sites for tonofilament orientation. The cells of the horny layer are cemented together to form a tough and flexible membrane, the superficial aspect of which is continuously being shed as large clusters of squames. The keratin layer prevents the loss of body fluids and influx of water into the skin by means of lipid deposits between the horny cells. The strength and integrity of the horny layer is believed to be due to the presence of disulphide bonds between adjacent keratin molecules.

Melanocytes

These cells are derived from the neural crest and are found only along the basal layers of the epidermis. They appear as clear cells on haematoxylin and eosin staining (Fig. 1.10, left). Melanin is readily identified by silver techniques such as the Masson-Fontanna reaction (Fig. 1.10, right) or by the dopa reaction. The ratio of melanocytes to basal cells varies considerably, 1:4 in the cheek to 1:10 in the arms. Melanocytes are dendritic cells and the melanin granules are transferred along the dendritic processes to adjacent keratinocytes where they are actively phagocytosed. In addition to skin and hair colouration, melanin pigment is of extreme importance as protection against the injurious properties of ultraviolet radiation. Electron-microscopically the melanocyte is characterized by pale cytoplasm and an absence of both tonofilaments and desmosomes (Fig. 1.11) but with the presence of electron-dense melanosomes. These tyrosinase-containing granules, believed to be formed in the Golgi apparatus, have an oval structure measuring about 400nm in its greatest dimension. Partially developed melanosomes show a lamellated internal structure (Fig. 1.12) which is obscured by a pigment production in the mature granule. The quantity of melanin determines colouration; the degree of skin colour is dependent upon the total number, size and distribution of melanin granules.

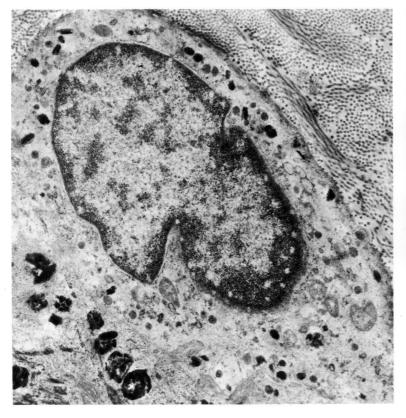

Fig. 1.11 Melanocyte typified by intracytoplasmic electron-dense melanosomes. EM, x 14,000.

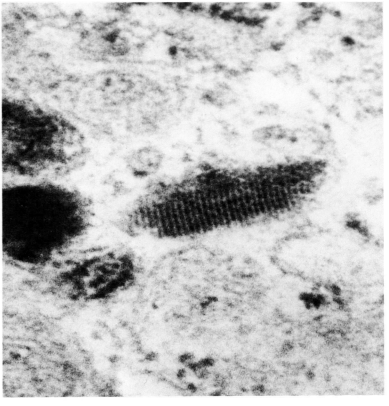

Fig. 1.12 Melanosomes from a case of malignant melanoma showing their lamellated internal structures. EM, x 200,000.

Langerhans Cells

These dendritic cells, present in the suprabasal layers of the epidermis, were first described in 1868 by Paul Langerhans, a Berlin medical student, using a gold chloride impregnation technique. They are difficult to identify with haematoxylin and eosin staining but can be demonstrated by a variety of techniques including supravital reactions with methylene blue, enzymatically by using adenosine triphosphatase and immunohistochemically by using anti-immune response-associated (anti-Ia) antibodies. Their dendritic processes extend between the keratinocytes up as far as the granular layer and down to the epidermodermal junction. Langerhans cells have also been found in the dermis. They have surface marker characteristics similar to those cells of the monocyte-macrophage series, bearing receptors for Fc-IgG and C3 and expressing Ia antigens. Electron-microscopically they can be distinguished from keratinocytes by the absence of desmosomes and tonofilaments; neither do they contain premelanosomes or individual melanosomes. The Langerhans cell typically has a lobulated nucleus (Fig. 1.13) and clear cytoplasm which contains the characteristic Langerhans granules (rod or racquet-shaped inclusions) (Fig. 1.14). As far as is known, these inclusions are quite specific for Langerhans cells.

At one time the Langerhans cell was believed to represent a worn out melanocyte but it is now thought to be a bone-marrow-derived immunocompetent cell functioning in delayed hypersensitivity and skin allograft reactions.

Merkel Cells

The Merkel cell is a distinctive, non-keratinocytic cell found in the epidermis of mammals. It is present in the basal layer of the epidermis, particularly on acral non-hairy skin, but also in association with hair follicles. Merkel cells are also found within the dermis in association with the Schwann cells of peripheral nerve endings. In the epidermis they are associated with intra-epidermal nerve endings. These cells cannot be distinguished on haematoxylin and eosin staining but their associated nerve fibres can be seen with the use of silver impregnation techniques.

The ultrastructure of the Merkel cell is distinctive. Unlike the melanocyte and the Langerhans cell, the Merkel cell is attached to adjacent keratinocytes by desmosomes but its basal cytoplasmic membrane is free from hemidesmosomes. It is typified by its clear cytoplasm, lobulated nucleus, specific granules and innervation. The granules measure 80-100nm in diameter, are membrane-bound and are located on the opposite side of the nucleus to the Golgi apparatus (Fig. 1.15). The function of these membrane-bound granules is disputed; although they resemble monoamine storage granules, at present catecholamines have not been demonstrated. The nerve associated with the Merkel cell is a myelinated fibre associated with touch reception; therefore, these cells are thought to function as slowly adapting sensory touch receptors (the Merkel disc and the tactile hair disc of Pinkus).

EPIDERMAL APPENDAGES
Sebaceous Glands

The sebaceous gland arises as a lateral protrusion of the outer root sheath of the developing hair follicle. It can be first clearly identified at the thirteenth to fifteenth week of gestation. During fetal life its secretory product, sebum, is partially responsible for the vernix caseosa, the other constituents being fetal hair and squames. Largely inactive during prepubertal life, it enlarges and becomes functionally active during and after puberty. Whilst fairly widespread in distribution they are not found on the palms or soles but are concentrated about the face and scalp, in the midline of the back and in the perineum. As can be imagined from their development they almost invariably drain into the follicular infundibulum. Exceptions do occur, however, including the Meibomian glands and Montgomery's tubercles of the areola. The largest sebaceous glands are associated with small vellus hairs in the specialized pilosebaceous units called sebaceous follicles.

The sebaceous gland is described as being holocrine in type because its secretion is dependent upon the complete degeneration of the acini. It consists of several lobules lying adjacent and connected to a hair follicle (Fig. 1.16), each lobule consisting of an outer layer of cuboidal basophilic cells from which arise the inner zone of lipid-laden vacuolated cells (Fig. 1.17). Its secretions drain into the sebaceous duct.

The mechanism of control of sebaceous activity is incompletely understood. Secretion appears to have a circadian rhythm, largely under the control of androgens and appearing to be inhibited by oestrogens. It, therefore, comes as no surprise that

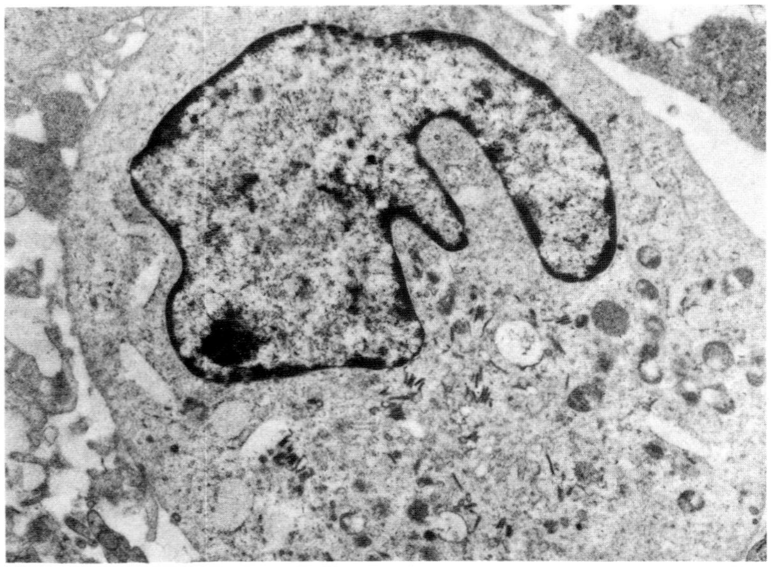

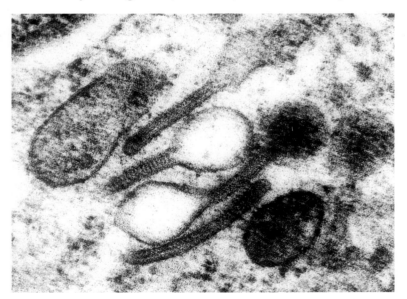

Fig. 1.13 Langerhans cell showing lobulated nucleus and clusters of Langerhans granules. EM, x 11,600.

Fig. 1.14 The 'handles' of the characteristic racquet-shaped inclusions of Langerhans cells have a trilaminar structure with cross-striations. EM, x 112,000.

male sebaceous glands are larger and more functionally active than those of females.

Sebum is an exceedingly complicated lipid mixture including triglycerides, wax esters and scalene. Its function in man, although uncertain, possibly includes waterproofing, control of epidermal water loss and a protective function inhibiting the growth of fungi and bacteria.

Apocrine Glands

Apocrine glands are found predominantly in the anogenital and axillary regions. They are derived from the epidermis and develop as an outgrowth of the follicular epithelium. Their function is unknown but in animals they are thought to be responsible for scent production. The fastidious twentieth century man might dispute this. Similar to sebaceous glands they are rather small in childhood, becoming larger and functionally active at puberty.

Apocrine glands consist of two distinct components, a secretory component situated in the lower reticular dermis or subcutaneous fat, and a tubular duct linking the gland with the pilosebaceous follicle at a site above the sebaceous duct. Microscopically the secretory portion comprises an outer layer of myoepithelial cells and an inner layer of cuboidal to columnar eosinophilic cells (Fig. 1.18). The duct portion consists of a double layer of cuboidal epithelium. The mechanism of apocrine secretion and control of apocrine glands is uncertain but they do receive adrenergic sympathetic innervation (consider the increased secretion in response to fear). The unpleasant odour of apocrine secretion which is itself odourless is due to breakdown products produced by the cutaneous bacterial flora.

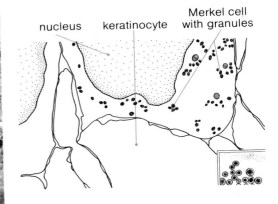

Fig. 1.15 Merkel cell typified by intracytoplasmic membrane-bound granules (inset). EM, x 16,000, (inset) x 40,000. By courtesy of Prof. A.S. Breathnach, Electron Microscopy of Cutaneous Nerves and Receptors, *The Journal of Investigative Dermatology*, **69**: 8–26, 1977; Williams & Wilkins Co.

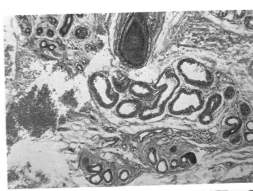

nucleus   keratinocyte   Merkel cell with granules

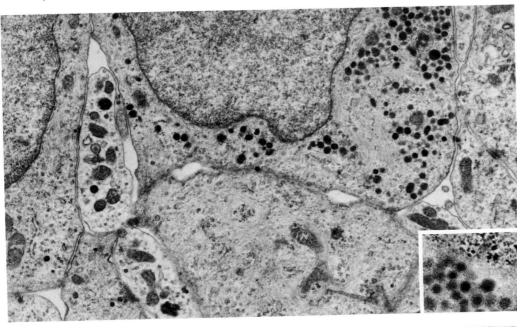

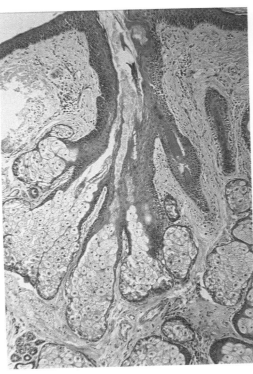

Fig. 1.16 Section from the nose showing numerous sebaceous lobules arising from a hair follicle. H & E stain.

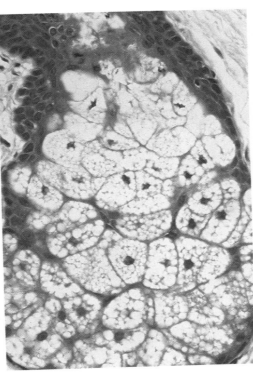

Fig. 1.17 Higher power view of sebaceous gland showing outer layer of basophilic germinative cells and inner lipid-laden mature cells. H & E stain.

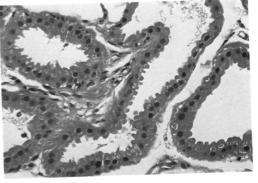

Fig. 1.18 Section from axilla showing prominent apocrine glands beneath a hair follicle (upper); higher power view showing apocrine (decapitation) secretion (lower). H & E stains.

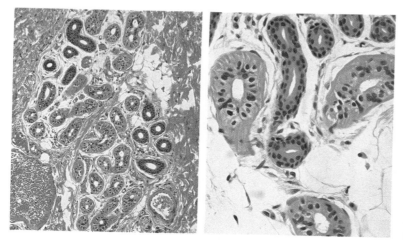

Fig. 1.19 Cross-section of normal eccrine gland with darker-staining ductal system (left); higher power view of three secretory coils amidst ducts (right). H & E stains.

Eccrine Sweat Glands

These are glands derived from a specialized downgrowth of the epidermis at about the fourth month of intrauterine life. They are found everywhere on the skin but are not present in the mucous membranes. Their sites of maximum distribution are the palms, soles, axillae and forehead. Histologically they are divided into four subunits: a coiled secretory gland; a coiled dermal duct; a straight dermal duct; and a coiled intraepidermal duct. The secretory component lies in the lower reaches of the reticular dermis or around the interface between the dermis and subcutaneous fat. It consists of an outer layer of contractile myoepithelial cells and an inner layer of secretory cells (Fig. 1.19). The latter consists of two cell types, large clear cells which appear to be responsible for its water secretions, and smaller darkly-staining mucopolysaccharide-containing cells. Between adjacent clear cells are canaliculi which open into the lumen of the tubule. The dermal duct components consist of a double layer of cuboidal basophilic cells. The duct is not just a conduit

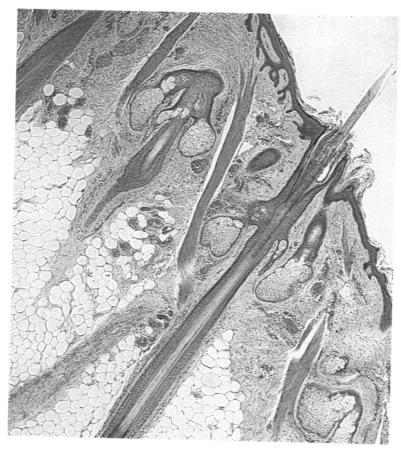

Fig. 1.20 Section of scalp showing several normal pilosebaceous units with adjacent arrector pili muscles. H & E stain. By courtesy of Dr. J.S. Dixon, University of Manchester.

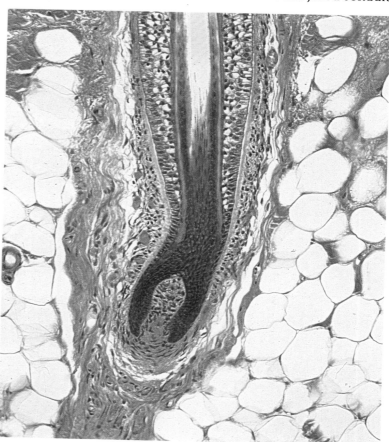

Fig. 1.21 Longitudinal section showing the various layers found in a normal hair. H & E stain. By courtesy of Dr. J.S. Dixon, University of Manchester.

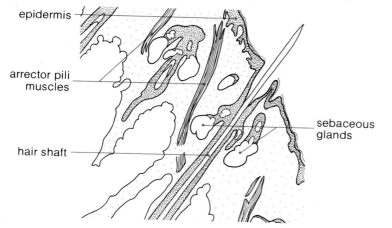

epidermis

arrector pili muscles

hair shaft

sebaceous glands

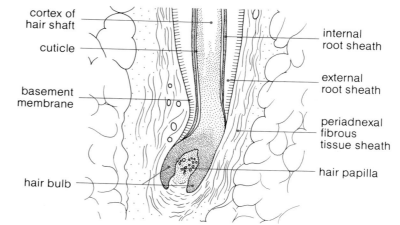

cortex of hair shaft

cuticle

basement membrane

hair bulb

internal root sheath

external root sheath

periadnexal fibrous tissue sheath

hair papilla

but has a biologically active function in modifying the composition of eccrine secretion, in particular, the reabsorption of water. The intraepidermal duct opens directly onto the surface of the skin.

Function of the eccrine gland is under the control of cholinergic postganglionic sympathetic nerve fibres. The activity of the secretory component is stimulated by thermal, mental and gustatory functions. Thermal sweating is dependent on an intact hypothalamus (activated by temperature changes of its perfusing blood). Thermoregulatory sweating occurs especially on the face and upper trunk. Mental sweating presumably is under the control of the limbic lobe. This induces particularly palmar sweating. Gustatory sweating of the lips, forehead and nose as after a hot spicy meal is of uncertain function and control. It is a particular complication of parotid gland resections.

Sweat of eccrine type has a basic similarity to the plasma from which it is derived, the duct appearing to be largely responsible for the modifications which occur. It is a clear hypotonic solution with a pH in the range of 4 to 6.8. In addition to water it contains sodium, chloride, potassium, urea and lactate.

HAIR

The hair follicle develops as an oblique or curved downgrowth of epidermal cells into the dermis or subcutaneous fat, becoming canalized to form the relatively immobile external root sheath of the hair. Proliferation of germinative cells at the base of the hair forms the inner root sheath and the hair shaft which lie within the follicular canal. In the region of the hair bulb, the external root sheath is continuous with the germinative cells of the hair matrix. Distally the enlarged hair bulb encloses the connective tissue hair papilla which is continuous with the periadnexal fibrous tissue sheath. The hair papilla is richly vascularized and contains abundant nerve endings, both myelinated and non-myelinated.

Hair covers all of the body except for the palms and soles, ventral aspects of the fingers and toes, inner aspect of the prepuce and glans penis and the inner parts of the female external genitalia.

By about the fifth to sixth month of intrauterine life the fetus is covered by a fine layer of very delicate lanugo hairs. This is lost before birth except for the scalp, the eyebrows and the eyelashes, where the hair becomes coarser and stronger. Shortly after birth a new growth of downy vellus hair covers the body of the infant. At around puberty, coarse pigmented hairs develop in the pubic and axillary regions and on the face and chest of males which are called terminal hairs. There are four main types of hair: straight, wavy, helical and spiral. Straight hair is predominantly found in the yellow or Mongoloid races, wavy hair in many races including Europeans and spiral hair in the Negroid races.

The fully developed hair has the following structure (Figs. 1.20 & 1.21). Enclosing the hair follicle is the vascular periadnexal fibrous tissue sheath which is separated from the cells of the external root sheath by a basement membrane. The external root sheath superficially consists of all layers of the epidermis whilst distal to the entrance of the sebaceous duct it consists only of the prickle cell layer. In this region the cells are markedly vacuolated due to the presence of glycogen. The germinative hair matrix cells, which give rise to all layers of the internal root sheath and hair shaft, have dark basophilic cytoplasm, large vesicular nuclei, and contain melanocytes. The internal root sheath consists of three concentric layers: Henle's layer which is one cell thick; Huxley's layer which is two cells thick; and the cuticle which consists of a layer of flattened scales. All of these cells undergo keratinization.

The shaft of the hair consists of a cuticle, a cortex and a medulla (the latter is absent from many hairs including all lanugo and vellus hairs). The cuticle consists of a single layer of flattened scales. The cortical cells undergo atypical keratinization in that keratohyalin granules are absent and the cells undergo a gradual transformation from living epidermal cells into keratin. The medulla, if present, consists of layers of polyhedral cells. The cuticle of the internal root sheath interlocks with the cuticle of the shaft so that they function as one structure during growth up the follicular canal.

The arrector pili muscle arises within the papillary dermis and passes obliquely downwards to its insertion into the perifollicular connective tissue sheath. Contraction of the arrector pili makes the hair 'stand on end' and brings on 'goose-pimples'.

Hair undergoes cyclical periods of growth divided into three phases: anagen, in which there is active hair growth; catagen, associated with involution; and telogen, the resting phase (Fig. 1.22). The cycle is variable in different regions of the body; for instance, the duration of eyelashes is about four months whilst that of scalp is about four years.

Hair colour depends on the number and type of melanosomes within the cortex of the hair shaft; thus, gray hair has a markedly diminished number of melanosomes whilst pure white hair has none at all. Blond hair has a diminished number of partially pigmented melanosomes and in red hair the melanosomes are chemically and structurally different from black hair.

The hair of mammals is of great importance in temperature conservation but in humans this function is largely subserved by the subcutaneous fat. Hair has some value as a touch receptor and is an obviously useful secondary sexual characteristic. The follicular epithelium is of immense value as a reserve of basal cells for epidermal regeneration following trauma.

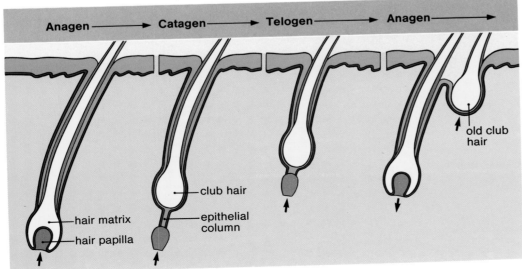

Anagen → Catagen → Telogen → Anagen

old club hair

club hair

hair matrix

epithelial column

hair papilla

Fig. 1.22 Growth cycle of hair: 1. During catagen, as the hair grows up the follicular canal its matrix is enclosed within a shortened, retracted external root sheath forming a club hair. A residual epithelial column (probably derived from both hair matrix and external root sheath) connects the club hair and the hair papilla. 2. During telogen the club hair progresses further towards the surface and the epithelial column contracts to form a nest of cells around the base of the club hair. The hair papilla also ascends to lie close to the epithelial nest. 3. With the onset of anagen a new hair matrix forms and, with the subjacent hair papilla, descends to its previous resting level. A new hair then develops which eventually dislodges the old club hair.

1.9

THE NAIL

Like hair, the nail is formed by an invagination of epidermis into dermis. The formed keratin is tough and densely adherent, rendering the nail plate a remarkably resilient structure.

Anatomically the nail consists of three distinct parts: the root, the nail plate and the free edge (Fig. 1.23). The root is overlapped by the proximal nail fold which is continuous at its margins with the lateral nail folds. Overlying the proximal portion of the nail plate is a thin cuticular fold, the eponychium, which partially or completely obscures the crescent-shaped lunula, the distal portion of the nail matrix. The lunula is usually completely visible in the thumbnail but is completely covered in the fifth nail. The undersurface of the free margin of the nail is continuous with the hyponychium, the thickened epidermis beneath it. The nail plate lies upon a richly vascularized nail bed which is continuous proximally with the nail matrix (Fig. 1.24); and the epithelia of both undergo keratinization which, like hair, occurs in the absence of a granular cell layer. The horny layers of the nail bed and the nail plate are firmly attached and forward movement of the nail plate is accompanied by forward movement of keratinized cells of the nail bed. On average, nails grow about 0.1mm per day, growth being faster in summer than in winter and fingernails growing faster than toenails.

THE DERMIS

The dermis is the supporting layer of the epidermis and consists of a fibrous component (collagen and elastin) together with the so-called ground substance. Lying within it are the epidermal appendages and the neurovasculature, and a cellular component including fibroblasts and various inflammatory cells. The dermis is divided into two layers: the papillary dermis (including a periadnexal component), and the reticular dermis. The papillary dermis is bounded superiorly by the epidermis, laterally by the epidermal ridges and inferiorly by the superficial vascular plexus and reticular dermis.

Collagen

Collagen gives the dermis its structural stability. In the papillary dermis it consists of fine fibres in haphazard arrangement whilst in the reticular dermis it consists of broad bundles lying roughly parallel to the epidermal surface (Fig. 1.25). Formed within the ribosomes of fibroblasts, the essential subunit of collagen is the monomer tropocollagen, which has a molecular weight of approximately 300,000 and is composed of 3 peptide chains. Each chain has a helical structure and the three chains are intertwined to form a superhelical molecule. The structural stability of collagen is increased by intra- and inter-molecular

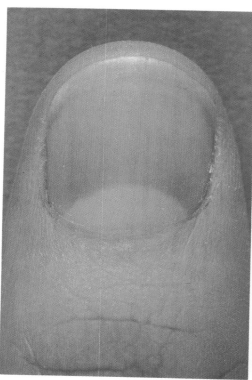

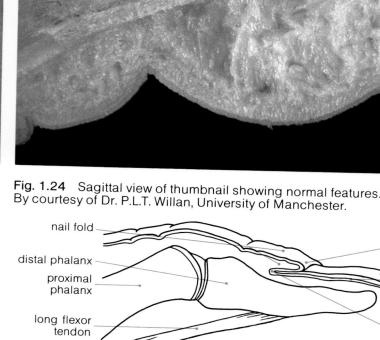

Fig. 1.23 Macroscopic view of thumbnail showing normal features.

Fig. 1.24 Sagittal view of thumbnail showing normal features. By courtesy of Dr. P.L.T. Willan, University of Manchester.

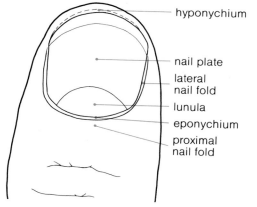

cross-linkages, the latter including side-to-side, end-to-end and overlapping types. This produces an enormously strong fibrillary structure. Collagen characteristically contains the amino acids hydroxyproline and hydroxylysine.

Collagen is not a homogeneous entity but consists of a variety of genetically distinct subtypes, designated Types I, II, III and IV according to morphology, amino acid composition and physical properties. In the dermis the broad bands of reticular collagen are Type I, the most common form, whilst the finer fibres (also known as reticulin) of the papillary dermis are Type III. When longitudinal sections of collagen are examined electronmicroscopically they exhibit cross-striations (Fig. 1.26) with a periodicity of approximately 64nm.

Elastic Tissue

Elastic fibres are intimately associated with collagen. They cannot be identified with haematoxylin and eosin staining but are easily demonstrated by a number of special stains such as elastic-van Gieson stain. In the papillary dermis the elastic fibres are thin and tend to run at right angles to the skin surface whilst those in the reticular dermis are thicker and tend to lie parallel to the skin surface (Fig. 1.27). Like collagen, elastic fibres are produced by fibroblasts. Ultrastructural examination shows elastic tissue to consist of an amorphous electron-dense component (elastin) in which are embedded microfibrils (Fig. 1.28). Elastic tissue characteristically contains the amino acids desmosine and isodesmosine. Whilst elastic fibres are responsible for cutaneous elasticity, they are also thought (in combination with ground substance) to be responsible for prevention of overextension.

Ground Substance

This is another product of fibroblasts and accounts for a large proportion of the volume of the dermis but cannot be visualized with routine stains, special stains such as alcian blue being necessary. Ground substance is not merely an amorphous material in which the fibrous components are embedded but can best be visualized as a gel-like substance existing in intimate chemical relationship with the fibrous components of the dermis. In addition to large quantities of water, it consists of glycosaminoglycans, hyaluronic acid, chondroitin-4-sulphate and dermatan sulphate.

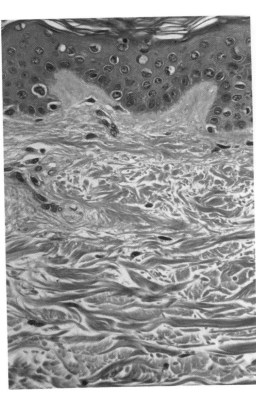

Fig. 1.25 High power view of normal skin showing broad bands of collagen in the reticular dermis. Masson's trichrome stain.

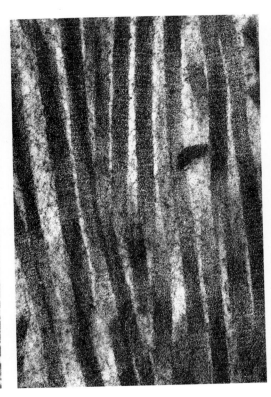

Fig. 1.26 Collagen showing typical cross-striations. EM, x 47,000.

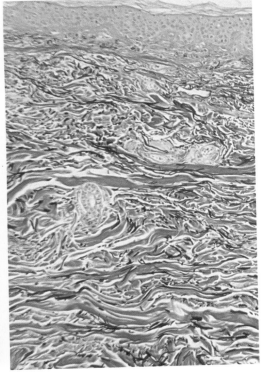

Fig. 1.27 Paucity of elastic fibres in the papillary dermis contrasts with their abundance in the reticular dermis. Elastic-van Gieson stain.

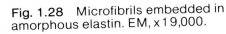

Fig. 1.28 Microfibrils embedded in amorphous elastin. EM, x 19,000.

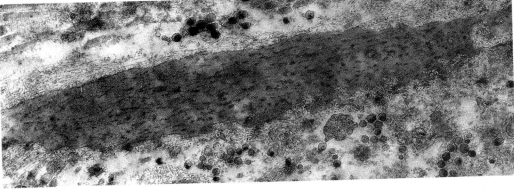

1.11

CUTANEOUS BLOOD VESSELS

The skin receives an extensive vascular supply from vessels within the subcutaneous fat. From these arise two vascular plexuses linked by intercommunicating vessels (Fig. 1.29); one, the deep vascular plexus, lies in the region of the interface between dermis and subcutaneous fat and the other, the superficial vascular plexus, lies in the superficial aspects of the reticular dermis and supplies the papillary dermis with a candelabra-like capillary loop system. Each loop consists of an ascending arterial limb and a descending venous limb. The collagenous component of the dermis receives only a limited blood supply, most of the capillary systems being associated with the metabolically active epidermis and its appendages.

A specialized cutaneous arteriovenous anastomosis, the Sucquet-Hoyer canal, is found in the dermis of the fingertips and to a lesser extent elsewhere on the body. The canal is surrounded by several layers of modified smooth muscle cells which function as a sphincter. These anastomoses enable the capillary networks of the superficial dermis to be bypassed, thus increasing the venous return from the extremities.

Cutaneous blood flow (under hypothalamic control) is of extreme importance in thermoregulation. Mediated by the systemic nervous system, heat loss can be increased or diminished by varying the volume of blood entering the superficial capillary systems. A higher outside temperature results in an increased blood flow to the papillary dermis accompanied by an increase in eccrine sweat gland secretion. Evaporation of sweat cools the outer parts of the body with a resultant diminution of the temperature of circulating blood. Thus temperature control depends upon a delicate interplay between both vascular and sweat gland function. The dermis also contains an extensive lymphatic system closely associated with the vascular plexuses.

CUTANEOUS NERVES

The skin receives a very extensive nerve supply, an efferent system responsible for control of the cutaneous vasculature and skin appendages derived from the sympathetic division of the autonomic nervous system, and an afferent system responsible for the appreciation of cutaneous sensation. Afferent receptors are of three types: free nerve endings; nerve endings in relation to hair; and encapsulated nerve endings. Free nerve endings, of both myelinated and non-myelinated types and of low conduction speed, are mainly responsible for the appreciation of temperature, itch and pain. Hair follicles are supplied by an intricate network of myelinated fibres, some of which ramify as free nerve endings in the periadnexal fibrous tissue while others enter the epidermis to terminate as expansions in intimate association with Merkel cells in the external root sheath, the so-called tactile discs, which function as touch receptors. Encapsulated nerve endings are of various types including in particular the specialized corpuscles of Meissner and Pacini. Pacinian corpuscles are responsible for the appreciation of deep pressure and possibly vibration and are found in the subcutaneous fat of the palmar aspect of the hand, the plantar aspect of the foot, the dorsal surfaces of the digits and around the genitalia. They are round or oval in shape and are quite large, measuring up to 2x0.5mm. They consist of a central core of packed lamellae lying around a nerve terminal surrounded by a cellular layer enclosed by a laminated capsule (Fig. 1.30) and have a myelinated nerve supply.

Meissner's corpuscles enable the appreciation of touch sensation and are especially found in the dermal papillae of hands and feet and on the front of the forearm. Oval in shape and measuring about 80x30μ, they consist of a perineural-derived lamellated capsule surrounding a core of cells and nerve fibres and are supplied by myelinated and non-myelinated nerve fibres.

SUBCUTANEOUS FAT

Fat is divided into lobules by fibrous septae and its cells are characterized by large quantities of lipid which compress the nucleus against the cytoplasmic membrane. Subcutaneous fat is of great importance in thermoinsulation and also functions as a nutritional store.

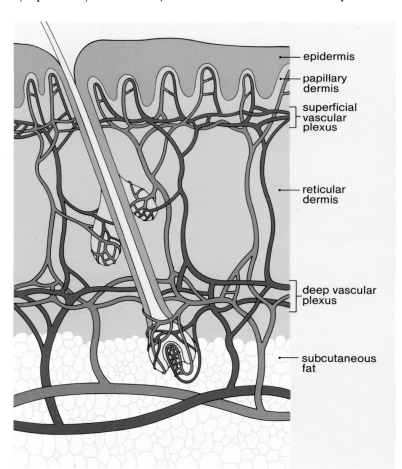

— epidermis

— papillary dermis

— superficial vascular plexus

— reticular dermis

— deep vascular plexus

— subcutaneous fat

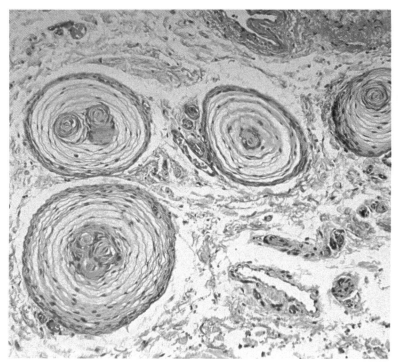

Fig. 1.29 Diagram showing the relationship of the superficial and deep vascular plexuses.

Fig. 1.30 Pacinian corpuscles showing their lamellated internal structure. H & E stain.

2 Eczema

Eczema is one of the commonest abnormalities of the skin. The diagnosis is made by eliciting certain symptoms in the history and observing certain signs on examinations. Eczema is not a disease entity in itself but, rather like anaemia, requires investigations to establish, if possible, a cause. There are a multiplicity of these, some of which are purely descriptive and others more precisely elucidated.

It exhibits three identifiable patterns which are related to the activity of the disease. These are termed acute, subacute or chronic and more than one form may be seen in a single patient at the same time. The patterns of eczema are best understood through the pathology. The blood vessels are dilated (seen clinically as erythema) and a predominantly perivascular infiltration of inflammatory cells is present. These cells migrate into the epidermis accompanied by oedema of the upper dermis and epidermis. Intercellular oedema (spongiosis) and intracellular oedema with consequent malfunctioning of epidermal cells occur. In an acute eczematous process vesicles and occasionally bullae are formed which are apparent on clinical (Fig. 2.1) and histological examination (Fig. 2.2). A serous exudate is observed (wet eczema).

More deeply situated spongiosis produces erythematous papules (Fig. 2.3) rather than vesicles. Subacute eczema is characterized by a glistening of serum (Fig. 2.4) rather than frank exudation. In chronic eczema only slight intercellular oedema is present but the epidermis is thickened (acanthosis) and there is excess production of keratin (hyperkeratosis) due to deranged epidermal cell function from intracellular oedema

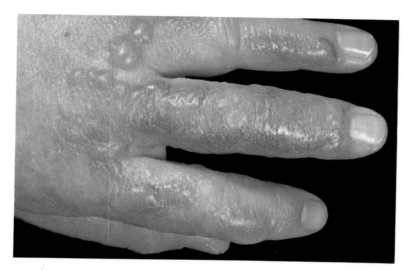

Fig. 2.1 Acute eczema due to an acute contact dermatitis. There are confluent vesicles on the backs of the fingers with some haemorrhage. By courtesy of St. Bartholomew's Hospital.

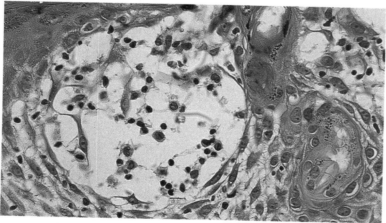

Fig. 2.2 Acute eczema. High power histological section of skin showing intercellular oedema (spongiosis) with vesicle formation. H & E stain. By courtesy of Dr. P.H. McKee.

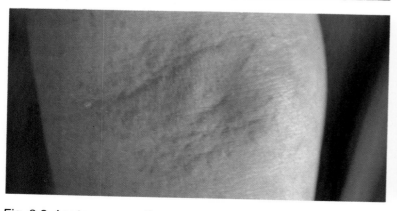

Fig. 2.3 Acute eczema. If spongiosis affects the epidermis at a deep level, erythematous papules may be observed.

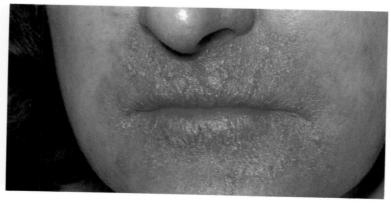

Fig. 2.4 Subacute eczema. There is glistening of serum rather than frank exudation. Crusting may also occur.

(Fig. 2.5). Clinically erythematous macules and papules coalesce; the skin is thickened, scaly and may fissure (dry eczema) (Fig. 2.6). Unlike psoriasis, the margins of an eczematous eruption are ill-defined (Fig. 2.7). Eczema is intensely pruritic. As a result of patient interference with the skin to relieve the pruritus, excoriation (Fig. 2.8) and lichenification (Fig. 2.9) occur. The latter is defined as thickened areas of the skin where the skin creases are exaggerated and is due to increased epidermal cell division. Postinflammatory hyperpigmentation (Fig. 2.9) and hypopigmentation (Fig. 2.10) are common consequences of eczema and in coloured races constitute a problem which may take a considerable time to return to normal.

Once a diagnosis of eczema has been made, it should, if possible, be classified. Some of the types are very well understood. For example, in contact dermatitis due to an allergen such as nickel a delayed hypersensitivity reaction modulated by thymus-derived lymphocytes and Langerhans' cells occurs and results in an eczematous response (see Fig. 2.20). On the other hand, the aetiology of seborrhoeic dermatitis (see Fig. 2.72), which consists of an eczematous pattern appearing in certain sites on the body where sebaceous gland function was erroneously thought to be abnormal, is quite obscure. Thus there are many forms of eczema, sharing a common cutaneous expression, but with widely differing aetiologies.

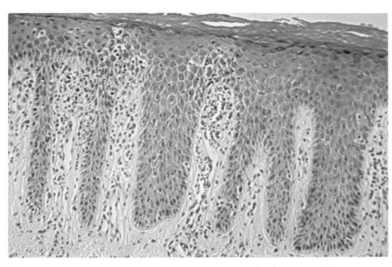

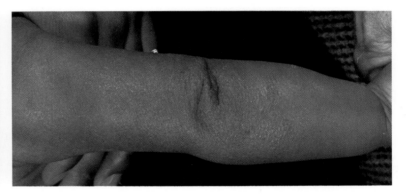

Fig. 2.5 Chronic eczema. Histological section of skin showing hyperkeratosis and marked acanthosis with prolongation of the epidermal ridges. Spongiosis can be seen. Within the dermis there is a lymphocytic infiltrate surrounding dilated blood vessels. H & E stain. By courtesy of Dr. P.H. McKee.

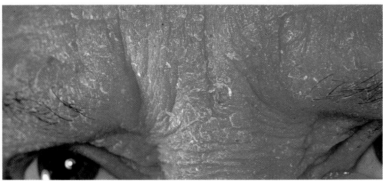

Fig. 2.6 Chronic eczema. The skin is red, scaly and dry.

Fig. 2.7 Eczema . The margins of an eczematous eruption are usually ill-defined.

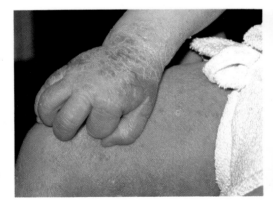

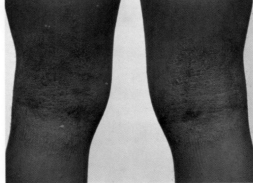

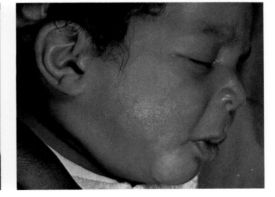

Fig. 2.8 Eczema. The eruption is extremely pruritic and excoriation resulting from patient interference occurs.

Fig. 2.9 Lichenification. The skin creases are thickened and exaggerated. Postinflammatory hyperpigmentation has occurred in this West Indian child with atopic eczema.

Fig. 2.10 Postinflammatory hypopigmentation. This developed as a result of atopic eczema on the face of this West Indian boy.

ATOPIC ECZEMA

Certain readily identifiable features make it possible to define this condition. Its first occurrence is often in infancy and frequently at about the age of three months. A family history of the disease or of a related condition such as asthma, allergic rhinitis or urticaria is common and there is a tendency for these conditions to develop in later life. A number of immunologically-mediated phenomena have been observed.

There is a predisposition to react positively to skin prick tests with various allergens. Raised levels of immunoglobulin E are present in serum. These patients are prone to bacterial and viral infections. It has been reported that the incidence of contact dermatitis is lower than expected. A transient immunoglobulin A deficiency may occur in early infancy, possibly permitting the entry of foreign allergens from the gastrointestinal tract so that

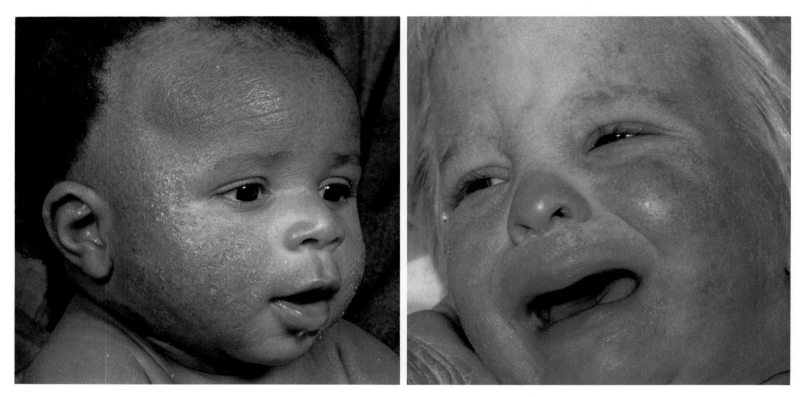

Fig. 2.11 Atopic eczema. This disease usually starts on the face in early infancy and classically at the age of three months. There is ill-defined redness and scaling.

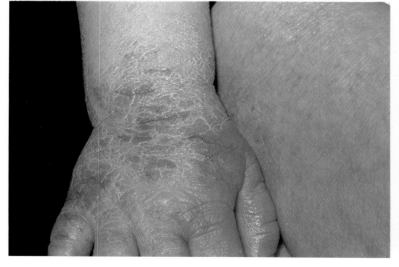

Fig. 2.12 Atopic eczema. The disorder is hereditary. Note that in the right of this picture eczema can also be seen on the back of the mother's wrist.

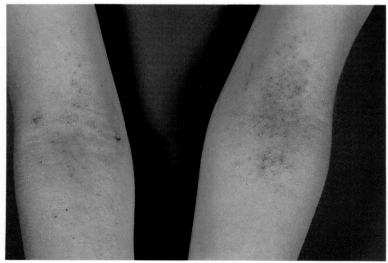

Fig. 2.13 Atopic eczema. This form of eczema has a predilection for the flexures.

strict dietary exclusion of foreign antigens by breast feeding is advocated by some authorities in an attempt to prevent the disease.

Clinically, the eruption begins on the face (Fig. 2.11) and subsequently spreads to the trunk and limbs. Here the sites of predilection are the flexures (Figs. 2.12 and 2.13), including obvious ones such as the elbows, wrists, knees, buttocks and ankles as well as the eyelids and neck. The eruption is symmetrical. The physical signs are typical of eczema and of the consequences of rubbing and scratching the skin in order to relieve pruritus. A particular variant is known as Besnier's prurigo in which itching is the dominant feature with the consequences of scratching overshadowing the eczematous lesion (Fig. 2.14).

Although most patients develop this disease in infancy it may occur for the first time in adulthood. The morphology and distribution of the eruption make the diagnosis clear. A significant proportion of patients have xeroderma, an inherited ichthyotic tendency. Secondary sepsis with staphylococci and/or streptococci is not uncommon particularly when the eczema is acute. Yellow pustules which crust (Figs. 2.15 – 2.17) indicate sepsis.

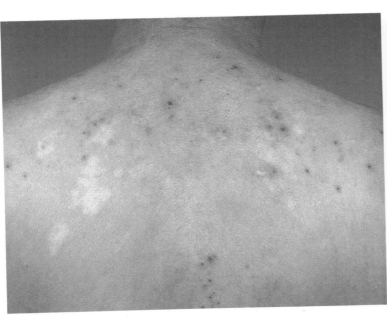

Fig. 2.14   Besnier's prurigo. Widespread excoriations overshadow the eczematous changes.

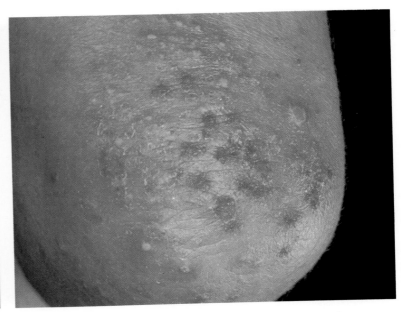

Fig. 2.15 Infected eczema. Yellow pustules are present, superimposed on the eczema.

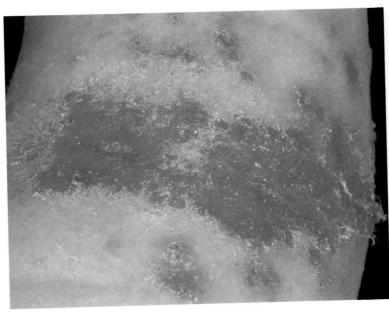

Fig. 2.16 Infected eczema. Yellow crusts are visible on this child's eczema. This appearance is sometimes termed impetigenized eczema.

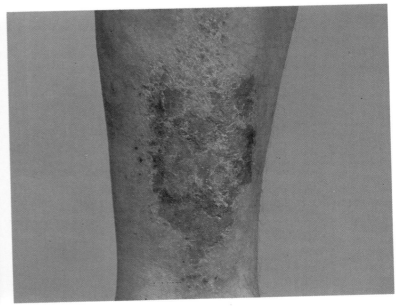

Fig. 2.17 Infected eczema. Staphylococcal and streptococcal infections are not uncommon. Yellow crusts may be seen on these eczematous lesions caused by allergy to nickel in the zip of the boots the patient had been wearing.

2.5

Superinfection with viruses occurs such as molluscum contagiosum (Fig. 2.18) and warts. These are frequently confused with the eczema and treated with glucocorticosteroids which aid their spread. A rare but dangerous consequence of secondary viral infection is Kaposi's varicelliform eruption. This occurs when a patient with eczema is infected with either the herpes simplex (eczema herpeticum, Fig. 2.19) or vaccinia virus (eczema vaccinatum). Viraemia and a life-threatening situation may develop. Clinically, distinct vesicles are observed surrounded by erythema on normal and eczematous skin. Patients with eczema should avoid contact with anyone with a cold sore and should never be routinely vaccinated nor exposed to siblings who have just been vaccinated.

DIFFERENTIAL DIAGNOSIS

SEBORRHOEIC DERMATITIS. In infancy seborrhoeic dermatitis (see Figs. 2.64–2.66) has to be considered and if the distinction is not clear initially, it will become so within a few weeks. Seborrhoeic dermatitis begins earlier and is likely to clear, whereas atopic eczema tends to localize, predominantly in the flexures.

CONTACT DERMATITIS. In eczema occurring for the first time in adolescence or later, contact dermatitis, particularly to nickel (Figs. 2.20 & 2.47), should be considered. This eruption occurs in areas such as the wrists, elbows, neck (from bracelets, necklaces, etc.), but the patient's history of sensitivity to metals, together with patch tests, will confirm the diagnosis.

SCABIES. Scabies is sometimes mistaken for eczema. However, papules between the fingers and elsewhere, with burrows (Fig. 2.21), no previous history of atopy, and similar symptoms in the patient's intimates, should suggest the diagnosis.

Management

There is no cure for atopic eczema but for the vast majority the disorder disappears with the passage of time. Management is thus an art aimed at keeping the patient comfortable with tar-containing preparations, emollients and systemic antihistamines and the judicious use of topical glucocorticosteroids. Some believe that inhaled antigens, such as those implicated in asthma, should be reduced. Substitutes for cow's milk and

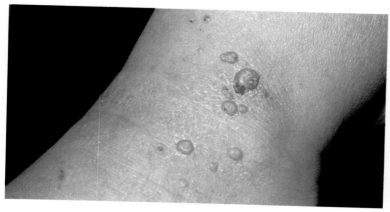

Fig. 2.18 Molluscum contagiosum superimposed upon eczema.

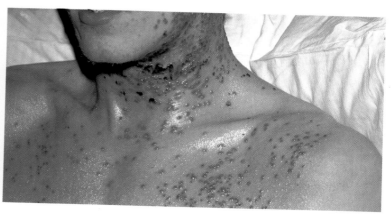

Fig. 2.19 Kaposi's varicelliform eruption. This patient who had suffered from atopic eczema all his life developed a widespread herpes simplex infection. This may have been transmitted to him by his girlfriend who had a herpes simplex infection on her lip.

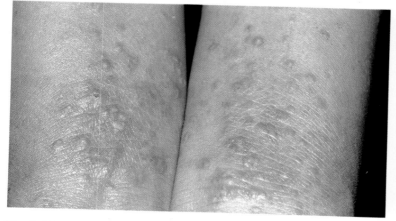

Fig. 2.20 Nickel dermatitis. This can be mistaken for atopic eczema of the wrists, but the disease begins during or after adolescence. Note the lichenoid nature of the eruption in the skin of a West Indian patient. Patch tests confirmed the diagnosis of nickel sensitivity.

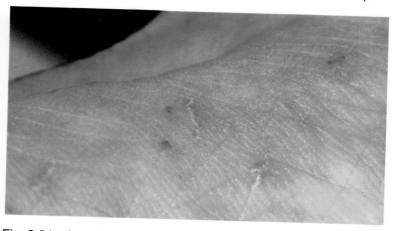

Fig. 2.21 Scabies. This is commonly mistaken for eczema. However, a lack of previous history of eczema and extreme irritation coupled with the finding of burrows such as those illustrated here confirms the diagnosis.

avoidance of other possible ingested antigens, particularly dairy products, may improve the eczema if standard topical therapies fail. Secondary sepsis should be recognized and treated appropriately. Frequently the disorder is more distressing to the parents than the child who often seems unaware of the condition until schoolmates make him or her conscious of it at a later age. Parental guidance is of great importance.

DISCOID ECZEMA (Nummular Eczema)

Because of its morphological appearance this is a highly distinctive variety of eczema and yet its aetiology is quite unknown. The lesions are well-defined, unlike most eczematous eruptions. They are disc or coin-shaped (Fig. 2.22). Discrete papulovesicles occur throughout the surface of the lesions and oozing and crusting may result. The lesions become dry and pink. Secondary bacterial infection is frequent. The eruption is largely found on the extensor surfaces of the limbs (Fig. 2.23) and is very pruritic.

There appears to be two varieties of this disease. Although it occurs in both sexes, in men it is predominantly an affliction of the middle and later years. In females it is a disorder of youth and is commonly seen on the backs of the fingers and hands (Fig. 2.24). The prognosis is variable and remissions and relapses are common. Ultimately the condition may resolve.

DIFFERENTIAL DIAGNOSIS

PSORIASIS. Although the lesions of discoid eczema and psoriasis are both well-defined, psoriasis does not weep and the lesions are red with a silvery scale (Fig. 2.25). Psoriatic lesions do occur on the limbs but, characteristically, the elbows and knees are also involved and there may be signs of the disorder elsewhere.

TINEA CORPORIS. The lesions of tinea corporis are asymmetrical in distribution, unlike discoid eczema, and occur anywhere on the body. Active scaling or vesiculation of the margin of the lesions with central clearing (Fig. 2.26) is characteristic of tinea and microscopic examination of scrapings confirms the diagnosis.

PARAPSORIASIS EN PLAQUES. Parapsoriasis en plaques is not a particularly common condition but may be confused with discoid eczema because the lesions are symmetrical, well-defined, and occur on the limbs (Fig. 2.27) and the trunk. However, they are dry, without much scale, have a wrinkled appearance and are not usually pruritic.

Management

Potent topical glucocorticosteroids are effective at controlling the condition. Combination with an antibiotic either topically or systemically may be necessary and antihistamines are helpful.

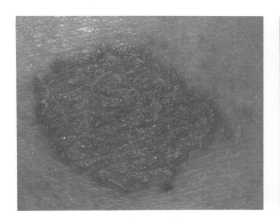

Fig. 2.22 Discoid eczema. The lesion is well-defined, unlike most eczematous eruptions. The eczematous change is seen over the entire surface of the lesion.

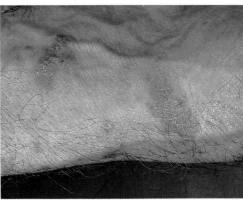

Fig. 2.23 Discoid eczema. This commonly occurs on the limbs.

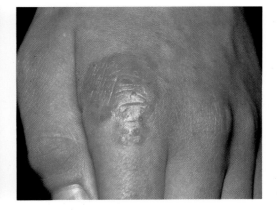

Fig. 2.24 Discoid eczema. In young patients this is often seen on the backs of the fingers.

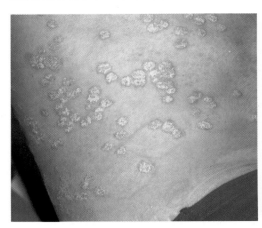

Fig. 2.25 Psoriasis. The lesions are well-defined and red with a pronounced silvery scale. They do not weep and should be readily differentiated from discoid eczema.

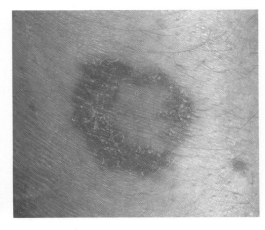

Fig. 2.26 Tinea corporis may be confused with discoid eczema. In tinea the margin of the eruption is most active with scaling or even vesiculation. There is central clearing, unlike discoid eczema.

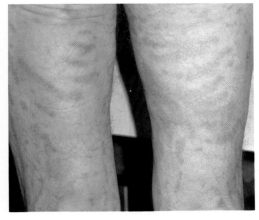

Fig. 2.27 Parapsoriasis en plaques. The lesions are symmetrical on the limbs but are dry without much scale and have a wrinkled appearance. Patients with this condition do not experience the intense pruritus of discoid eczema.

ECZEMA OF THE HANDS AND FEET (Pompholyx)

Eruptions on the hands and feet are common and their differential diagnosis is important in terms of prognosis and management.

A distinctive entity is the so-called cheiro (hand) and/or podo (foot) pompholyx, which is also known as dyshydrotic eczema, because hyperhidrosis is a frequent finding in those suffering from this disease. Pompholyx means a blister and in the acute stage, because the stratum corneum is so thick in these areas, the vesicles do not rupture but appear as tense fluid-containing swellings of various sizes (Fig. 2.28), lasting for several days. One or several attacks lasting from two to four weeks occur in the summer months, sometimes year after year. Pompholyx eczema is a disease of the first half of adult life. The vesicles are itchy and are found on the sides of the fingers and toes, and on the palms and soles (Fig. 2.29). The eruption tends to be symmetical. As the vesicles dry, redness and scaling with raw, painful fissuring result (Figs. 2.30 & 2.31). The condition may become chronic (Fig. 2.32). The aetiology of the condition is unknown although there is a theory that the vesicles represent retained

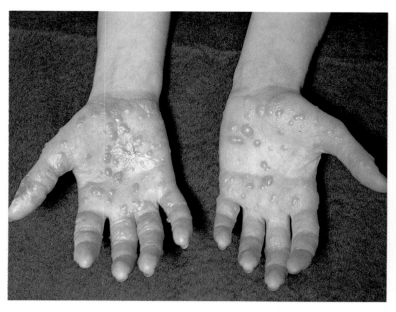

Fig. 2.28 Acute pompholyx. Tense vesicles or blisters, which are intensely pruritic, occur on the palms or soles.

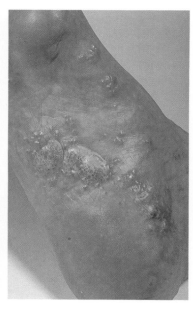

Fig. 2.29 Podopompholyx. Many vesicles and bullae are present. Both soles and palms were affected.

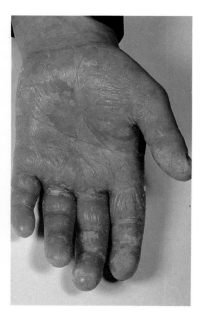

Fig. 2.30 Eczema of the hand. The blistering process results in a painful, raw, red, exudative eruption which may be quite persistent.

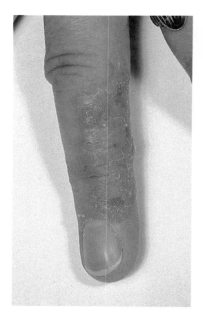

Fig. 2.31 Eczema of the hand. As the vesicles dry, painful fissures occur. The sides of the fingers are commonly affected.

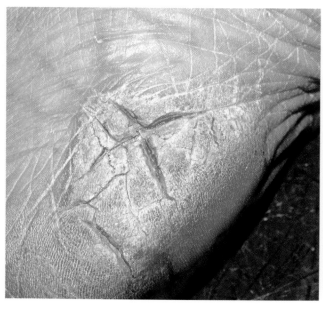

Fig. 2.32 Chronic podopompholyx. In the chronic variety of pompholyx, hyperkeratosis and painful fissuring are the predominant features.

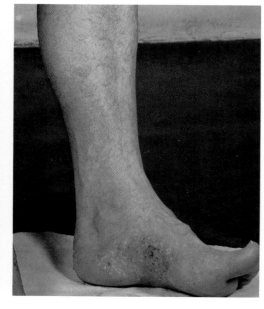

Fig. 2.33 Infected pompholyx. Lymphangiitis may occur as a result of secondary infection of hand or foot eczema. A linear erythema progressing up the leg is evident.

sweat secondary to hyperhidrosis. When this form of eczema is found on the hands it is important to examine the feet in particular because occasionally patients will be found to have tinea pedis or a contact dermatitis. In such a case the eruption on the hands is a secondary phenomenon, and treatment of the feet will result in the disappearance of the hand lesions.

A common complication of pompholyx is secondary infection (and occasionally lymphangiitis) in which the vesicles become pustular and a linear erythema is seen (Fig. 2.33).

DIFFERENTIAL DIAGNOSIS

CONTACT DERMATITIS. In contact dermatitis the dorsa of the hands or feet are involved as well as the wrists and ankles. It is at these sites that the irritant or allergen is able preferentially to penetrate the thin epithelium (Figs. 2.34 – 2.37) rather than the thick stratum corneum of the palms and soles which are usually spared. Patch testing is essential. Many patients with primary irritant eczema and negative patch tests have a personal or family history of atopic eczema.

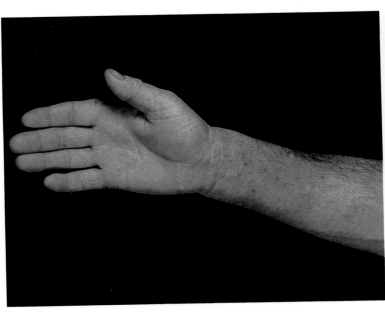

Fig. 2.34   Contact dermatitis of the hands due to rubber gloves. The wrists and backs of the hands are affected more than the palms.

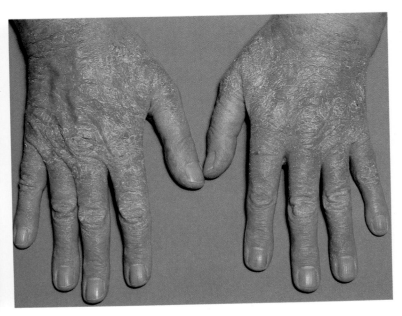

Fig. 2.35   Contact dermatitis due to lanolin. The eczematous process predominantly affects the backs of the hands and fingers. Patch tests were positive.

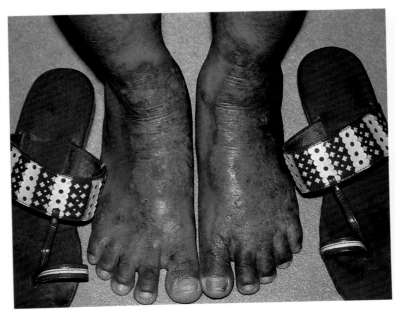

Fig. 2.36   Contact dermatitis of the feet. This can be distinguished from pompholyx by the fact that the lesions are found predominantly on the dorsal rather than the ventral surfaces. This patient had developed a contact dermatitis to her sandals.

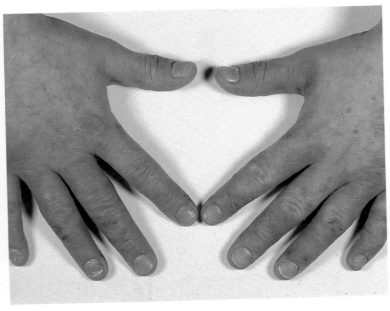

Fig. 2.37   Primary irritant dermatitis in a junior hairdresser. The backs of the hands and fingers were most affected. The shampooing had irritated her skin. She was also an atopic.

2.9

PSORIASIS. Psoriasis of the hands (Fig. 2.38) and feet may occur in the absence of psoriasis elsewhere. The eruption is very well-defined and red with characteristic silver scales. The lesions occur in plaques and symmetry is the hallmark of this condition. The palmar and plantar surfaces are most often affected. The resistance of the disease to therapy, nail involvement and a positive family history are useful diagnostic pointers.

PUSTULAR PSORIASIS. Pustular psoriasis may occur in the presence or absence of, and may or may not be related to, typical psoriatic lesions elsewhere on the patient's skin. Pustular psoriasis presents as well-defined symmetrical red and scaling plaques on palmar or plantar surfaces with pustules of a white or yellow colour which go brown as they resolve (Fig. 2.39).

TINEA MANUUM AND TINEA PEDIS. It is relatively easy to diagnose tinea on the hands because the fungus has a remarkable and quite unexplained propensity for one hand only and rarely the other (Fig. 2.40). The skin creases are filled with a fine powdery scale and there is scaling elsewhere. The nails are also usually involved. Tinea on the feet, however, can cause confusion particularly when *Trichophyton mentagrophytes* var, *interdigitale* or *Epidermophyton floccosum* are involved since vesicle formation similar to that of a pompholyx occurs on the instep. However, the eruption is usually unilateral. Tinea should be suspected if toe webs or nails are affected. In the non-blistering forms of tinea, the marginated nature of the eruption with scaling and a tendency to central healing is characteristic (Fig. 2.41).

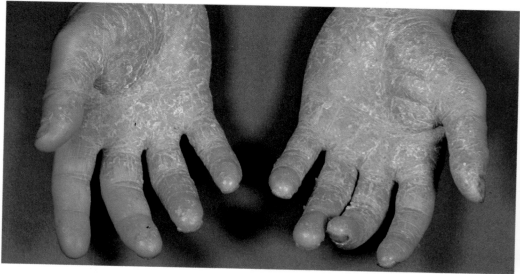

Fig. 2.38 Psoriasis of the palms. This is extremely well-defined and red with characteristic silvery scales. The eruption is symmetrical and can be extremely resistant to treatment.

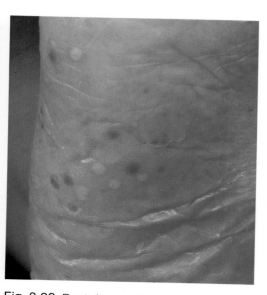

Fig. 2.39 Pustular psoriasis. Well-defined yellow pustules which go brown as the lesions age are found on the palmar or plantar surfaces.

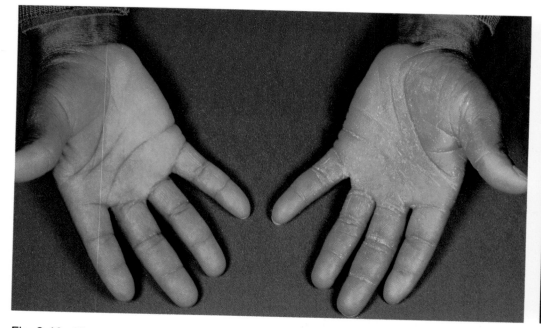

Fig. 2.40 Tinea of the hand. Fungal infections can be distinguished from eczema of the hand because they have a predilection for one hand only with sparing of the other. The skin creases are filled with a fine powdery scale and there is scaling elsewhere. The nails may be involved.

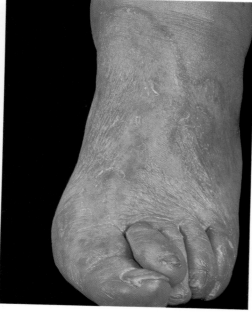

Fig. 2.41 Tinea of the foot. There is a well-defined active red margin with scaling and a tendency to central healing.

CONTACT DERMATITIS

The term dermatitis is an arbitrary and unsatisfactory one. It is synonymous with eczema but it is accepted by most dermatologists as indicating an exogenous cause. Unfortunately, other skin diseases which do not have an eczematous nature have this term incorporated in their title (eg., dermatitis herpetiformis and exfoliative dermatitis), and this causes confusion. To the patient, the term dermatitis often implies a reaction to agents encountered at work and the possibility of litigation which may or may not be justified.

A division may conveniently be made into primary irritant and true allergic contact dermatitis. The possibility of contact dermatitis must be considered in any patient exhibiting the features of an eczematous eruption. The distribution of the eruption should be carefully noted because this information may give a clue to the agent involved. The diagnosis of a contact factor is important because elimination of this agent may lead to eradication of the eruption.

Primary Irritant Dermatitis

An irritant dermatitis can occur in any individual provided that the irritant agent is sufficiently concentrated and exposure to it is sufficiently prolonged. Irritant dermatitis is not the result of an immunological reaction and the susceptibility of individuals varies enormously. The stratum corneum and the film of sebum from the sebaceous glands combined with sweat protect against external noxious substances. Substances or events which defat, dehydrate or damage the stratum corneum may cause primary irritant dermatitis.

Strong irritants such as caustics can, of course, produce dermatitis on first exposure but in such cases the diagnosis is obvious and is not within the framework of the common primary irritant condition.

In infants the continual drooling of saliva and food around the mouth will in some susceptible individuals result in a primary irritant dermatitis. Saliva caught under a dummy further compounds the problem (Fig. 2.42).

Primary irritant dermatitis of the napkin area in infancy (Fig. 2.43) is a result of constant and prolonged immersion of the skin of susceptible patients in urine and faeces. The occlusive nature of the sodden napkin which is frequently covered by plastic pants compounds the problem. The eruption is found on the area covered by the napkin with sparing of the flexures. Occasionally a manifestation similar to a chemical burn (Jacquet's dermatitis) may arise. The condition clears with better handling techniques and especially if the child is kept dry.

Housewives are particularly vulnerable to primary irritant dermatitis. It occurs on the backs of the hands, often starting under the wedding ring shortly after the birth of a baby, and later spreads to other areas on the backs of the fingers and hands (Fig. 2.44). Although washing the baby's napkins and clothing, constant cleaning of the infant and performing household chores, and repeated exposure to detergents are all factors in pathogenesis, there is no doubt that many individuals have a personal or family history of atopic eczema.

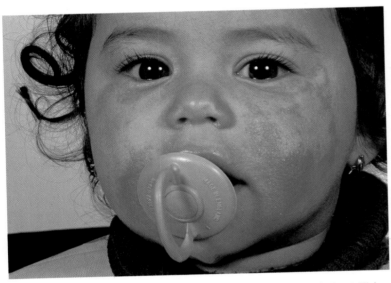

Fig. 2.42 Primary irritant dermatitis on the face of an infant. This was caused by the continual drooling of saliva and food around the mouth and cheeks. The dummy compounds the problem by occluding the area.

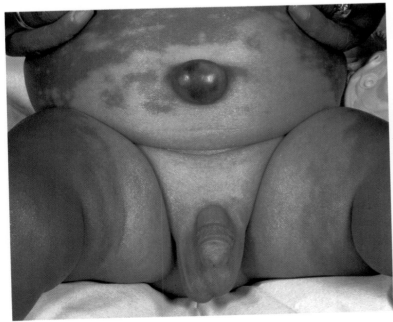

Fig. 2.43 Primary irritant dermatitis of the napkin area. This results from constant and prolonged immersion of the skin of susceptible babies in urine and faeces. In this West Indian child postinflammatory hypopigmentation has resulted.

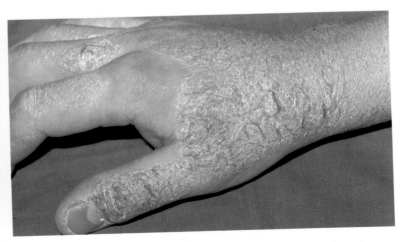

Fig. 2.44 Primary irritant dermatitis of the backs of the hands. This is most commonly seen in housewives and in those whose occupation requires their hands to be repeatedly immersed in water and in contact with irritant substances. This patient worked as a garage mechanic.

Occupation is important. For example, trainee hairdressers are initially employed in continuous shampooing while learning the skills of the profession. Many develop a primary irritant dermatitis of the hands. The intense cold of winter combined with a low relative humidity and dry atmosphere may be responsible for exacerbating primary irritant dermatitis and may produce 'chapping' in susceptible individuals. Overzealous bathing of the elderly in the low humidity environment of centrally-heated hospitals tends to dry out the skin and produces a condition known as asteatotic eczema. It usually begins on the lower legs and is easily recognizable from the cracked 'crazy-paving' appearance it produces (Fig. 2.45).

Allergic Contact Dermatitis

This is an immunological reaction to an external agent. It is unusual in childhood. It is a manifestation of a Gell and Coombes Type IV delayed hypersensitivity response and is lymphocyte-mediated. The antigen is frequently a low molecular weight chemical (e.g. nickel) known as a hapten, which links with protein and passes to lymph glands where thymus-derived (T) lymphocytes are primed. 24 to 72 hours after subsequent exposures to the allergen an eczematous response occurs. This form of contact dermatitis differs from the primary irritant type in that only those with a predisposition react in this way.

Once a patient has developed this type of allergic reaction susceptibility is usually life-long. The complete cutaneous surface is vulnerable. It is in this type of dermatitis that patch testing is useful (Fig. 2.46). There are many chemicals which have been incriminated in allergic dermatitis but there are about thirty which are commonly encountered. These have been incorporated into a 'battery' of allergens which are applied to the skin of the back under patches. These sites are examined for evidence of an eczematous response 48 and 96 hours later. They can be used to confirm a suspected allergen as responsible for the eruption or to indicate an allergen when the history has been unrevealing. Some examples of agents which commonly cause allergic contact dermatitis are:

Apparel
Nickel is a metal which is a constituent of jewellery which is not solid gold or silver, and is found in zips, fasteners, money and ornamental accessories to such articles as handbags. The diagnosis is to be suspected when an eczematous eruption is observed at sites covered by bracelets (see Fig. 2.20), earrings, necklaces, brassiere clips, etc. A common site is under a jeans stud just below the umbilicus (Fig. 2.47). This has become the modern equivalent of the formerly commonly encountered suspender dermatitis which is now seen rarely owing to the widespread adoption of tights. The presence of clothing between the allergen and the skin does not necessarily prevent the dermatitis (Fig. 2.48). Nickel dermatitis (Fig. 2.49) is more common in women and frequently the eczematous eruption is found at sites such as the eyelids and antecubital fossa, which are remote from the point of direct contact. This is known as an autosensitization reaction. This underlines the dermatological axiom of the importance of examining the complete surface if diagnostic signs are not to be missed.

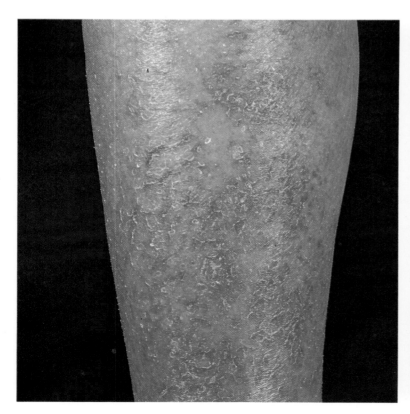

Fig. 2.45 Asteatotic eczema. The elderly are particularly susceptible to this primary irritant eczema over the lower legs and, in particular, the shins. This form of eczema is very dry and fissured producing a 'crazy-paving' appearance.

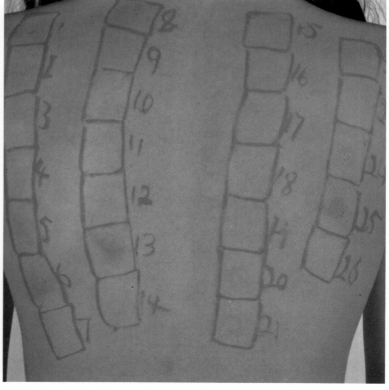

Fig. 2.46 Patch tests. Various commonly encountered allergens are put onto the skin of the back and examined 48-72 hours later for the production of an eczematous response. Three positive reactions can be seen (patches 6, 13 and 25).

As well as being an industrial source of sensitization, rubber in gloves, elasticated clothing, condoms and shoes is a commonly encountered allergen. The sharply demarcated margins of the eruption suggests the diagnosis; for example, the cut off at the wrists in rubber glove dermatitis. Also it is the dorsa of the hands or feet rather than the palms or soles which are particularly susceptible in rubber glove or shoe dermatitis. Presumably the thick stratum corneum of the palms and soles makes penetration of these areas by the allergen difficult. A similar distribution is seen in contact dermatitis caused by chromium which is used to tan leather shoes or gloves. Chromates are also found in cement where they are a common industrial cause of dermatitis. It should be noted that when sensitivity to a substance has occurred in one situation cross-sensitivity to the same substance in a different form is inevitable.

Dyes present in clothing such as trousers or stockings may cause allergic contact dermatitis. In such cases the areas most affected are those in closest contact with the material. These are the inner thighs, the popliteal fossa and the dorsa of the feet. In the case of blouses, it is usually the borders rather than the vault of the axilla and those areas of skin not protected by underwear which are affected. Dyed nylon hairnets may produce an eruption of the upper forehead, above the ears and on the nape of the neck. Hair dyeing may produce a very acute dermatitis caused by paraphenylenediamine. This reaction tends to affect the face and may even cause closure of the eyes. The scalp seems less pervious to allergens. Pigments may produce a contact dermatitis when used for tattoos (Fig. 2.50). A granulomatous response may also occur.

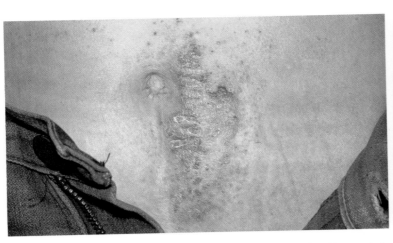

Fig. 2.47 Nickel dermatitis. The patient has reacted to the metal of the zip and the stud of her jeans. This propensity will persist throughout her life and such patients should avoid skin contact with nickel.

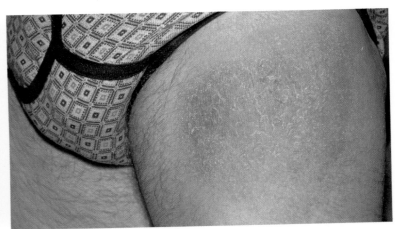

Fig. 2.48 Contact dermatitis. This patient had reacted to the phosphorus sesquisulphide in the striking part of a match box which he kept in his pocket. Clothing material between the allergen and the skin does not necessarily prevent dermatitis.

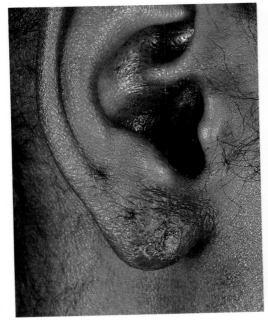

Fig. 2.49 Contact dermatitis to metal earrings. Post-inflammatory pigmentation is a common sequel in pigmented skin.

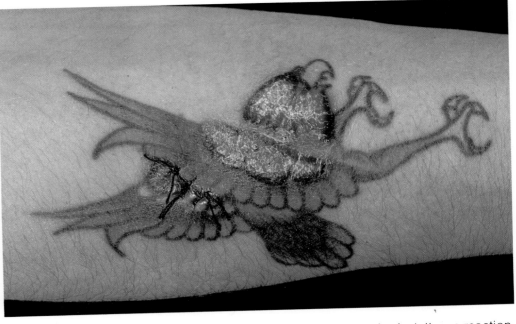

Fig. 2.50 Contact dermatitis. Some years after this patient acquired a tattoo, a reaction to the red, mercury-containing dye occurred. In such cases excision of the area affected is the only treatment.

Cosmetics

The incidence of true allergic contact dermatitis caused by cosmetics is low considering their widespread usage. Many suspected incidences are probably due to primary irritation. Where it occurs this type of contact dermatitis is commonly due to such allergens as preservatives (such as parabens and formaldehyde), perfumes (Fig. 2.51), and lanolin. The diagnosis of lipstick dermatitis, caused by the dye eosin, is not difficult. Lipstick dermatitis manifests itself as a dry eczema on the vermilion of the lips. Nail varnish dermatitis (Fig. 2.52) is a more subtle problem since the varnish is normally applied to the nails very carefully and the fingers themselves tend to be unaffected. However, patches of eczema are seen on areas such as the eyelids, cheeks, jaw, and upper chest, which are touched by the varnished nails.

Medicaments

Certain drugs so frequently produce a dermatitis when applied to the skin that their use topically has been or should be abandoned. These include antibiotics such as penicillin, the sulphonamides and streptomycin, local anaesthetics such as benzocaine, amethocaine and procaine (but not lignocaine) and some antihistamines, particularly mepyramine maleate (Fig. 2.53). Also incriminated but not so commonly as to preclude their use are neomycin, chloramphenicol and hydroxyquinoline. These preparations are frequently used in treatment either alone or in combination with topical glucocorticosteroids. If a condition which ordinarily responds to such treatment either fails to improve or deteriorates then the possibility of sensitivity to the medication should be considered. This observation also applies to preservatives and vehicles which are involved in formulations of medicaments.

Dermatitis medicamentosa most commonly develops during ophthalmic treatment (chloramphenicol eye drops), during treatment for pruritus ani (local anaesthetics), and the most frequently of all during treatment for varicose eczema. In the latter case the eczema fails to respond and subsequently an autosensitization eczema develops. This is the development of an eczema at sites distal to the initial point of entry of the allergen. Thus the face and particularly the eyelids (Fig. 2.54), the upper torso and the arms, become extremely pruritic and eczematous.

INDUSTRIAL DERMATITIS

The exact elucidation of the chemical involved in dermatitis in a work environment is often complicated and may require a visit to the patient's place of work, so that this field has become a sub-speciality within dermatology. Resins in the plastics industry,

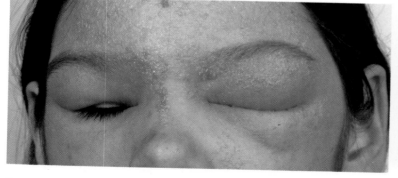

Fig. 2.51 Contact dermatitis. Perfume dermatitis is seen at the sites of application and in particular on the sides of the neck.

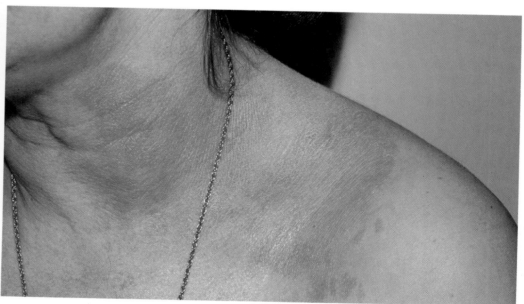

Fig. 2.52 Contact dermatitis. Nail varnish dermatitis does not occur on the nails but on those areas of skin which are touched by the nail varnish, in particular, on the face and sides of the neck.

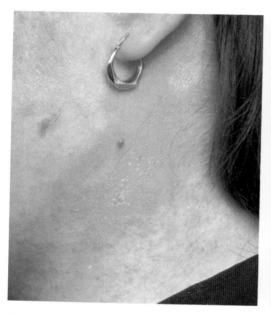

Fig. 2.53 Contact dermatitis. A reaction may occur to drugs applied to the skin and, in this case, mepyramine maleate has resulted in severe dermatitis with closure of the eyelids.

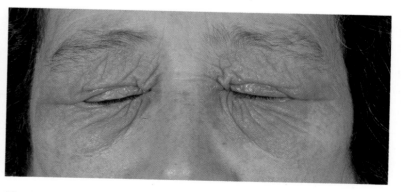

Fig. 2.54 Contact dermatitis. Eczema around the eyes should always suggest the possibility of contact dermatitis. This patient was sensitive to rubber in her elasticated garments and developed a secondary autosensitization phenomenon around her eyes.

rubber, dyes, glues and cement are common allergens. The diagnostic clues are eruptions in exposed areas of skin, a tendency to heal when the patient is away from work at the weekend or on holiday, and the observation that other workers are similarly affected. Because this diagnosis may lead to unemployment and litigation, expert advice is essential.

PLANTS

Primula (Fig. 2.55) and chrysanthemums are common culprits. The eruption is distinctive. It is acute with vesiculation, sometimes bullae, oedema and weeping in those parts such as the fingertips which are exposed to the leaves of the plants (Fig. 2.56). Areas of the skin which are touched by the fingers may also be affected. An eruption on the face may be so severe that the eyes are closed. Patch testing with a compressed leaf once the reaction has settled will confirm the diagnosis.

In North America, poison ivy or poison oak are such common sources of acute contact dermatitis that this is common knowledge. These weeds do not, however, occur in the United Kingdom.

A dry eczema which is largely hyperkeratotic and fissured is sometimes seen on the tips of the fingers and thumbs of those who have been handling bulbs of garlic, tulips, or onions but this condition is not particularly common.

PHOTOCONTACT DERMATITIS

An eruption caused by the interaction of a chemical and ultraviolet light is known as a photocontact dermatitis. It may either be of the primary irritant variety (phototoxic reaction) or a true immunological photoallergic reaction. Often it is difficult to categorize such eruptions precisely. The diagnosis of any photosensitization reaction is based on finding the eruption in those parts of the individual which have been exposed to ultraviolet irradiation. Normally this will include the face (Fig. 2.57), the V of the neck, the backs of the hands (Fig. 2.58) and, in females, the legs. A useful feature is sparing of those areas of the face shielded from ultraviolet light, such as the eyelids (shielded by the eyebrows), the upper lip (shielded by the nose), the front of the neck (shielded by the chin) and behind the ears.

Phototoxic Reactions

These are non-immunological and as in primary irritant reactions, are dose-related responses which can arise in any individual depending on susceptibility and simultaneous interaction of the chemical with ultraviolet light of the appropriate wavelength. The clinical picture is that of an acute and often severe sunburn. There is burning, redness and swelling, followed by hyperpigmentation.

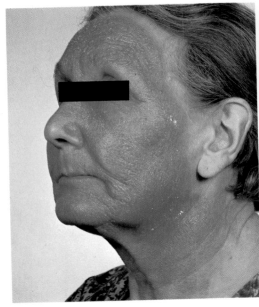

Fig. 2.55 *Primula obconica*. This is the commonest cause of plant dermatitis in the United Kingdom.

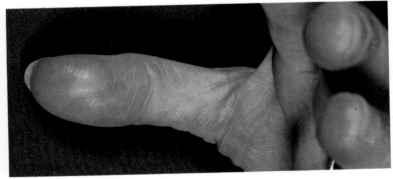

Fig. 2.56 Contact dermatitis to primula. A vesicular or bullous eruption occurs on the fingertips and those areas of the body touched by the contaminated fingers, notably the face.

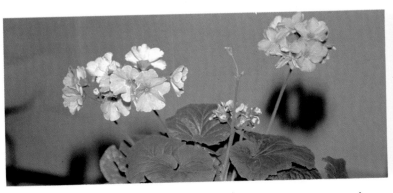

Fig. 2.57 Photocontact dermatitis. This occurs on those areas of skin exposed to ultra-violet light irradiation. Note sparing of the scalp (protected by hair) and skin underneath the nose.

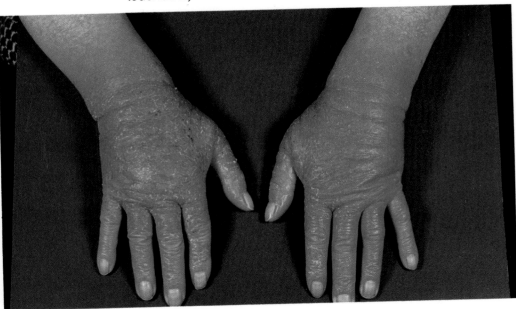

Fig. 2.58 Phototoxic contact dermatitis. Well-defined erythema and oedema has occurred on the backs of the hands in a light-exposed distribution in this patient secondary to a thiazide diuretic.

Blistering sometimes occurs (Fig. 2.59). Common examples of phototoxic reactions are as follows:

Phytophotodermatitis

This is due to an interaction of furocoumarins, notably psoralens, and longwave ultraviolet light. They are present in various plants, particularly those of the umbelliferae, rutaceae,

leguminosae and moraceae families. The clinical picture is distinctive. Linear blistering on an erythematous base is seen distributed in a bizarre streaky (Fig. 2.60) and criss-cross distribution. A history of having been lying in a meadow on a bright day, or having had some other similar exposure to the weeds can usually be elicited from the patient.

Berloque Dermatitis

This is a disorder of a similar mechanism but due to the interaction of oil of bergamot, which contains 5-methoxy-psoralen, and longwave ultraviolet light. Oil of bergamot is present in many colognes and perfumes. The acute sunburn phase may not always be seen. Sometimes only postinflammatory hyperpigmentation is observed. Typically this is seen on the neck and the odd configurations observed are due to the spattering of the perfume in this area (Fig. 2.61).

Other substances which may produce a phototoxic reaction are pitch and coal tar which are encountered industrially and as medicaments.

Photoallergic Contact Dermatitis

These eruptions occur only in a small number of persons who must have been previously sensitized and is based on the immunological principles of a delayed hypersensitivity response (Fig. 2.62). The eruption is largely eczematous in contrast to the intense erythema and inflammatory response of the phototoxic reaction. Occasionally, even though the contact factor is eliminated the condition becomes intractable (the 'persistent light reaction'). The halogenated phenols were formerly popular chemical additives as antiseptic agents to perfumes, soaps, cosmetics and deodorants. An epidemic of photoallergic dermatitis occurred in the United Kingdom in the early 1960's due to the addition of tetrachlorsalicylanilide to Lifebuoy soap.

Certain drugs, which include chlorpromazine, promethazine hydrochloride and the sulphonamides, can cause photocontact dermatitis in patients if applied to the skin, in medical personnel administering the drugs and in those involved in the manufacture of these preparations. They should not be used to treat skin diseases and care should be exercised in their use in other situations.

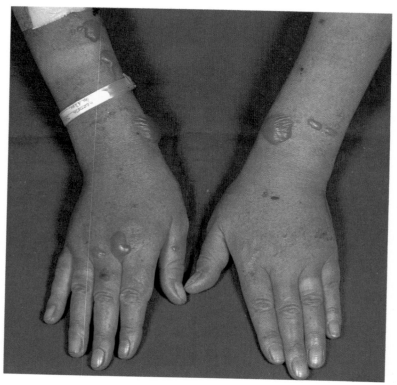

Fig. 2.59   Phototoxic eruption. Blistering on the skin may result. This patient had been taking nalidixic acid.

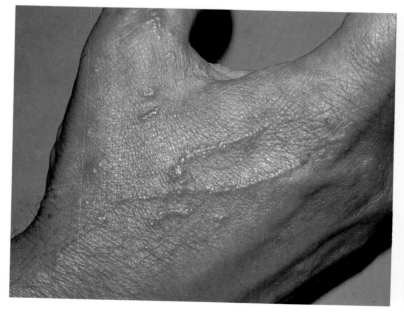

Fig. 2.60   Phytophotodermatitis. This is due to an interaction of furocoumarins and ultraviolet light. This man had been cutting back his parsnips in high summer. Bizarre linear blistering is characteristic of this eruption.

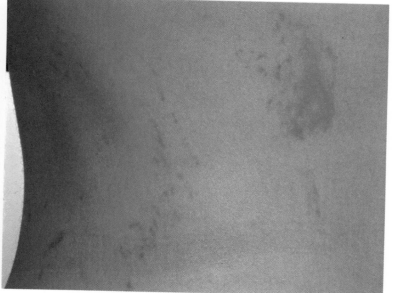

Fig. 2.61   Berloque dermatitis is a reaction between psoralens in perfumes or colognes and ultraviolet light. Frequently the inflammatory phase is not seen but only postinflammatory hyperpigmentation. This patient had spilled drops of cologne onto her abdomen whilst sunbathing.

Systemic Drug Photosensitization Reactions

The previous discussion has centred around chemicals in direct contact with the skin and their interaction with ultraviolet light. In a number of instances, patients have developed drug eruptions following systemic therapy when they have been previously allergically sensitized by a topical route. This type of reaction has been documented with promethazine hydrochloride cream.

Chloropromazine produces an exaggerated sunburn (phototoxic) response in patients, whereas factory workers manufacturing the drug can be shown to develop true allergic contact dermatitis. Thus the picture is unclear in many cases but the tetracycline group of drugs (and in particular demethylchlortetracycline), frusemide, nalidixic acid, chlorpromazine, psoralens, chlorthiazides, chlorpropamide, tolbutamide, trimeprazine tartrate, promethazine hydrochloride and thioridazine are all known photosensitizers.

Photo-onycholysis

Separation of the distal nail plate from the nail bed may occur after strong sunlight exposure and the ingestion of tetracyclines or the non-steroidal anti-inflammatory drug benoxaprofen (Fig. 2.63). There may be pain and intense erythema of the digits and, if exposed, the toes preceding the eruption.

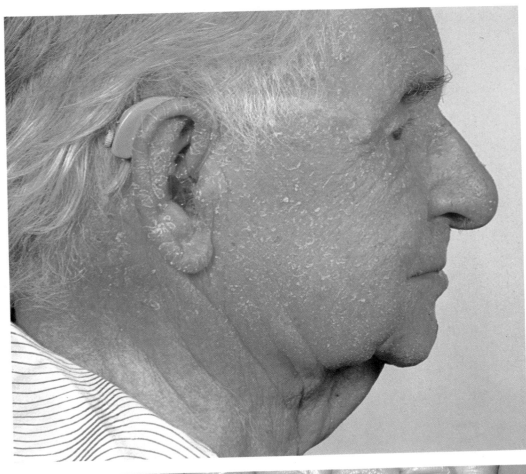

Fig. 2.62 Photoallergic contact dermatitis. This is a true allergic dermatitis and the eruption is usually eczematous rather than an intense erythema. The distinction between the two is not always clear as the same drugs may cause both the toxic and the allergic variety of photodermatitis.

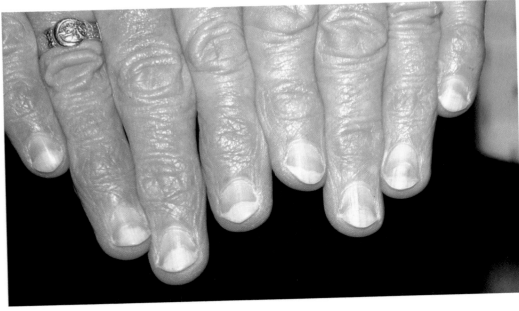

Fig. 2.63 Photo-onycholysis. Separation of the distal nail plate from the nail bed may occur after ultraviolet light irradiation and the ingestion of certain drugs. This patient had been taking benoxaprofen.

SEBORRHOEIC ECZEMA

This term is a misnomer. The dry yellow scales associated with the disease were thought to represent dried sebum but they are in fact exfoliated cells of the stratum corneum. Although the eruption occurs in areas such as the head and neck, which are associated with a large number of sebaceous glands, it is also encountered at sites with few sebaceous glands such as the groins and axillae. However, the term is retained for want of a better one. It refers to an eczematous condition which is easily recognized by its distribution.

The disease occurs in infancy and in adult life and these two forms appear to be distinct. There is no concrete evidence to indicate that those who suffer from seborrhoeic eczema in infancy have increased vulnerability to the adult form.

Seborrhoeic Eczema of Infancy

This is a common self-limiting condition occurring within the first few months of life. The simplest form occurs on the scalp as yellow-brown greasy scales and is known colloquially as 'cradle cap' (Fig. 2.64). The face is involved, particularly the eyebrows (Fig. 2.65) and the ears (Fig. 2.66). A more troublesome disorder is the napkin eruption. There is no uniform agreement on the pathogenesis or even nomenclature of this condition. Some dermatologists divide napkin eruptions into those occurring as part of a seborrhoeic diathesis, those secondary to candidosis, those due to the primary irritant effect of urine or the chemical burn effect of ammonia and those due to psoriasis. In practice it can be difficult to distinguish some of these entities from one another and for this reason all forms of napkin eruption are included in this discussion.

Seborrhoeic Dermatitis

In this condition eczema occurs in the napkin areas but unlike primary irritant dermatitis it is not confined to the area covered by the napkin (Fig. 2.67).

Secondary involvement (Fig. 2.68) may occur in the axillae, on the trunk, on the face, on the neck, on the scalp and behind the ears; occasionally erythroderma is encountered (Fig. 2.69).

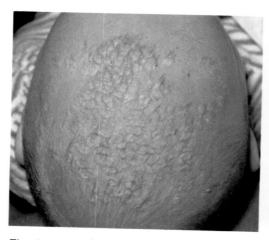

Fig. 2.64   Cradle cap. This is one of the first signs of seborrhoeic eczema of infancy.

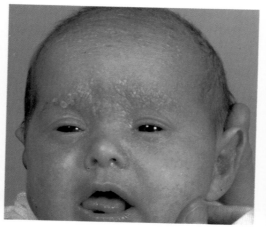

Fig. 2.65   Seborrhoeic eczema of infancy. This starts at an earlier age than atopic eczema and, as well as involving the face, particularly affects the eyebrows.

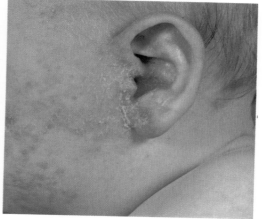

Fig. 2.66   Seborrhoeic eczema of infancy. The ears are commonly affected.

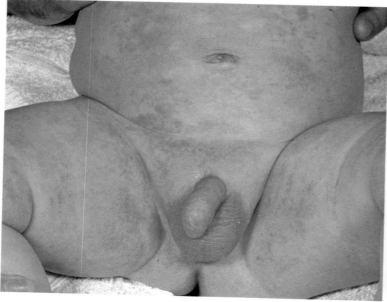

Fig. 2.67   Seborrhoeic dermatitis. This occurs in the napkin area but has a tendency to spread. This is in contrast to a primary irritant dermatitis which is specifically caused by a sodden napkin and which remains limited to the area covered by the napkin.

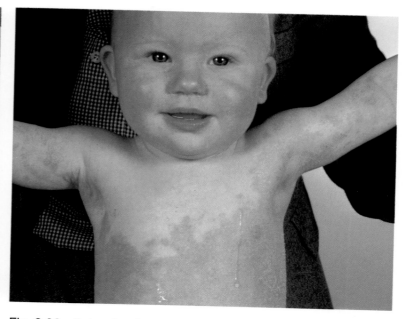

Fig. 2.68   Seborrhoeic dermatitis of infancy. The trunk and axilla are often involved.

Candida Intertrigo of Infancy

True primary candidosis may be diagnosed upon finding well-defined areas which are moist and macerated with satellite pustules located away from the main eruption. This condition is not as common as secondary contamination of a seborrhoeic eczema with candida.

Primary Irritant Dermatitis of Infancy

On examination eczema is found to be limited to those areas covered by the napkin (Fig. 2.43). Thus the lower lumbar region, the buttocks, upper thighs, pubic area and genitalia are involved but the flexures which are not touched by the napkin (the genitocrural folds and the natal cleft) are spared.

Ammoniacal (Jacquet's) Dermatitis

This is the result of inexperienced or neglectful care of an infant. The sodden and soiled napkin is left in contact with the skin for prolonged periods resulting in blisters and well-defined erosions similar to chemical burns (Fig. 2.70).

Napkin Psoriasis

This is a morphological diagnosis in that the eruption is very well-defined, red and has a silvery scale as in psoriasis (Fig. 2.71). The condition always resolves either spontaneously or as a result of treatment, but it would appear that some patients will develop psoriasis in later life. Scattered psoriasiform lesions may occur away from the napkin area. The condition may represent a Koebner phenomenon in reaction to the irritant effect of urine and faeces.

Atopic Eczema

It can be difficult to distinguish atopic eczema from seborrhoeic eczema and primary irritant eczema at the first consultation. Atopic eczema tends to appear somewhat later (at about the age of 3 months) than the other two conditions. It begins on the face and then spreads, and is highly pruritic (Figs. 2.11 & 2.13). It is perhaps surprising that the infant with seborrhoeic eczema seems little troubled by irritation no matter how extensive the eruption. This is an exception to the rule that eczema is always pruritic. In this condition the eruptions start within the first six weeks of life and the prognosis is excellent. In the case of atopic eczema the future is uncertain and the disease is certainly more prolonged. A positive family history and the flexural distribution favour the diagnosis of atopic eczema.

Management

Primary irritant, seborrhoeic and ammoniacal dermatitis all resolve as the infant becomes dry. Attention to local skin care is of the greatest importance. Early changing of soiled napkins, periods free of the napkin and the reduction of the wearing of occlusive rubber or plastic pants to a minimum are beneficial measures. Topical mildly potent glucocorticosteroids combined with anti-infectives if necessary are very effective. Candidosis is treated with nystatin or an imidazole but usually candida is a secondary invader and combination with a topical steroid is essential.

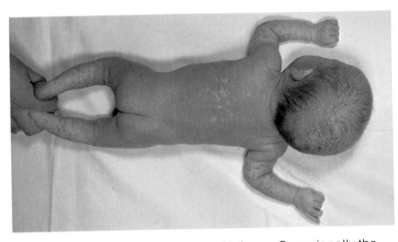

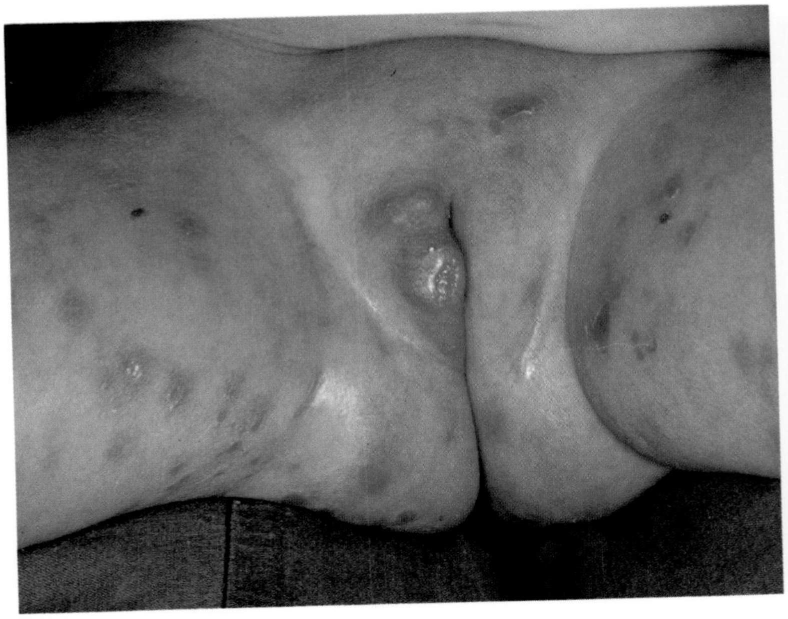

Fig. 2.69 Seborrhoeic dermatitis of infancy. Occasionally the entire body surface may be involved, producing an erythroderma.

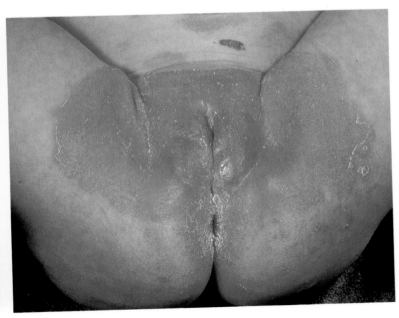

Fig. 2.70 Jacquet's dermatitis. This is usually the result of neglectful or inexperienced care of an infant in such a way that a sodden or soiled napkin is left in contact with the skin for prolonged periods. Blistering and erosions in the napkin area result.

Fig. 2.71 Napkin psoriasis. This morphological diagnosis is based on the presence of a well-defined red eruption often with a silvery scale. There is some question as to whether or not it is a separate entity from seborrhoeic dermatitis. The solitary, deep red lesion on the abdomen is an incidental strawberry naevus.

2.19

Adult Seborrhoeic Dermatitis

This is a very common condition. It arises after puberty and usually disappears in later life. Complete remissions are frequent but relapses are not uncommon. It is thought to be more often encountered in those of Celtic racial background. Many believe it to be precipitated by stressful events and certainly its incidence was markedly increased during the two world wars. An association with Parkinsonism suggests a role of the nervous system in pathogenesis. An eczematous eruption in a characteristic distribution is the main diagnostic feature.

The scalp is most commonly involved. In this area seborrhoeic dermatitis is to be distinguished from the dry white scales of dandruff, which are the result of an exaggeration of the normal process of exfoliation of stratum corneum cells. Seborrhoeic dermatitis, unlike dandruff, is characterized by the presence of an inflammatory component in the form of erythema. Erythema may indeed be the sole and persistent component.

The central areas of the face are next most commonly affected. The eyelid margins, the nasolabial folds, the cheeks, the eyebrows, the forehead (Figs. 2.72 & 2.73), the chin and the upper lip may be involved totally or in part. Inflammation behind and within the ears (otitis externa, Fig. 2.74) is part of the same clinical picture. The manifestations are those of an eczema with ill-defined redness and scaling but the conditions may sometimes be more acute, in which case, secondary bacterial sepsis may supervene.

The interscapular and presternal sites (Fig. 2.75) are less frequently involved but, like the sites mentioned above, they are

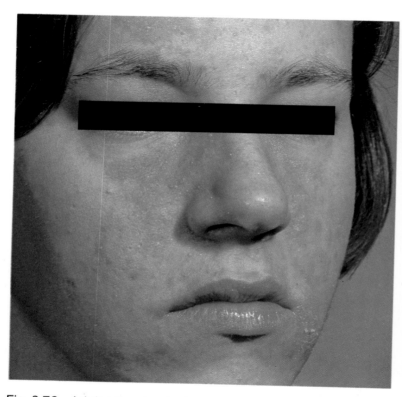

Fig. 2.72 Adult seborrhoeic dermatitis. This occurs particularly on the face around the forehead and spreading from the cheeks onto the ala nasi folds.

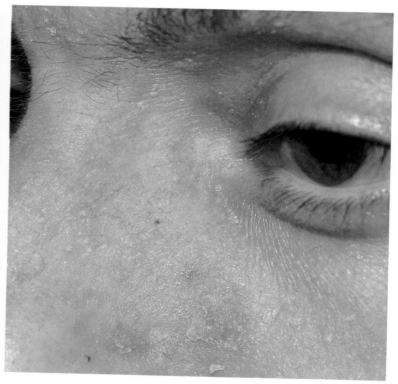

Fig. 2.73 Seborrhoeic dermatitis. The glabella, eyebrows and ala nasi are characteristically affected.

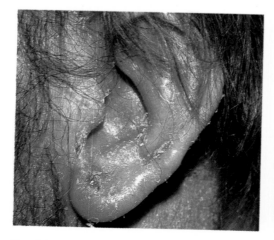

Fig. 2.74 Otitis externa. Secondary bacterial infection may occur.

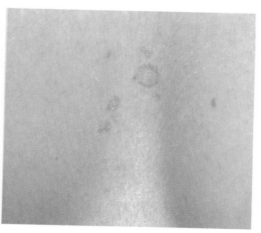

Fig. 2.75 Seborrhoeic dermatitis. Although a relatively minor disease, this can give rise to considerable anxiety. These small red patches on the chest are characteristic. They are frequently mistaken for pityriasis versicolor in which the lesions are brown rather than red.

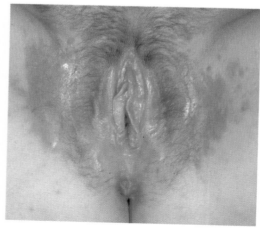

Fig. 2.76 Seborrhoeic dermatitis around the vulva. The eruption may be severe but responds well to potent topical corticosteroids. Note the symmetry of the eruption and involvement of the folds.

areas in which sebaceous glands are most abundant and active. On the other hand, this is not so for the intertriginous variety of seborrhoeic dermatitis. Here the axillae, groin, and perineum (Fig. 2.76) may be affected. Folds of skin which become particularly apposed such as those secondary to obesity, over the abdomen, under pendulous breasts and in the umbilicus are prone to this disease.

DIFFERENTIAL DIAGNOSIS
1. SEBORRHOEIC DERMATITIS OF THE SCALP
PSORIASIS. The lesions are more palpable, well-defined and red. Usually individual plaques are distributed symmetrically. There may be lesions elsewhere.

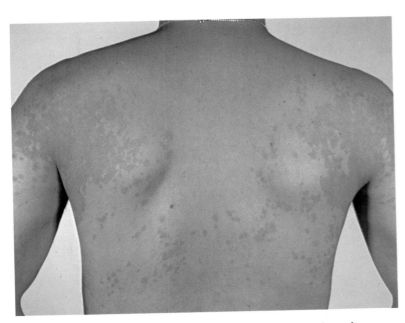

Fig. 2.77 Pityriasis versicolor of the trunk may produce fawn-coloured macules on the skin but not the red lesions of seborrhoeic dermatitis.

PITYRIASIS AMIANTACEA. This is a distinctive condition in which yellow scales are found attached to the lower portions of the hair follicles. The aetiology is unknown but it may be a form of seborrhoeic dermatitis possibly altered by the use of topical glucocorticosteroids.

Other common conditions of the scalp such as ringworm, alopecia areata and lupus erythematosus are distinguished by loss of hair.

2. SEBORRHOEIC DERMATITIS OF THE TRUNK
PITYRIASIS VERISCOLOR. The lesions are individual fawn-coloured macules (Fig. 2.77) which subsequently coalesce on the trunk as opposed to the red and scaling lesions of seborrhoeic eczema or psoriasis.

PSORIASIS. The lesions are well-defined and red with a characteristic silvery scale (Fig. 2.25).

3. SEBORRHOEIC INTERTRIGO
PSORIASIS. The lesions are very well-defined, symmetrical and erythematous. The characteristic silvery scale may be absent but there may be areas of typical psoriasis elsewhere.

TINEA. This is a largely postpubertal male disorder when it occurs in the groin and the physical signs are of an eruption with a well-demarcated, active, slightly raised red margin away from the body fold and with a tendency to central healing and postinflammatory hyperpigmentation. Asymmetry is a feature of fungus disorders (Fig. 2.78).

ERYTHRASMA. This is an infection due to *Corynebacterium minutissimum* and presents as well-defined red lesions which turn brown and develop a fine scale with a wrinkled appearance (Fig. 2.79). Examination under Wood's rays reveals a red fluorescence.

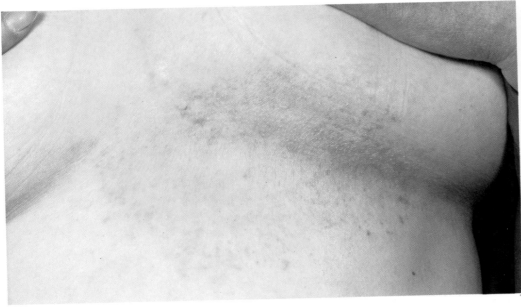

Fig. 2.78 Tinea intertrigo. This patient had an eruption under one breast only which did not respond to topical glucocorticosteroids. Microscopic examination of scrapings showed the skin to be invaded by fungal hyphae. Tinea is usually asymmetrical.

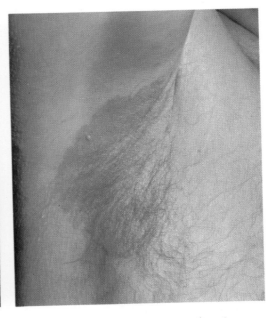

Fig. 2.79 Erythrasma. Well-defined reddish-brown lesions occur in the axilla or groin. The surface has a finely wrinkled appearance.

HYPOSTATIC (VARICOSE) ECZEMA

This form of eczema occurs secondary to venous hypertension in the lower limbs. The cause of this hypertension is either congenital absence of the valves in the perforating vessels ('primary varicose veins') or damage to the valves following deep venous thrombosis. Venous drainage of the leg is via the superficial veins which clear the skin and subcutaneous tissues, and the deep veins which are enclosed in muscles and the fascia lata. As the muscles contract, particularly when walking, the blood is pumped upwards in the deep vessels. Consequently, blood is drawn into them from the superficial veins via the perforating vessels which contain the valves whose proper functioning is essential to the health of the skin. Primary varicose veins are hereditary and occur in early youth. Secondary varicosities occur as a result of venous thrombosis after childbirth, prolonged immobilization or injury. The majo-

rity of sufferers are female and are often overweight.

The results of venous hypertension are oedema of the lower leg, tortuous veins and particularly the venous flare seen around the medial border of the foot (Fig. 2.80). Pigmentation due to haemosiderin from extravasated red blood cells is also a sign of venous hypertension. This leads to eczema, panniculitis and ulceration (Fig. 2.81).

The physical signs of this type of eczema are similar to those found elsewhere on the body. The eruption is ill-defined, red and scaly and is found on one or both sides of the lower half of the leg (Fig. 2.82). At this site eczema has a marked tendency to develop contact sensitization to medicaments used in the treatment of infections. Infection particularly of the associated ulcer is a common problem in this condition. Topical antibiotics such as neomycin and its cross-sensitizers, soframycin and framycetin, used in the form of ointments or impregnated in

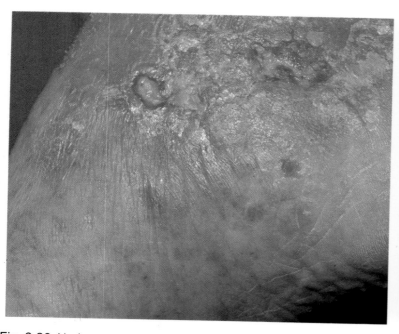

Fig. 2.80 Varicose eczema around the medial malleolus with ulceration. The venous flare around the medial border of the foot indicates venous hypertension which is an important factor in the aetiology of varicose eczema.

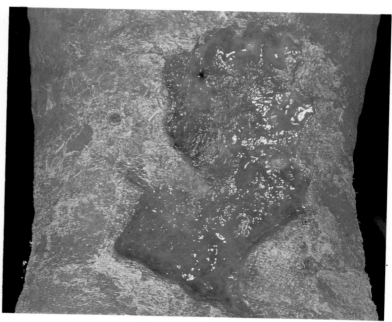

Fig. 2.81 Venous ulceration. This is the advanced stage of venous hypertension.

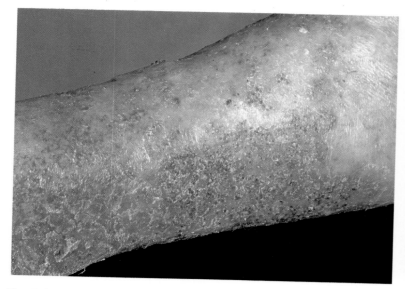

Fig. 2.82 Varicose eczema. Patches of eczema occur in association with varicosities. They may become secondarily infected.

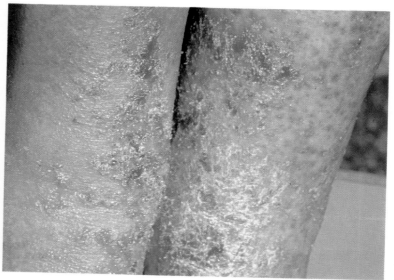

Fig. 2.83 Dermatitis medicamentosa. This is a common occurrence during the treatment of varicose eczema. An acute eczematous process is seen. Antibiotic ointments are among the most common allergens in this condition.

tulle, are common sensitizers. Local anaesthetics and anti-histamines should never be applied to the skin. Various ingredients of the bases of ointments, for example lanolin or the preservative parabens and even the rubber of elasticated stockings or bandages may cause dermatitis medicamentosa (Fig. 2.83). This diagnosis should be suspected if a varicose eczema fails to heal or deteriorates during treatment. Often the eczema becomes acute with vesiculation and is well-defined, conforming to the distribution of the sensitizer. Autosensitization may then occur with eczema appearing on the face, especially around the eyes, on the neck and on the arms. When this happens the patient may present as an emergency and frequently will not connect the eruption with the varicose eczema. If the physician is unaware of this phenomenon and treats the autosensitization eczema without stopping the allergen, the condition will deteriorate further.

LICHEN SIMPLEX (Localized Neurodermatitis)

This is a dermatological form of habit tic. The patient tends to scratch an area of skin which results in a lichenified eczematous reaction. Hyperpigmentation may also be a feature. It is a response to stress and relevant factors should be sought and discussed with the patient. The appearance is an isolated well-defined patch of lichenification found in one of several locations. These are the back of the neck, the area just below the elbow, the hand, the inner aspect of the thigh, the area around the anus, the outer aspect of the lower leg (Fig. 2.84) and ankle and the genitalia (Fig. 2.85). The patch is unilateral (Fig. 2.86) corresponding usually to the handedness of the patient. Occasionally lesions are multiple. The condition is extremely pruritic. It responds to potent topical glucocorticosteroids and systemic antihistamines.

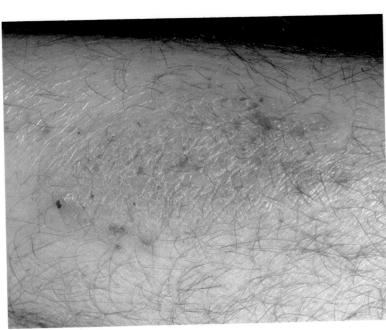

Fig. 2.84 Lichen simplex. An isolated well-defined patch of lichenification is found in one of several characteristic locations. This patient was in the habit of scratching the outer aspect of his lower leg.

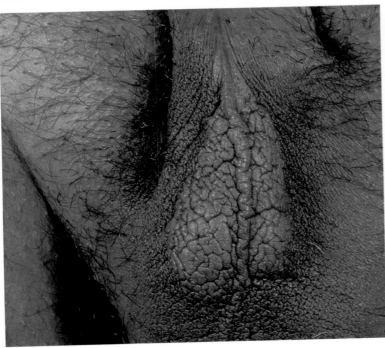

Fig. 2.85 Lichen simplex of the scrotum.

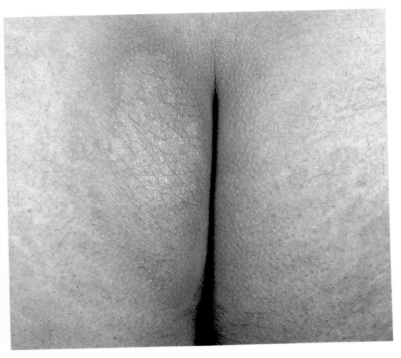

Fig. 2.86 Lichen simplex. The patch is well-defined and unilateral. The skin creases are exaggerated and the skin is thickened.

MISCELLANEOUS FORMS OF ECZEMA

Lichen Striatus

This is a distinctive condition which is occasionally seen in children. It is a self-limiting linear form of eczema which occurs relatively suddenly along a limb (Fig. 2.87) or across the trunk. The histopathology is eczematous but the cause is unknown. It resolves in a number of months.

Pityriasis Alba

This is a very common condition of childhood. It occurs on the face, particularly the cheeks (Fig. 2.88), and is most often seen in pigmented skin, producing a striking hypopigmentation of the skin. Sometimes a pink scaling eczema is seen which is believed to cause the loss of pigmentation. The cause is unknown and treatment with topical steroids is of little avail. The condition ultimately resolves.

Juvenile Plantar Dermatitis

This condition is seen in childhood. It is a well-defined eczema with a somewhat glazed and sometimes fissured appearance which affects the plantar surfaces symmetrically sparing the instep (Fig. 2.89). It is not a contact dermatitis but may well be related to the occlusive effect of the modern track shoe or 'trainer' footwear interfering with normal sweating in the area. It resolves with changing to cotton socks and leather shoes.

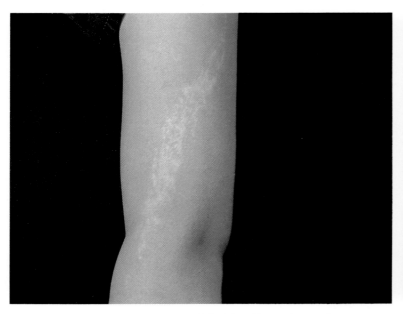

Fig. 2.87 Lichen striatus is a self-limiting linear form of eczema. The aetiology is quite unknown and in this case has left behind a postinflammatory hypopigmentation which eventually resolved spontaneously.

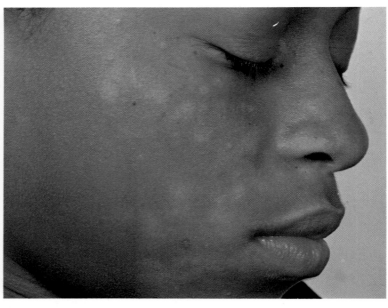

Fig. 2.88 Pityriasis alba of the cheeks. This condition possibly begins as an eczematous eruption and may leave behind post-inflammatory hypopigmentation which can take years to resolve.

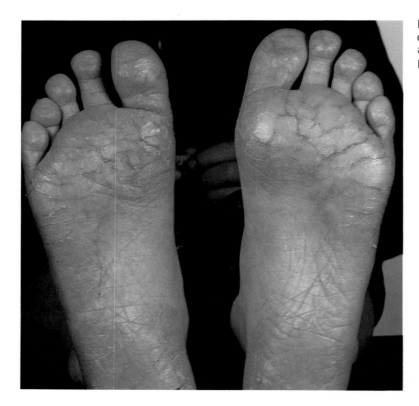

Fig. 2.89 Juvenile plantar dermatosis. This is a well-defined condition with a somewhat glazed and sometimes fissured appearance on the plantar surfaces sparing the instep. It is probably related to modern 'trainer' footwear.

3 Psoriasis

Psoriasis is one of the most common non-infectious disorders of the skin. It is frequently inherited, often chronic and may affect the nails and joints. Diagnosis is usually straightforward because the physical signs are distinctive. The eruption is characterized by well-defined, slightly raised, erythematous lesions (Fig. 3.1) which in the chronic state are covered by a silver scale (Fig. 3.2). The lesions vary in size from small papules (so-called guttate lesions; Fig. 3.3) to large plaques (Fig. 3.4) which are sometimes circular but generally more irregular in outline. They tend to heal centrally (Fig. 3.5), thus appearing as rings (Fig. 3.6). Gentle

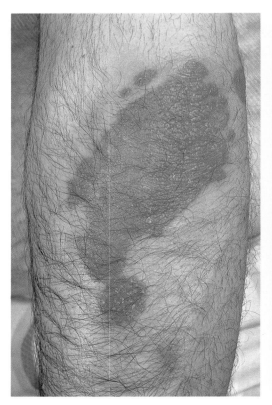

Fig. 3.1 Psoriasis. The plaque is well-defined, slightly raised and red. The silver scale is absent following treatment with a topical steroid and dithranol (anthralin).

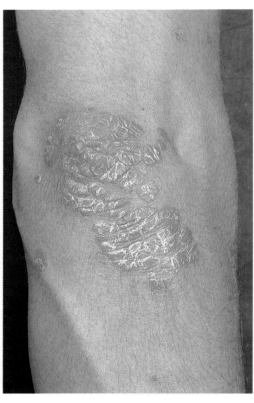

Fig. 3.2 Psoriasis. Chronic plaques are covered by a silvery scale. The points of the elbows are characteristically involved.

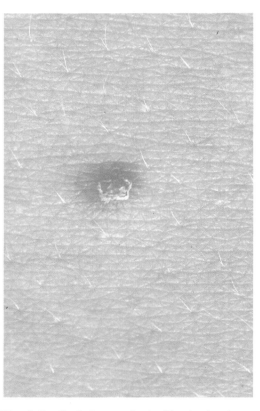

Fig. 3.3 Guttate psoriasis. The lesion is like a 'drop' of psoriasis on the skin. The basic characteristic of a red, extremely well-defined lesion covered with a silvery scale is retained.

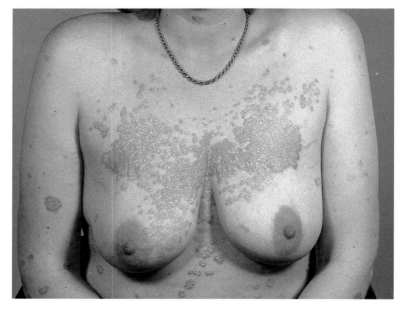

Fig. 3.4 Psoriasis. These lesions, some of which have become confluent forming a large plaque, followed burning of the skin with a sun lamp (Koebner phenomenon).

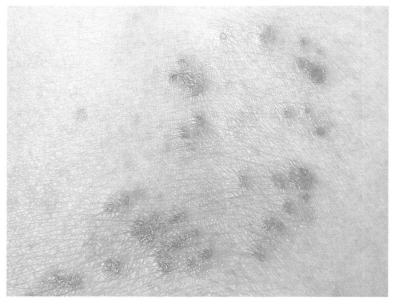

Fig. 3.5 Healing psoriasis. The disease clears from the centre. This sign frequently indicates imminent remission.

scratching of the surface of the lesion reveals minute bleeding points, which is an almost specific diagnostic sign. In the patient whose psoriasis is itchy and consequently excoriated, raw areas of psoriasis can be seen (Fig. 3.7).

The distribution of the eruption is especially helpful in the diagnosis, as psoriasis has a predilection for certain sites; these are the scalp (Fig. 3.8), knees, elbows (Fig. 3.9) and lumbosacral regions. Also, it is remarkable how lesions occurring on one side of the body are reduplicated on the other (Fig. 3.9); this

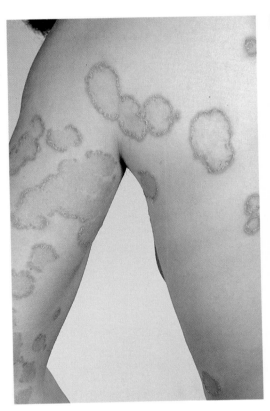

Fig. 3.6   Annular psoriasis. This results from central healing.

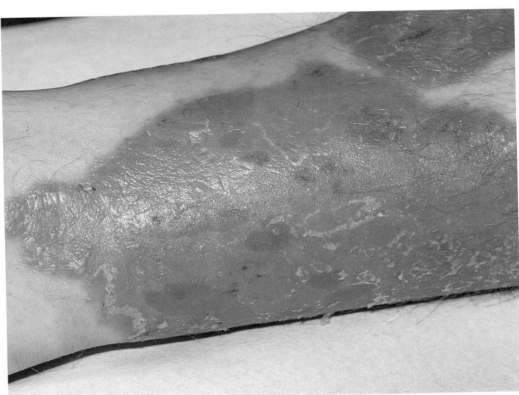

Fig. 3.7   Psoriasis. The raw areas are due to scratching of this plaque on the leg.

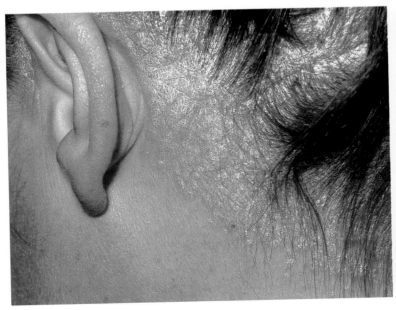

Fig. 3.8   Psoriasis in the scalp. This can be distinguished from dandruff by the red scaly plaques which are well-defined and extend to or beyond the hair margin.

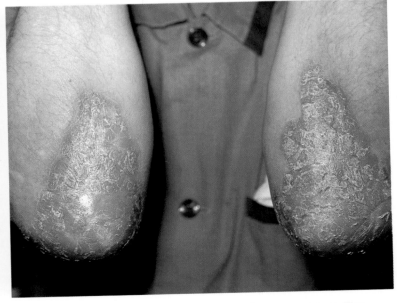

Fig. 3.9   Psoriasis. The lesions are usually symmetrical. The elbows are a characteristic site.

3.3

symmetry is so characteristic that the diagnosis based on a unilateral patch is likely to be erroneous (Figs. 3.10 – 3.12).

Psoriasis is recorded in all races but is more common in temperate climes and rare in the tropics. Fair-skinned persons are affected more than the dark-skinned and there is a definite familial tendency, probably inherited as an autosomal dominant with incomplete penetrance. Both sexes are affected equally. It may start at any time in life from infancy to old age but most frequently in the second and third decades. It waxes and wanes in intensity throughout life, but prolonged and occasionally permanent remissions do occur. Although some patients learn to tolerate it, the majority find it an accursed affliction, whatever the degree of their conditions. This varies from minor involvement to a debilitating disorder when it is widespread (Fig. 3.13). It may interfere with important areas of function such as the hands (Fig. 3.14) or feet (Fig. 3.15), or be visible and therefore disfiguring (Fig. 3.16). It is a social disability such that most patients limit their activities accordingly. If left untreated the skin feels uncomfortable and sometimes can be very pruritic.

The course of psoriasis is influenced by a variety of factors.

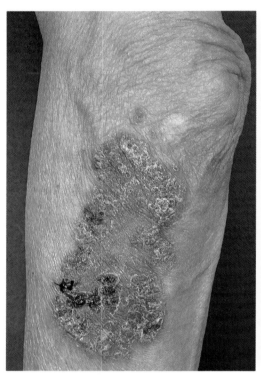

Fig. 3.10 Tertiary syphilis. This scaly plaque could well have passed for psoriasis but the solitary nature of the lesion raised the possibility of the great mimic, syphilis.

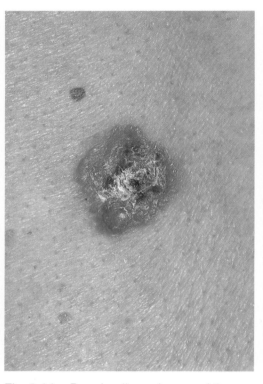

Fig. 3.11 Basal cell carcinoma of the trunk. Although the lesion is red and well-defined with a silvery scale, it is solitary and has a raised rolled margin. The adjacent brown lesions are seborrhoeic warts and a Campbell de Morgan spot is present.

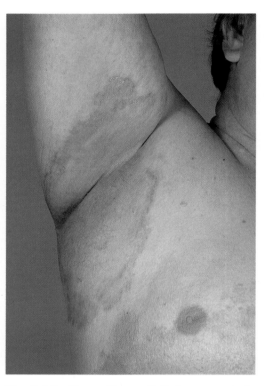

Fig. 3.12 Tinea. The activity is present at the margin, with central clearing and pigmentation. The lesion was unilateral.

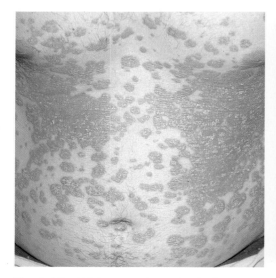

Fig. 3.13 Widespread psoriasis. The lesions are of different sizes but the symmetry and the sharp borders of the red scaly lesions are diagnostic.

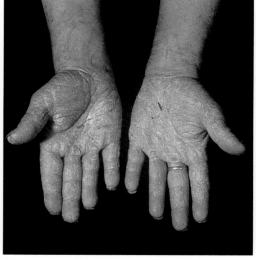

Fig. 3.14 Psoriasis of the hands. This may be socially isolating. All the physical signs of redness, scaling and definition are here. In addition, there are fissures which may be painful and interfere with manual dexterity.

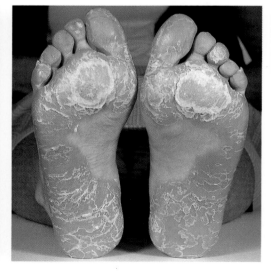

Fig. 3.15 Psoriasis of the soles. Note the symmetry, silver scale and well-defined nature of the condition. The patient found walking painful and difficult.

Physical illness and emotional stress can make it worse, while sunshine and rest can improve it. Trauma to the skin may precipitate development of the disease (Figs. 3.4 & 3.17). This curious and unexplained phenomenon was described by Koebner and is also seen in lichen planus and plane warts. Certain drugs, particularly lithium and antimalarials, may exacerbate the condition. A psoriasiform eruption associated with serious eye, peritoneal and pericardial complications was seen with practolol (a beta-blocker) before it was withdrawn. Frequently, however, the factors are not identifiable.

HISTOLOGICAL FEATURES

The histology is characteristic (Figs. 3.18 & 3.19). There is an immature epidermis with parakeratosis (retention of the nuclear remnants in the stratum corneum), acanthosis (thickening of the epithelium), loss of the granular cell layer and increased activity in the basal cell layer. The dermal capillary loops are dilated and tortuous. Inflammatory cells are found in the dermal papillae and, in acute cases, polymorphs migrate into the epidermis forming microabscesses.

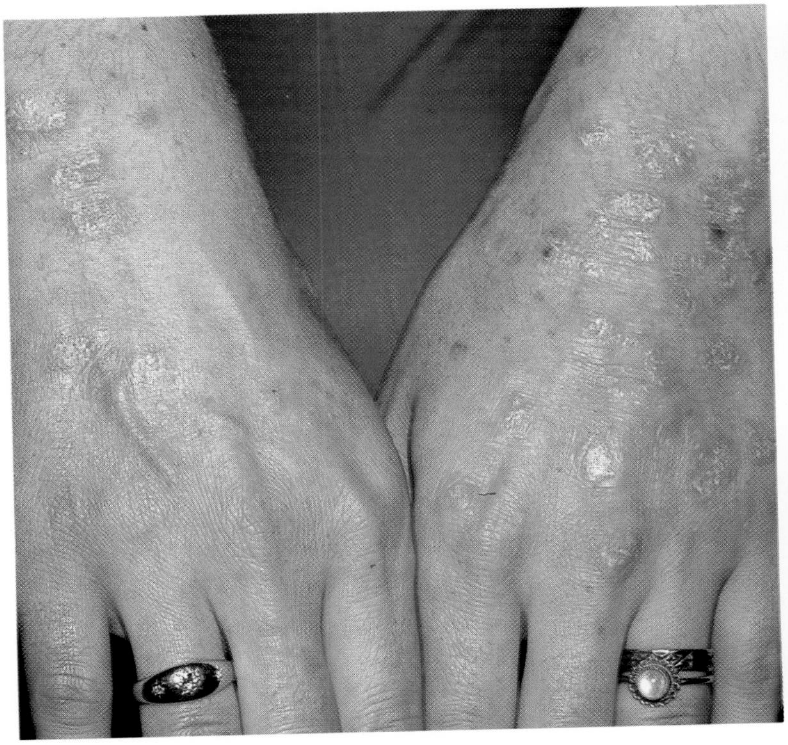

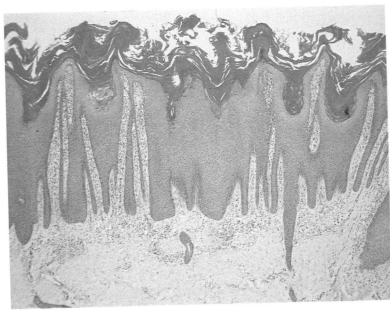

Fig. 3.16 Psoriasis of the backs of the hands. Fortunately, psoriasis is usually not present on exposed sites.

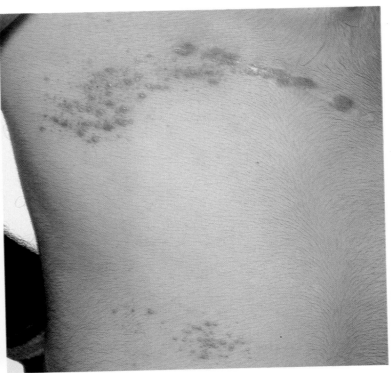

Fig. 3.17 The Koebner phenomenon. This represents an eruption following trauma to the skin. This patient developed psoriasis around a recent operation scar.

Fig. 3.18 Psoriatic plaque. Low power view showing hyperkeratosis with parakeratosis overlying a grossly acanthotic epidermis. The epidermal ridges are elongated, clubbed and fused at their lower borders. H&E stain. By courtesy of Dr. P.H. McKee.

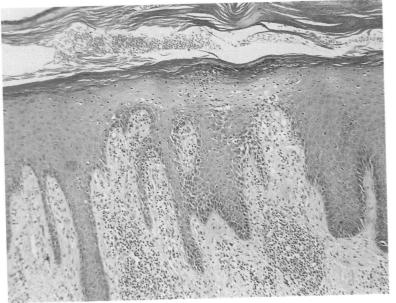

Fig. 3.19 Medium power view of a psoriatic plaque. Polymorphs migrating through the epidermis have formed a small collection (Munro microabscess) within the greatly thickened, partially parakeratotic stratum corneum. The dermal papillae are widened and contain dilated capillaries. An appreciable lymphohistiocytic infiltrate is seen in the dermis. H&E stain. By courtesy of Dr. P.H. McKee.

AETIOLOGY

The aetiology of psoriasis is unknown. There is epithelial hyper-proliferation and studies of cell transit through the epidermis indicate that cell replacement occurs roughly seven times faster than in normal skin. A basal cell in psoriasis is shed in about four days as opposed to the twenty-eight in normal skin. The scale which is shed so freely from psoriatic skin is the result of this overactivity. The erythema of the skin is due to the dilated dermal capillaries and the pustules of pustular psoriasis are due to the invading inflammatory cells. Some authorities believe that the inflammatory cells, be they neutrophils or lymphocytes, are of prime importance. Numerous biochemical and immunological abnormalities have been described but it is not known whether they are primary events or represent secondary responses.

CLINICAL FEATURES

Although psoriasis is a relatively easy condition to diagnose, it is helpful to consider certain forms of the disorder which have different prognostic and therapeutic implications. Also, psoriasis on certain sites can give rise to diagnostic confusion and particular therapeutic difficulties. Differential diagnosis is integrated into the following text. The list is not exhaustive and certain problems in diagnosis are discussed in other chapters.

FORMS OF PSORIASIS
Psoriasis Vulgaris

The most stable form of psoriasis, this responds most readily to treatment with topical agents. The patches are red, well-defined and covered with a silver scale (see Fig. 3.2).

DIFFERENTIAL DIAGNOSIS

LICHEN SIMPLEX. Like psoriasis, the lesions are well-defined. However, the patches are asymmetrical, often solitary and at sites readily available for scratching, such as the nape of the neck, the forearm and the lateral border of the lower leg or ankle (Fig. 3.20). Lichenification (thickening of the skin with pronounced surface markings) is the distinguishing feature.

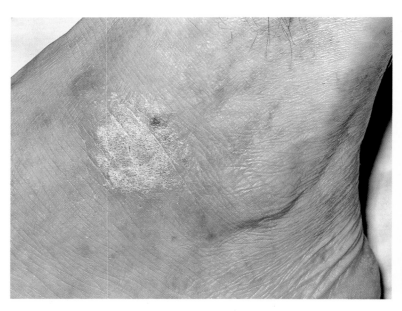

Fig. 3.20 Lichen simplex of the lateral malleolus. This was a solitary lesion and lichenification is present.

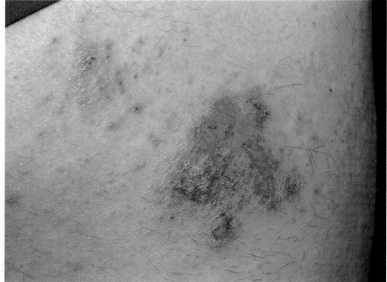

Fig. 3.21 Discoid eczema. This lesion is red and relatively well-defined but there is vesiculation and weeping of the skin.

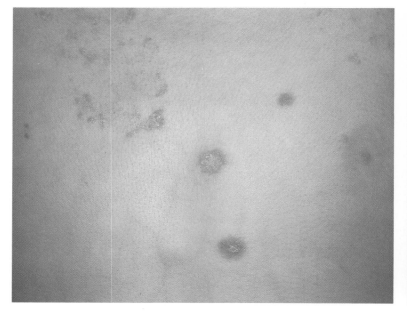

Fig. 3.22 Tinea corporis due to cat ringworm. The lesions are asymmetrical and show redness and scaling predominantly at the margin with a tendency to clear centrally.

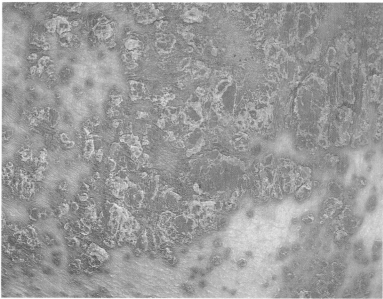

Fig. 3.23 Unstable psoriasis. This term refers to a red, inflamed and sore form which requires careful management as erythroderma or pustular psoriasis may supervene.

DISCOID ECZEMA. The lesions (Fig. 3.21) are also well-defined (unlike most other forms of eczema) but they are papulovesicular, causing oozing and crusting, with a predilection for the limbs.

TINEA CORPORIS. The lesion is often well-defined with an active, slightly raised, red scaling margin and a central healing area (Fig. 3.22) which sometimes shows postinflammatory hyperpigmentation. The distribution is usually asymmetrical.

Subacute or Acute Psoriasis

Psoriasis may become inflamed, sore and unstable (Fig. 3.23). There is often no obvious reason for this change but sometimes injudicious treatment may be the cause. The application of dithranol (anthralin) to a sensitive site, such as the flexures, or in too high a concentration for the skin type of the patient may have occurred. Bland therapy or topical steroids are required until there is a return to the stable state. If involvement is extensive, the use of systemic agents may be warranted.

Guttate Psoriasis

This occurs following a streptococcal throat infection in a person predisposed to psoriasis (Fig. 3.24). Tiny lesions appear suddenly and explosively all over the skin, particularly on the trunk (Fig. 3.25) and limbs. The small size of the lesions distinguishes it from psoriasis vulgaris (Fig. 3.26). It is seen in the younger age groups and usually remits spontaneously within three months, often permanently. It may, however, remain as a few chronic plaques. Tar baths followed by ultraviolet light is a useful therapy.

DIFFERENTIAL DIAGNOSIS

PITYRIASIS ROSEA. This disease (Fig. 3.27) erupts quickly in a manner similar to guttate psoriasis and is also mostly truncal in distribution. It is a condition of approximately six weeks duration, starting with a patch that is larger than subsequent lesions and which heralds the onset of the disease. Although the patches are well-defined, they are pinker than psoriasis and have a fine scale towards the periphery (Fig. 3.28), unlike the diffuse silvery thick scale of psoriasis. The lesions are much larger than those of guttate psoriasis.

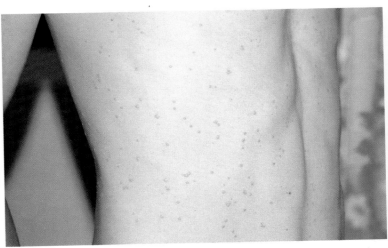

Fig. 3.24 Guttate psoriasis. Small drop-like lesions occur in a shower-like distribution over the trunk and limbs.

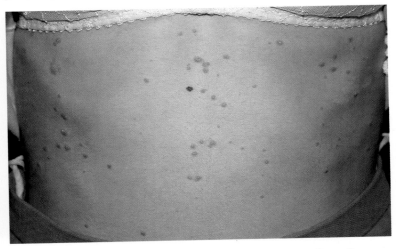

Fig. 3.25 Guttate psoriasis. This erupts suddenly, often after a throat infection. It is usually associated with a good prognosis.

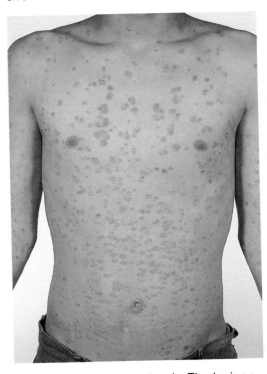

Fig. 3.26 Psoriasis vulgaris. The lesions are larger than those of guttate psoriasis.

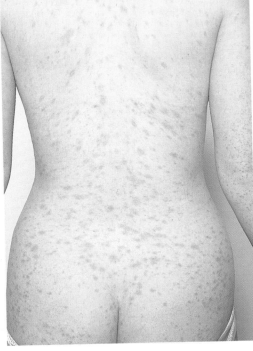

Fig. 3.27 Pityriasis rosea. The eruption is usually limited to the trunk, upper arms and thighs.

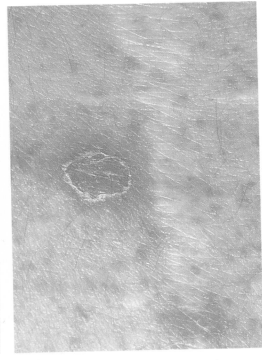

Fig. 3.28 Pityriasis rosea. The lesions are more pink than red and have a fine scale towards the periphery of the lesion.

3.7

SECONDARY SYPHILIS. This disease is still the great mimic and may present as a psoriasiform eruption on the trunk (Fig. 3.29). However, the patient usually feels unwell, lymphadenopathy is present and lesions are found on the palms, soles (Fig. 3.30), face and genitalia. Other mucous membrane stigmata may be present and, in cases of the slightest doubt, the serology should be done.

LICHEN PLANUS. This disease can be differentiated from psoriasis by its violaceous or purple colour (Fig. 3.31). The lesions are papular but they are polygonal in shape, flat-topped and shiny. Their distribution, although symmetrical, differs from psoriasis, being found in particular on the fronts of the wrists (Fig. 3.32), backs of the hands, forearms, ankles and shins. Involvement of the mouth is characteristic.

Pustular Psoriasis

LOCALIZED PUSTULAR PSORIASIS confined to the palms (Fig. 3.33) and soles (Fig. 3.34) is an intractable variant. Yellow pustules, which turn brown as they age, appear on a background of erythema. They occur especially on the thenar or hypothenar eminences and on the central and medial aspects of the soles. It might be difficult to accept the appearances as psoriasis were it not for typical plaques often being found elsewhere.

GENERALIZED PUSTULAR PSORIASIS (Figs. 3.35 & 3.36) is a rare and sometimes lethal variant of the disease. Extensive waves of small sterile pustules cover the skin and during each crop the patient's life is in danger. There is toxaemia, high fever and leucocytosis. The skin is fiery red and sore, causing much distress and

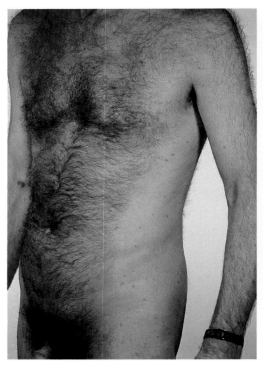

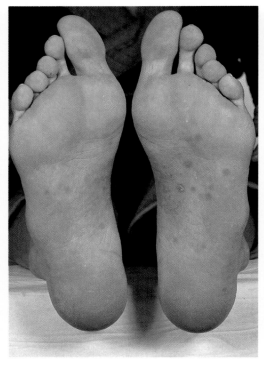

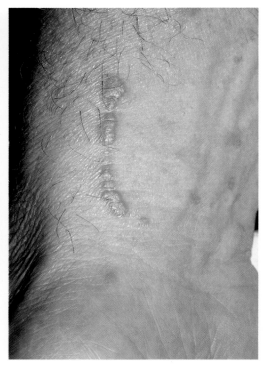

Fig. 3.29 Secondary syphilis. This may easily be mistaken for psoriasis. Other factors have to be considered for a correct diagnosis.

Fig. 3.30 Secondary syphilis. Involvement of the palms and soles is a characteristic finding (same patient as in Fig. 3.29).

Fig. 3.31 Lichen planus. The papules are purple rather than red in colour.

Fig. 3.32 Lichen planus. The violaceous colour helps to distinguish it from psoriasis. The white patterning of the surface of the lesions and distribution on the fronts of the wrists are typical.

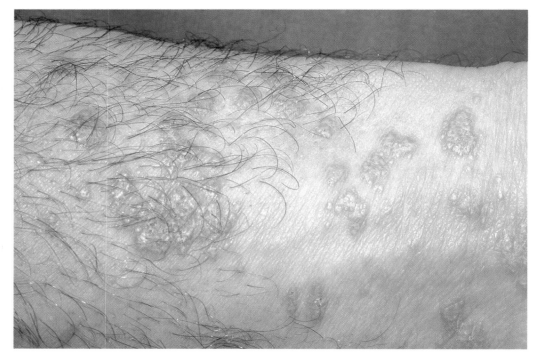

prostration. The danger includes secondary bacterial infection of the skin, urinary tract and lungs, septicaemia, electrolyte imbalance, dehydration, hypocalcaemia and hypoalbuminaemia. The change to pustulation may occur without obvious cause in a patient with previous psoriasis vulgaris; occasionally localized palmar or plantar pustular psoriasis may become generalized. However, pustular psoriasis is usually due to mismanagement. Steroids, usually systemic but occasionally certain potent topical forms (for example, clobetasol propionate) may precipitate the disease. Systemic steroids should not be used specifically to treat psoriasis but they are sometimes given for coexisting conditions and, if reduced quickly by a physician unaware of the danger, may result in pustulation. Similar cases have been seen with patients withdrawn suddenly from using potent topical steroids.

The disease may remit spontaneously but systemic agents are usually necessary and must be used with great caution and under specialist supervision. Methotrexate is probably the drug of choice but should be administered in much smaller amounts than for other forms of psoriasis because of the increased likelihood of bone marrow toxicity. Etretinate is also proving to be an effective agent.

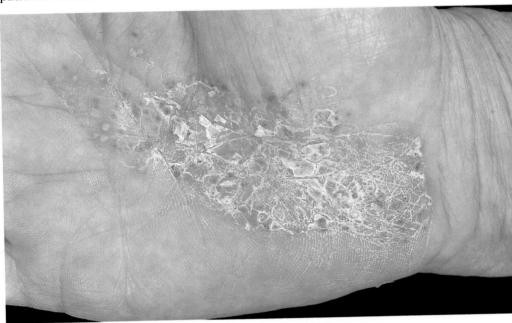

Fig. 3.33 Pustular psoriasis of the palms is characterized by yellow pustules, which become brown, on a background of well-defined scaling and erythema.

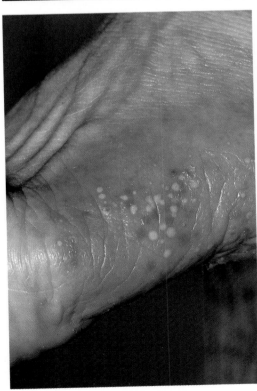

Fig. 3.34 Pustular psoriasis of the foot. Small sterile yellow pustules which turn brown are found symmetrically on a red base. The condition responds very poorly to topical therapy.

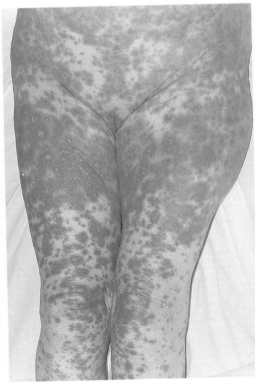

Fig. 3.35 Generalized pustular psoriasis of von Zumbusch. Sheets of small sterile pustules erupt on red inflamed skin. By courtesy of St. Mary's Hospital.

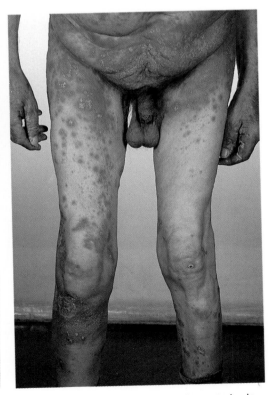

Fig. 3.36 Generalized pustular psoriasis of von Zumbusch. The skin is fiery red and sore and studded with white or yellow sterile pustules.

DIFFERENTIAL DIAGNOSIS

There should be no confusion as long as true bacterial infection of the skin (folliculitis) is ruled out (Fig. 3.37).

Erythrodermic Psoriasis

Psoriasis is one of the more common causes of erythroderma or exfoliative dermatitis (Fig. 3.38), these terms being synonymous for universal involvement of the skin. The diagnosis may be made because typical silver scales are present on the background erythema, because nail or joint changes are present or because the patient is known to have had ordinary psoriasis. Again, the patient is dangerously unwell, although not usually to the degree seen in generalized pustular psoriasis. The skin is very red due to vasodilatation and there is considerable loss of heat; the patient feels cold, shivers and requires many blankets. Increased cardiac output because of the increased cutaneous blood flow may precipitate cardiac failure. There is dehydration due to cutaneous water loss and hypoproteinaemia and anaemia from loss of protein, iron and folic acid in the scales. If the patient is debilitated from another general medical condition, erythrodermic psoriasis may be the final straw.

Although the disease may start without a preceding history of psoriasis, this is unusual. More often, psoriasis vulgaris becomes erythrodermic because of an infection, drug allergy or adverse reaction to topical therapy. Systemic treatment is almost always required. Occasionally, generalized pustular psoriasis may develop. Drug reactions, eczema, pityriasis rubra pilaris, mycosis fungoides and its variant, the Sézary syndrome, may all present as an erythroderma, so differential diagnosis may not be easy based on physical signs alone. However, the history, a skin biopsy and specialized investigations usually clarify the situation.

Psoriatic Arthropathy

This disease of the joints occurs in a minority of patients, who usually also have the stigmata of psoriasis elsewhere on the skin or in the nails (Fig. 3.39). However, it can be seen in patients with no dermatological features although a family history of the disease may be present. It is beyond the scope of this text to detail the changes but various patterns are recognizable. The hands and feet may be affected but characteristically involving the distal interphalangeal joints with sparing of the proximal ones (Fig. 3.40). This serves to differentiate it from rheumatoid arthritis along with absence of the serological abnormalities found in the latter disease. A monarticular, often asymmetrical, arthritis of larger joints, such as the knees and elbows, may occur. Sacroiliitis and ankylosing spondylitis are unusual but distinctive and, rarely, a mutilating form occurs. All forms of the arthritis may precede and follow the onset of psoriasis.

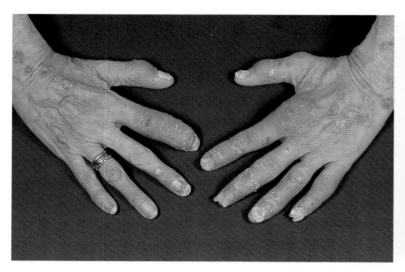

Fig. 3.37 Folliculitis. The pustules are yellow and follicular in distribution. Culture of the purulent material is necessary.

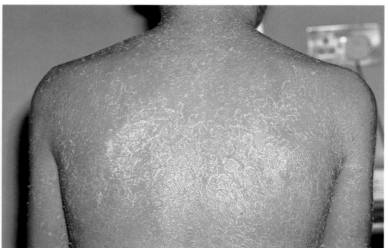

Fig. 3.38 Erythrodermic psoriasis. The skin is universally involved. In some areas it is red (erythrodermic) and in others scaling (exfoliating).

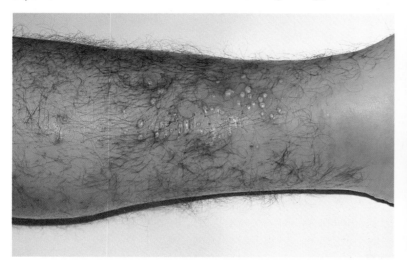

Fig. 3.39 Psoriasis of the skin, nails and joints. The distal interphalangeal joints and nails are characteristically affected.

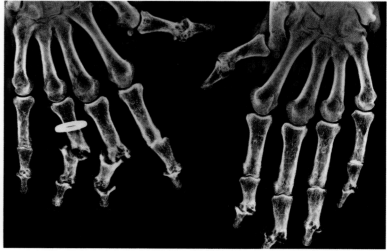

Fig. 3.40 Psoriatic arthropathy. The arthritis which accompanies psoriasis is similar to rheumatoid arthritis. A distinguishing feature is pronounced involvement of the distal interphalangeal joints in psoriasis. By courtesy of Dr. P. Gishen, King's College Hospital.

SITES OF PSORIASIS
Scalp
The scalp is very commonly affected and indeed may be the only site involved. Discrete symmetrical red plaques with considerable scaling are found and there is a tendency for the disease to extend beyond the hair-bearing areas onto the adjacent skin (Fig. 3.41). Remarkably, the condition rarely results in hair loss.

Psoriasis of the scalp is particularly difficult to treat. Local steroids are easy to use but only suppress symptoms and not very well at that. Coconut oil compound ointment (60% coconut oil, 13% emulsifying wax, 12% coal tar solution, 9% yellow soft paraffin, 4% precipitated sulphur, 2% salicylic acid) is probably the most effective treatment but unpleasant to use and may require the help of a dermatologically trained nurse.

DIFFERENTIAL DIAGNOSIS
SEBORRHOEIC DERMATITIS. The scalp is pink; the lesions are less well-defined and the scales finer than those of psoriasis.

PITYRIASIS AMIANTACEA. This condition (Fig. 3.42) may be a manifestation of psoriasis but is more usually a short-lived condition of the scalp and hair, probably related to seborrhoeic eczema. It is a disorder of youth. Sticky thick scales are found on the scalp and characteristically attach to the hair shafts. Although the affected hairs usually fall out, they do regrow. The condition responds to tar-containing preparations but not to topical steroids.

TINEA CAPITIS. Seen rarely after puberty, this is a disorder of childhood (Fig. 3.43). Although, as in psoriasis, varying degrees of erythema and scaling occur, unlike psoriasis the patches are asymmetrical and hair loss, which recovers after treatment, is the rule.

LUPUS ERYTHEMATOSUS. Redness and an adherent scale lead to hair loss and scarring (Fig. 3.44).

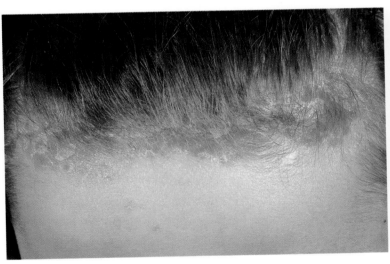

Fig. 3.41 Psoriasis of the scalp. This often extends beyond the hair margin onto the skin. Hair loss is most unusual. Therapy is difficult.

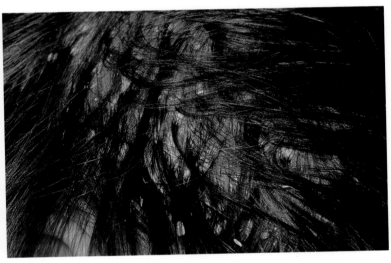

Fig. 3.42 Pityriasis amiantacea. Thick scales are found on the scalp and attached to the hair shafts. It sometimes results from psoriasis, but more commonly, it is a manifestation of seborrhoeic eczema and is short-lived, responding rapidly to tar-containing ointments. Hair loss occurs but is followed by complete recovery.

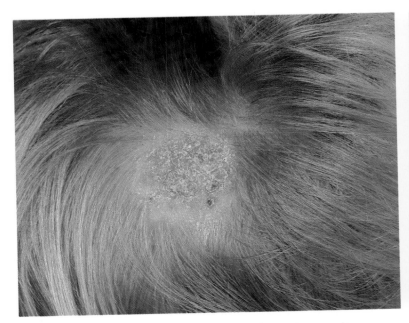

Fig. 3.43 Tinea capitis. Scaling and erythema is seen in ringworm of the scalp but is accompanied by hair loss. This disease is rare after puberty.

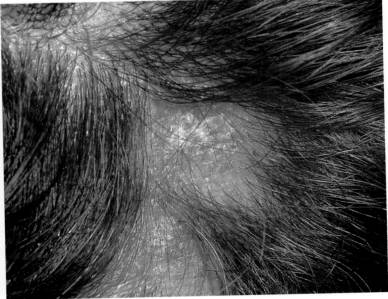

Fig. 3.44 Lupus erythematosus of the scalp. Erythema and scaling is present with hair loss, usually permanent due to scarring.

Ears

The ears (Fig. 3.45) are frequently involved together with the scalp. Occasionally the condition may be misdiagnosed as otitis externa (Fig. 3.46).

Face

Fortunately, the face (Fig. 3.47) is usually spared but, when involved, gives rise to embarrassment. It does not respond well to hydrocortisone, the treatment for facial seborrhoeic eczema,

and is the exception to the rule that powerful steroids should not be used on the face. Dithranol can be used but the staining is often unacceptable, as is the burning which can occur unless used with caution.

DIFFERENTIAL DIAGNOSIS

SEBORRHOEIC ECZEMA. The lesions are ill-defined and pink (Fig. 3.48) as opposed to being well-defined and red as in psoriasis. Also the scale is thicker and whiter.

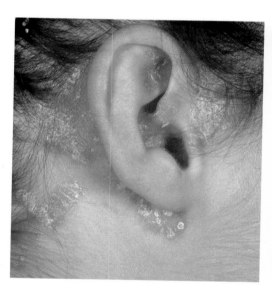

Fig. 3.45 Psoriasis of the ear. The adjacent scalp and skin are also involved and the thick silver scale is obvious.

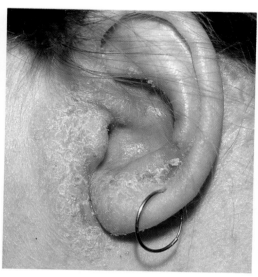

Fig. 3.46 Otitis externa (seborrhoeic eczema of the ear). Psoriasis is often mistaken for this because the adjacent scalp or other areas of the skin are not examined for involvement. Otitis externa may weep and crust (as here) and the scale is finer and the colour less red than in psoriasis.

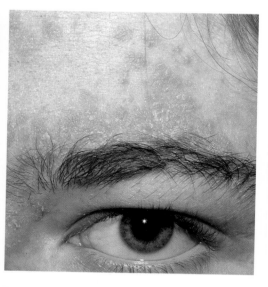

Fig. 3.47 Psoriasis of the face. There is usually enough evidence of psoriasis elsewhere on the body to make the diagnosis clear. However, the eruption is redder, more well-defined and scaly than seborrhoeic eczema and does not respond well to hydrocortisone.

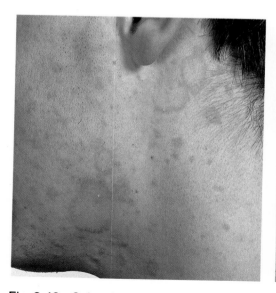

Fig. 3.48 Seborrhoeic eczema of the face. The patches are pink and have a finer scale.

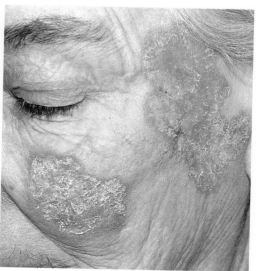

Fig. 3.49 Lupus erythematosus of the face. The lesions are well defined and the scale is tenacious. Scarring may be present.

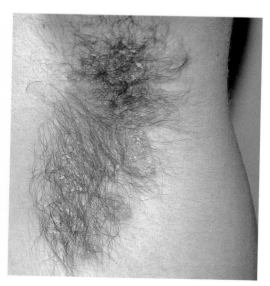

Fig. 3.50 Axillary psoriasis. Potent topical steroids are indicated as dithranol aggravates psoriasis in the flexures.

LUPUS ERYTHEMATOSUS. Well-defined plaques occur (Fig. 3.49) but the scales are tenacious. There is a tendency to scarring. Skin biopsy will aid differentiation from psoriasis.

Flexures

A variant of psoriasis occurring predominantly in the flexures (Figs. 3.50 – 3.53) is one of the causes of intertrigo and may represent a Koebner phenomenon. It is seen in middle-aged and elderly patients, especially women (Fig. 3.54) and often in those who are obese. The skin is red and the plaques well-defined, but the characteristic silver scale is absent. It is often resistant to local therapy. Dithranol aggravates the condition and topical steroids are only partially successful. In widespread intractable cases, systemic therapy should be considered.

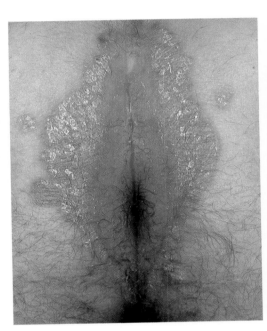

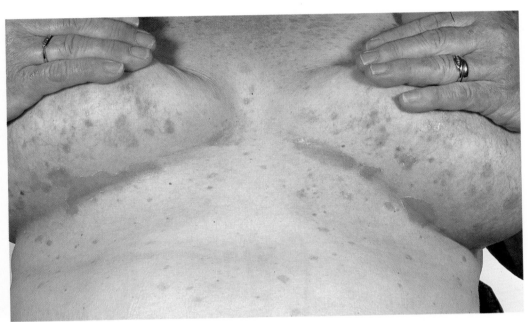

Fig. 3.51 Perianal psoriasis. The symmetry, deep red colour and silver scale are characteristic.

Fig. 3.52 Submammary psoriasis. The plaques are well-defined and red. It is always wise to take scrapings to exclude a fungal disorder.

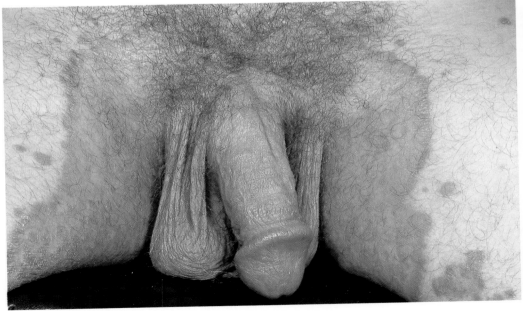

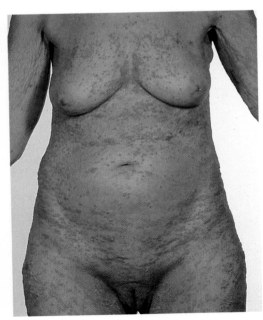

Fig. 3.53 Psoriasis in the groin. Scrapings were negative. The deep red colour, symmetry and involvement of the penis, scrotum and adjacent skin is suggestive of psoriasis.

Fig. 3.54 Flexural psoriasis. Widespread psoriasis, predominantly in intertriginous areas particularly in the elderly, responds poorly to topical therapy.

3.13

DIFFERENTIAL DIAGNOSIS

The differential diagnosis and management of intertrigo is considered elsewhere but fungal disorders must always be considered and scrapings taken for mycology. It is not unusual for tinea (Fig. 3.55) to occur in addition to psoriasis elsewhere.

Hands and Feet

The visibility of psoriasis on the hands is a serious social disability and, in addition, may interfere with manual dexterity. Involvement of the feet can make walking painful and difficult. Therapeutically, palmar and plantar psoriasis are exceedingly troublesome because the thickness of the stratum corneum in these areas makes penetration by topical remedies difficult. The affected areas are symmetrical, red and scaly (Fig. 3.56) but are frequently fissured and easily mistaken for eczema, particularly if there is no evidence of psoriasis elsewhere. Its resistance to local therapy and the lack of pruritus should suggest that the disorder is not eczema. Also, there are no vesicles or exudates (Fig. 3.57). Distinction is important because systemic cytotoxic therapy, which is inappropriate to eczema, may be very beneficial in the treatment of psoriasis of these areas (Fig. 3.58). The differential diagnosis is considered in the chapter on hand eczema.

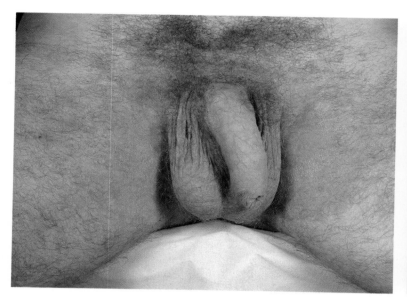

Fig. 3.55 Tinea cruris. Fungal hyphae were found in scrapings taken from the skin which had been treated with topical steroids. Tinea and psoriasis may coexist. The usual inflammatory margin has been suppressed by the steroids.

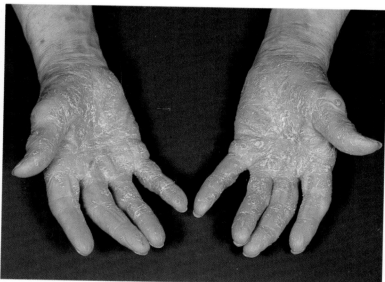

Fig. 3.56 Psoriasis of the palms. This may be difficult to differentiate from eczema in the absence of lesions elsewhere. The condition is dry, red and well-defined with a thick silver scale. Painful fissures are common.

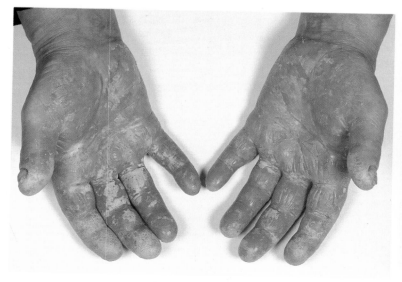

Fig. 3.57 Eczema of the palms. Vesiculation and consequent weeping are characteristics of eczema not found in psoriasis. Eczema is pruritic which psoriasis usually is not.

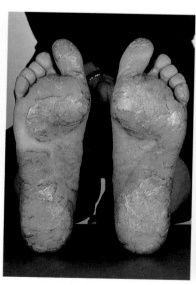
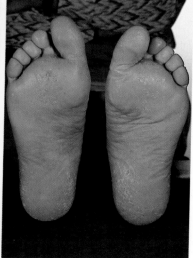

Fig. 3.58 Psoriasis of the feet. Topical therapy is frequently ineffective, and because the disorder may make walking difficult, systemic therapy may be necessary. Methotrexate has been invaluable in preserving function in this case.

Lower Legs

If psoriasis is present elsewhere the diagnosis is obvious; but if only the lower limbs are affected (Fig. 3.59), certain other disorders should be considered.

LICHEN PLANUS. In this site the characteristic violaceous colour (Fig. 3.60) may be difficult to discern from the more livid red of psoriasis. Examination of the mucous membranes and skin elsewhere thus becomes very important.

LICHEN SIMPLEX. The plaque (Fig. 3.61), although well-defined, is unilateral and lichenified.

TINEA. Activity at the margin of the plaque (Fig. 3.62) with central clearing is characteristic.

VARICOSE ECZEMA. The eruption is red with fine scales and is ill-defined (Fig. 3.63). Unlike psoriasis it may weep and associated varicosities and ulceration may be found.

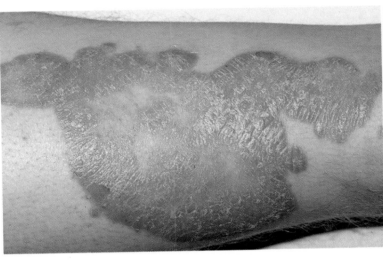

Fig. 3.59 Psoriasis of the leg. The eruption is red and the silver scale is present.

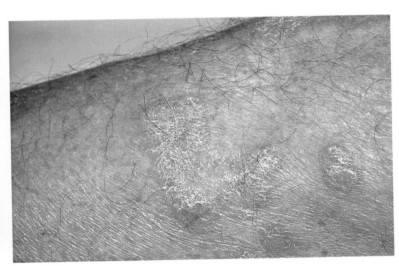

Fig. 3.60 Lichen planus. The lesions have a violaceous colour.

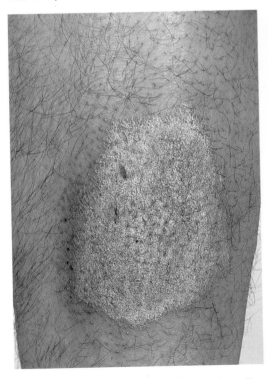

Fig. 3.61 Lichen simplex. Although well-defined the plaque is usually solitary and unilateral with pronounced skin markings

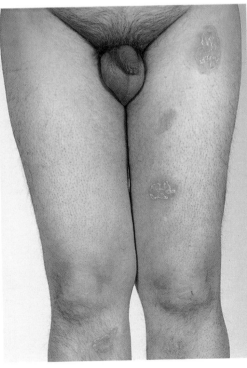

Fig. 3.62 Tinea. Activity at the margin of the plaque suggests tinea. The lesions are asymmetrical, unlike psoriasis.

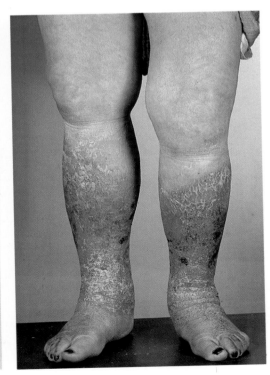

Fig. 3.63 Varicose eczema. The eruption is largely confined to the lower legs and shows features of eczema.

3.15

Genitals

Since genital psoriasis (Fig. 3.64) rarely occurs in the absence of psoriasis elsewhere, diagnosis is generally not difficult. There are usually one or more plaques which are red, well-defined and symmetrical but the silver scale is absent. Treatment with topical steroids is effective.

The differential diagnosis is considered elsewhere. However, lichen planus (Fig. 3.65) is often mistakenly diagnosed but its shiny flat-topped violaceous papules are distinctive.

Nails

Involvement of the nails occurs with or without psoriasis of the skin. The features are multiple small pits (Fig. 3.66) and onycholysis (Fig. 3.67), caused by separation of the nail plate from the nail bed by subungual disease; but these features are not exclusive to psoriasis. Severe dystrophy (Fig. 3.68) and even temporary loss of nails are the result of subungual hyperkeratosis secondary to epidermal hyperplasia. Nail involvement is usually symmetrical, distinguishing it from tinea (Fig. 3.69). In its erythrodermic and pustular forms, psoriasis of the skin overlying the posterior nail fold may cause destructive changes (Fig. 3.70), leading some surgeons to resort to amputation, which is unwise as the disease will return (Fig. 3.71). The differential diagnosis of nail disorders is dealt with in its own section.

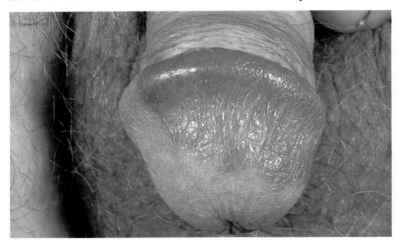

Fig. 3.64 Genital psoriasis. Although frequently no scale is visible, the plaque is slightly raised, red and well-defined.

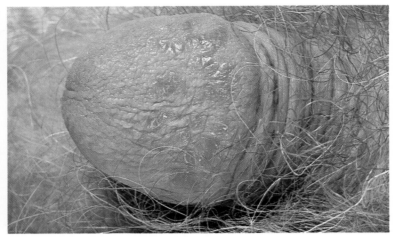

Fig. 3.65 Lichen planus. Shiny purple flat-topped papules are distinctive.

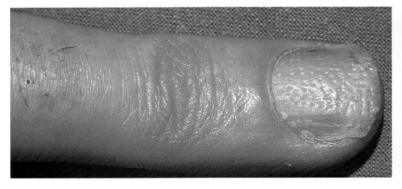

Fig. 3.66 Psoriasis of the nail. This fingernail is covered by multiple small pits and some onycholysis is present.

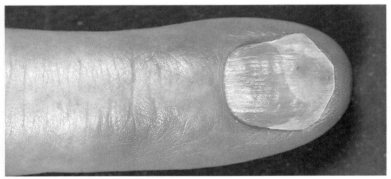

Fig. 3.67 Onycholysis. The distal end of the nail has separated from the nail bed. The nail has a creamy yellow appearance.

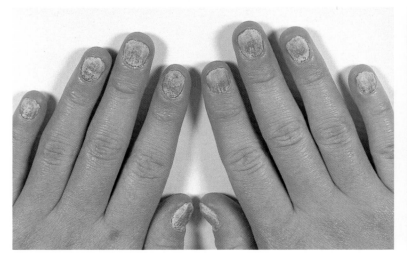

Fig. 3.68 Psoriasis of the nails. The involvement is characteristically symmetrical and considerable dystrophy has resulted from subungual hyperkeratosis.

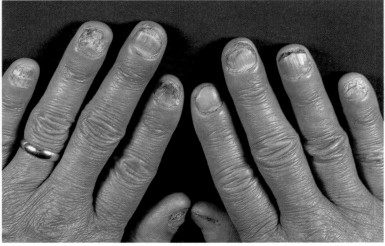

Fig. 3.69 Tinea of the nails. The involvement is asymmetrical. For example, the nail of the index finger of the right hand is barely involved whereas that of the left hand is grossly affected.

TREATMENT OF PSORIASIS

Since this is a chronic disorder of unknown aetiology, treatment must never in the long run be of more harm than good to the patient. Explanation and support are of paramount importance and topical preparations the mainstay of therapy. Potent gluco-corticosteroids are cosmetically acceptable and can be remark-ably effective, but more often the response is short-lived and results in little more than removal of the surface scale (see Fig. 3.1). However, even this is helpful to the patient because psoriasis is uncomfortable if left untreated. As itching can be extremely distressing, antihistamines are useful. On the other hand, the side-effects from overuse of local and systemic therapies are hazards. Secondary sepsis or folliculitis (Fig. 3.72) occasionally occurs. Topical steroids may produce atrophy of the dermis and epidermis; the resultant thinned skin appears red from increased visibility of dilated blood vessels (telangiectasia) no longer protected by collagen, and purpura may result (Fig. 3.73). Striae (Fig. 3.74) are common, especially in flexural areas. Excessive application and enhanced percutaneous absorption have been known to lead to Cushing's syndrome and, if the applications are abruptly discontinued, adrenal failure and generalized pustular psoriasis may sometimes result (Fig. 3.75).

Tar is messy, malodorous and unpleasant to use but is undoubtedly effective, especially in combination with

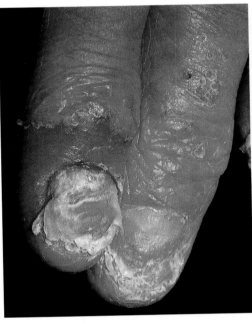

Fig. 3.70 Psoriasis of the nails. Localized pustular psoriasis involving periungual skin has produced dystrophy of the nail.

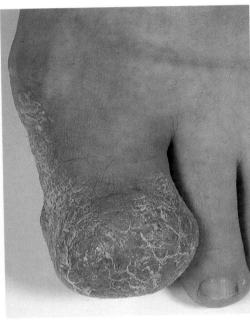

Fig. 3.71 Psoriasis of the toe. Nails and even digits are sometimes unnecessarily removed. In this case the psoriasis recurred in the amputation stump.

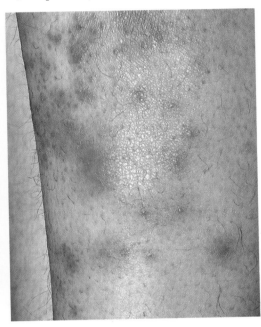

Fig. 3.72 Folliculitis. This may result from treatment of psoriasis with potent topical glucocorticosteroids.

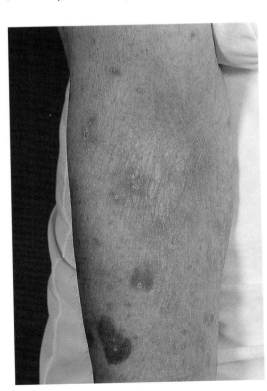

Fig. 3.73 Atrophy of the skin and purpura may occur from excessive use of potent topical glucocorticosteroids.

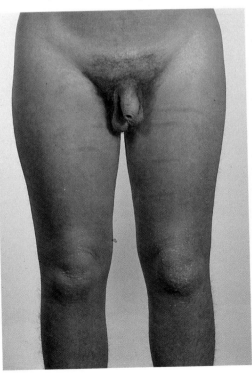

Fig. 3.74 Striae due to excessive use of topical steroids. This man has severe erythrodermic psoriasis and systemic therapy was ultimately necessary.

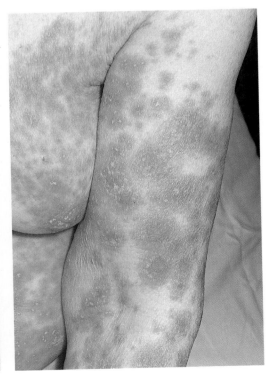

Fig. 3.75 Generalized pustular psoriasis. This may be precipitated if very potent steroids are abruptly discontinued. By courtesy of St. Mary's Hospital.

ultraviolet light. Dithranol is most effective (Fig. 3.76, upper) but stains the skin temporarily (Fig. 3.76, lower) and clothing permanently and must be used with caution to avoid burning (Fig. 3.77). It is the standard in-patient therapy for psoriasis, in combination with tar baths and ultraviolet light irradiation. Rest and relaxation must not be neglected.

In debilitating forms such as erythroderma, pustular psoriasis and psoriasis of the hands and feet, systemic therapy may be justifiable, in particular methotrexate, if one bears in mind that in the long term it may cause cirrhosis of the liver. Recently, photochemotherapy (PUVA) which involves a psoralen (P) drug taken orally, followed by exposure to long wave ultraviolet (UVA) light for activation (Fig. 3.78), has given excellent results (Fig. 3.79). Other drugs are also used, particularly azathioprine, hydroxyurea and etretinate and undoubtedly more will become available. The majority of these agents appear to act by inhibiting epithelial cell division. All have attendant hazards and should only be administered by those with dermatological training.

The treatment of psoriasis represents one of the most important dermatological failures of the present day. The disease affects over one percent of the European and North American populations, causes considerable suffering and is still of unknown causation. Topical therapy has not seen an advance for many years and tar, dithranol and ultraviolet light have been in use for over fifty years.

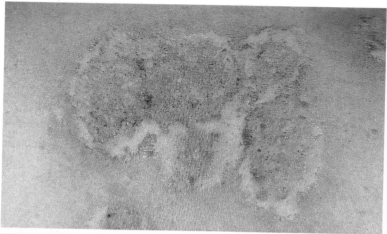

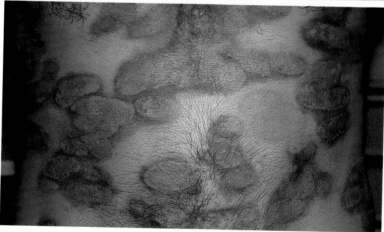

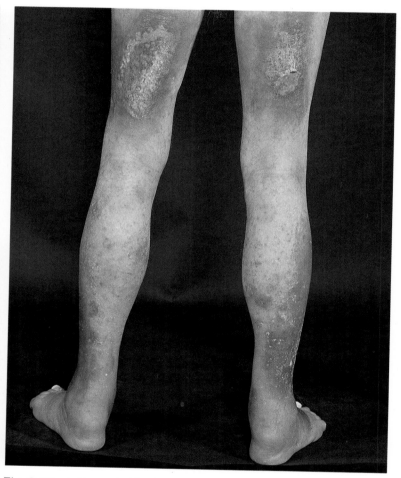

Fig. 3.76 Dithranol staining: (upper) of a plaque of psoriasis through which healed skin can be seen; (below) of psoriasis on the trunk. Compare with the lesion which has been left untreated.

Fig. 3.77 Inflamed skin due to injudicious use of dithranol.

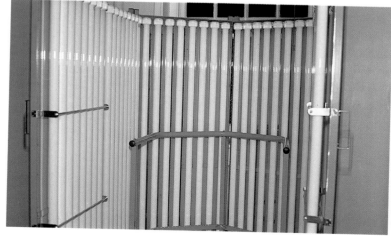

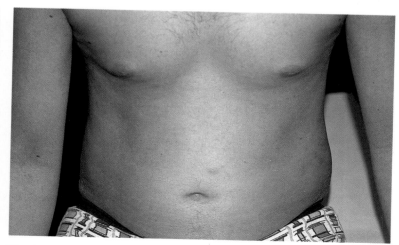

Fig. 3.78 PUVA machine. The tubes emit long wave ultraviolet light (UVA) which photoactivates psoralen (P).

Fig. 3.79 Complete clearing with photochemotherapy of the psoriasis shown in Fig. 3.13. Note the pronounced tanning.

4 Pityriasis Rosea, Lichen Planus and Pityriasis Rubra Pilaris

The only justification for grouping these three conditions together in one chapter is the fact that they are specific skin disorders of unknown aetiology. Pityriasis rosea and lichen planus are two of the easiest dermatological conditions to diagnose, and they demonstrate clearly the dermatological principles of precise description of the eruption's morphology and proper observation of its distribution. Some authorities classify pityriasis rosea under viral infections, for which there is no evidence, and lichen planus under immunological disorders, for which there is some evidence. Pityriasis rubra pilaris is an extremely rare disorder and is sometimes classified on its own or under disorders of keratinization; most texts of this level leave it out completely. Its inclusion here is largely a matter of convenience, but it does have specific physical signs and is an important differential diagnosis of erythroderma.

PITYRIASIS ROSEA

Pityriasis rosea is a common self-limiting skin disorder of young people. A single attack is the rule but recurrences are occasionally reported. The disease is seen more frequently in the spring and autumn and, occasionally, a cluster of cases occurs within institutions and family groups. The rarity of second attacks, suggesting the development of immunity, and the recognition of the occasional clustering of cases have led to the theory that the disorder is of an infectious nature, possibly viral. However, sophisticated viral techniques have been applied to the disorder with no positive results. The histopathology of the rash is that of an eczema.

Clinical Features

The onset of the eruption is heralded by a single patch (Fig. 4.1) which is present for a few days, and sometimes a few weeks,

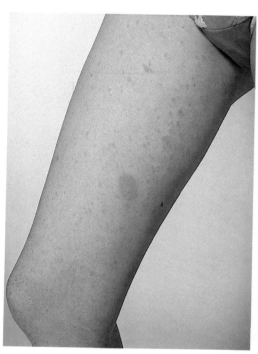

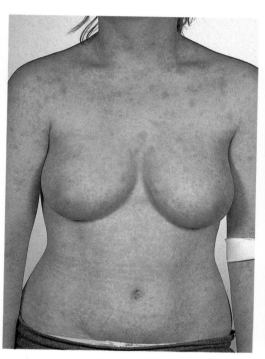

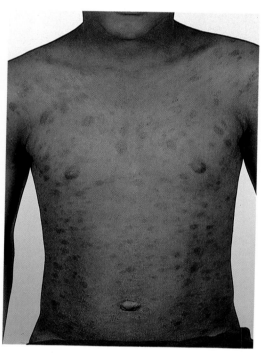

Fig. 4.1 Pityriasis rosea. The herald patch is the first lesion and is larger than subsequent lesions. This eruption is on the patient's thigh and later spread to her trunk. By courtesy of St. Mary's Hospital.

Fig. 4.2 Pityriasis rosea. This disorder predominantly affects the trunk.

Fig. 4.3 Pityriasis rosea. In the pigmented skin, the pink colour is often indiscernible, but the lesions are still oval and found predominantly on the trunk.

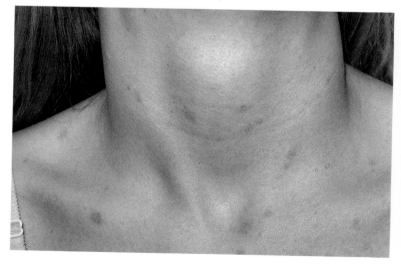

Fig. 4.4 Pityriasis rosea. The face is rarely involved but the neck is characteristically affected.

Fig. 4.5 Pityriasis rosea. The earliest lesions are pink papules, which rapidly become oval patches.

before the rest of the rash appears. It is at this stage that the diagnosis is most difficult since the ring-shaped lesion can easily be confused with ringworm. The subsequent eruption (Fig. 4.2) develops rapidly over a few days on the neck, trunk, upper arms and upper thighs, in what has been described as the rugger shirt and shorts distribution. It is remarkable how the brunt of the eruption almost always falls within this area (Fig. 4.3), affecting the forearms and lower legs only sparsely, if at all. The face is rarely involved but the neck almost always is (Fig. 4.4). The herald patch occurs at any site within this distribution and is larger than any of the subsequent lesions.

The earliest lesions are pink papules (Fig. 4.5) which are occasionally mistaken for insect bites but which rapidly become oval macules. These macules are particularly characteristic, having a fine scale which forms a collarette towards, but not at, the periphery of the lesions (Figs. 4.6 and 4.7). These lesions are pink and oval-shaped and vary in size from 1 to 3 cm, in contrast with the herald patch (Fig. 4.8) which is often 5 or 6 cm in size, making it easily distinguishable. The rash persists for approximately six weeks, then disappears. In the vast majority of patients it never returns. The patient feels perfectly well throughout and, although itching may be severe enough to require treatment, in the majority the rash is asymptomatic.

In most patients, the history of a single patch followed by a widespread, though essentially truncal eruption makes the diagnosis fairly obvious even before the patient is examined. However, there is a variant of pityriasis rosea in which the eruption following the herald patch is limited either to the area immediately around the herald patch or to the sun-spared areas of the axillae, breasts and groins (Fig. 4.9). Also, in a significant minority of patients, no herald patch can be found.

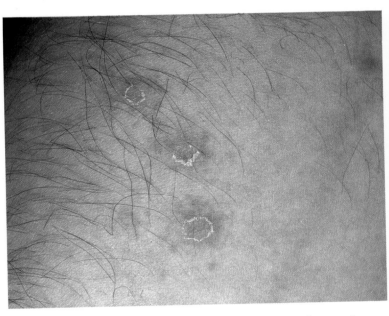

Fig. 4.6 Pityriasis rosea. Oval pink macules with a fine scale towards the periphery are characteristic.

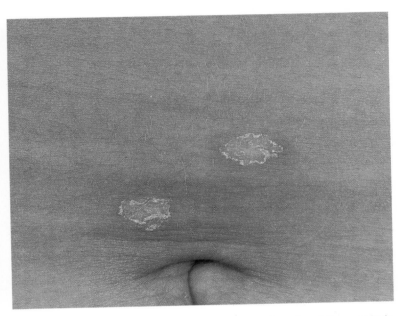

Fig. 4.7 Pityriasis rosea. The peripheral collarette of the scale is obvious.

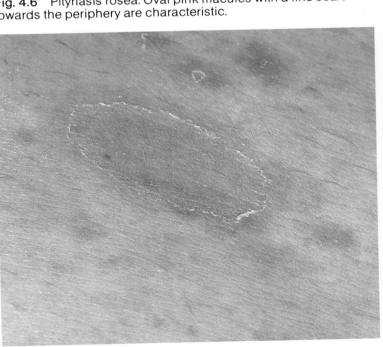

Fig. 4.8 Pityriasis rosea. The herald patch is larger than subsequent patches. By courtesy of St. John's Hospital for Diseases of the Skin.

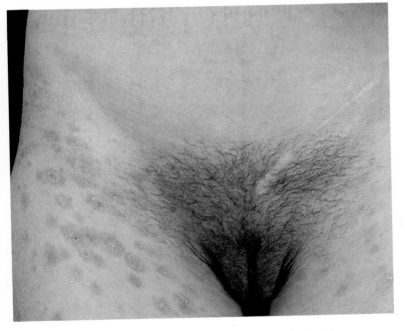

Fig. 4.9 Pityriasis rosea. Occasionally, this is limited to sun-spared areas such as the groin. By courtesy of St. John's Hospital for Diseases of the Skin.

4.3

Another variant which occurs in negroes is called an eczematide; in this case the herald patch may or may not be present. The eruption is more widespread, especially on the limbs, and the course is more protracted, taking many months before ultimately resolving. Post-inflammatory hyperpigmentation (Fig. 4.10) is a consequence of the eruption, as in all inflammatory skin disorders occurring in pigmented skin. The pinkness of the lesions may be difficult to discern but the oval shape and peripheral collarette of scale make it possible to identify this disorder.

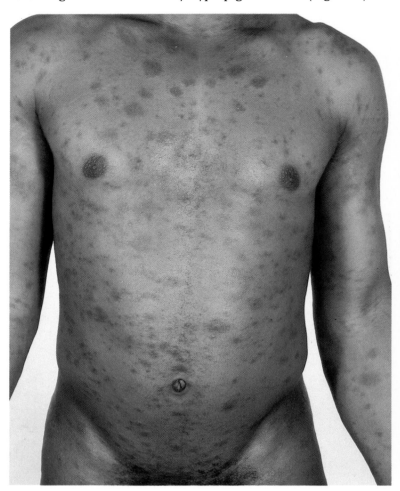

Fig. 4.10 Pityriasis rosea. Post-inflammatory pigmentation is the rule in pigmented skins. This will clear, but often slowly in the darkest skins.

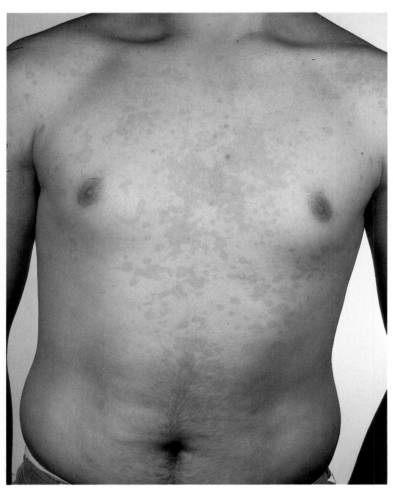

Fig. 4.11 Pityriasis versicolor. The lesions, although favouring the trunk as in pityriasis rosea, are brown not pink in colour.

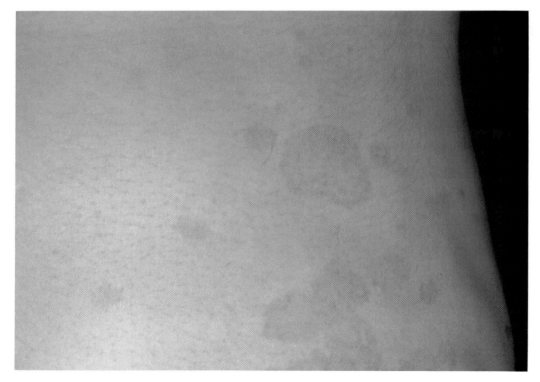

Fig. 4.12 Pityriasis versicolor. The lesions may be various sizes and shapes.

DIFFERENTIAL DIAGNOSIS

PITYRIASIS VERSICOLOR. This disease occurs in a distribution similar to pityriasis rosea; the trunk and neck are favoured, the face is spared and sometimes in severe cases the limbs are involved. However, the lesions are hyper- (Fig. 4.11) or hypo-pigmented instead of pink and the scale is seen over the entire surface of the lesion rather than only peripherally as in pityriasis rosea. Also, the lesions of pityriasis versicolor are asymmetrically distributed and are of varying sizes (Figs. 4.12 and 4.13) as a result of coalescence of the initial small lesions. There is no herald patch and the evolution of the disease is slow in contrast with the rapid onset of pityriasis rosea.

GUTTATE PSORIASIS. This condition is sometimes confused with pityriasis rosea because of its rapid development. However, the lesions are tiny and coloured a deeper red than the pink of pityriasis rosea. Each lesion has a thick silvery scale throughout its surface (Fig. 4.14). Again, no herald patch is present, this sign being specific for pityriasis rosea.

PSORIASIS VULGARIS OF THE TRUNK. This may produce lesions of a similar size to those of pityriasis rosea (Fig. 4.15) but the morphology of psoriasis is obvious and other lesions are likely to be found, particularly on the scalp, elbows and knees.

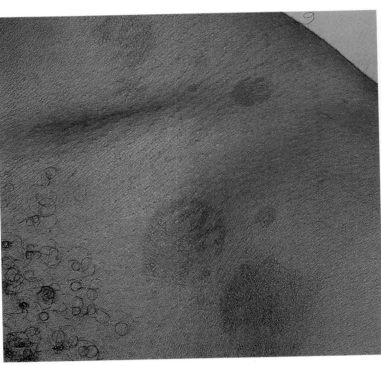

Fig. 4.13   Pityriasis versicolor. In pigmented races, colour differences are not so easily discernible, but these pigmented patches do not have the peripheral scale of pityriasis rosea as seen in Fig. 4.7.

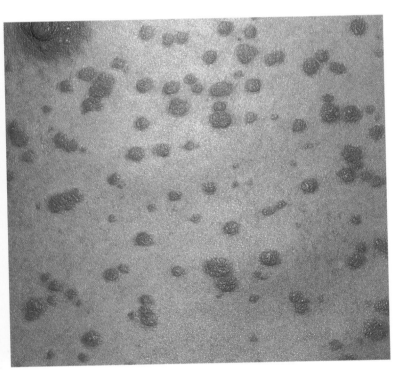

Fig. 4.14   Guttate psoriasis. The eruption develops rapidly over the trunk, as does pityriasis rosea, but in guttate psoriasis the lesions are a deeper red and no herald patch is found.

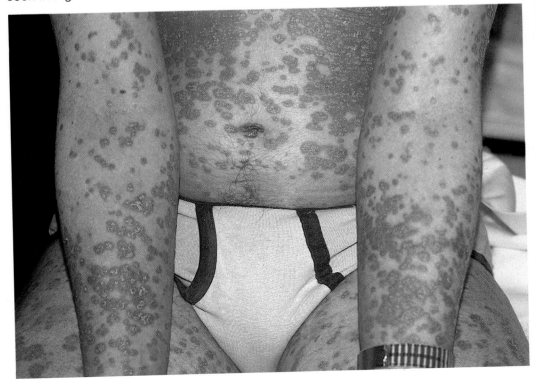

Fig. 4.15   Psoriasis vulgaris. Although the lesions may be of a similar size and distributed symmetrically as in pityriasis rosea, the colour is a deep red and the scale is thicker and covers the lesion.

4.5

SECONDARY SYPHILIS. This disease must be considered whenever there is an eruption which is widespread (Fig. 4.16). The lesions have a copper colour (Fig. 4.17) and involvement of the mucous membranes, genitalia, palms, soles and face, coupled with lymphadenopathy in a generally unwell patient, should raise the suspicion of syphilitic disease.

DRUG ERUPTION. This is usually more florid because it is more widespread (Fig. 4.18), involving the face and rest of the skin surface, unlike the limited distribution of pityriasis rosea. The lesions are usually itchy and maculopapular (Fig. 4.19) with a tendency to confluence (Fig. 4.20). However, gold (Figs. 4.21 and 4.22) can produce an eruption not unlike pityriasis rosea in

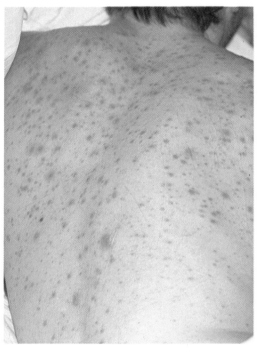

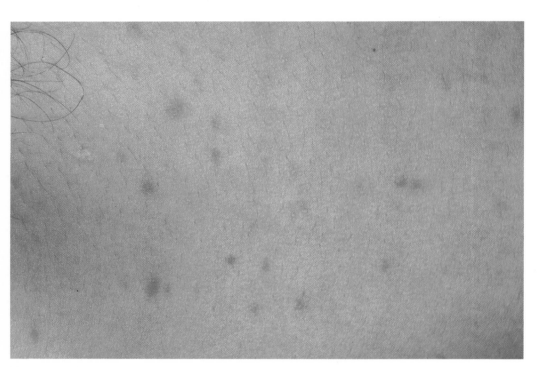

Fig. 4.16   Secondary syphilis. This is a very important differential diagnosis because syphilis will simulate many skin disorders, including pityriasis rosea. The distribution is more widespread, however, including involvement of the face, genitalia, palms and soles. The eruption does not itch and the patient is generally unwell. By courtesy of St. Mary's Hospital.

Fig. 4.17   Secondary syphilis. The lesions often have a brown copper-coloured hue. By courtesy of St. Mary's Hospital.

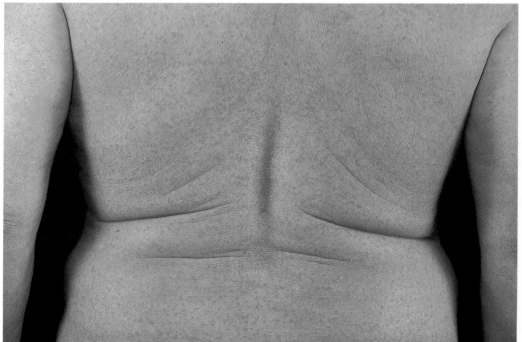

Fig. 4.18   Drug eruption. Although involving the trunk the eruption is usually generalized unlike pityriasis rosea (see Fig. 4.19 for close-up). By courtesy of St. John's Hospital for Diseases of the Skin.

Fig. 4.19   Drug eruption. The lesions are maculopapular. By courtesy of St. John's Hospital for Diseases of the Skin.

morphology, so a history should be taken for present or prior drug ingestion.

SEBORRHOEIC ECZEMA. This should not produce confusion because, although it does occur in the trunk, it is largely limited to the central areas of the front and back of the chest (Fig. 4.23).

Also, the lesions are not as well-defined as the oval patches of pityriasis rosea, and may be found on the face, scalp, axilla and groin.

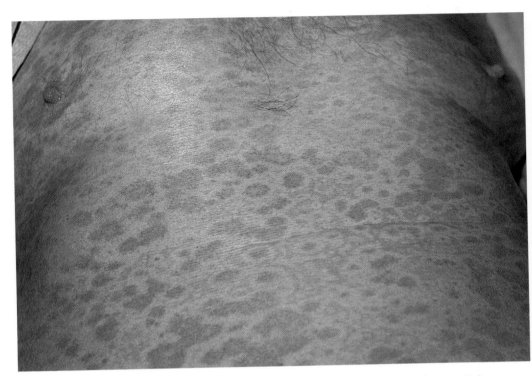

Fig. 4.20   Drug eruption. There is a tendency for confluence of the lesions. This eruption was caused by ampicillin.

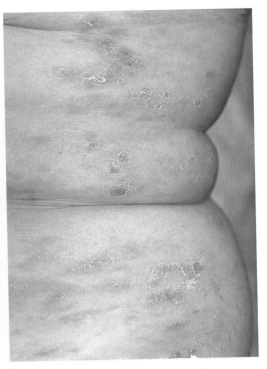

Fig. 4.21   Gold eruption. Pityriasis rosea may be simulated by a reaction to gold injections. The history will differentiate the conditions.

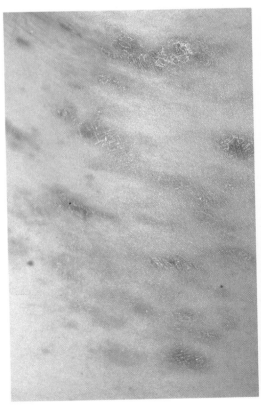

Fig. 4.22   Gold eruption. A closer view shows the lesions to be less than uniform unlike pityriasis rosea.

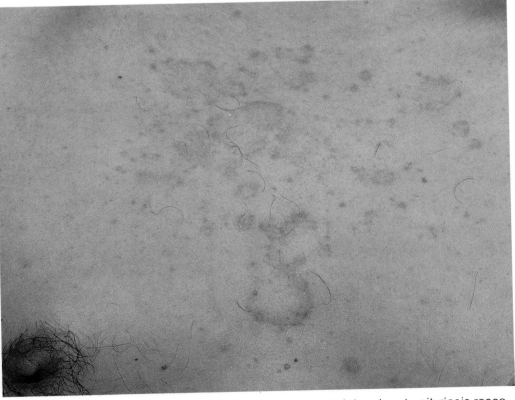

Fig. 4.23   Seborrhoeic eczema. The lesions are a similar pink colour to pityriasis rosea but favour the central areas of the front and back of the chest. They may be annular but are chronic not acute in nature.

TINEA CORPORIS. This condition can be confused with the herald patch of pityriasis rosea. However, the activity of tinea is at the margin of the lesion with a tendency to central healing (Fig. 4.24) so that the scale is truly peripheral. The lesions are asymmetrical (Fig. 4.25) and animal ringworm produces marked inflammation (Fig. 4.26). Scraping the lesion and examining the scales in potash will show the hyphae.

ROSACEA. Although quite different from pityriasis rosea, this has a passing similarity in name to rosea and the conditions may become confused. Rosacea, however, is a papulopustular eruption (Fig. 4.27) occurring on the face.

Treatment
It is important to explain to the patient that the eruption will disappear without a trace shortly and to give reassurance that it is not infectious and, in particular, that it is highly unlikely to appear on the face. However, in this author's experience, the prescription of bland therapy proposed in most textbooks will often lead the patient who is suffering from irritation to seek a second opinion. Since topical corticosteroids of medium potency are effective in alleviating the itch, practitioners should not hesitate to prescribe them.

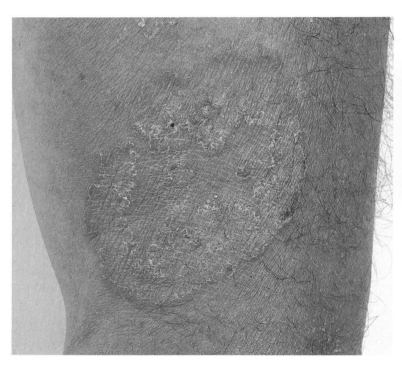

Fig. 4.24 Tinea corporis. The herald patch of pityriasis rosea is often mistaken for tinea. The margin of the ringworm lesion is the most active with a tendency for central healing.

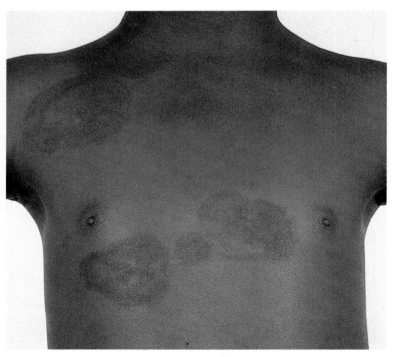

Fig. 4.25 Tinea corporis. The lesions are asymmetrical in distribution.

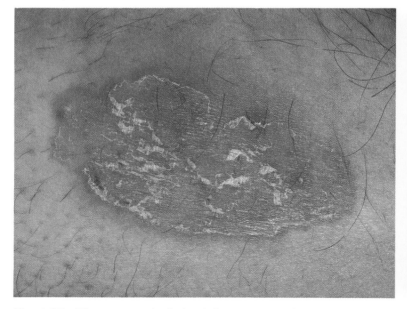

Fig. 4.26 Tinea corporis. Animal ringworm (cat in this patient) is inflamed and the margins are more active.

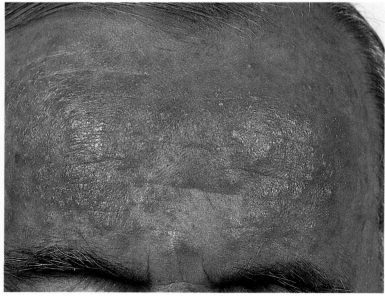

Fig. 4.27 Rosacea. This disorder is a papulopustular eruption involving only the face. Frequently the word rosea is mistaken for rosacea.

LICHEN PLANUS

This relatively common disorder of the skin and mucous membranes accounts for approximately one percent of dermatological consultations. The eruption has a distinct colour (Fig. 4.28) and characteristic distribution, so diagnosis is usually quite simple. The condition is frequently very pruritic but is amenable to treatment with corticosteroids, the majority of cases disappearing within 18 months. Second attacks occur only rarely. It is largely a disorder of adults and the cause is unknown in all but a small proportion of cases.

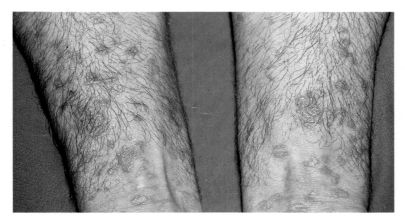

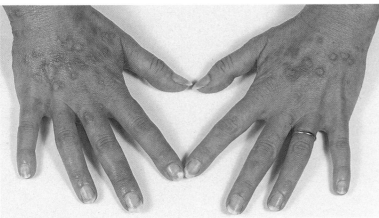

Fig. 4.28 Lichen planus. The eruption has a characteristic purple or violaceous colour and tends to be symmetrical.

Aetiology

Although diabetics seem to develop lichen planus more frequently than chance would indicate, and cases have been described in association with primary biliary cirrhosis and chronic active hepatitis, for the vast majority lichen planus is an isolated event. However, eruptions similar to lichen planus, so-called lichenoid reactions, are well described in certain situations; for example, about one-third of patients undergoing bone marrow transplantation develop an eruption with similar clinical, pathological and direct immunofluorescent findings to those of idiopathic lichen planus. It occurs as part of the graft versus host immunological reaction between donor immunocompetent cells and recipient tissues. Certain drugs, in particular penicillamine (especially when prescribed for primary biliary cirrhosis), arsenic, gold, methyldopa and para-aminosalicylic acid produce lichenoid eruptions. Antimalarials, especially mepacrine hydrochloride, were responsible for a certain morbidity among troops taking the drug during the Second World War. The eruption was similar to that of lichen planus except that it had a tendency to last longer and to produce more scarring. Finally, a lichenoid eruption is seen on the backs of the hands and around the wrists of certain individuals who develop a contact dermatitis to colour developer. Although contact dermatitis ordinarily implies an eczematous response to an external allergen, this particular eruption is the exception. The condition responds to removal of the allergen.

Pathology

The histopathology of lichen planus is as characteristic as the clinical features (Figs. 4.29 and 4.30). There is an intense infiltration of the epidermis by thymus-derived lymphocytes in a band-like distribution immediately below the epidermis. This pushes the epidermis upwards, forming a papule. The basement membrane and basal cell layer of the epidermis are destroyed by the lymphocytes, producing liquefaction necrosis of the basal cells. The rete pegs are flattened outwards, giving an appearance similar to the teeth of a saw. Some of the degenerating epidermal cells stain pink with eosin and are known as colloid bodies; these are highly characteristic of the disorder. Immunoglobulins and, in particular, IgM are found in these bodies. Macrophages in the upper dermis contain pigment lost from the destruction of the lower epidermis. In the epidermis itself there is an increase in the granular cell layer and stratum corneum.

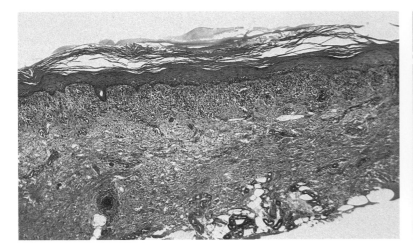

Fig. 4.29 Histopathology of lichen planus – scanning view. This section shows hyperkeratosis, irregular acanthosis and a lichenoid chronic inflammatory cell infiltrate. Haematoxylin and eosin stain. By courtesy of Dr. P.H. McKee.

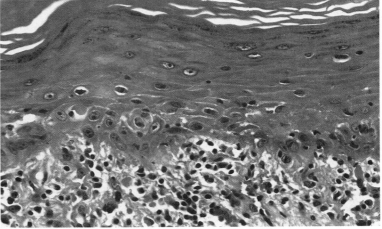

Fig. 4.30 Histopathology of lichen planus – high power view. In this view there is hyperkeratosis, prominence of the granular cell layer and acanthosis. Hydropic degeneration of the basal layer of epidermis is present and scattered, irregular, eosinophilic cytoid bodies are seen in both the epidermis and dermis. The inflammatory cell infiltrate comprises predominantly lymphocytes and histiocytes. Haematoxylin and eosin stain. By courtesy of Dr. P.H. McKee.

Clinical Features

Lichen planus can affect virtually any part of the skin and mucous membranes (Fig. 4.31) but manifests a predilection for the fronts of the wrists and forearms, the backs of the hands (Fig. 4.32), ankles (Fig. 4.33) and shins, and lumbar regions (Fig. 4.34). The eruption is remarkably symmetrical and usually intensely pruritic. Each lesion is a small papule which is polygonal in outline with a flat surface, which tends to shine when viewed in a good light. The colour of the eruption is highly characteristic, being purple or violaceous.

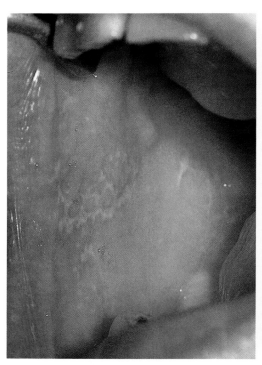

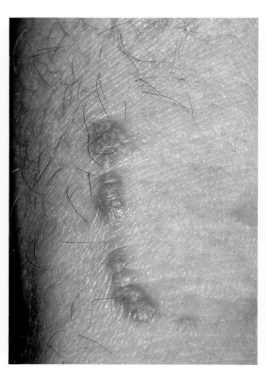

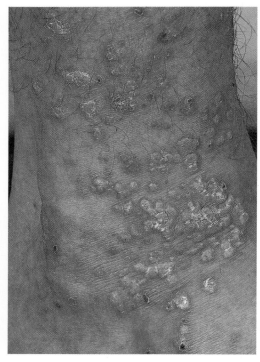

Fig. 4.31 Lichen planus. A white lace-like, reticulate patterning of the buccal mucous membranes is a common, often asymptomatic finding.

Fig. 4.32 Lichen planus. The lesions are purple. The linear arrangement illustrates the Koebner phenomenon.

Fig. 4.33 Lichen planus. Purple polygonal papules, some of which have coalesced to form plaques, are seen on this man's ankles. Wickham's striae are present.

Fig. 4.34 Lichen planus. The lumbar region is often involved. The lesions tend to have a shiny surface. Even in pigmented skins, the purple colour is obvious during the active phase.

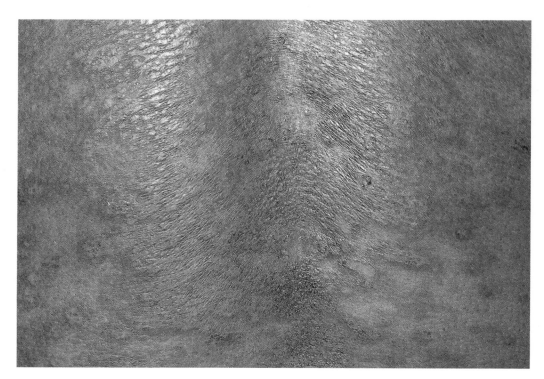

White lines are found on the surface of many of the papules and are known as Wickham's striae (Fig. 4.35). Dabbing a lesion with mineral oil will highlight the striae. Individual papules frequently coalesce so that superficially it appears as if large plaques have formed, but close examination reveals that they consist of collections of these papules. As the papules heal, a brown pigmentation is left behind in all cases. In the Caucasian this disappears after a number of weeks or months. In pigmented skins the pigmentation can last for many years and may be disfiguring (Fig. 4.36). The eruption may occur at sites of trauma

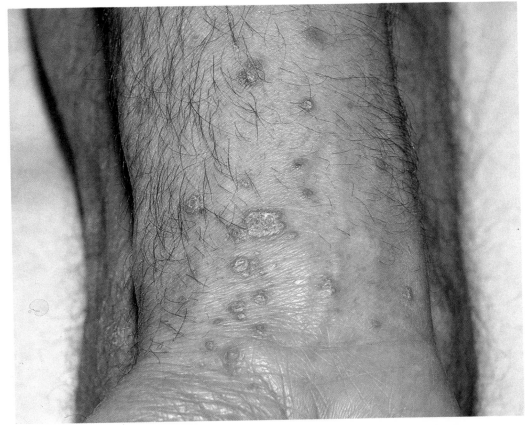

Fig. 4.35 Lichen planus. White lines, known as Wickham's striae are found on the surface of many of the papules.

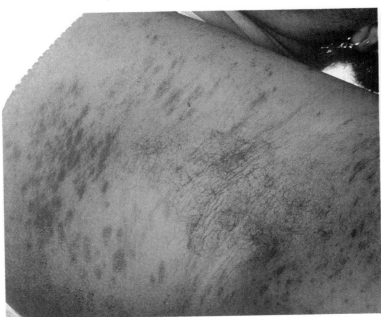

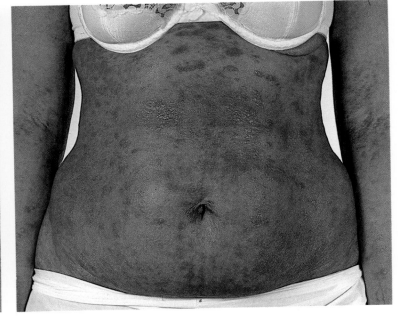

Fig. 4.36 Lichen planus. In pigmented races, the post-inflammatory hyperpigmentation may be extremely persistent and disfiguring, as in these two patients.

4.11

(Fig. 4.37 and 4.38) as happens in psoriasis; this is known as the Koebner phenomenon. The mouth may or may not be involved but the finding of either a lace-like network of white striae or dots on the buccal mucosa (Fig. 4.39) helps to confirm the diagnosis. The gingiva, tongue (Fig. 4.40) and lower lip may also be involved.

These oral lesions are usually asymptomatic.

Occasionally, involvement of the mouth is the sole manifestation and often mistakenly diagnosed as candidosis (Fig. 4.41). In these cases it is a painful condition with ulcers on the tongue, lips (Fig. 4.42), buccal mucous membranes (Fig. 4.43),

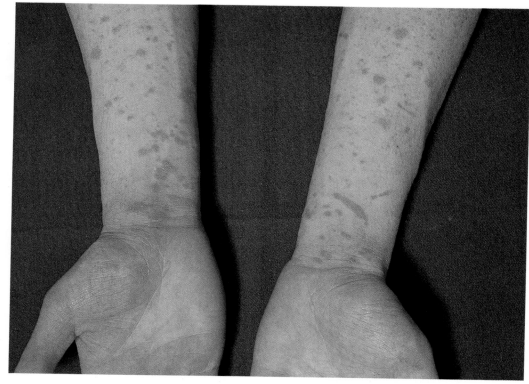

Fig. 4.37 Lichen planus. Linear lesions are present on the wrists secondary to scratching: the so-called Koebner phenomenon. Lichen planus is extremely pruritic. By courtesy of St. Mary's Hospital.

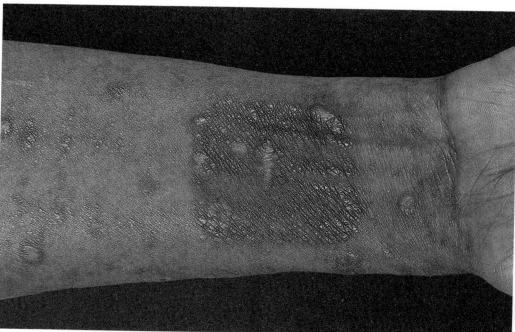

Fig. 4.38 Lichen planus. This patient had burnt her wrist. Purple papules and post inflammatory hyperpigmentation are present.

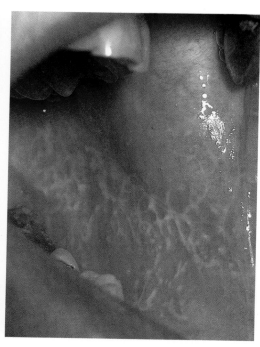

Fig. 4.39 Lichen planus. Patients are often unaware of the involvement of buccal mucous membranes.

floor of the mouth and palate, and can cause great distress (Fig. 4.44). Actinic cheilitis and squamous cell carcinoma (Fig. 4.45) may simulate white patches, and biopsy may be necessary. Rarely, malignant change occurs in chronic oral lichen planus.

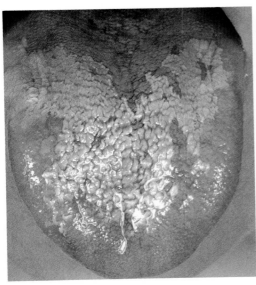

Fig. 4.40 Lichen planus. White patches may occur on the tongue in this disorder.

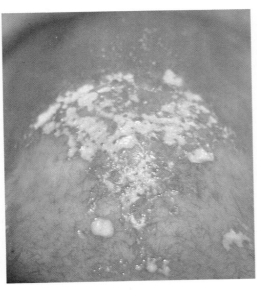

Fig. 4.41 Candida of the mouth. The lesions are pustular and, unlike lichen planus, can be scraped away with a spatula, leaving a raw mucosa. By courtesy of St. Mary's Hospital.

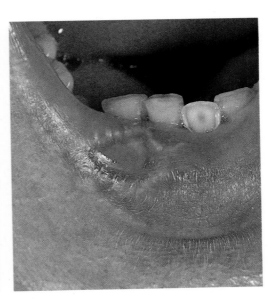

Fig. 4.42 Eroded lichen planus. The lips may be involved, with white streaks, and erosion may be present. This must be differentiated from premalignant white patches. Occasionally malignant change occurs in lichen planus of the mucous membranes.

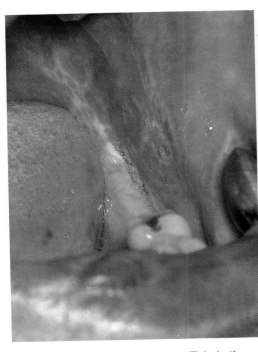

Fig. 4.43 Oral lichen planus. This is the same patient as in Fig. 4.42 and the characteristic reticulate pattern is seen on the buccal mucous membrane.

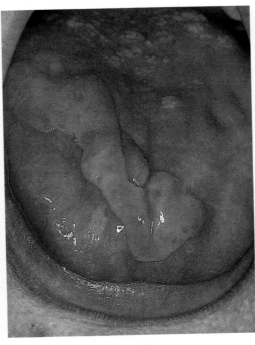

Fig. 4.44 Oral lichen planus. Painful erosions and ulcers may occur. By courtesy of Dr. J.J.H. Gilkes.

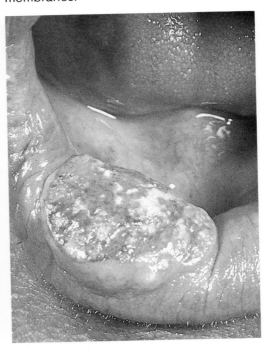

Fig. 4.45 Squamous cell carcinoma of the lower lip. Although this lesion has a white surface at the rim, it is heaped up and is an ulcerated nodule. By courtesy of St. Mary's Hospital.

Variations

The average case of idiopathic lichen planus presents no diagnostic difficulty, but there are certain variations that occur often enough to warrant separate description.

Annular Lichen Planus

This simply refers to the configuration of the eruption. It may be seen in addition to the usual pattern of lichen planus, particularly when the eruption involves the penis (Fig. 4.46). There is a variety, however, with only a few large, scattered, annular lesions (Fig. 4.47). This eruption is frequently not recognized clinically but the histopathology is characteristic.

Genital Lichen Planus

The genitalia are frequently involved in lichen planus (Figs. 4.48–4.50) and occasionally genital or oral lesions may be the only manifestations. The individual violaceous papules with their shiny surfaces and lace-like white streaks are characteristic. In the female, the latter are sometimes mistaken for carcinoma in situ (sometimes called leukoplakia) and unnecessary vulvectomy is performed.

Acute Generalized Lichen Planus

This is a rare exanthem of lichen planus with sudden onset and may involve most of the cutaneous surface (Fig. 4.51). Initially

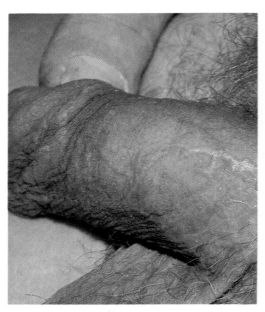

Fig. 4.46 Annular lichen planus. The eruption is often annular on the penis.

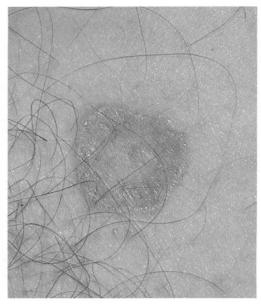

Fig. 4.47 Annular lichen planus. Scattered annular lesions may occur, which may be seen to be purple in colour and to be made up of individual shiny papules. The diagnosis is often missed clinically but discovered after biopsy.

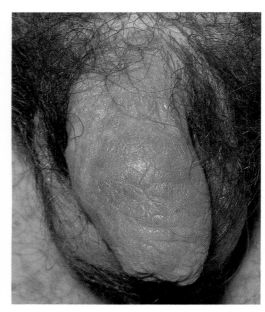

Fig. 4.48 Genital lichen planus. The purple colour is very characteristic.

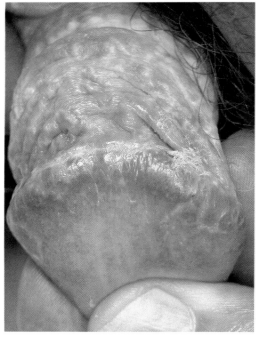

Fig. 4.49 Genital lichen planus. The white reticulate pattern of lichen planus is evident here.

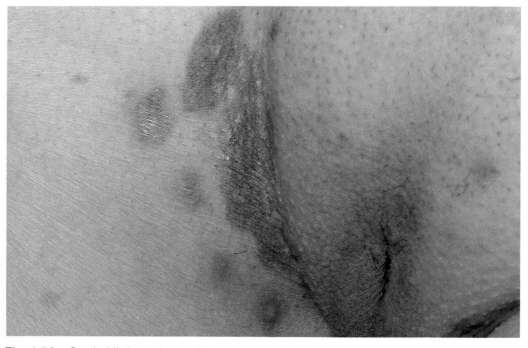

Fig. 4.50 Genital lichen planus. The purple colour, annular configuration and post-inflammatory pigmentation are shown in this vulval eruption.

the eruption is red but becomes purple as it progresses. Scrutiny of the individual lesions reveals the shiny, flat-topped papules.

Hypertrophic Lichen Planus
Although the vast majority of patients who suffer from lichen planus are free of the disease within two years, a few are left with raised plaques, particularly on the lower legs (Fig. 4.52). The surface of the lesions often feels rough and appears warty. In pigmented races the violaceous colour is not so easy to discern (Fig. 4.53). These lesions may be heavily pigmented and may persist indefinitely, and treatments are only partially effective. At this stage the condition can be difficult to distinguish from lichen simplex chronicus, although a preceding history of lichen planus facilitates the diagnosis. A biopsy may be necessary.

Atrophic Lichen Planus
Atrophic patches of skin occasionally result as the active lesions of lichen planus resolve (Fig. 4.54).

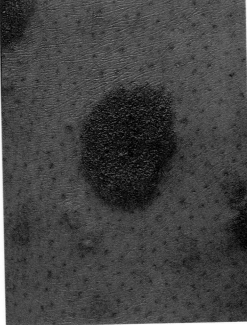

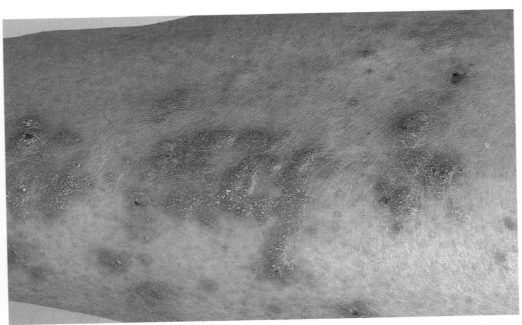

Fig. 4.51 Acute generalized lichen planus. Rarely, lichen planus erupts as an exanthem and the papules are red initially. Biopsy may be required to establish the diagnosis.

Fig. 4.52 Hypertrophic lichen planus. On the lower legs in particular, the lesions may be thickened, extremely difficult to treat and extremely persistent, remaining long after the rest of the eruption has cleared. The lesions retain their purple colour. Intralesional steroids are the treatment of choice.

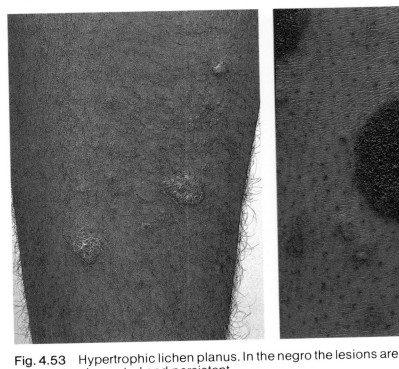

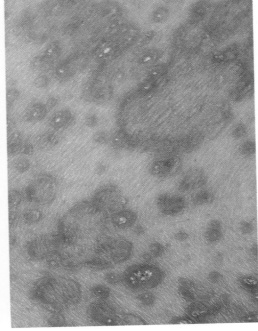

Fig. 4.53 Hypertrophic lichen planus. In the negro the lesions are very warty, pigmented and persistent.

Fig. 4.54 Atrophic lichen planus. Atrophy has occurred within these lesions of lichen planus.

4.15

Linear Lichen Planus

This is a rather rare condition in which the individual morphology is that of lichen planus but the distribution is linear (Fig. 4.55) although not corresponding to a dermatome. It is often seen in childhood and later may be followed by an attack of ordinary lichen planus.

Lichen Planopilaris

In this variation the lesions of lichen planus occur predominantly around the hair follicles (Fig. 4.56). If this occurs in the scalp, scarring may result in permanent loss of hair unless systemic steroids are given early in the course of treatment.

Actinic Lichen Planus

As already stated, the Koebner phenomenon, an eruption in a traumatized area of skin, occurs in lichen planus (Fig. 4.57). Ultraviolet light irradiation may thus aggravate the disease. There is also a variety which seems to be a separate entity and is seen in Mediterranean and Middle Eastern countries, particularly in children and predominantly on light-exposed areas of skin.

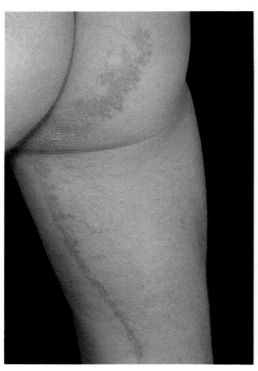

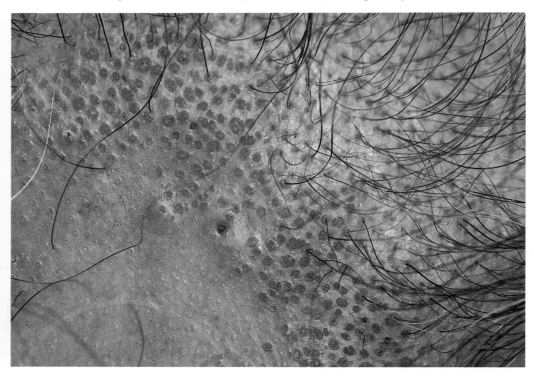

Fig. 4.55   Linear lichen planus. This is a rare condition. The individual papules are lichenoid and ordinary lichen planus may follow.

Fig. 4.56   Lichen planopilaris. Lichen planus predominantly involving the hair follicles may result in scarring alopecia. By courtesy of St. John's Hospital for Diseases of the Skin.

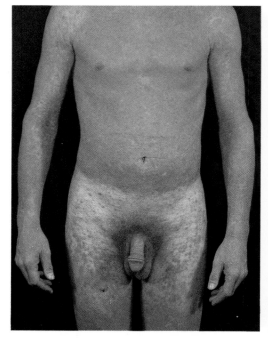

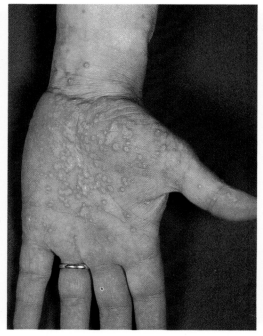

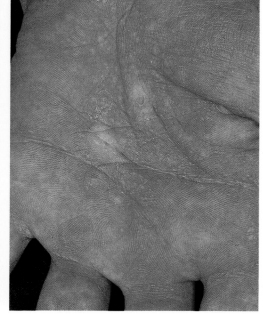

Fig. 4.57   Actinic lichen planus. Lichen planus has occurred on sunburnt skin. The purple colour is well illustrated. By courtesy of St. John's Hospital for Diseases of the Skin.

Fig. 4.58   Lichen planus of the palms. In the absence of lesions elsewhere, the diagnosis may be difficult, because the usual purple colour may be obscured by the thickness of the stratum corneum in the area. Yellow papules result.

Lichen Planus of the Palms and Soles

It is unusual for the palms and soles to be the only areas of involvement (Fig. 4.58) and, if this is so, the diagnosis is difficult. The lesions are papular or nodular and rather warty, tending to be yellow rather than purple probably because of the thickness of the stratum corneum in the affected area.

Lichen Nitidus

In this distinctive variant of lichen planus, most frequently seen in the coloured races (Fig. 4.59), the morphology of the lesion is a minute version of ordinary lichen planus (Fig. 4.60), although the purple colour is usually not discernible. It has the same distribution.

Bullous Lichen Planus

It is not uncommon for blisters to be seen during the course of lichen planus, particularly on the lower legs (Fig. 4.61). Rarely, the eruption is predominantly bullous (Fig. 4.62).

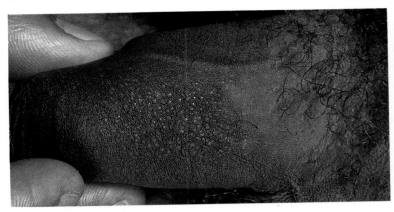

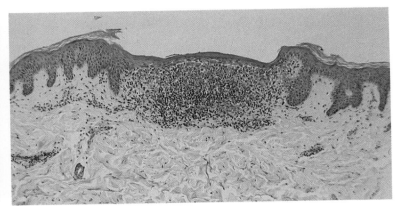

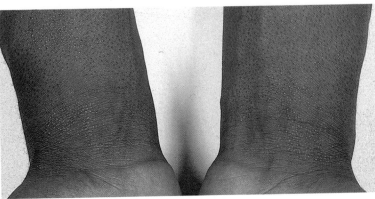

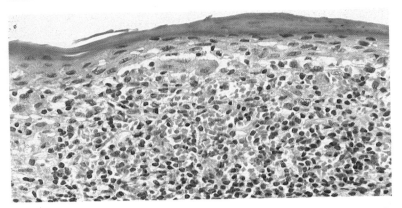

Fig. 4.59 Lichen nitidus. The lesions are minute replicas of ordinary lichen planus. The shiny surface of the papules, so characteristic of lichen planus, is striking here (top). The distribution of the eruption is similar to that of lichen planus. This disorder is more common in negroes.

Fig. 4.60 Lichen nitidus. The low power view (top) shows a small papule bordered by angulated epidermal ridges. There is hyperkeratosis, epidermal atrophy and a circumscribed lichenoid infiltrate. The high power view (bottom) shows effacement of the dermo-epidermal junction, pigmentary incontinence and a lymphohistiocytic infiltrate. Purpura is also present. Occasionally a granulomatous component can be observed. By courtesy of Dr. P.H. McKee.

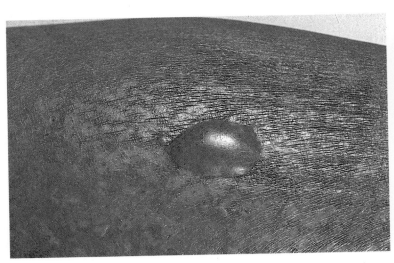

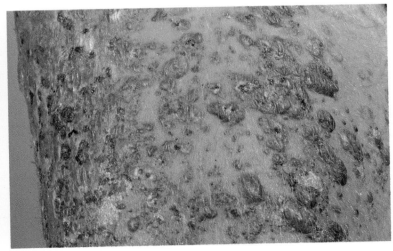

Fig. 4.61 Bullous lichen planus. Blisters may occur during the course of lichen planus, especially on the lower legs.

Fig. 4.62 Bullous lichen planus. Rarely the eruption is predominantly bullous but the characteristic purple colour is still present and biopsy confirmed the diagnosis. By courtesy of Dr. A.C. Pembroke.

Nail Involvement

Occurring in only a minority of patients, the most common changes are longitudinal lines (Fig. 4.63) or depressions in the nail plate. Occasionally, however, severe damage occurs to the nails, leading to permanent destruction (Fig. 4.64). A characteristic feature is an adhesion between the epidermis of the posterior nailfold and the nail bed, a change known as pterygium formation (Fig 4.65).

DIFFERENTIAL DIAGNOSIS

PSORIASIS. The lesions of psoriasis are red not purple as in lichen planus. There is a silver scale, whereas there is no scaling in lichen planus. This is largely because, in the latter, the brunt of the pathology is in the dermis, whereas in psoriasis it is in the epidermis. Guttate psoriasis (Fig. 4.66) may cause confusion but, although the lesions are tiny papules like those of lichen planus, again the redness and the silver scale should serve to differentiate the two.

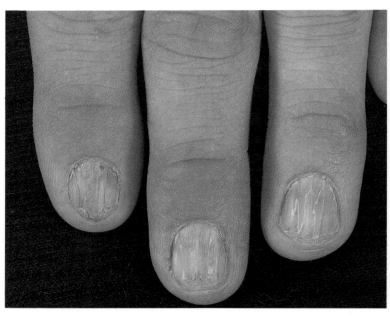

Fig. 4.63 Lichen planus of the nails. Longitudinal lines sometimes occur in the nail plates with lichen planus. By courtesy of St. John's Hospital for Diseases of the Skin.

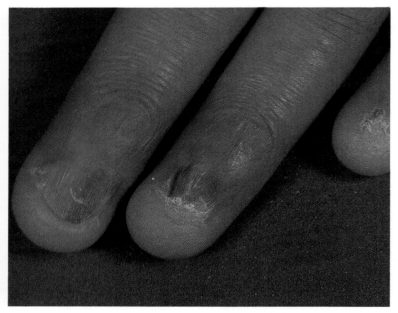

Fig. 4.64 Lichen planus of the nails. Permanent destruction of the nails may occur.

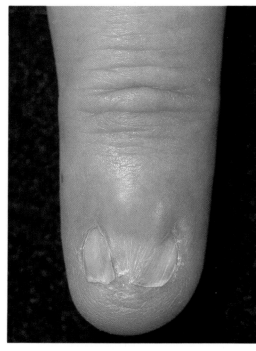

Fig. 4.65 Lichen planus of the nails. Adhesion may form between the epidermis of the posterior nail fold and the nail plate. The result is known as pterygium formation. By courtesy of St. John's Hospital for Diseases of the Skin.

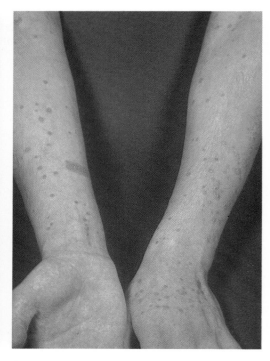

Fig. 4.66 Guttate psoriasis. The lesions are papules red in colour with a silver scale. Lichen planus does not scale. Note the Koebner phenomenon, a feature of both disorders.

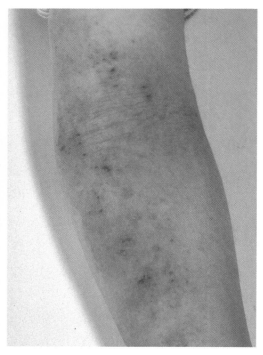

Fig. 4.67 Atopic eczema. Redness, scaling and excoriations are features of eczema. Lichenification secondary to continued rubbing of the skin is notable in the flexures.

ECZEMA. Lichenification is a common feature of eczema, occurring predominantly in the flexures of patients with atopic eczema (Fig. 4.67) and should present no great difficulty. Lichenification is thickening of the skin with exaggeration of the skin creases, resulting from continual rubbing. However, localized areas of lichenification can occur in eczema, particularly in pigmented races, producing lichenoid papules but lacking the purple colour of lichen planus (Figs. 4.68 and 4.69).

LICHENOID CONTACT ALLERGY TO COLOUR DEVELOPER. The eruption is remarkably similar in colour to true lichen planus. It is however limited to the site of contact, viz. the backs of the hands and forearms (Fig. 4.70).

LICHEN SIMPLEX CHRONICUS. This eruption is usually unilateral, corresponding to the handedness of the patient, and is well-defined and lichenified (Fig. 4.71) secondary to scratching. Multiple patches may occur.

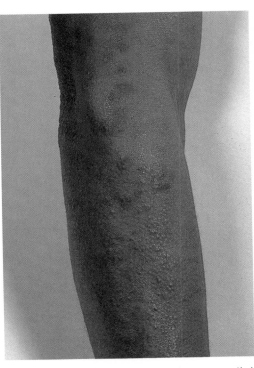
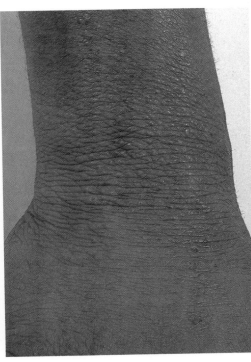
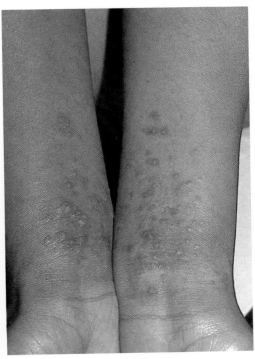

Fig. 4.68 Atopic eczema. In the negro, lichenoid papules commonly result from rubbing atopic eczematous skin. The violaceous colour of lichen planus is absent however. A family and personal history of atopy is a feature and the disorder usually commences in infancy.

Fig. 4.69 Contact dermatitis to nickel. Pigmented lichenoid papules frequently occur in eczema in negroes. This lady has metal allergy.

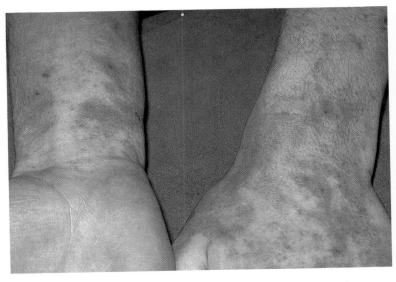
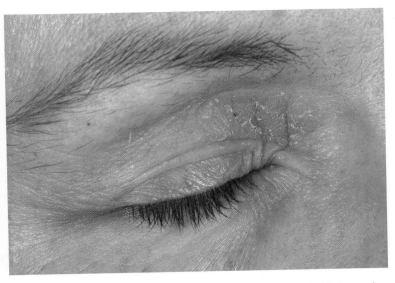

Fig. 4.70 Lichenoid contact allergy to colour developer. An eruption remarkably similar to lichen planus is occasionally seen as a delayed hypersensitivity reaction to colour developer. The backs of the hands and wrists are involved, with sparing of the thick palmar skin.

Fig. 4.71 Lichen simplex. The lesion is well-defined, thickened and the skin creases are pronounced. It results from continued rubbing of the skin, often secondary to anxiety or depression. Confusion with lichen planus may arise because of its name.

PRURIGO. This is a chronic disorder which is particularly pruritic. Persistent scratching induces excoriated papules (Fig. 4.72) on the limbs and buttocks. This may progress to nodules and plaques (Fig. 4.73). The lesions are rarely purple and the typical shiny, flat-topped papules of lichen planus are not present. The patient is otherwise well, without a trace of systemic disturbance.

SCABIES. Lichen planus and scabies are both eruptions that are intensely itchy but there the resemblance ends. The burrows of scabies, from which the acarus can be extracted, are characteristic and specific findings. Papules do occur in scabies, especially on the trunk, between the fingers (Fig. 4.74), on the genitalia, in the axillae and on the buttocks, but they lack the violaceous colour and the flat-topped nature of the papules of lichen planus (Fig. 4.75).

SYPHILIS. The rash of secondary syphilis is not itchy, unlike lichen planus. Occasionally lichenoid changes occur but other physical signs (referred to previously) and the serology will distinguish the two diseases.

Treatment

Lichen planus is a steroid-responsive disorder such that in the majority of patients, only topical steroids are required. However, it should be noted that the disease responds only to the most potent topical steroids. It does not respond to hydrocortisone, responds only slightly to moderately potent steroids such as betamethasone valerate (betnovate), but responds well to the most potent steroids such as clobetasol propionate (dermovate). Sometimes, polythene occlusion is nessary in order to enhance the penetration of this steroid, particularly on the lower legs. Occasionally, injection of steroids such as triamcinolone acetonide into the lesions is necessary and, in severe cases, systemic steroids are required. Antihistamines are useful for their antipruritic action. However, a very important part of management is reassurance of the patient that it is not an infectious disease and that it is highly likely to clear permanently within a couple of years.

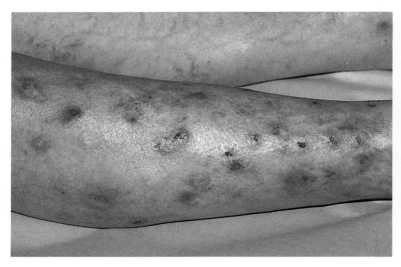

Fig. 4.72 Prurigo. Excoriations secondary to scratching are seen.

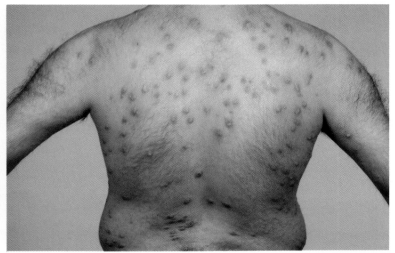

Fig. 4.73 Nodular prurigo. Excoriated papules and nodules are present. Skin biopsy confirmed the diagnosis. The condition is particularly chronic.

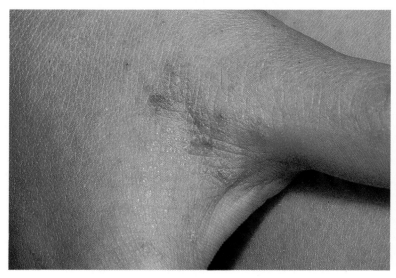

Fig. 4.74 Scabies. Excoriated papules occur between the fingers, especially between the thumb and index finger. The finding of a burrow is diagnostic.

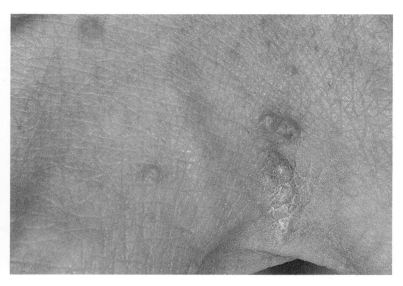

Fig. 4.75 Lichen planus. The hands are often involved in lichen planus but the lesions are discrete purple papules which may be readily distinguished from the papules of scabies.

PITYRIASIS RUBRA PILARIS

This condition is exceedingly rare and is included here only because of its distinctive clinical pictures and because it represents one of the differential diagnoses of erythroderma. It occurs most commonly in adults in the fifth decade but there is a juvenile type occurring in the first decade.

Aetiology and Histopathology

The aetiology is unknown, but it has been suggested that there may be an abnormality of vitamin A metabolism since some patients show a clinical response to therapy with vitamin A and its derivatives. The histology is not specific, but there is hyperkeratosis around follicular orifices and a mild inflammatory cell infiltrate in the dermis.

Clinical Features

Adult Form of Pityriasis Rubra Pilaris

This is an acute disorder of rapid evolution, beginning with a red scaly patch on the back, followed by redness on the face and severe scaling in the scalp. The palms and soles become erythematous and thickened and appear yellow (Fig. 4.76). Sometimes over a period of a few months following this, the eruption extends to involve the entire skin, causing an erythroderma (Fig. 4.77). In other patients, islands of normal skin can be seen (Figs. 4.78 and 4.79). A characteristic finding is redness around the pilosebaceous follicular orifices which are plugged with keratin, producing a skin texture sometimes likened to that of a nutmeg grater. The backs of the fingers are particularly involved in this manner.

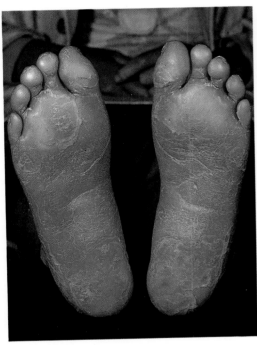

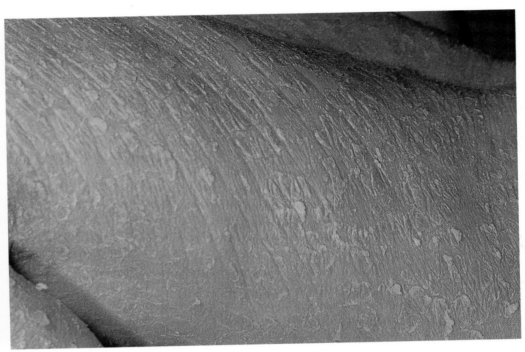

Fig. 4.76 Pityriasis rubra pilaris. The soles are grossly thickened. By courtesy of St. John's Hospital for Diseases of the Skin.

Fig. 4.77 Pityriasis rubra pilaris. Erythema and scaling of the entire cutaneous surface (erythroderma) may result.

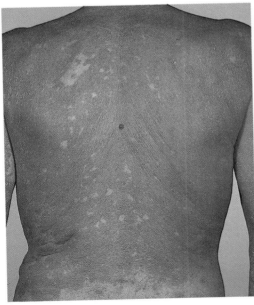

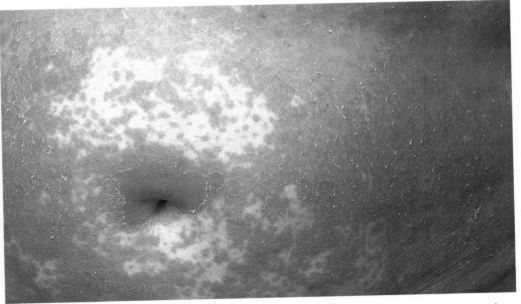

Fig. 4.78 Pityriasis rubra pilaris. Islands of normal skin occur within the erythroderma. By courtesy of St. John's Hospital for Diseases of the Skin.

Fig. 4.79 Pityriasis rubra pilaris. A curious and unexplained feature of the disease is the sparing of areas of skin. By courtesy of St. John's Hospital for Diseases of the Skin.

4.21

The name of this condition essentially describes the prominent scaling (pityriasis), redness (rubra) and follicular involvement (pilaris) (Fig. 4.80) of the disease. The involvement of the palms and soles is not included in the title of the disease, but is nonetheless a constant and characteristic feature. In the initial stages, the disease may be extremely itchy, a feature which may persist or resolve as the disorder progresses. In many patients there is spontaneous resolution within two to three years without recurrence.

Juvenile Form of Pityriasis Rubra Pilaris
The onset of this disorder is more gradual than that of the adult form. It is not present at birth but usually develops around the age of two or three years. The thickening of the palms and the soles, fine scaling in the scalp and follicular plugging aid diagnosis. Erythroderma does not seem to occur and, interestingly, about one-third of the patients have a positive family history of the disorder.

Juvenile Variant of Pityriasis Rubra Pilaris
This is a more common condition which is localized around the knees (Fig. 4.81) and elbows. It occurs in childhood and is frequently mistaken for psoriasis. The eruption is very well-defined and the plaques consist of follicular plugging.

DIFFERENTIAL DIAGNOSIS
SEBORRHOEIC ECZEMA. In the initial stages aof the disease the involvement of the face and scalp simulates seborrhoeic dermatitis, and distinction may be impossible until involvement of the hands and feet occurs, followed by the more widespread involvement of the body. The redness and excess keratin around the follicles and palmar or plantar hyperkeratosis will determine the diagnosis.

ERYTHRODERMA. A small proportion of patients with pityriasis rubra pilaris become erythrodermic; but other causes of erythroderma such as psoriasis, eczema, drug eruptions, mycosis fungoides and Sézary syndrome have to be considered. The history of the evolution of the eruption, past history of skin disease, skin biopsy and other more sophisticated investigations may be necessary.

PSORIASIS. In psoriasis there are well-defined plaques but they are red with a characteristic silvery scale and show no tendency towards being more prominent around hair follicles.

ECZEMA. This disorder is common and much more likely to be the correct diagnosis; but the appearance of follicular derangement, redness and scaling with palmar and plantar involvement must be suggestive of pityriasis rubra pilaris.

Treatment
The adult form of pityriasis rubra pilaris usually clears within three years, but for the juvenile form the diagnosis is more guarded. Specific treatment is not forthcoming but cytotoxic drugs, particularly methotrexate, and vitamin A and its derivatives have their advocates. The juvenile circumscribed variant rarely gives rise to symptoms but topical vitamin A acid may be of benefit.

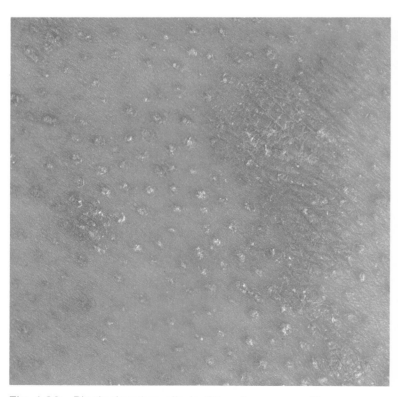

Fig. 4.80 Pityriasis rubra pilaris. Pilosebaceous orifices are plugged with keratin and surrounded by erythema. By courtesy of St. John's Hospital for Diseases of the Skin.

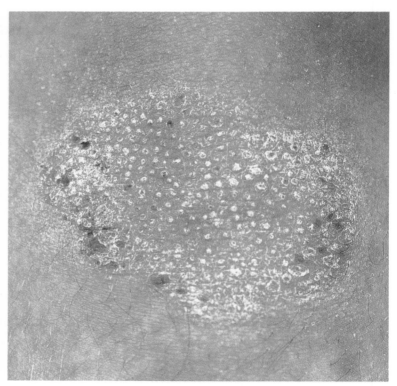

Fig. 4.81 Juvenile variant of pityriasis rubra pilaris. This more common variant occurring most commonly on the elbows and knees and frequently mistaken for psoriasis, is distinguished by its follicular nature. By courtesy of Dr. A. Griffiths, St. John's Hospital for Diseases of the Skin.

5 Naevi

Anthony du Vivier MD, FRCP

Phillip H. McKee MB BCh, BaO, MRC Path

Localized abnormalities of the skin are so common that virtually every individual has at least one variant (Fig. 5.1). Most can be diagnosed by simple inspection of the skin or, if necessary, by biopsy and histological examination. The medical importance of accurate clinical diagnosis lies in their distinction from malignant lesions. However, in the majority of cases, patients request advice because they find their naevi unsightly. Correct diagnosis allows the physician to predict whether the lesion will resolve spontaneously, should be simply excised, requires the special skills of a plastic surgeon or should be best left alone.

The term naevus [L.blemish] means a benign proliferation of a tissue element, which may be present at birth or appear within the first decades of life. Although often loosely used to refer to moles, that is pigmented malformations of melanocytes, it is preferable to qualify this latter type of naevus as a pigmented melanocytic naevus.

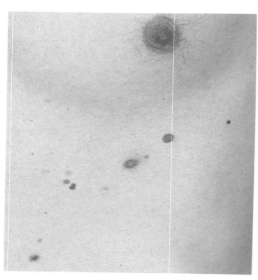

Fig. 5.1 Localized abnormalities of the skin. These are very common. Moles, haemangiomata and an accessory nipple are present here.

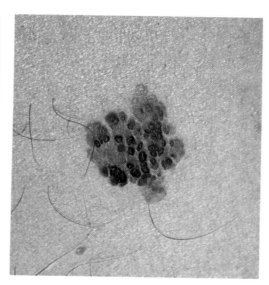

Fig. 5.2 Epidermal naevus. This lesion was present at birth. It has a rough warty surface.

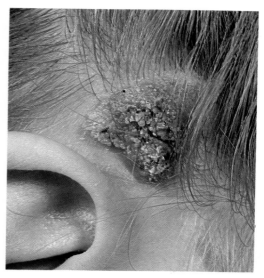

Fig. 5.3 Epidermal naevus. The lesion is well defined and has a rough and fissured surface resembling a wart, but it was present at birth.

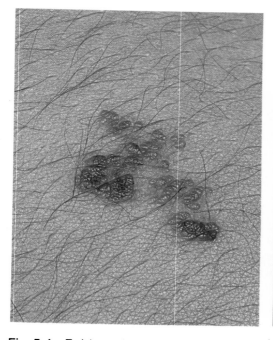

Fig. 5.4 Epidermal naevus. Sometimes epidermal naevi are arranged in a linear manner.

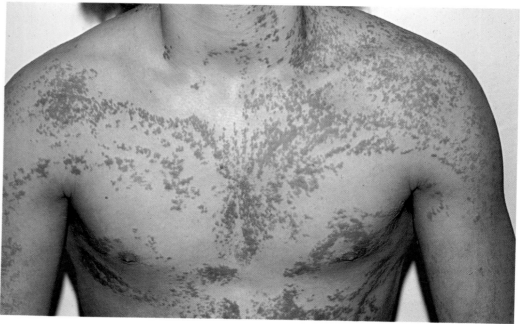

Fig. 5.5 Systematized epidermal naevi. Disfiguring widespread epidermal naevi occasionally occur in a zosteriform manner.

Epidermal Naevus

This lesion is present at birth or appears within the first decade of life. It has a warty (Figs. 5.2 and 5.3) or psoriasiform surface. It is sometimes arranged in a linear (Fig. 5.4) or zosteriform manner. Occasionally systematized naevi occur (Fig. 5.5). Rarely an inflammatory component is present (Fig. 5.6) in which instance confusion with psoriasis or eczema may occur (inflammatory linear verrucous epidermal naevus – ILVEN). The development of a basal cell or squamous cell carcinoma is an exceedingly rare complication. Epidermal naevi may be excised.

Histology

Epidermal naevi may show a variety of patterns. Most often they present as simple squamous papillomata showing hyperkeratosis, papillomatosis and acanthosis (Fig. 5.7). Some variants show seborrhoeic wart-like features (Fig. 5.8) and an occasional example may show the presence of epidermolytic hyperkeratosis (Fig. 5.9). This consists of massive hyperkeratosis overlying an acanthotic epidermis showing marked vacuolation and containing abundant irregular keratohyalin-like material.

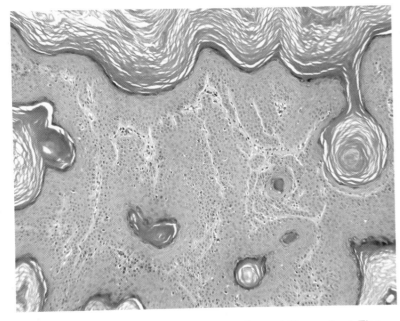

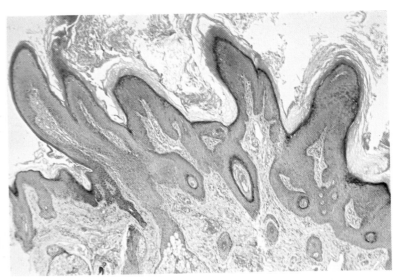

Fig. 5.6 Inflammatory linear verrucous epidermal naevus. A red inflammatory component may accompany an epidermal naevus.

Fig. 5.7 Epidermal naevus: papillomatous variant. The lesion, which is sharply demarcated from the normal skin (left), shows marked papillomatosis with a prominent granular cell layer and hyper (ortho) keratosis. The epidermal ridges are accentuated and partly fused.

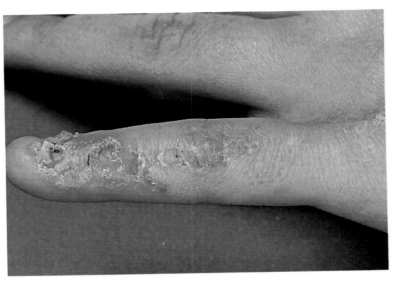

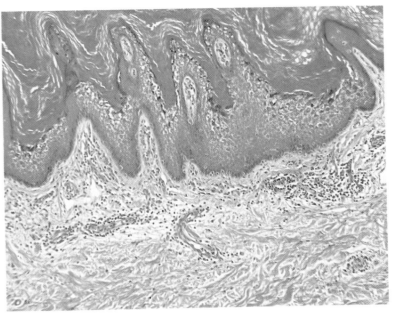

Fig. 5.8 Epidermal naevus: seborrhoeic wart-like variant. The histological features of hyperkeratosis, acanthosis and a variable mixture of small basaloid cells and squamous cells with horn cyst formation are indistinguishable from a seborrhoeic wart.

Fig. 5.9 Epidermal naevus: epidermolytic variant. This uncommon sub-type shows the features of epidermolytic hyperkeratosis. There is massive hyperkeratosis, papillomatosis, generalized peri-nuclear vacuolation and clumps of irregular keratohyalin-like material. Similar histological changes are seen in the rare condition – congenital bullous ichthyosiform erythroderma. By courtesy of Dr. D. McGibbon, St. Thomas' Hospital.

Pigmented Hairy Epidermal Naevus (Becker's Naevus)

This lesion, which is more common in men, is not present at birth but usually appears in adolescence. It is unilateral and consists of a hyperpigmented lesion situated predominantly on the chest (Fig. 5.10) or shoulder (Fig. 5.11) and often covered with coarse hairs. The lesion is permanent but remains entirely benign.

Histology

The histological features of a Becker's naevus may be quite difficult to discern, but in an established example the changes are those of mild hyperkeratosis with slight increase in the granular cell layer and perhaps an accentuation of the epidermal ridge pattern (Fig. 5.12). There is marked pigmentation of the basal layer associated with increased numbers of melanocytes

and pigmentary incontinence (Figs. 5.13 and 5.14). The hair follicles appear normal and there is no evidence of melanocytic naevus formation. A not uncommon association found with the epidermal changes is the presence of abundant smooth muscle bundles in the dermis.

Sebaceous Naevus

This is a relatively common tumour occurring in the head and neck region and particularly affecting the scalp. It is well circumscribed, raised, yellow and consists of many small rounded elevations (Fig. 5.15). When present in the scalp there is no hair growth within the area of the tumour. It becomes smaller after the first year of life, just as normal sebaceous glands decrease in size at this time, since they are no longer under the influence of maternal androgens, but the naevus enlarges

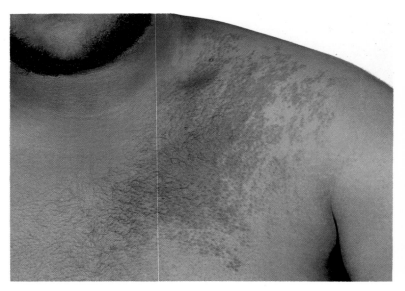

Fig. 5.10 Becker's naevus. The lesion is unilateral, occurs more commonly in men and involves the front or back of the upper chest.

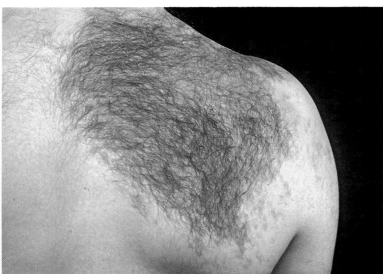

Fig. 5.11 Becker's naevus. This pigmented hairy epidermal naevus usually presents in adolescence and characteristically affects the back of the shoulder.

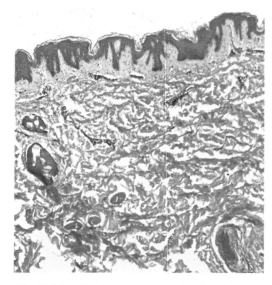

Fig. 5.12 Becker's naevus. In this low power view the changes are easily missed. There is slight hyperkeratosis with focal acanthosis (right of field) and a little accentuation of the epidermal ridge pattern.

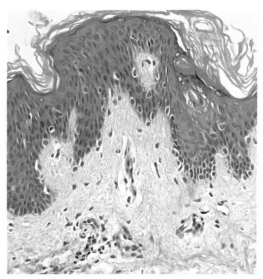

Fig. 5.13 Becker's naevus. A high power view shows increased numbers of melanocytes and conspicuous epidermal pigmentation.

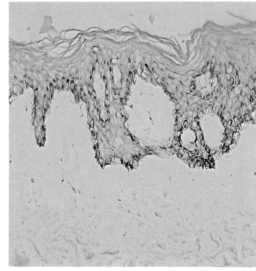

Fig. 5.14 Becker's naevus. A silver reaction highlights the abundant pigmentation of the basal cells and also demonstrates focal pigmentary incontinence (Masson-Fontanna).

permanently at puberty. A significant proportion of these lesions develop neoplasms, especially basal cell carcinoma (Fig. 5.16) and since excision is usually very simple, this is the treatment of choice.

Histology

The histological features can be quite variable, but in the fully established plaque of naevus sebaceous the squamous epithelium is acanthotic and frequently papillomatous (Fig. 5.17). Sebaceous glands are increased in number, appear hypertrophied and, of particular diagnostic importance, are situated abnormally high in the dermis where they appear distorted and sometimes communicate directly with the surface epithelium (Fig. 5.18). A common finding is the presence of small, immature hair follicles (hair germs) situated close to or apparently arising from the surface epithelium or sebaceous glands (Fig. 5.19). Mature hair follicles are reduced in number or absent. A frequent manifestation of naevus sebaceous is the presence of ectopic apocrine glands situated deeply in the dermis or subcutaneous fat (Fig. 5.20).

In some instances, particularly in the pre-pubertal, histology may show a diminution in the number of glands, with diagnosis depending upon the presence of other features particularly hair germ formation and the occasional superficially located, distorted sebaceous gland.

Naevus sebaceous can be complicated by the development of a variety of tumours including basal cell carcinoma and syringocystadenoma papilliferum, a benign tumour of probable apocrine derivation.

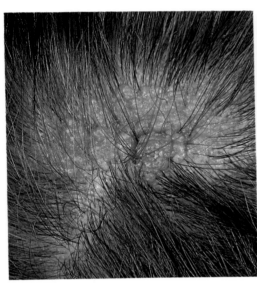

Fig. 5.15 Naevus sebaceous. This is a well-circumscribed, raised yellow plaque occurring most commonly in the scalp.

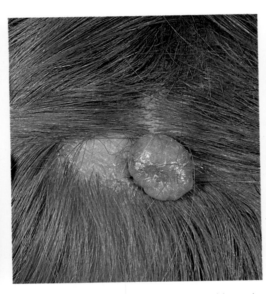

Fig. 5.16 Naevus sebaceous and basal cell carcinoma. Basal cell carcinoma does develop relatively commonly in naevus sebaceous such that prophylactic excision is advisable.

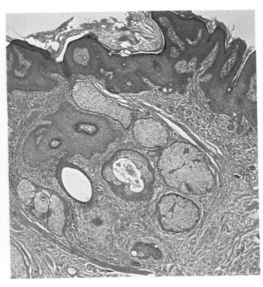

Fig. 5.17 Naevus sebaceous. The epidermis is irregular, hyperkeratotic and has a rather verrucous surface. Abundant abnormal sebaceous glands are present.

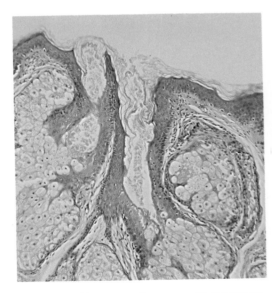

Fig. 5.18 Naevus sebaceous. Sebaceous glands are encroaching upon the papillary dermis and appear to be communicating directly with the surface.

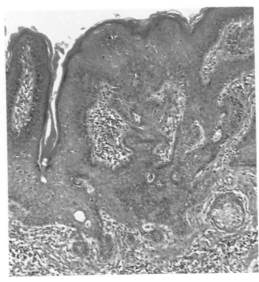

Fig. 5.19 Naevus sebaceous. A common finding is the presence of marked proliferative changes of basal epithelium giving rise to hair-germ structures. Exaggeration of this process may result in the development of a basal cell carcinoma.

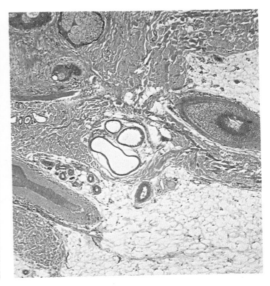

Fig. 5.20 Naevus sebaceous. In the centre of the field are three cystically dilated ectopic apocrine glands.

Connective Tissue Naevus

Connective tissue naevi are hamartomatous lesions of dermal elastic fibres and collagen. Many variants are inherited and they may present at birth or appear in the first two decades. Included under the designation are familial cutaneous collagenoma, the shagreen patch of tuberous sclerosis (Bourneville's disease) and the cutaneous manifestations (dermatofibrosis lenticularis disseminata) of the Buschke-Ollendorff syndrome.

In familial cutaneous collagenoma, a disorder with an autosomal dominant mode of inheritance, multiple indurated, smooth, skin-coloured nodules are present on the thighs, buttocks and particularly the back (Fig. 5.21). Lesions usually appear in the second decade and there is an increased incidence of hypertension and cardiomyopathy in patients with this disorder. Isolated collagenoma may occasionally present as an acquired lesion.

Tuberous sclerosis, a congenital disease with an autosomal dominant mode of inheritance, comprises a complex of developmental abnormalities including cerebral cortical astrocytic sclerotic foci (tubera), retinal abnormalities (phakomata), cardiac hamartomata and renal angiomyolipomata. Patients may suffer from mental retardation and epilepsy. The cutaneous manifestations include periungual fibromata (Fig. 5.22), facial adenoma

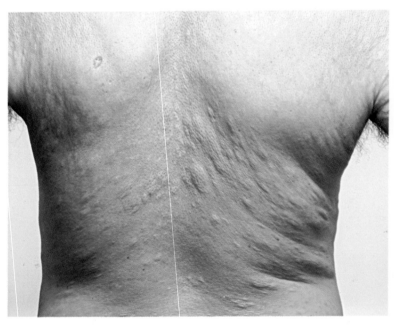

Fig. 5.21 Connective tissue naevus. Flesh-coloured raised plaques occur on the trunk. By courtesy of St. Mary's Hospital.

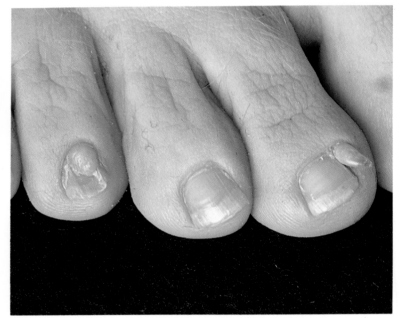

Fig. 5.22 Connective tissue naevus. Periungual fibromata are features of tuberous sclerosis.

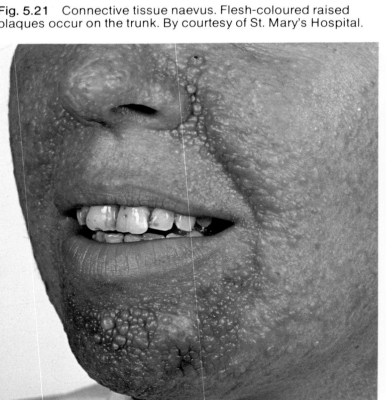

Fig. 5.23 Tuberous sclerosis. Facial angiofibromata occur in association with connective tissue naevi in tuberous sclerosis. By courtesy of Dr. A.C. Pembroke.

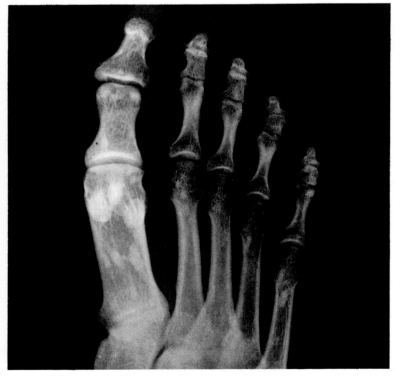

Fig. 5.24 Osteopoikilosis. Multiple dense radio-opaque spots are present. By courtesy of Dr. P. Gishen, King's College Hospital.

sebaceum (Fig. 5.23) (a misnomer as the lesions are angio-fibromata) and shagreen patches. The latter consist of irregular thickened plaques, usually situated on the lower back.

The Buschke-Ollendorff syndrome, which has an autosomal dominant mode of inheritance, consists of osteopoikilosis (Fig. 5.24) (asymptomatic, irregular, radio-opaque lesions situated particularly within the long bones, pelvis, hands and feet) associated with a widespread connective tissue naevus predominantly involving the thighs, buttocks, trunk and proximal extremities. The lesions are asymmetrically grouped, skin-coloured papules and plaques.

Histology

The histopathology of the collagenoma (inherited or acquired) consists essentially of increased dermal collagen (Figs. 5.25 and 5.26). Elastic fibres may appear diminished but whether this represents a real or apparent phenomenon is uncertain (Fig. 5.27). Similarly the shagreen patch represents an increase in collagen within the dermis.

The skin lesions of the Buschke-Ollendorff syndrome consist of excess thickened elastic fibres in the mid and lower dermis. Fragmentation and calcification as seen in pseudoxanthoma elasticum (a generalized congenital disease of elastic tissue) is not a feature. Isolated lesions with identical histology are known as juvenile elastoma (naevus elasticus).

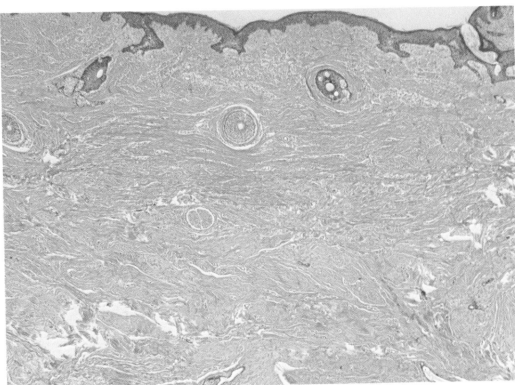

Fig. 5.25 Connective tissue naevus. The dermis is expanded by variably orientated broad bundles of collagen.

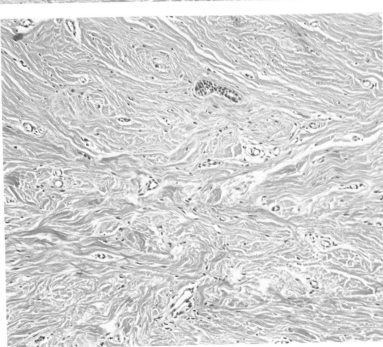

Fig. 5.26 Connective tissue naevus. The fibrous tissue is relatively acellular. An obliquely cut eccrine duct is seen in the lower centre of the field.

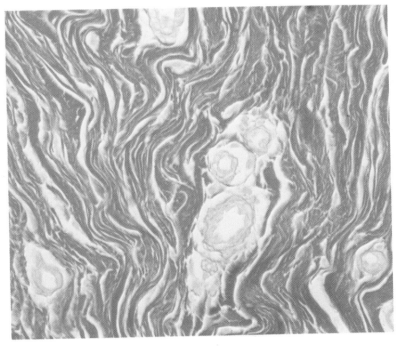

Fig. 5.27 Connective tissue naevus. There is complete absence of elastic fibres (elastic van Gieson).

MELANOCYTIC (PIGMENTED) NAEVI

These are very common skin tumours, being evident in almost all Caucasians (Fig. 5.28). Some are present at birth. These are permanent and are usually a couple of centimetres or more in diameter. Most melanocytic naevi, however, develop gradually during childhood, rapidly during adolescence, fairly slowly during adult life and subsequently disappear so that it is uncommon to be able to find evidence of melanocytic naevi in the elderly. The pigmented naevus arises from melanocytes which are derived early in fetal life from the neural crest. Melanocytic naevi are classified as junctional, compound, dermal or blue depending on the position of the naevus cells in the skin.

Junctional Naevus

The naevus cells are found in nests at the dermo-epidermal junction. The lesions are either flat or slightly raised, pigmented and vary in size from about 1mm to 1cm (Figs. 5.29-5.33). They are well defined and either oval or round. The colour varies from light tan to dark brown. The distribution of the pigment within the lesion is orderly, regular and even and frequently the central area is darker than the periphery. They have a smooth surface and the skin lines are preserved. Any lesion which has junctional activity has potential for malignant change but this is rare in comparison with the frequency of the lesions, for it is estimated that the average Caucasian has at least 25 such lesions. Quite probably too, the majority of malignant melanomas develop on

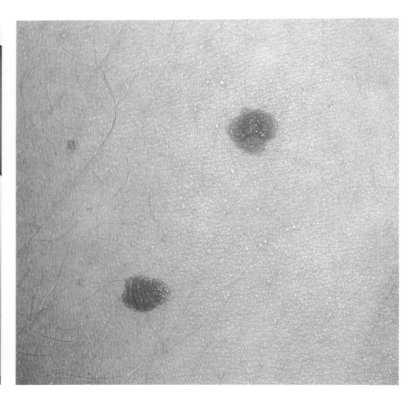

Fig. 5.28 Melanocytic naevi. Virtually all Caucasians have moles, which develop during childhood and early adult life and disappear with advancing years.

Fig. 5.29 Junctional naevi. These two moles are regular in both outline and colour.

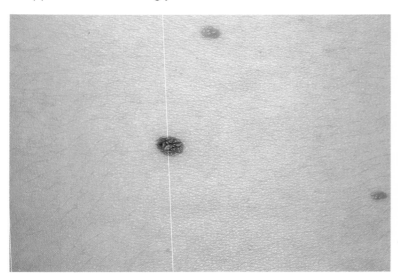

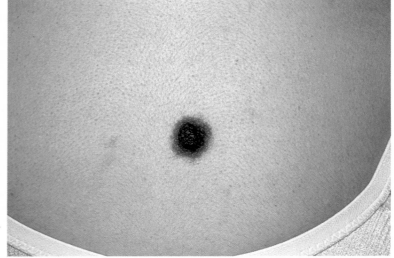

Fig. 5.30 Junctional naevus. This mole is quite dark but the pigment is distributed evenly and there is no indentation or notching in the outline.

Fig. 5.31 Junctional naevus. Although centrally this lesion is very dark, the overall pattern of colour is regular, as is the outline.

skin which has previously appeared perfectly normal. However, junctional naevi are a source of anxiety to patients and doctors and the question of prophylactic excision is a common problem in practice. An experienced observer should be able to differentiate a benign from a malignant mole but if there is doubt, excision and histological examination is the wisest course.

Histology

This is the earliest stage in the evolution of the melanocytic naevus. Melanocytes proliferate to form discrete collections (nests) of naevocytes in the lower aspect of the epidermis usually situated within the epidermal ridges. The individual cells are uniform, have pale or clear cytoplasm and often show rather evenly dispersed fine granules of melanin pigment (Fig. 5.34). In heavily pigmented variants, melanin may be found within the cytoplasm of histiocytes (melanophages) within the papillary dermis (Fig. 5.35). The natural history of a benign junctional naevus is towards dermal involvement – the compound melanocytic naevus. Infiltration of the upper layers of the epidermis by naevocytes is not usually a feature of the junctional naevus. Its presence therefore should be viewed with suspicion and great care taken to exclude the possibility of malignancy.

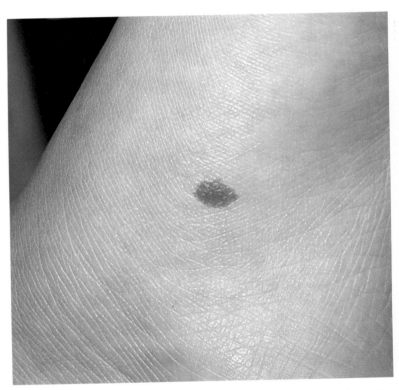

Fig. 5.32   Junctional naevus. Moles commonly occur on the sole of the foot. Provided they are benign there is no need to remove them prophylactically.

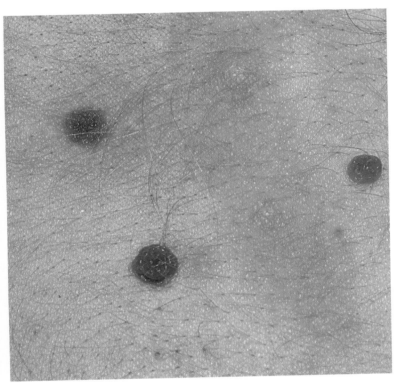

Fig. 5.33   Junctional naevi. These moles are pedunculated but quite even. The patient also has marked dermatographia.

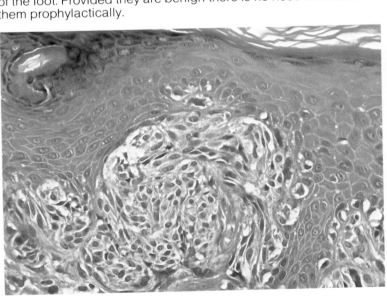

Fig. 5.34   Junctional naevus. A typical nest of uniform melanocytes is seen in the centre of the field. Note the pale cytoplasm and regular oval nuclei with prominent nucleoli.

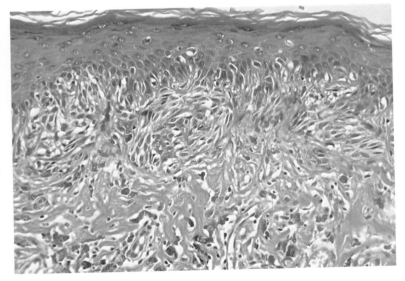

Fig. 5.35   Junctional naevus. In this example there is much pigment present both within the melanocytes and also in macrophages (melanophages) in the underlying dermis (pigmentary incontinence).

Compound Naevus

The naevus cells are found both at the dermo-epidermal junction and also in the dermis and this change represents a departure of naevus cells from the epidermis. The lesion is a raised, smooth-surfaced and well-defined round papule or nodule (Fig. 5.36). It feels soft or firm and pigment is still visible on the surface. Coarse hairs may project from the surface of compound naevi.

Histology
The compound melanocytic naevus shows collections (theques) of naevocytes within the dermis in addition to the junctional zone (Fig. 5.37). Areas may show nests appearing to 'drop off' into the papillary dermis. Superficially melanin production may be retained but typically the deeper aspect of the naevus shows little or no pigmentation (Fig. 5.38). The dermal component often appears compact consisting of uniform, somewhat smaller cells with darker staining nuclei. Mitotic activity is not present. Compound naevi may be associated with quite marked squamous epithelial proliferation which may result in a warty or verrucous gross appearance. Ordinarily benign melanocytic proliferations are not associated with a lymphocytic infiltrate in the dermis (cf. Sutton's naevus and malignant melanoma).

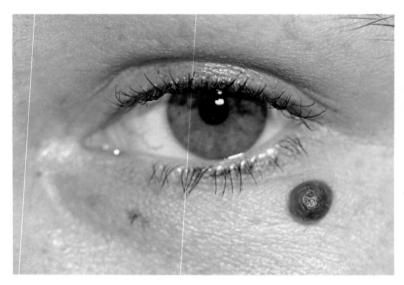

Fig. 5.36 Compound naevus. This lesion is pigmented and raised indicating the presence of naevus cells at the dermo-epidermal junction and within the dermis. It is well-defined, has a smooth surface and is round in outline.

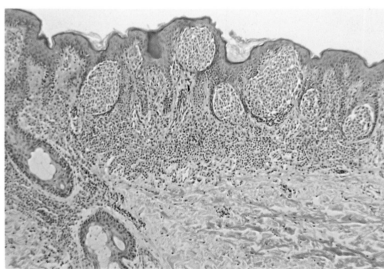

Fig. 5.37 Compound naevus. The surface of this specimen has a somewhat warty appearance. In addition to a junctional component, numerous melanocytes are present in the dermis.

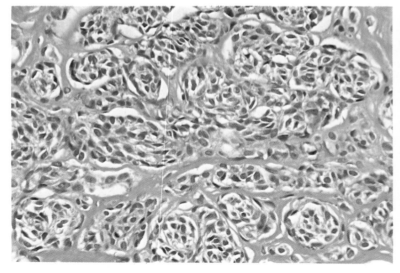

Fig. 5.38 Compound naevus. The dermal component shows diminished pigmentation with increasing depth of the lesion.

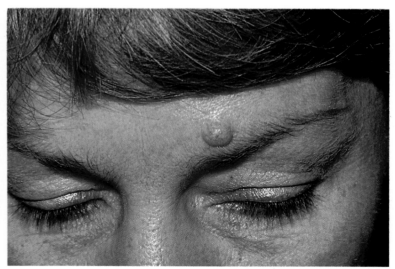

Fig. 5.39 Intradermal naevus. The lesion is raised, regular in outline and smooth-surfaced. The naevus cells are solely in the dermis.

Dermal Naevus

In this situation, the naevus cells are entirely within the dermis and they present as flesh-coloured, raised, dome-shaped lesions (Fig. 5.39). They are commonly seen on the face (Fig. 5.40) and are quite benign and have no malignant potential. The smaller ones can be dealt with safely and effectively by shaving them off flush with the surface and cauterizing the base.

Histology
Intradermal Naevus

As the lesion matures the junctional component is lost leaving an entirely intradermal naevus (Fig. 5.41). With increasing depth of the lesion, the naevocytes become progressively smaller with darkly staining nuclei and little cytoplasm. They may adopt a spindle cell form and not infrequently show 'neural' features (Fig. 5.42). Involuting naevi quite often contain bizarre multinucleate giant cells (Fig. 5.43).

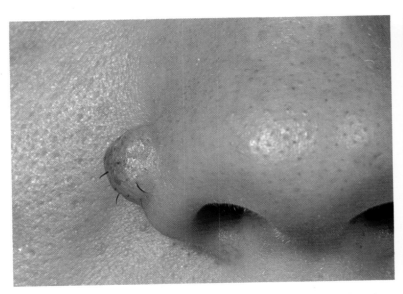

Fig. 5.40 Intradermal naevus. These naevi lack pigment and are flesh-coloured.

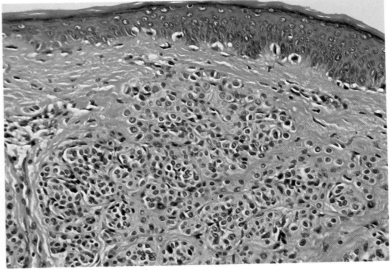

Fig. 5.41 Intradermal naevus. The epidermis is flattened over the surface of the lesion. Scattered melanocytes are seen but there is no evidence of junctional activity. In the dermis are collections of non-pigmented melanocytes, many of which have rather hyperchromatic nuclei.

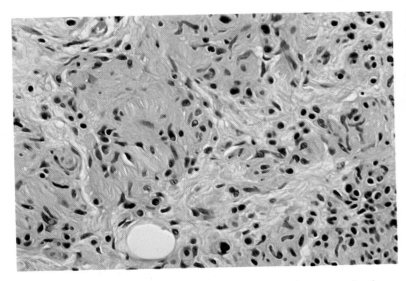

Fig. 5.42 Intradermal naevus. The specimen shows marked neural features including a number of 'Meissner-like corpuscles'. So-called neurotization is often seen in regressing naevi.

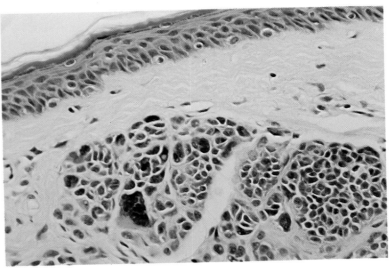

Fig. 5.43 Intradermal naevus. Giant cells as seen in this field are frequently a feature of regression.

Blue Naevus

The blue naevus is regarded as a failure of melanocytes from the neural crest to arrive at the dermo-epidermal junction. The melanocytes are found in the lower dermis and the refraction of light at this level gives rise to the blue appearance (Fig. 5.44). They are usually found on the hands and feet or head and neck and are quite benign.

Histology

The histological hallmark of the simple blue naevus is the heavily pigmented dendritic melanocyte (Fig. 5.45) which may be found singly or arranged in interlacing fascicles (Fig. 5.46). They are typically elongated, irregular and often branched and their pigment content is such that all cellular details are obscured. Associated with the melanocytes are melanin containing macrophages and a variable degree of scarring. Except in those instances where a co-existent epidermal derived melanocytic naevus (combined naevus) is present, the epidermis is normal. The simple blue naevus is *not* associated with any tendency for malignant transformation.

Mongolian Blue Spot

This is a dermal naevus of a greater size than the blue naevus. The lesions are usually located on the buttocks or sacrum (Fig. 5.47). They are seen quite commonly in mongoloid or negroid babies but may rarely be found in Caucasians. The Mongolian blue spot usually disappears in early childhood.

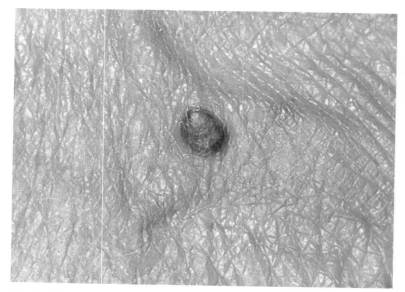

Fig. 5.44   Blue naevus. The lesion is raised and appears blue in colour. The naevus cells are deep in the lower dermis and incident light refracts blue.

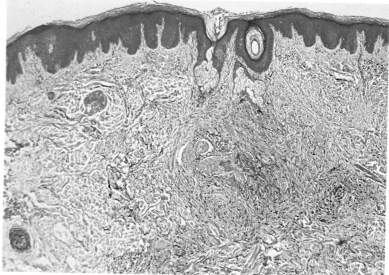

Fig. 5.45   Blue naevus. No junctional or upper dermal component is present. Situated within the reticular dermis is an irregular, heavily pigmented spindle cell lesion.

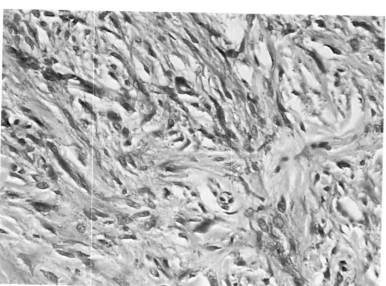

Fig. 5.46   Blue naevus. Numerous heavily pigmented spindle cells are seen with elongated, tapering cytoplasmic processes.

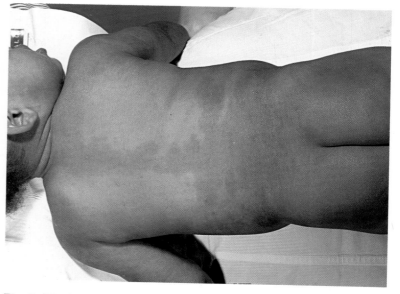

Fig. 5.47   Mongolian blue spot. These blue pigmented patches occur most commonly in negroes or mongoloid babies over the lower back and buttocks. They disappear spontaneously.

Histology

In this lesion dendritic, pigmented melanocytes are still present in the deeper layers of the reticular dermis representing a migratory arrest. Disappearance of the lesion is related to gradual reduction of melanogenesis.

Naevus of Ota

This is a bluish hyperpigmentation affecting one side of the face in the areas supplied by the ophthalmic and maxillary divisions of the trigeminal nerve (Fig. 5.48). Often the sclera is involved (Fig. 5.49). It is most common in the Japanese. There is a similar condition affecting the areas supplied by the posterior supra-clavicular and lateral brachial cutaneous nerves and is known as the naevus of Ito.

Histology

The histology of the naevi of Ota and Ito is indistinguishable from that of the Mongolian blue spot.

Naevus Achromicus

A solitary unilateral white patch may be present at birth (Fig. 5.50). The lesion is of no significance although occasionally associated retardation and epilepsy have been recorded. The naevus is permanent.

Histology

The achromic naevus is characterized by reduced numbers of (functionally abnormal) melanocytes.

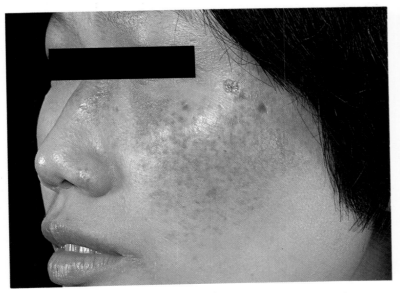

Fig. 5.48 Naevus of Ota. This blue blemish occurs most commonly in Orientals. The face is affected unilaterally and the stain is permanent.

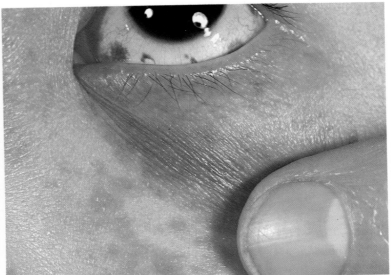

Fig. 5.49 Naevus of Ota. The sclera may be involved in addition to the face.

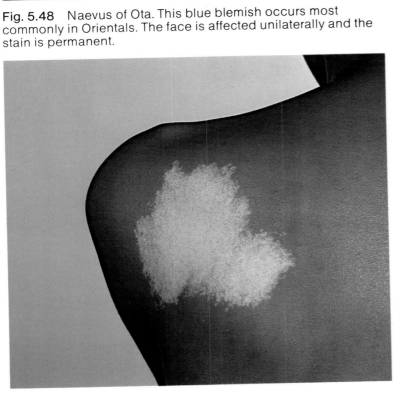

Fig. 5.50 Naevus achromicus. These naevi are unilateral, congenital and permanent.

Café au Lait Macule

A single well-circumscribed pale brown patch (Fig. 5.51) may occur as a solitary birthmark in up to 10% of the normal population. Several lesions, however, may suggest a systemic disturbance such as neurofibromatosis (Fig. 5.52) (von Recklinghausen's disease) or Albright's syndrome.

Histology

The café au lait macule is characterized by increased numbers of functionally hyperactive melanocytes.

Congenital Pigmented Naevus

These naevi are present at birth and are usually several centimetres in size (Figs. 5.53 and 5.54). They may be various shades of brown, be flat or have mamillary projections, and sometimes they are hairy. Congenital melanocytic naevi can appear anywhere on the body and usually have no systemic significance. Those occurring over the vertebral column, however, may be associated with spina bifida or meningocoele. There is an increased incidence of malignant melanoma developing in

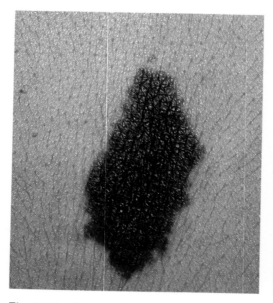

Fig. 5.51 Café au lait patch. Single patches are common in otherwise healthy individuals.

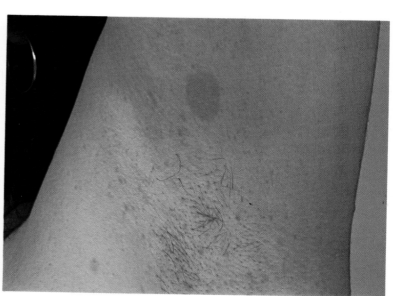

Fig. 5.52 Von Recklinghausen's disease. Café au lait patches and axilliary freckling are characteristic pigmentary features of this disorder.

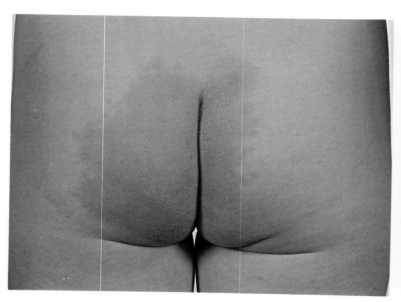

Fig. 5.53 Congenital pigmented naevus. This lesion was present since birth and is larger than an acquired melanocytic naevus. The pigment is evenly distributed throughout the naevus.

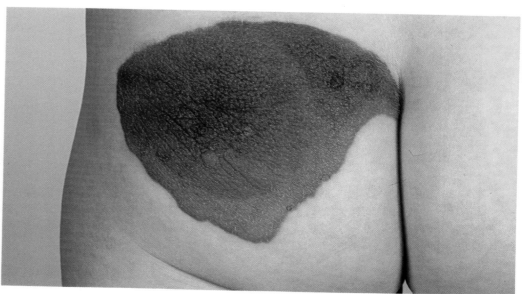

Fig. 5.54 Congenital pigmented naevus. These naevi are present at birth and are usually several centimetres in size. They may be various shades and sizes. Very occasionally malignant change occurs after many years.

these lesions although this is not very common. If it is practicable, prophylactic excision is worthwhile.

Histology

These are either compound or intradermal melanocytic naevi and although they have many features in common with their acquired counterparts there are a number of points of distinction. Congenital naevi tend to involve the deeper aspects of the reticular dermis and characteristically spread into the fibrous septae and adipose tissue of the subcutaneous fat (Figs. 5.55 and 5.56). Typical of these lesions is involvement of the adnexae (Fig. 5.57) — sebaceous glands, hair follicles, arrector pili muscles and eccrine glands and also permeation of naevus cells into nerves, lymphatics and especially blood vessels (involvement of the latter three structures should not be regarded as a sinister feature). In the congenital naevus, single cell and Indian-file arrangements of the melanocytes is typical (Fig. 5.58).

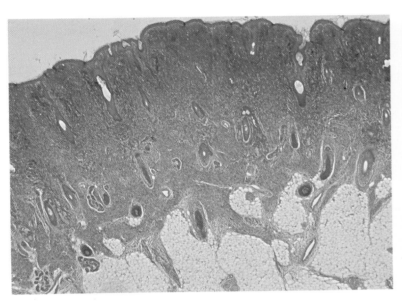

Fig. 5.55 Congenital pigmented naevus. In this scanning view massive melanocytic proliferation extends from the epidermis into the subcutaneous fat. All of the appendage structures appear surrounded by a mantle of naevus cells. The surface of the lesion has a warty appearance.

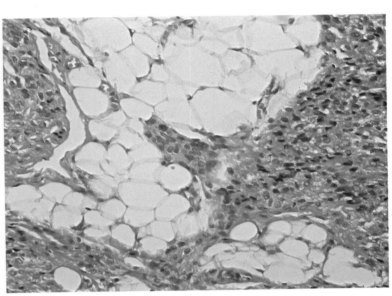

Fig. 5.56 Congenital pigmented naevus. The septae of the subcutaneous fat contain large numbers of small melanocytes with oval hyperchromatic nuclei and indistinct cell borders.

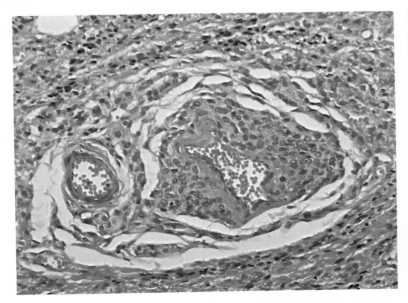

Fig. 5.57 Congenital pigmented naevus. This field taken from the deep aspect of the lesion shown in Fig. 5.55 shows involvement of the media of a large arteriole. In tumours such as this, infiltration of blood vessel walls is not uncommon and should *not* be regarded as having any sinister implication.

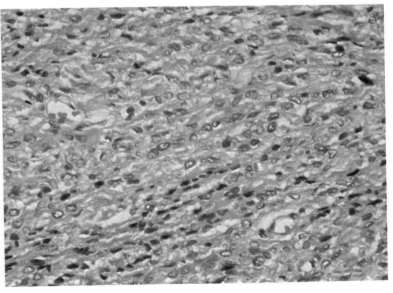

Fig. 5.58 Congenital pigmented naevus. Single cells and Indian-file arrangement are often a feature of congenital naevi.

Giant Hairy 'Bathing Trunk' Naevi

This condition is fortunately rare. The infant is born with extremely extensive involvement of the skin with large pigmented naevi (Fig. 5.59), some of which are hairy (Fig. 5.60) and many are raised, becoming more so with time. Some have papillomatous projections and the skin may become quite redundant in areas. The lesions are various shades of brown. The condition is so named because the bathing trunk area (Fig. 5.61) is usually extensively involved. Malignant melanoma does occur in this condition, including during childhood. The exact incidence is not known due to the rarity of the condition and the tendency to report only those cases which do eventuate in malignant melanoma and metastasis.

Histology

The histological features of the congenital giant naevus are variable but may be similar to those of the more usual congenital lesion. In addition, however, neurotization is often marked (Fig. 5.62) and other appearances include neurofibromatous foci, blue naevi and even juvenile melanoma-like areas.

Halo Naevus (Sutton's Disease)

These are common particularly in adolescence and present a striking picture of a melanocytic naevus surrounded by a white halo (Fig. 5.63). There may be several of these in any one patient and they are usually found on the trunk. With the passage of time, the pigmented naevus disappears and the halo completely

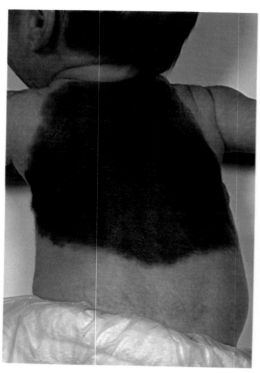

Fig. 5.59 Giant hairy 'bathing trunk' naevus. This extensive pigmented naevus is present from birth.

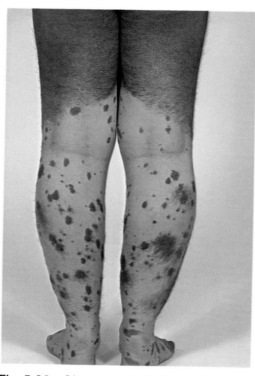

Fig. 5.60 Giant hairy 'bathing trunk' naevi. These naevi are often multiple and sometimes hairy.

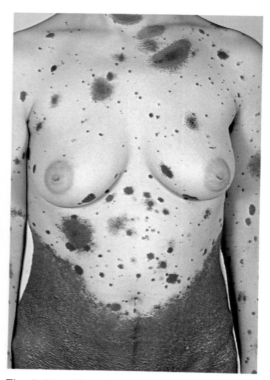

Fig. 5.61 Giant hairy 'bathing trunk' naevi. Malignant melanoma can occur in these naevi, but the exact incidence is unknown.

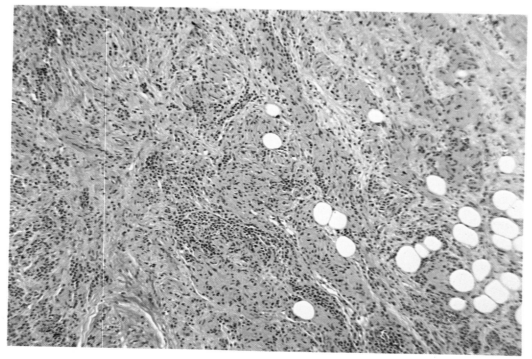

Fig. 5.62 'Bathing trunk' naevus. Neurotization (neural features) as shown in this field is a very common phenomenon.

re-pigments. Halo naevi are thought to be an auto-immune phenomenon and antibodies found in the circulation of affected patients have been demonstrated to be directed towards the cytoplasm of malignant melanoma cells *in vitro*. The condition is entirely benign. There is an increased incidence of vitiligo associated with the condition.

Histology

The halo naevus phenomenon is usually, although not invariably, based upon a compound melanocytic naevus (it may rarely occur in relation to a blue naevus, a juvenile melanoma and even a malignant melanoma). The established lesion presents as a circumscribed raised dermal nodule in which there is an intense chronic inflammatory cell infiltrate (Fig. 5.64). The latter may have a lichenoid distribution and consists predominantly of lymphocytes and histiocytes although occasional plasma cells and mast cells may also be present. At an early stage melanocytes may be easily seen both as nests and as individual cells (Fig. 5.65), but with progression of the lesion they become increasingly difficult to identify (Fig. 5.66). With destruction of pigment-containing naevus cells the released melanin is taken up by macrophages which in old resolving lesions may be all that is left to mark the scene of the previous battleground. The histology of the surrounding halo is characterized by an absence of any visible melanin pigment associated with a negative dopa reaction.

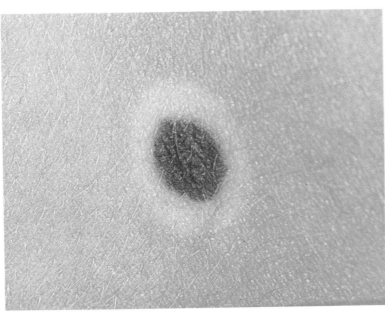

Fig. 5.63 Sutton's 'halo' naevus. A melanocytic naevus is surrounded by a white halo. This harmless phenomenon is quite common in the first or second decade. The naevus ultimately may disappear and the area repigment.

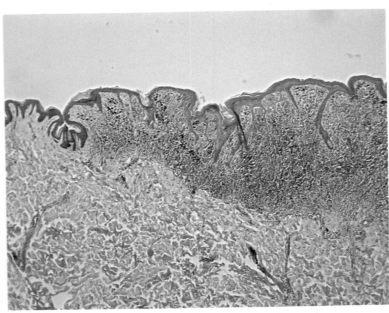

Fig. 5.64 Halo naevus. The lesion, which is sharply demarcated from the normal skin (left), shows a dense lichenoid inflammatory cell infiltrate.

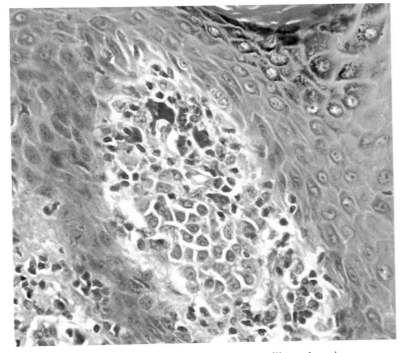

Fig. 5.65 Halo naevus. In this view the papillary dermis contains a cluster of obvious melanocytes. The deeply pigmented cells are melanophages.

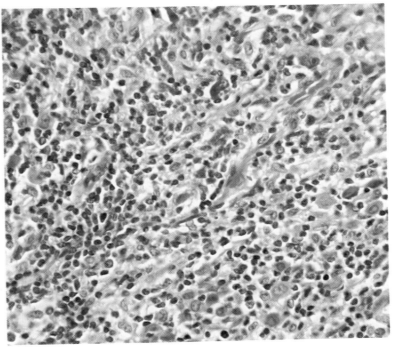

Fig. 5.66 Halo naevus. In this field the melanocytic nature of the lesion is difficult to detect, the few naevus cells that are present are obscured by the intense chronic inflammatory cell infiltrate.

Juvenile Melanoma (Spitz's Naevus)

This is an important lesion because the histology is frequently reported by those unaware of the condition as being that of a malignant melanoma (Fig. 5.67). However, the average age of the patients presenting with this tumour is about ten years, which is very rare for a malignant melanoma. The lesion is a dome-shaped red or red-brown papule(Fig. 5.68)which does not look at all like a malignant melanoma. It is commonly seen on the face, particularly the cheeks, and is usually raised and grows quite rapidly initially and the patient or the patient's mother can usually be quite accurate as to the time of its onset. The juvenile melanoma is quite benign.

Histology
Recognition of the histological features of the juvenile melanoma is of great importance in order to avoid confusion with a truly malignant lesion. It is an uncommon, benign variant of a compound naevus characterized by its pleomorphic appearance. The tumour shows a striking symmetry with melanocytic proliferation confined within the lateral borders of the lesion.

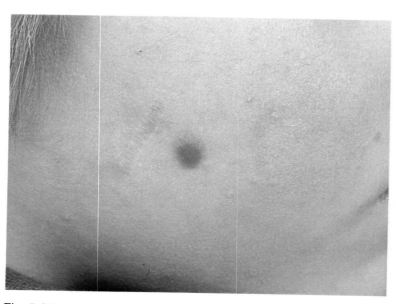

Fig. 5.67   Juvenile melanoma (Spitz's naevus). Commonly occurring on the cheek of a young child, the lesion is a red-brown papule. The adjacent scar is from one removed previously. Originally reported as a malignant melanoma, an authoritative second opinion confirmed the clinical diagnosis of a benign juvenile melanoma.

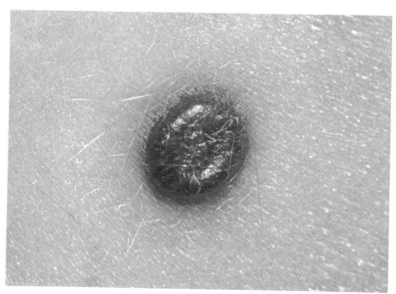

Fig. 5.68   Juvenile melanoma. The lesion has a red-brown colour and commonly occurs on the cheek of a young child.

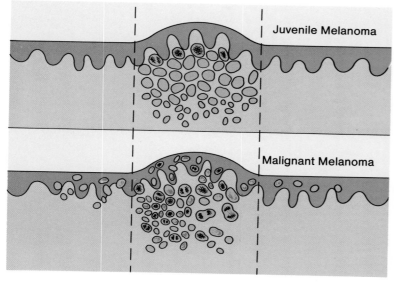

Fig. 5.69   A comparison between juvenile melanoma and malignant melanoma.

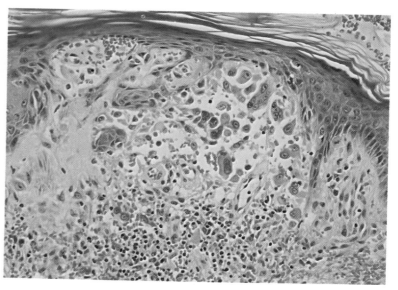

Fig. 5.70   Juvenile melanoma. In the centre of the field scattered 'epithelioid' melanocytes are seen, characterized by abundant eosinophilic cytoplasm, large vesicular nuclei and prominent nucleoli.

This is in contrast to the 'juvenile melanoma-like' malignant melanoma in which junctional and/or dermal involvement typically is present on either side of the main tumour mass (Fig. 5.69). The cells of the superficial aspect of the juvenile melanoma may have an epithelioid or more commonly a spindle cell appearance and characteristically have abundant eosinophilic cytoplasm with rather large but typically uniform nuclei (Figs. 5.70 and 5.71). Mononuclear and multinucleate giant cells may be present which show little nuclear pleomorphism in

contrast to the tumour giant cells of a malignant melanoma (Fig. 5.72). Juvenile melanoma usually has little pigment present, its pink coloration being due to the ectatic blood vessels which are often found in its stroma (Fig. 5.73). Mitotic activity may be seen but only in the superficial component of the tumour. The deeper aspect of the lesion shows evidence of maturation as would be expected in a benign compound naevus. Differentiating features between juvenile melanoma and malignant melanoma are shown in Fig. 5.74.

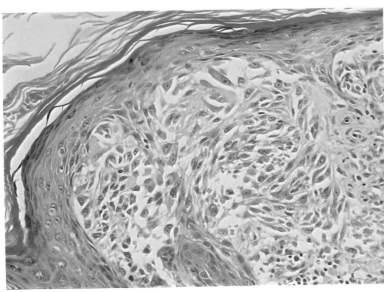

Fig. 5.71 Juvenile melanoma. In this view the melanocytes are mainly of the spindle cell type. Note the absence of melanin pigment – a typical feature of this lesion.

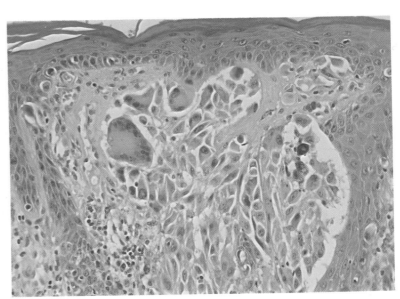

Fig. 5.72 Juvenile melanoma. Several giant cells are seen in this example. Nuclear pleomorphism and hyperchomatism, which would be anticipated in a malignant tumour, are absent.

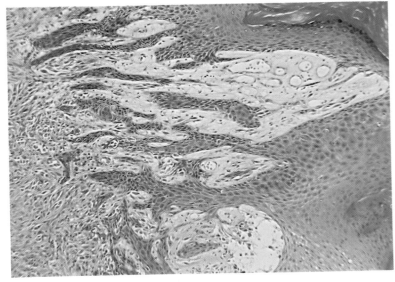

Fig. 5.73 Juvenile melanoma. In this low power view several ectatic blood vessels are present in the papillary dermis in the upper right quadrant. In this interesting example there is striking *pseudo*-epitheliomatous hyperplasia.

Feature	Juvenile Melanoma	Malignant Melanoma
Symmetry	Usually present	Usually absent
Involvement of over-lying epidermis by single naevus cells	Infrequent	Common
Pleomorphism Cytoplasmic Nuclear	Present Absent	Present Present
Giant cells	Uniform nuclei	Pleomorphic nuclei
Mitotic activity	Usually inconspicuous, never atypical	Often conspicuous, frequently atypical
Melanin pigment	Usually absent	May often be conspicuous
Vascular ectasia	Often present	Usually absent
Maturation with depth of lesion	Present	Absent

Fig. 5.74 Histological distinction between juvenile melanoma and 'juvenile melanoma-like' malignant melanoma.

VASCULAR NAEVI
Strawberry Naevi

These are quite common, usually occurring as a single lesion, often on the face (Fig. 5.75), a month or so after birth. Occasionally they are multiple. They grow rapidly and cause great concern and difficulties for the parents because of their appearance. They occasionally bleed and sometimes temporarily ulcerate (Fig. 5.76). It is important to appreciate that most disappear spontaneously by the age of about seven (Fig. 5.77). Thus it is incorrect to embark on treatment such as radiotherapy or surgery which will result in scarring (Fig. 5.78), when the lesion is highly likely to disappear without trace on its own accord (Fig. 5.79). If there is any residual lesion, it can always be dealt with by a plastic surgeon at a later date. The only indications for active intervention are when the lesion is interfering with a vital structure such as the eye, where closure

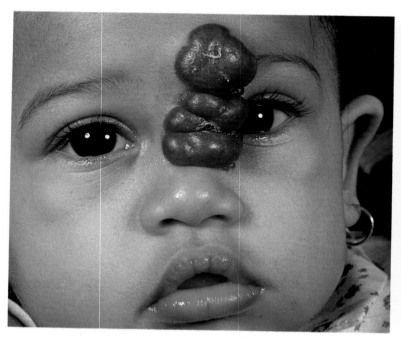

Fig. 5.75 Strawberry naevus. The naevus appears shortly after birth and is red and raised. Lesions on the face are a great trial to the parents whereas the child is oblivious until older. At this stage, however, the naevus begins to show signs of resolution.

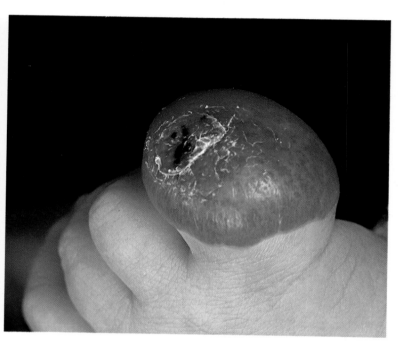

Fig. 5.76 Strawberry naevus. Necrosis of part of the surface occasionally occurs. By courtesy of St. John's Hospital for Diseases of the Skin.

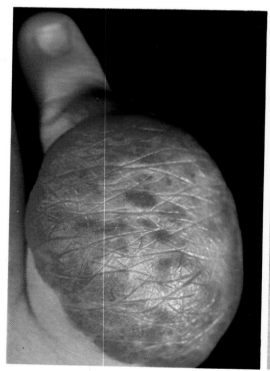
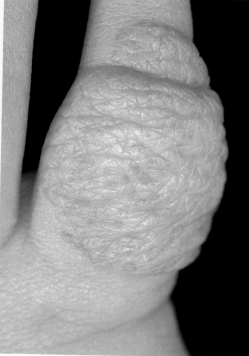

Fig. 5.77 Strawberry naevus. The red colour lessens first, before the lesion fractures. These pictures were taken 18 months apart.

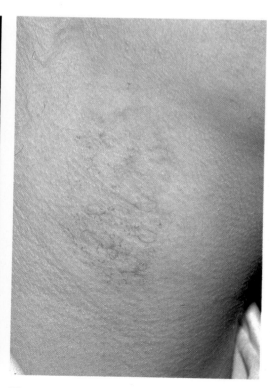

Fig. 5.78 Irradiation of a strawberry naevus. Radiotherapy and surgery result in unnecessary permanent scarring.

5.20

may result in failure to develop binocular vision, or over the mouth where it might interfere with feeding. High doses of systemic corticosteroids may be indicated in these situations to shrink the naevus. The lesions are easy to diagnose, being well-defined red tumours. They vary in size but usually stop growing by about 18 months of age. As they begin to involute, the surface becomes paler. Very occasionally, large haemangiomas may trap platelets leading to consumption of clotting factors.

Histology
The histological features of the strawberry naevus are those of a capillary haemangioma. It appears as an exuberant proliferation of small vascular channels (Figs. 5.80 and 5.81).

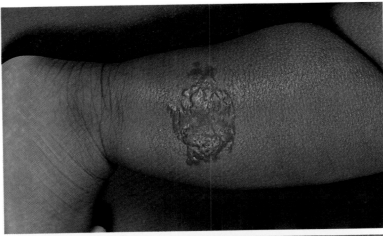

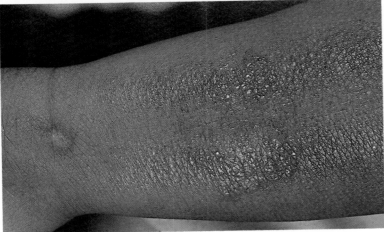

Fig. 5.79 Strawberry naevus. Most lesions disappear completely, without trace. Involution is occurring.

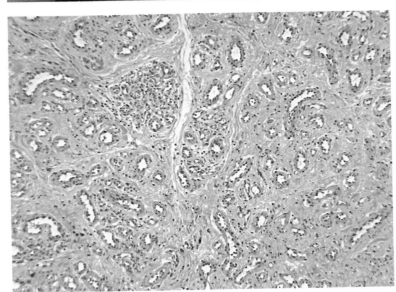

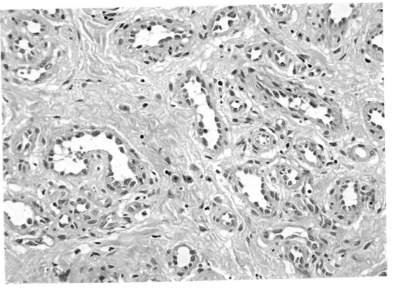

Fig. 5.80 Strawberry naevus. This biopsy taken from a relatively early lesion shows aggregates of blood vessels dispersed in a fibrous stroma.

Fig. 5.81 Strawberry naevus. The vascular channels are lined by plump endothelial cells. Scattered mast cells with eosinophilic cytoplasm are scattered throughout the tumour.

Port Wine Stain (Naevus Flammeus)

This vascular malformation is present at birth. It is a flat lesion varying in colour from pink to deep red. It is usually several centimetres in size and although it may occur anywhere on the body it is most commonly situated on the face (Fig. 5.82) or nape of the neck. Regrettably, these lesions are permanent and those on the face are most disfiguring. There has been no successful treatment up until the present time, although lasers are being used experimentally.

The majority of patients with these haemangiomas are perfectly well in every other respect but the following two syndromes are occasionally associated with these naevi.

Sturge-Weber Syndrome

Intracranial angiomas are associated with vascular naevi involving the skin, predominantly in the distribution of the trigeminal nerve (Fig. 5.83). The conjunctivae and oral mucosa are often involved. The condition may present with epilepsy, mental retardation or contralateral hemiparesis. Radiography of the skull may reveal streaks of calcification (Fig. 5.84) in the angioma on the same side as the naevus. The lesions may well be operable.

Klippel-Trenaunay-Weber Syndrome

In this condition, the cutaneous haemangioma is associated with a vascular malformation of the underlying soft tissue and bone such that hypertrophy occurs (Fig. 5.85).

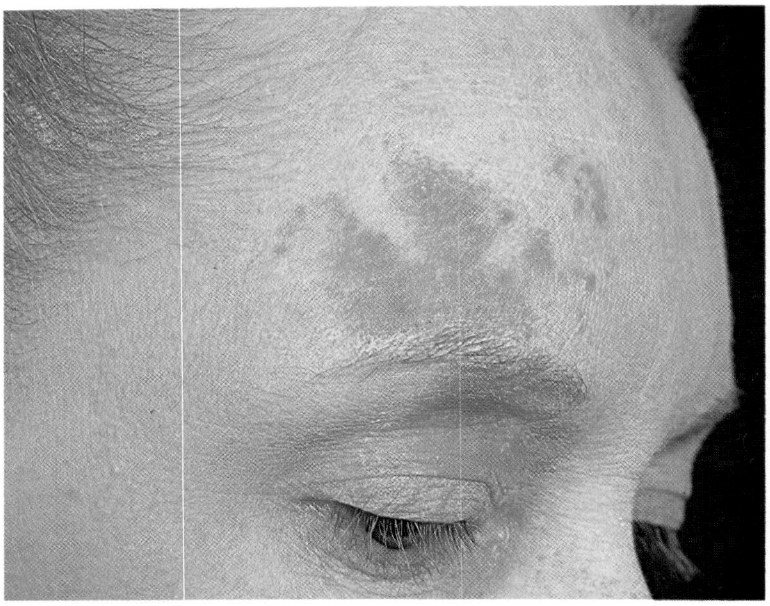

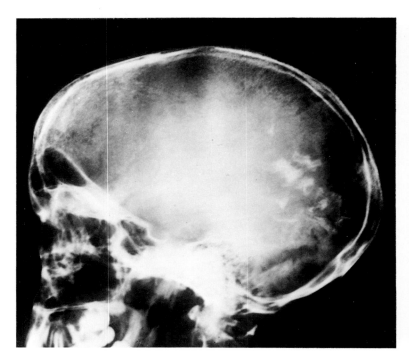

Fig. 5.82 Capillary naevus. The port wine stain is present at birth and is disfiguring and permanent.

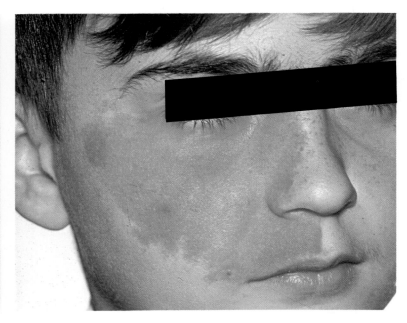

Fig. 5.83 Sturge-Weber syndrome. A port wine stain in the distribution of the trigeminal nerve may indicate the presence of an ipsilateral cranial angioma. By courtesy of St. Mary's Hospital.

Fig. 5.84 Sturge-Weber syndrome. Intracranial calcification of the angioma may be seen at X-ray. By courtesy of St. Bartholomew's Hospital.

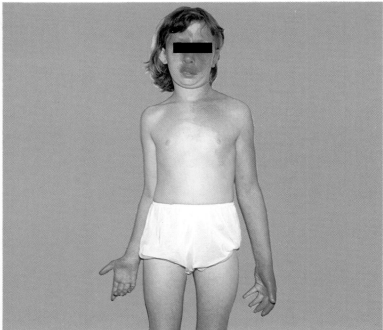

Fig. 5.85 Klippel-Trenaunay-Weber syndrome. Vascular malformation of soft tissues and bones resulting in limb hypertrophy occurs in association with the port wine stain. By courtesy of St. Bartholomew's Hospital.

Histology

The lesion consists of widespread dilated blood filled vascular channels showing no proliferative features (Fig. 5.86).

Salmon Patches

There are also capillary naevi but the prognosis is usually excellent. The lesions are much paler pink and are found on the mid-forehead (Fig. 5.87) and over the eyelids. They usually fade sometime after the first year.

Spider Naevus

This is a very common and normally innocent lesion. It is an arterial dilatation and can occur anywhere in the distribution of superior vena cava but is particularly seen on the face (Fig. 5.88). More than one lesion may be present. In pregnancy they may subsequently resolve. Spider naevi are one of the cutaneous features of liver disease (Fig. 5.89). A good cosmetic result can be obtained by cauterizing the central vessel.

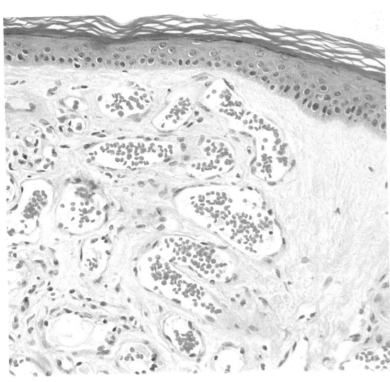

Fig. 5.86 Port wine stain. The lesion is characterized by numerous dilated thin-walled capillaries.

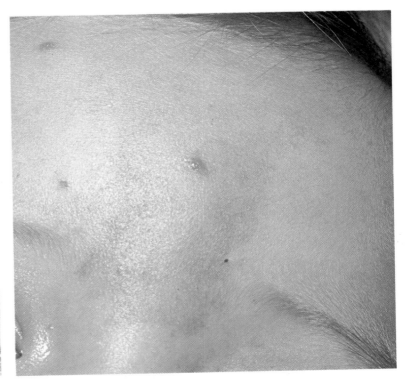

Fig. 5.87 Salmon patch. These pale pink patches often found over the forehead in infants fade soon after the first year.

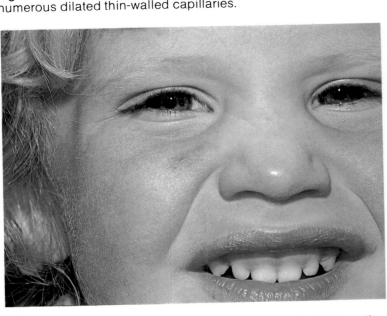

Fig. 5.88 Spider naevus. These are common particularly on the faces of healthy young people.

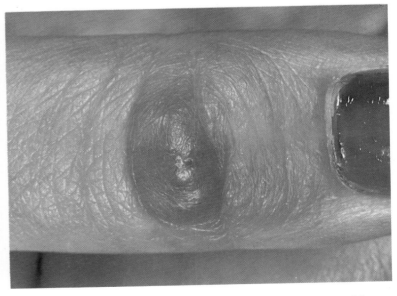

Fig. 5.89 Spider naevus. Spider naevi may be stigmata of liver disease. Giant naevi may occur as in this patient. Spider naevi occur anywhere within the distribution of the superior vena cava.

Hereditary Haemorrhagic Telangiectasia (Osler-Weber-Rendu Syndrome)

This condition which has an autosomal dominant mode of inheritance is a disorder of blood vessels which are dilated (ectatic) and found in the skin, mucous membranes and viscera. Discrete small red lesions are found characteristically on the fingers, face, lips (Fig. 5.90) and oral and nasal mucous membranes. Spider naevi and telangiectases are also found. They are associated with arteriovenous fistulae in the lungs and vascular abnormalities in the liver. The danger of the condition is haemorrhage from the mucous membranes, for example of the nose or gastrointestinal tract or from the lungs.

Angiokeratoma

This is a small red papule with a hyperkeratotic surface – a disorder of blood vessels with associated overlying epidermal changes. A single lesion, which may bleed, usually occurs on a limb in childhood or adolescence. Multiple lesions may occur particularly on and around the genitalia (Fig. 5.91) and are quite harmless. Multiple lesions of angiokeratoma become significant in Anderson-Fabry disease (angiokeratoma corporis diffusum) (Figs. 5.92 and 5.93). As the name implies, the angiokeratomas are widespread but have a particular predilection for the genitalia, lower trunk and thighs. The condition affects males primarily because it has a sex-linked recessive mode of inheritance but angiokeratomas may occur in heterozygote female carriers. Anderson-Fabry disease is a condition of sphingolipid metabolism in which patients have a deficiency of the lysosomal enzyme alpha galactosidase A (ceramide trihexosidase) with resultant accumulation of the glycolipid ceramide trihexoside within the cytoplasm of cells of a variety of tissues including blood vessels, smooth muscle, heart, kidney and the central nervous system. Death is commonly due to renal failure but myocardial infarct and cerebrovascular lesions may also occur. An unexplained but typical symptom of the disease is periodic attacks of excruciating burning pain in the extremities associated with fever. The typical skin lesions associated with eye changes (conjunctival vessel dilatation and tortuosity, corneal opacities

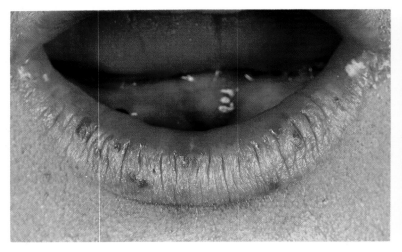

Fig. 5.90 Hereditary haemorrhagic telangiectasia (Osler-Rendu-Weber disease). Vascular malformations occur in the skin, mucous membranes, liver and lungs. Uncontrolled bleeding is the danger of this condition.

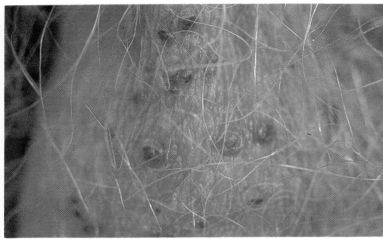

Fig. 5.91 Angiokeratoma. Small red papules with a hyperkeratotic surface are common on and around the genitalia and are quite harmless.

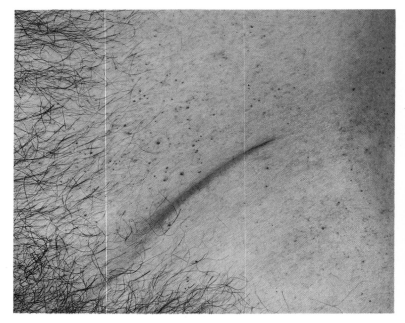

Fig. 5.92 Angiokeratoma. Papules may occur in association with alpha galactosidase A deficiency. A serious sex-linked systemic condition known as Anderson-Fabry disease results.

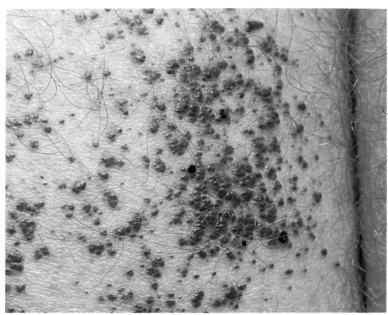

Fig. 5.93 Anderson-Fabry disease. A myriad of discrete purple papules are present on the skin. By courtesy of Dr. R. Holmes, St. Thomas' Hospital.

revealed by slit lamp observation and dilatation and tortuosity of the retinal veins) should enable a clinical diagnosis to be made. Confirmation can be established by the estimation of alpha galactosidase A levels in circulating leucocytes and cultured fibroblasts.

Anderson-Fabry disease is a serious condition with many male mortalities in the fifth decade. Female carriers have a normal life expectancy.

Histology

The histological features of the angiokeratoma are those of dilated thin-walled blood vessels situated within the upper, particularly papillary dermis often appearing to be located within the epidermis. There is a variable degree of associated hyperkeratosis (Figs. 5.94 and 5.95).

In Anderson-Fabry disease, the appearances are similar but the presence of small vacuoles in the media of cutaneous blood vessels is of diagnostic importance. They may also be seen in the endothelial cells and are strongly diastase-PAS positive. The

deposits can also be stained on frozen sections using Sudan black. Similar vacuoles may also be seen in the arrector pili muscles and smooth muscle elsewhere in the body including the myocardium. Vacuolation of the renal glomeruli and tubular system is conspicuous although at a late stage of the disease severe glomerulosclerosis is found.

With electron microscopy characteristic lamellar bodies (periodicity 5nm) and dense bodies (lipid inclusions) may be detected.

Naevus Anaemicus

This is a single well-circumscribed patch of pale skin which otherwise appears normal (Fig. 5.96) It is quite indistinguishable from the surrounding skin if the area is blanched by a microscopic slide. The pallor is due to an increased reactivity of the blood vessels to catecholamines and can be reversed by blocking the sympathetic nerves. It is most commonly found on the chest. Patients with von Recklinghausen's disease have a higher incidence of naevus anaemicus.

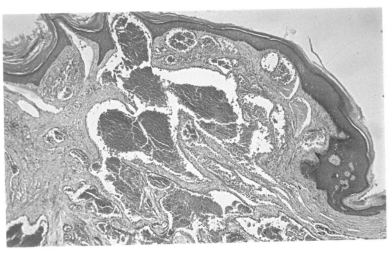

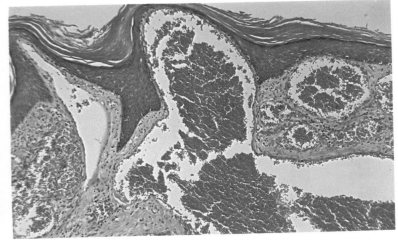

Fig. 5.94 Angiokeratoma. This low power view taken from the middle of a papule (normal epithelium on far right) shows conspicuous thin-walled vascular spaces in both the papillary and reticular dermis. Note the overlying hyperkeratosis.

Fig. 5.95 Angiokeratoma. A large blood-filled dilated blood vessel is causing marked attenuation of the overlying squamous epithelium.

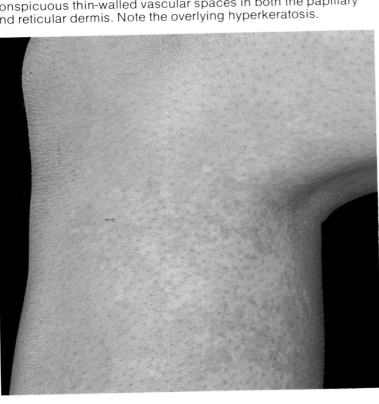

Fig. 5.96 Naevus anaemicus. The lesion is off white, well-defined with irregular margins. It becomes indistinguishable from surrounding skin with pressure from a glass slide. By courtesy of St. John's Hospital for Diseases of the Skin.

LYMPHATIC NAEVI
Lymphangioma

These lesions are usually present at birth as a cluster of vesicles from which clear fluid may discharge. A common site is the buttocks or lower abdomen (Fig. 5.96). They occasionally become secondarily affected. They are quite benign but require specialized surgical skills if they are to be excised successfully, for they frequently recur.

Histology

Superficial cutaneous lymphangioma, sometimes known as lymphangioma circumscriptum histologically, appears as a collection of dilated, thin-walled lymphatic channels usually but not always containing lymph (Fig. 5.97). The surrounding epidermis is acanthotic and in many instances the lymphatic spaces within the papillary dermis simulate an intra-epidermal location. Of particular importance to the diagnosis of lymphangioma circumscriptum is the knowledge that if the 'feeder' vessels in the reticular dermis or subcutaneous fat are not adequately treated then recurrence of the lesion is very likely (Fig. 5.98).

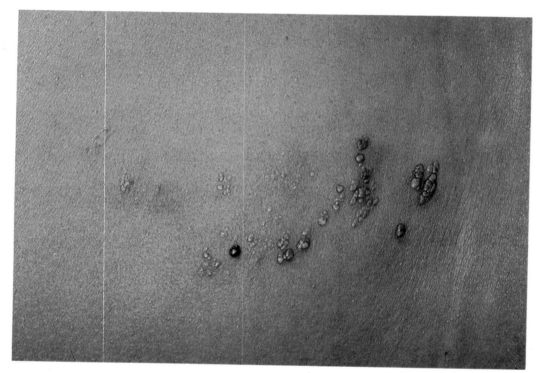

Fig. 5.97 Lymphangioma circumscriptum. Usually present at birth, a cluster of vesicles occurs from which clear fluid may discharge. The lower abdomen is a common site.

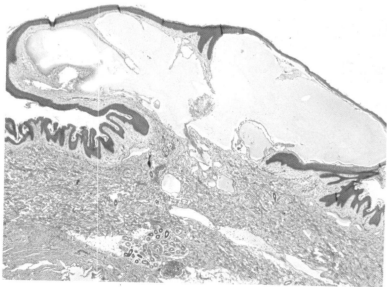

Fig. 5.98 Lymphangioma circumscriptum. This scanning view shows a polypoid lesion composed of greatly dilated lymphatic channels. Scattered smaller vessels are also present in the reticular dermis.

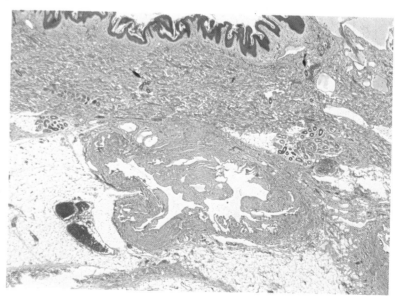

Fig. 5.99 Lymphangioma circumscriptum. In the centre of the field is a large irregular muscular lymphatic trunk.

6 Benign Tumours of the Skin

Anthony du Vivier MD, FRCP

Phillip H. McKee MB BCh, BaO, MRC Path

EPIDERMAL LESIONS

Cysts

There is a tendency among clinicians to refer to cutaneous cysts as sebaceous cysts but in the majority this terminology is inaccurate; there is no evidence that they develop from sebaceous glands, except in the case of sebocystomatosis (steatocystoma multiplex). Most cysts in fact can be divided histologically into epidermoid and pilar types, but clinically they are often indistinguishable (Fig. 6.1).

Epidermoid Cyst

This lesion, which is derived from squamous epithelium, presents as a smooth, mobile, cutaneous or subcutaneous lump often with a central punctum (Fig. 6.2) through which its contents may be expressed as cheese-like material. It is commonly found on the trunk. Some epidermoid cysts result from implantation of squamous epithelium due to injury from a sharp instrument e.g. a needle. Epidermoid cysts are also frequently associated with acne vulgaris, particularly acne conglobata (nodulo-cystic acne), in which there may be one or more cysts on the face (Fig. 6.3) or trunk. They are often inflamed (Fig. 6.4)

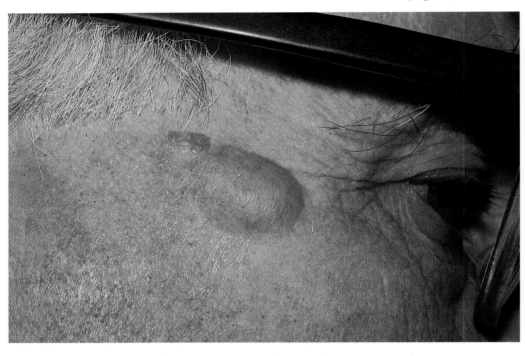

Fig. 6.1 Epidermal cyst. Clinically, epidermoid and pilar cysts are often indistinguishable and are known as epidermal cysts or 'wens'.

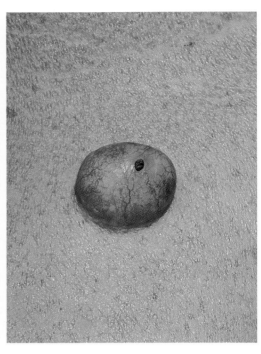

Fig. 6.2 Epidermoid cyst. The cyst is a round and smooth-surfaced swelling. A central punctum is present, through which the contents may be expressed.

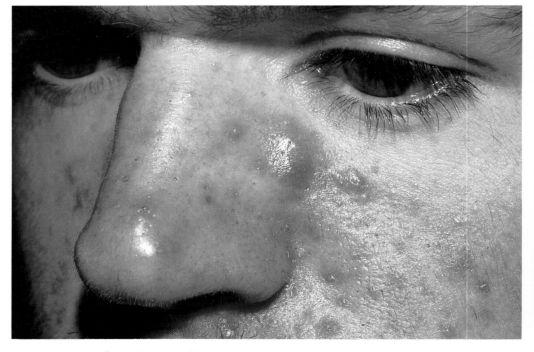

Fig. 6.3 Nodulo-cystic acne. The histology of the cysts in nodulo-cystic acne (acne conglobata) is that of an epidermoid cyst.

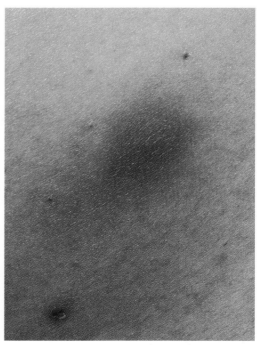

Fig. 6.4 Cystic acne. Acne cysts are often inflamed. They eventually subside spontaneously.

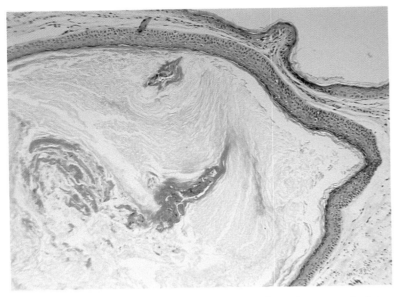

Fig. 6.5 Epidermoid cyst. This low power view shows part of a discrete cyst located below the surface epithelium. In this instance there was a past history of trauma suggesting an implantation pathogenesis.

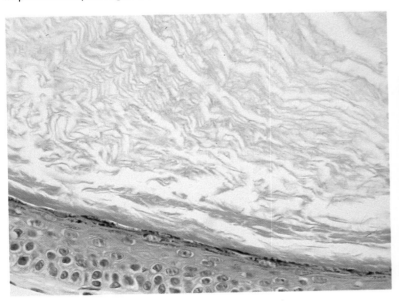

Fig. 6.6 Epidermoid cyst. The cyst wall is composed of mature, keratinizing squamous epithelium. Note the prominent granular cell layer and keratin lamellae in the lumen (upper).

Histology

The cyst wall is composed of keratinizing stratified squamous epithelium and it contains abundant, well-defined keratin lamellae (Figs. 6.5 and 6.6). Rupture of the cyst is not uncommon and results in a foreign body giant cell reaction.

Pilar (Tricholemmal) Cyst

Less common than the epidermoid cyst, this lesion is derived from the external root sheath of the hair follicle and is not associated with a punctum. They are most common on the face, neck and scalp (Fig. 6.7), where they may be multiple and are often referred to as 'wens'. Sometimes the family history is associated with an autosomal dominant mode of inheritance. Histological examination is often required to distinguish between epidermoid and pilar cysts.

Histology

The pilar cyst epithelium is derived from the external root sheath of the hair follicle and thus undergoes tricholemmal keratinization — an abrupt transition from epithelium to keratin in the absence of a granular cell layer. The cyst wall is composed of an outer palisaded layer of small basal cells which merge with larger eosinophilic cells. The latter are in turn desquamated resulting in the granular contents of the pilar cyst (Figs. 6.8 and 6.9). Calcification commonly occurs and a foreign body giant cell reaction is sometimes seen following rupture.

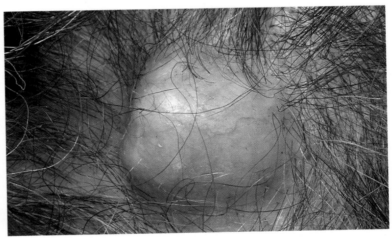

Fig. 6.7 Pilar cyst. The scalp is a common site for this type of epidermal cyst. They may be multiple and are sometimes hereditary.

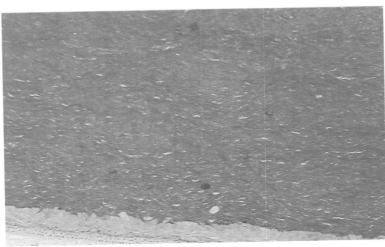

Fig. 6.8 Pilar cyst. This low power view shows a portion of a typical pilar cyst. The lining epithelium is seen in the lower field. Note the homogenous eosinophilic contents.

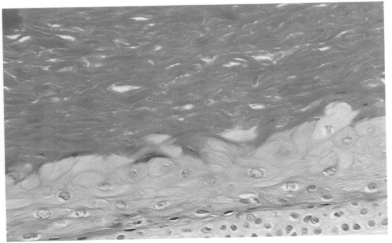

Fig. 6.9 Pilar cyst. The cyst wall consists of an outer layer of small cuboidal cells which merge with an inner zone of much larger, irregular pale cells. The latter merge imperceptibly with the cyst contents.

Dermoid Cyst

These lesions are often present at birth. They are mobile flesh-coloured swellings (Fig. 6.10) found at foci of embryonic fusion resulting from inclusion of embryonic epithelium. They are found most commonly on the face e.g. in the skin adjacent to the upper outer corner of the eye.

Histology

The wall of the dermoid cyst is composed of squamous epithelium accompanied by adnexal structures such as hair follicles and sebaceous glands. The cyst often contains hair shafts. (Fig. 6.11).

Milia

Milia are very small white or cream-coloured cysts which may occur spontaneously at any age, including infancy. They occur particularly in association with acne (Fig. 6.12) but may also be induced by sun damage, both acute after erythema and chronic, especially on the face. They develop as an end result of blistering disorders (Fig. 6.13) which affect the epidermo-dermal junction e.g. bullous pemphigoid, porphyria cutanea tarda (Fig. 6.14) or epidermolysis bullosa. In youth they may disappear spontaneously but they can be easily removed by breaking the surface with a needle and scraping out the small cyst.

Histology

A milium represents a minute epidermoid cyst. Situated within the upper dermis it consists of a thin wall of stratified squamous epithelium surrounding keratin lamellae (Fig. 6.15).

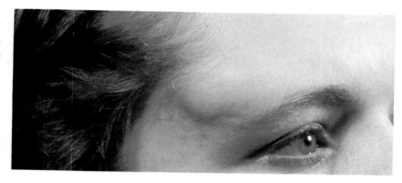

Fig. 6.10 Dermoid cyst. The dermoid cyst is present at birth and results from inclusion of embryonic epithelium. By courtesy of Queen Victoria Hospital, East Grinstead.

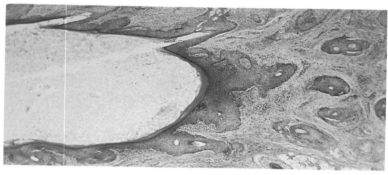

Fig. 6.11 Dermoid cyst. The cyst wall is composed of keratinizing squamous epithelium from which numerous hair follicles and sebaceous glands arise.

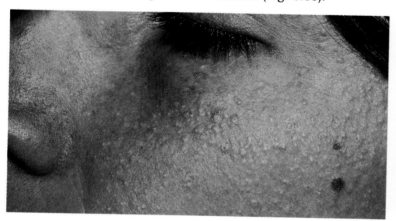

Fig. 6.12 Milia. These tiny white cysts are commonly seen on the face, often in association with acne. They are also induced by trauma e.g. from ultra-violet light.

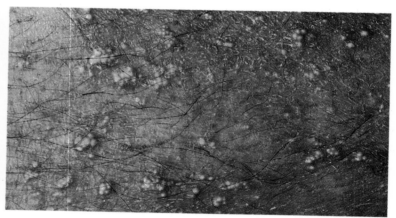

Fig. 6.13 Milia. A myriad of white cysts is seen over the shin. The patient had had blistering following profound oedema of the legs, secondary to the nephrotic syndrome.

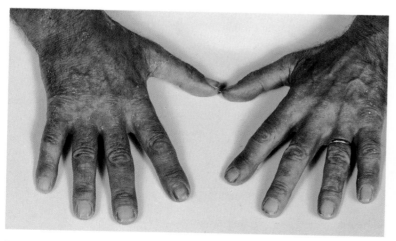

Fig. 6.14 Milia. Milia often occur as an end result of a blistering process of the skin, which involves the dermo-epithelial junction. This patient had porphyria cutanea tarda.

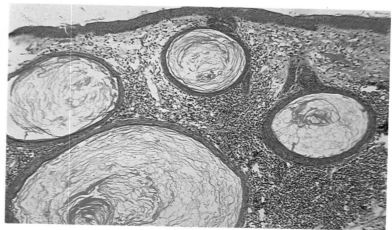

Fig. 6.15 Milia. Four small milia (mini-epidermoid cysts) are present in the superficial dermis. Two of them (upper right) are related to eccrine sweat ducts.

Seborrhoeic Wart (Seborrhoeic Keratosis, Basal Cell Papilloma)

This is an extremely common skin tumour in white-skinned races, which occurs with increasing frequency with advancing years. It may be a solitary lesion but more often it is multiple and occurs on areas of the body that have been exposed to ultra-violet light. Seborrhoeic warts are thus most commonly found on the face, on the backs of the hands, and on the forearms and trunk. The condition is due to a failure of keratinocyte maturation which results in the accumulation of immature, yet benign cells within the epidermis. Neighbouring melanocytes may transfer melanin to the abnormal keratinocytes and thus the lesions are often pigmented, varying in colour (Fig. 6.16) from light tan to a dark brown or black (Fig. 6.17). The seborrhoeic wart is usually raised and gives an appearance of having been stuck on to the skin. It has a rough surface and close examination may reveal fine fissures (Fig. 6.18). Sometimes the lesions are pedunculated, especially those around the eyelids or in the flexures. At other sites, particularly on the backs of the hands and on the face, they may be quite flat, lack-lustre and difficult to distinguish from simple lentigines (Fig. 6.19), although tiny fissures, present on the surface, may be a distinguishing factor. Seborrhoeic warts are of no clinical significance but are unsightly and often itchy (Fig. 6.20). They may be easily removed by curettage and cautery or by freezing with liquid nitrogen, with excellent cosmetic results. Although this condition is largely confined to Caucasians who tend to burn in the sun, there is a variety known as *dermatosis papulosis nigra* (Fig. 6.21) which is seen in negroes and has the same histology as seborrhoeic warts. It occurs on the cheeks and there does seem to be a hereditary tendency.

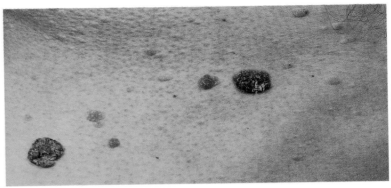

Fig. 6.16 Seborrhoeic warts. The lesions vary in colour and size. Multiple lesions are common.

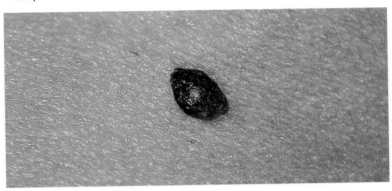

Fig. 6.17 Seborrhoeic wart. The lesion may be very large and can be mistaken for a malignant melanoma.

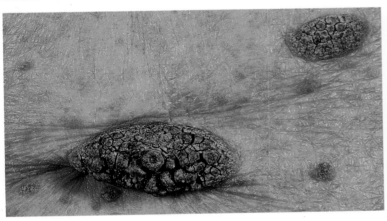

Fig. 6.18 Seborrhoeic wart. The lesion is well-defined, raised and has a rough and fissured surface.

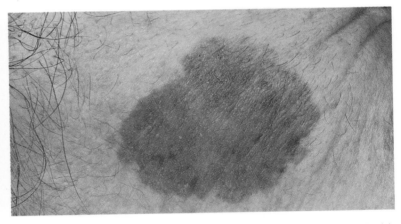

Fig. 6.19 Lentigo. This lesion is flat but may become raised with time. The histopathology is often similar to that of a seborrhoeic wart.

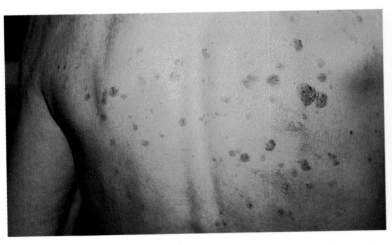

Fig. 6.20 Seborrhoeic wart. The lesion may be very itchy and the surrounding skin becomes inflamed.

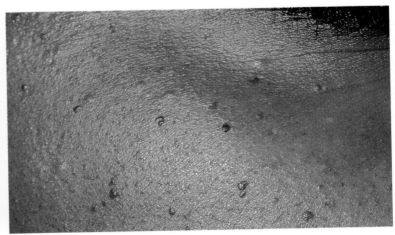

Fig. 6.21 Dermatosis papulosa nigra. There are multiple pigmented lesions on the face. This condition is common in negroes and the tendency is inherited.

6.5

Histology

Seborrhoeic warts, composed of an admixture of small basal cells and keratinocytes may display a variety of patterns. Commonly the keratotic (papillomatous) type is seen, which is characterized by hyperkeratosis, acanthosis, papillomatosis and horn cyst formation (Figs. 6.22 and 6.23). The acanthotic variant typically has a smooth surface and is often heavily pigmented (Fig. 6.24). A less common form is the adenoid seborrhoeic wart which is characterized by a downgrowth of thin proliferating epidermal strands (Fig. 6.25). The irritated seborrhoeic wart (inverted follicular keratosis) is characterized by the development of conspicuous squamous whorls – so-called squamous eddies (Fig. 6.26).

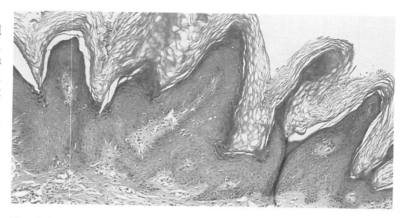

Fig. 6.22 Seborrhoeic wart (papillomatous variant). The appearances are those of a simple squamous papilloma, consisting of hyperkeratosis, papillomatosis, acanthosis with some fusion of the epidermal ridges.

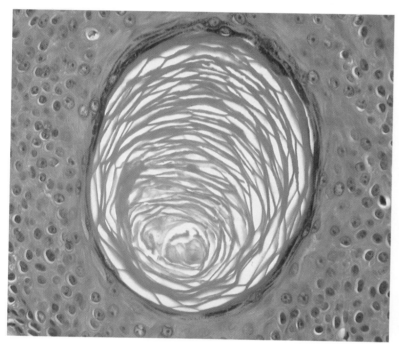

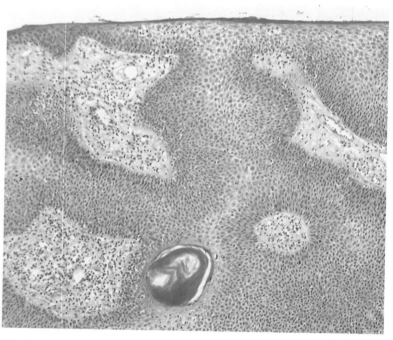

Fig. 6.23 Seborrhoeic wart (horn cyst). Sharply defined concentric lamellae of keratin, surrounded by a conspicuous granular cell layer typify the horn cysts so characteristic of the seborrhoeic wart.

Fig. 6.24 Seborrhoeic wart. This variant is composed of broad anastomosing bands of small basaloid cells. Note the smooth surface.

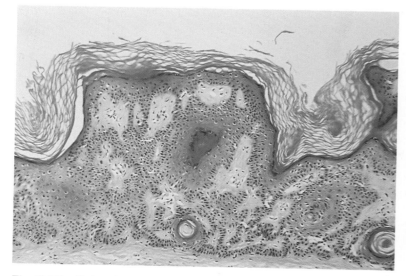

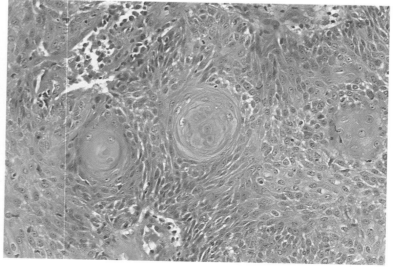

Fig. 6.25 Seborrhoeic wart (adenoid variant). Arising from the surface epithelium are thin strands of highly pigmented basaloid cells. Note the typical horn cysts in the lower field.

Fig. 6.26 'Irritated' seborrhoeic wart. *'Differentiation'* with the formation of whorls of squamous cells – so-called eddies, is typical.

CONNECTIVE TISSUE TUMOURS
Skin Tags (Fibroepithelial Polyps)
These are extremely common, particularly with increasing age, and occur on the eyelids, neck or in the axillae and groin (Fig. 6.27). They may also erupt during pregnancy. They are pedunculated, either flesh-coloured or slightly pigmented, with a rough or smooth surface (Fig. 6.28). They are of cosmetic significance only and can easily be removed by cautery.

Histology
The appearances of a skin tag (fibroepithelial polyp) consist of stratified squamous epithelium overlying a fibrovascular core, and are thus rather non-specific.

Hypertrophic Scars and Keloids
These represent hyperproliferative responses of fibrous tissue to inflammation, infection or trauma (Fig. 6.30). The clinical

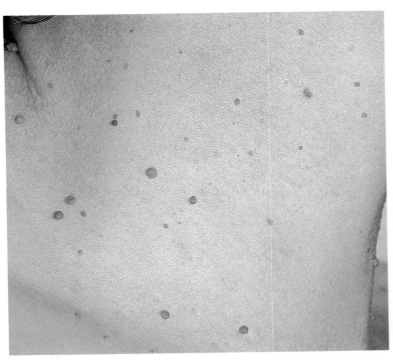

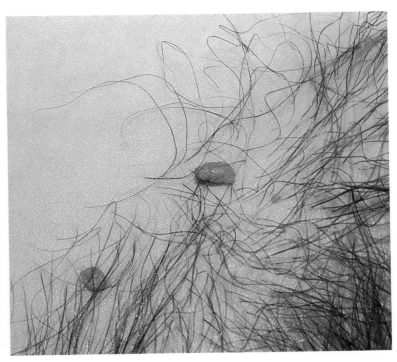

Fig. 6.27 Skin tags. These common lesions occur particularly on the neck or in the axillae and groins. They are flesh-coloured or pigmented.

Fig. 6.28 Skin tag. Pedunculated lesions sometimes occur.

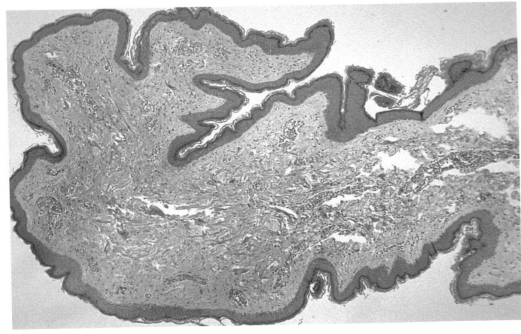

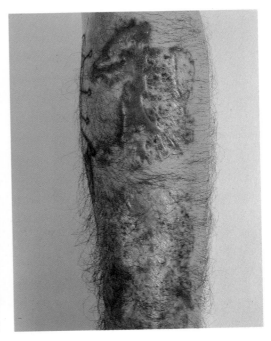

Fig. 6.29 Fibroepithelial polyp. The polyp is composed of mature keratinizing squamous epithelium overlying a fibrovascular core.

Fig. 6.30 Hypertrophic scar. Scarring has occurred secondary to sepsis following an amateur attempt to remove this tattoo. The scar will eventually flatten.

6.7

difference between these two lesions is that a hypertrophic scar is confined to the site of the initiating factor whereas a keloid spreads beyond it. The lesions have a smooth, shiny surface, are raised and firm to touch (Fig. 6.31). They are most commonly found on the upper chest, shoulders and back, which are thus poor operative sites. Keloids are particularly seen in dark-skinned races (Fig. 6.32) and are common after ear-piercing and in association with acne and folliculitis. Keloids tend to recur and often increase in size following surgery. They respond only to a limited extent to intralesional corticosteroids and radiotherapy.

Histology
Both hypertrophic scars and keloids are composed of dense fibrous tissue but in the latter the lesion consists predominantly of broad hyalinized bundles of collagen (Figs. 6.33 and 6.34).

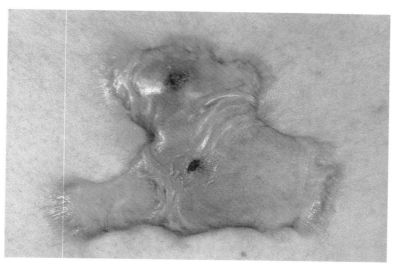

Fig. 6.31   Keloid. A keloid scar is raised, firm and has a smooth surface. It spreads beyond the site of the initiating factor.

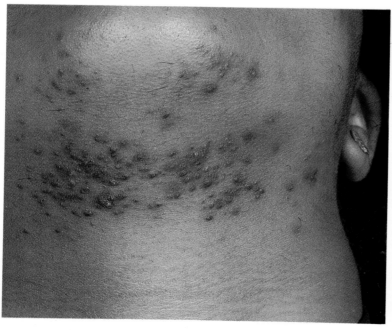

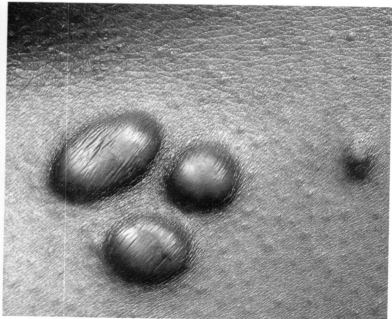

Fig. 6.32   Keloids in negroes. These are a common problem and are very difficult to treat successfully. They occur secondary to inflammation for example following acne.

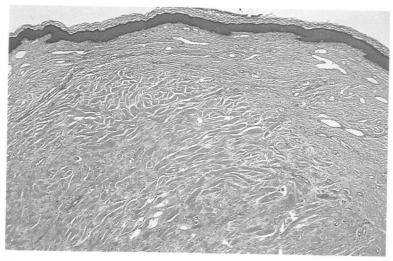

Fig. 6.33   Keloid. This specimen comes from the shoulder of an 18 year old African girl who suffered severe burns at this site as a child. The epidermis is unremarkable. The dermis is greatly expanded by dense, acellular fibrous tissue. Note the superficially located ectatic vessels.

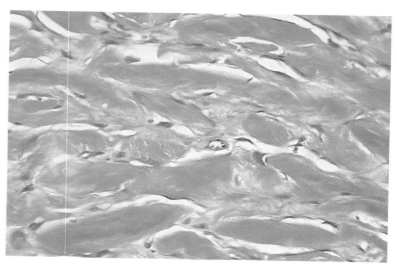

Fig. 6.34   Keloid. High power view showing broad bundles of hyalinized collagen.

Dermatofibroma (Histiocytoma, Sclerosing Haemangioma)

This is a common tumour (Fig. 6.35). It occurs more often in women than in men and is found especially on the lower legs. One or several lesions may be present. Dermatofibromata are firm, raised, usually hyperpigmented and round, varying in size from a few millimetres to a couple of centimetres in diameter. The lesion is adherent to the overlying skin but is easily moved in the underlying tissue. They are thought by some to be a response to some long-forgotten injury, particularly insect bites. The firmness and circumscribed nature of the lesion should serve to make the diagnosis obvious but if there is any doubt, an excision biopsy is indicated. Other than for cosmetic reasons, typical lesions need no treatment.

Histology

The dermatofibroma, a tumour of presumed fibrohistiocytic derivation, has a variable histological appearance depending upon the relative proportions of fibroblasts, histiocytes and collagen. It is a spindle-cell neoplasm which predominantly occupies the reticular dermis and is often separated from an acanthotic epidermis by a grenz-zone of sparing (Fig. 6.36). The lateral margins of the tumour are typically indistinct, blending imperceptibly into the adjacent tissues. It is composed of variably cellular, interlacing fascicles of spindle-cells with plump, elongated nuclei and indistinct cytoplasmic margins (Fig. 6.37).

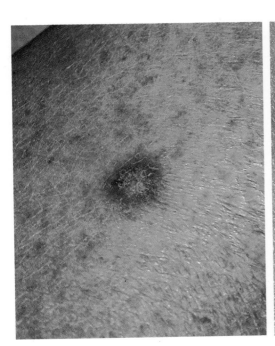 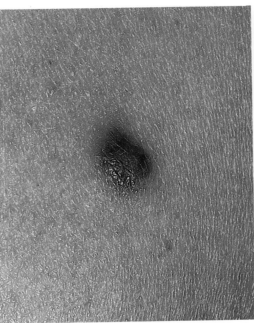 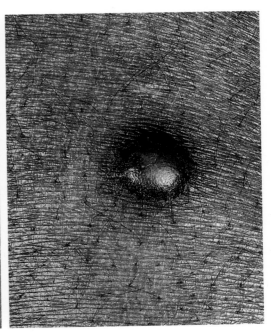

Fig. 6.35 Dermatofibroma. The lesion may be solitary or multiple. It is firm, round and attached to the overlying skin. It is frequently pigmented. The legs are the most common site.

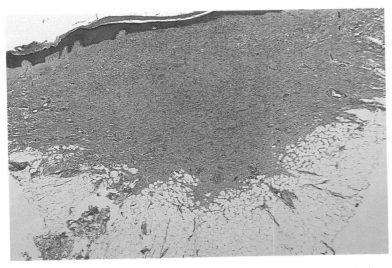

Fig. 6.36 Dermatofibroma. In this scanning view the dermis is completely replaced by a connective tissue neoplasm. Note the highly irregular lateral margins and the involvement of the superficial aspect of the subcutaneous fat.

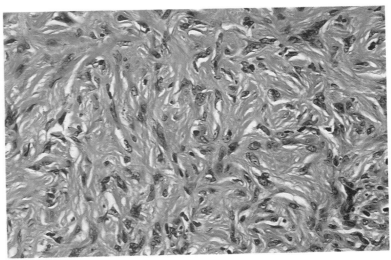

Fig. 6.37 Dermatofibroma. High power view showing irregular spindle cells dispersed in an abundant collagenous stroma. Note the absence of pleomorphism, nuclear hyperchromasia and mitotic figures.

A storiform pattern is sometimes present. The dermato-fibroma characteristically lacks pleomorphism and shows minimal or no mitotic activity. Admixed with the fibroblasts are histiocytes, inflammatory cells and often xanthoma cells (Fig. 6.38). When there is a histiocytic predominance, the tumour is sometimes called a fibrous histiocytoma. Some tumours which are excessively vascular and accompanied by marked haemosiderin deposition (Fig. 6.39) are known as sclerosing haemangiomas and are of particular importance because macroscopically they may be mistaken for malignant melanomas.

Myxoid Cyst

This localized lesion is found over the dorsal surface of the distal phalanx of a finger. It usually indents the nail, producing a characteristic longitudinal furrow (Fig. 6.40). It is a smooth, well-circumscribed, firm, flesh-coloured nodule and results from overproduction of connective tissue mucopolysaccharides in the region of the finger joint. These cysts are benign but frequently recur after excision.

Histology

The cyst is associated with irregular angulated fibroblasts dispersed in a myxoid stroma (Figs. 6.41 and 6.42).

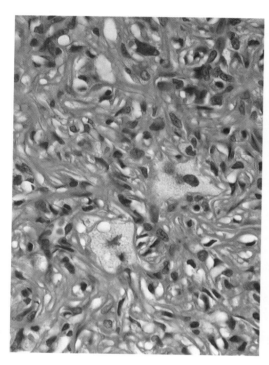

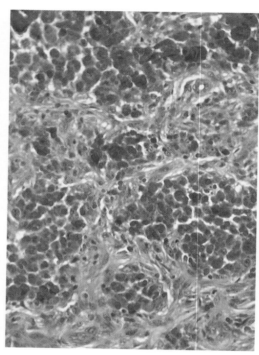

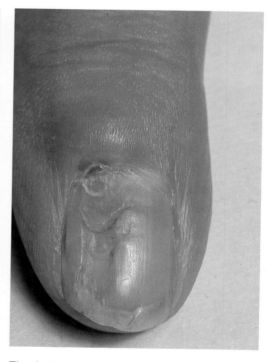

Fig. 6.38   Dermatofibroma (fibrous histiocytoma). In the centre of the field are two typical foamy xanthomatous cells.

Fig. 6.39   Dermatofibroma (sclerosing haemangioma). This tumour has a conspicuous vascular component and haemosiderin is abundant.

Fig. 6.40   Myxoid cyst. A localized swelling occurs over the dorsal surface of the distal phalanx. The nail is indented and a longitudinal furrow is apparent.

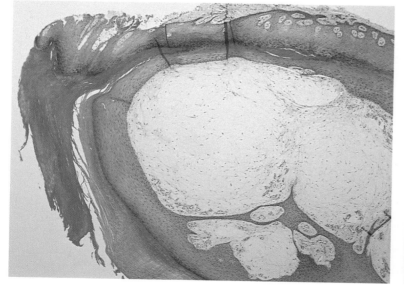

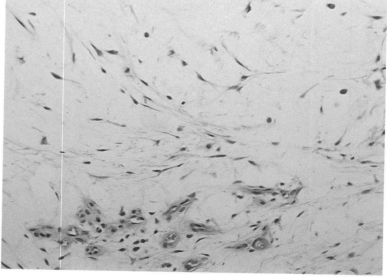

Fig. 6.41   Myxoid cyst. The dermis is expanded and largely replaced by abundant myxoid tissue giving rise to a multi-loculated 'cystic' lesion.

Fig. 6.42   Myxoid cyst. The lesion is composed of irregular stellate cells dispersed in a pale staining myxoid stroma.

Lipoma

This benign tumour of adipose tissue arises in the subcutaneous fat (Fig. 6.43). There may be one or several lesions, which are easily diagnosed because they are soft, sometimes lobulated and have a normal skin surface. They can be of quite large size (Fig. 6.44) and are commonly situated on the arms, back of the neck and trunk.

Histology

The lipoma is a discrete lesion composed of mature adult fat cells (Fig. 6.45). Sometimes there is an excessive vascular component – the so-called angiolipoma (Figs. 6.46 and 6.47).

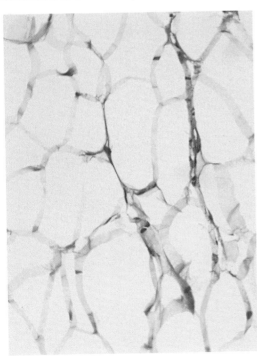

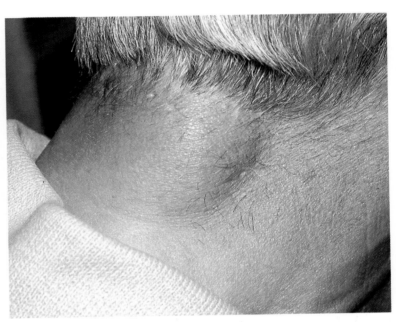

Fig. 6.43 Lipoma. These subcutaneous swellings are often lobulated and relatively soft. The skin surface is quite normal.

Fig. 6.44 Lipoma. The swelling may attain a large size.

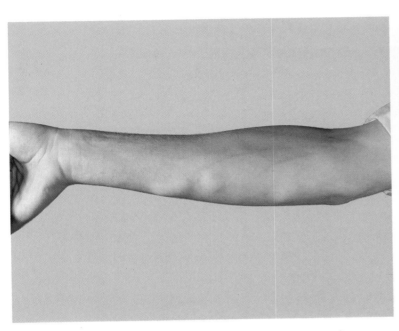

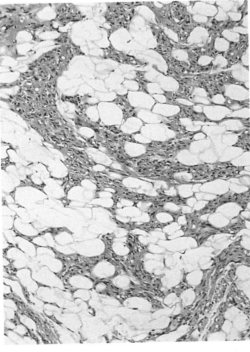

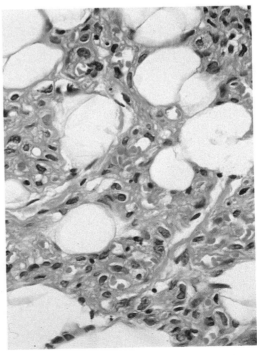

Fig. 6.45 Lipoma. The lesion is composed of adult fat cells. A portion of the capsule is seen on the far right.

Fig. 6.46 Angiolipoma. In this tumour in addition to adult fat there is a variable admixture of proliferating blood vessels thereby mimicking the normal embryogenesis of adipose tissue.

Fig. 6.47 Angiolipoma. High power view showing foci of small vessels.

6.11

VASCULAR TUMOURS

Pyogenic Granuloma

This is a common benign tumour consisting of newly formed capillaries with surrounding oedema, possibly initiated by trauma. The lesion, which occurs at any age, particularly childhood, is usually solitary and often arises on the face or the side of the finger (Fig. 6.48), but may be found anywhere on the body including mucosal surfaces. It is a red nodule initially and can grow quite rapidly. It is friable and bleeds easily. It can most readily be treated by curettage and cautery. Occasionally the lesion may recur.

Histology

The pyogenic granuloma is a benign vascular tumour of uncertain histogenesis. It is a raised lesion, often ulcerated and inflamed and sometimes bordered laterally by an epidermal collarette (Fig. 6.49). It consists of a number of longish muscular vascular trunks from which numerous small capillary vessels arise – the lesion thus has a rather lobulated appearance (Fig. 6.50). Sometimes these typical changes are obscured by marked stromal oedema.

Haemangioma

This is a common vascular tumour (Fig. 6.51). It is well-defined, raised and has a smooth surface. Its red colour suggests the diagnosis (Fig. 6.52).

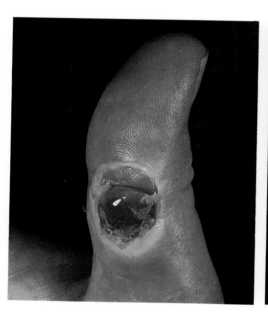

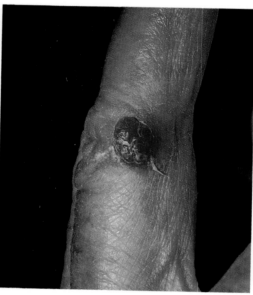

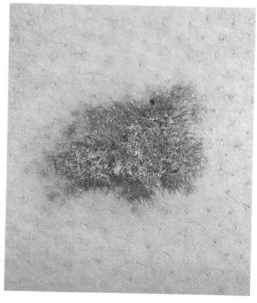

Fig. 6.48 Pyogenic granuloma. A localized red swelling erupts quite rapidly. The tissue is friable and bleeds easily. The finger is a common site. The lesion may arise secondary to injury.

Fig. 6.49 Pyogenic granuloma. This low power view shows the typical scanning appearances of a pyogenic granuloma. The surface is ulcerated and on the far right the epidermal collarette can be seen.

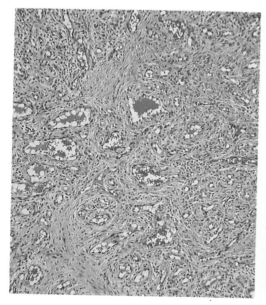

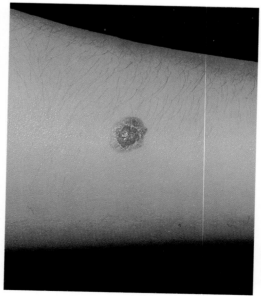

Fig. 6.50 Pyogenic granuloma. Widely dilated blood-filled vascular channels are surrounded by small proliferating capillary buds. Fibrous septae inpart a nodularity to the lesion.

Fig. 6.51 Haemangioma. The red colour suggests the vascular nature of this well-circumscribed benign tumour.

Fig. 6.52 Haemangioma. Haemangiomata are red. This lesion also has a warty surface.

Campbell de Morgan Haemangioma (Senile Haemangioma)

These are very common and are usually multiple on the trunk (Fig. 6.53). They may start to appear quite early in adult life but are particularly common in elderly patients. They appear to have no medical significance. They are small, bright red spots which may be flat or slightly raised.

Histology

The lesion is a simple capillary haemangioma.

Venous Varix

This is a benign blue nodule which is made up of dilated thick-walled blood vessels and is found particularly on the face and lips of the elderly (Fig. 6.54).

Glomus Tumour

This small flesh-coloured or red nodule is usually found on the hands (Fig. 6.55) (particularly beneath the nails), but may occur elsewhere. The tumour is characterized by paroxysmal pain, often without any apparent cause. It is an uncommon benign neoplasm derived from the arteriovenous shunts which occur quite normally in the body, and may occur at any age, including childhood when multiple lesions are sometimes present. The latter is associated with an autosomal dominant mode of inheritance. Leiomyomas of the skin may also be paroxysmally painful and may cause diagnostic confusion. Complete excision is essential, for otherwise recurrence is frequent.

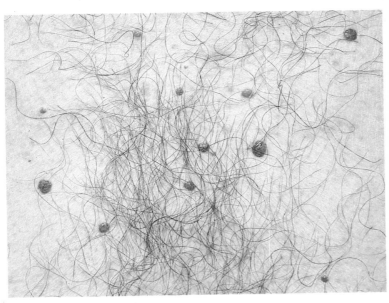

Fig. 6.53   Campbell de Morgan spots. Although often known as senile haemangiomata, these spots may appear quite early in adult life. They are usually multiple and are discrete, red, smooth-surfaced papules. They are of no medical significance.

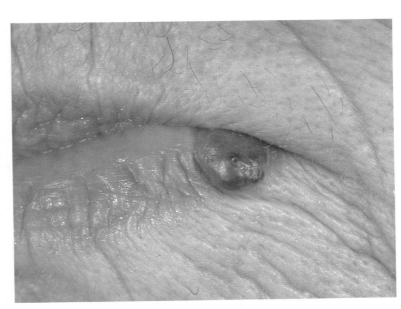

Fig. 6.54   Venous varix. A purple papule is present on the lower lip.

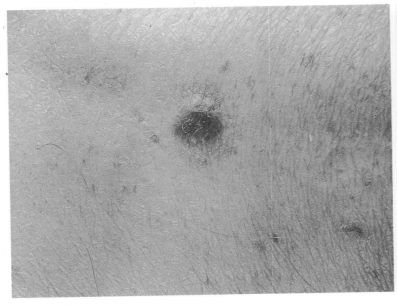

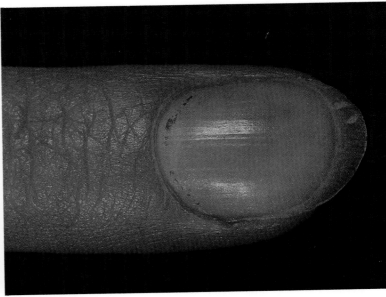

Fig. 6.55   Glomus tumour. The lesion is solitary and rarely greater than a centimetre in diameter. It may be red in colour. Paroxysmal pain is the most suggestive clinical feature of the diagnosis. By courtesy of St. John's Hospital for Diseases of the Skin.

Histology

The glomus tumour is a benign vascular neoplasm arising from the cells of the Sucquet-Hoyer canal – an arteriovenous coiled shunt composed of an arterial and a venous segment united by a vascular channel, the media of which contains cuboidal modified smooth muscle (glomus) cells.

The solitary glomus tumour is composed of dilated blood-filled vascular channels lined in part by endothelial cells but also by cuboidal cells with eosinophilic cytoplasm (glomus cells) (Fig. 6.56). The latter component is often multi-layered. In many areas the wall of the vessel contains large numbers of glomus cells (Fig. 6.57) Glomus tumours are richly innervated. The lesions from patients with multiple glomus tumours are characterized by larger vascular channels with much less conspicuous glomus cells.

SWEAT GLAND TUMOURS
Syringomata

These are multiple, small (1–3 mm diameter), usually flesh-coloured, smooth-surfaced papules that occur on the face particularly around the eyelids (Fig. 6.58), on the chest, neck and axillae. The tumours are of cosmetic importance only.

Histology

The syringoma, a benign tumour of eccrine origin is composed of small, irregular, cleft-like glandular spaces situated within the dermis (Fig. 6.59). The spaces are usually lined by a double layer of epithelium, and tangential cutting gives rise to the characteristic 'tadpole' appearance of this tumour (Fig. 6.60). Knowledge of the existence of this tumour is of importance because occasionally it may be mistaken for a breast duct carcinoma.

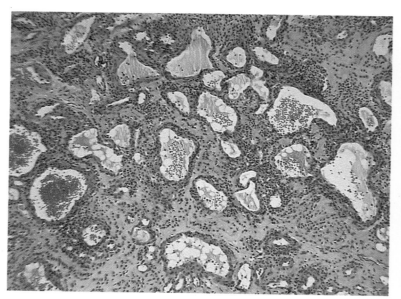

Fig. 6.56 Glomus tumour. Low power view showing dilated vascular channels surrounded by a mantle of small eosinophilic cells.

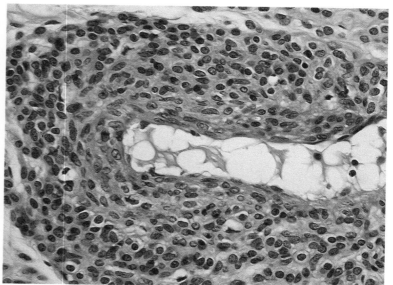

Fig. 6.57 Glomus tumour. The endothelial lined vessel is surrounded by a broad sheath of regular 'glomus' cells with uniform nuclei and indistinct cytoplasmic margins.

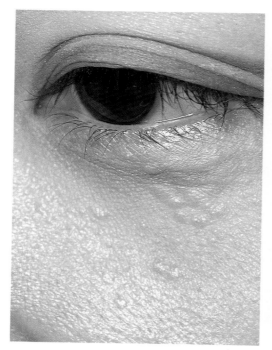

Fig. 6.58 Syringomata. Multiple small, flesh-coloured and smooth-surfaced papules develop, especially around the eyes.

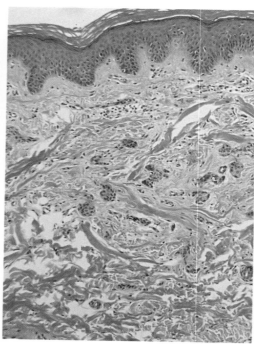

Fig. 6.59 Syringoma. A small number of glandular spaces occupy the mid-dermis.

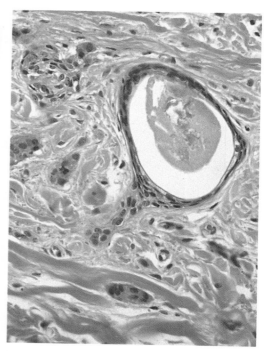

Fig. 6.60 Syringoma. In the right side of the field is a 'tadpole' gland – so typical of syringomata. Elsewhere the epithelial islands are not canalized.

Eccrine Poroma

This occurs as a solitary nodule and may be difficult to diagnose prior to excision, although its favoured site of the palm or sole (Fig. 6.61) may suggest the diagnosis. It is not common.

Histology

The eccrine poroma is a benign tumour which arises from the intra-epidermal component of the sweat duct. It is composed of islands of uniform darkly-staining cuboidal cells (Figs. 6.62 and 6.63) and regularly forms small duct-like structures (Fig. 6.64).

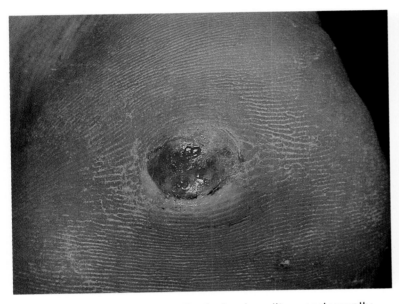

Fig. 6.61 Eccrine poroma. The lesion is solitary and usually occurs in the palm or sole. It may be red in colour and may ulcerate.

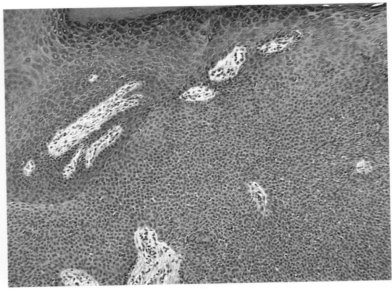

Fig. 6.62 Eccrine poroma. Arising from the squamous epithelium (seen on the left) is a highly cellular tumour. Note the absence of horn cyst formation as would be seen in an acanthotic seborrhoeic wart. The hyperkeratosis of the surface is unremarkable as this lesion arose on the sole of the foot.

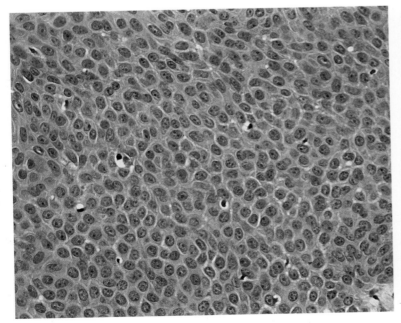

Fig. 6.63 Eccrine poroma. The tumour is composed of very uniform cells with vesicular nuclei and basophilic cytoplasm.

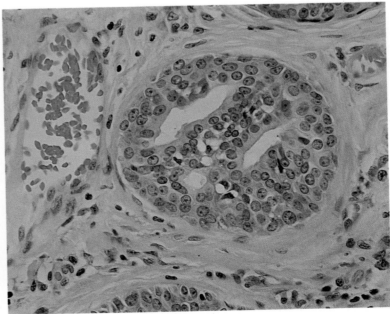

Fig. 6.64 Eccrine poroma. Ducts, as seen in the centre of the field, are characteristic of eccrine poroma. Sometimes a periodic acid Schiff reaction is necessary for their demonstration.

APOCRINE GLAND TUMOURS
Cylindroma

This tumour, which may occur as a solitary nodule of varying size on the scalp or face in adult life, has a smooth surface with noticeable telangiectasia (Fig. 6.65). Multiple lesions may develop on the scalp as a dominantly inherited disorder. In some instances there may be so many lesions that the entire scalp is covered as if by a turban (turban tumours) (Fig. 6.66).

Histology

The cylindroma has a very distinctive histological appearance, being composed of multiple lobules surrounded by an intensely eosinophilic hyaline mantle (Fig. 6.67). Within the lobules are two cell types. Situated predominantly peripherally are palisaded small cells with oval, dark nuclei and negligible cytoplasm (Fig. 6.68). Within the lobule are larger cells with prominent vesicular nuclei and in places associated with hyaline material similar to the mantle. Intra-lobular duct formation may be conspicuous (Fig. 6.69). The cylindroma, a tumour of uncertain histogenesis, is quite benign.

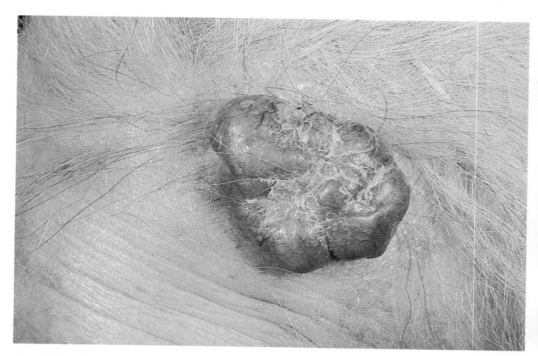

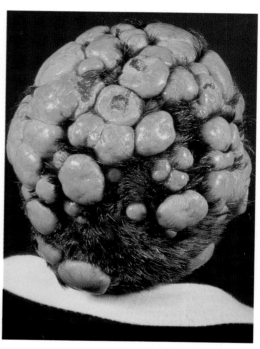

Fig. 6.65 Cylindroma. The scalp is a common site for this benign nodule. It has a smooth surface and telangiectasis may be present.

Fig. 6.66 Turban tumour. Multiple disfiguring lesions occur. These are often inherited as an autosomal dominant. By courtesy of Queen Victoria Hospital, East Grinstead.

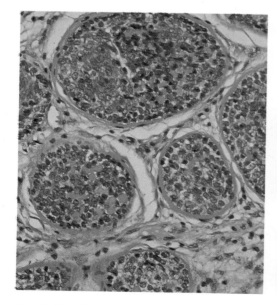

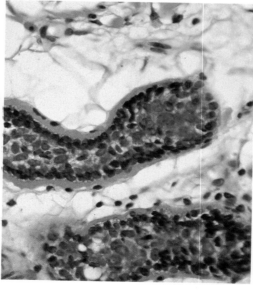

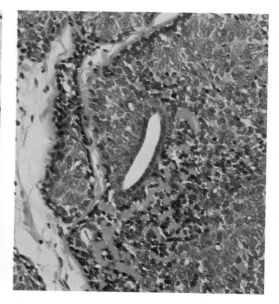

Fig. 6.67 Cylindroma. In this view, cords of small basophilic cells surrounded by a thick eosinophilic hyaline mantle can be seen. Similar material is also present admixed with the tumour cells.

Fig. 6.68 Cylindroma. In this high power view the dual cell population is clearly seen.

Fig. 6.69 Cylindroma. An intralobular duct is seen in the centre of the field.

HAIR FOLLICLE TUMOURS

Trichofolliculoma

This lesion which is not particularly common presents on the face or neck as a small, dome-shaped, flesh-coloured nodule. The diagnosis is not usually made until the lesion is excised but often there is a central pore from which delicate hairs protrude (Fig. 6.70) and this may suggest the diagnosis.

Histology

The trichofolliculoma which may or may not communicate with the surface epidermis consists of a cystic cavity lined by keratinizing stratified squamous epithelium and from which numerous primordial hair follicles arise (Figs. 6.71 and 6.72). Many of these are well-developed and contain a central hair shaft which can be particularly well visualized when the section is viewed with polarized light (Fig. 6.73). The follicles are surrounded, as might be expected, by concentric lamellae of fibrous tissue (perifollicular connective tissue sheaths).

Multiple Trichoepithelioma

This is a dominantly inherited disfiguring condition usually affecting the face (Fig. 6.74) and sometimes neck and upper trunk. It may be associated with cylindromata. Multiple skin-coloured or pink papules and nodules appear after puberty and gradually increase in number and enlarge. Because there may be telangiectasia on the surface of the lesions, they may be mistaken for basal cell epitheliomata.

Histology

The trichoepithelioma is histologically similar to a keratotic basal cell carcinoma. Often distinction depends upon the clinical information. It is composed of islands of small basophilic cells showing peripheral palisading and central, conspicuous keratin cyst formation (Fig. 6.75). Occasionally abortive hair forms are present.

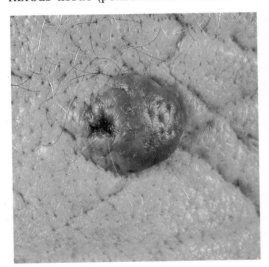

Fig. 6.70 Trichofolliculoma. A dome-shaped nodule is present with a central pore from which hair may protrude. The neck is a common site.

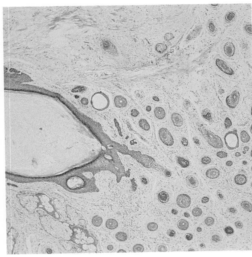

Fig. 6.71 Trichofolliculoma. In this low power view numerous small hair germ structures can be seen adjacent to and arising from a cystically dilated pre-existent follicle.

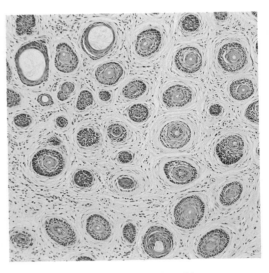

Fig. 6.72 Trichofolliculoma. Numerous immature hair structures are present, each surrounded by a well-developed layer of connective tissue.

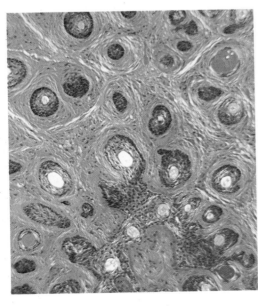

Fig. 6.73 Trichofolliculoma. The presence of hair shafts is highlighted with the use of polarized light.

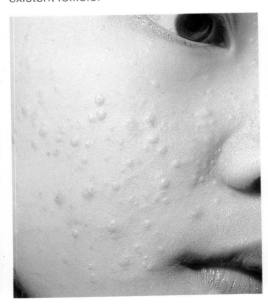

Fig. 6.74 Multiple trichoepithelioma. Multiple disfiguring papules appear on the face after puberty. The condition is dominantly inherited. By courtesy of St. Mary's Hospital.

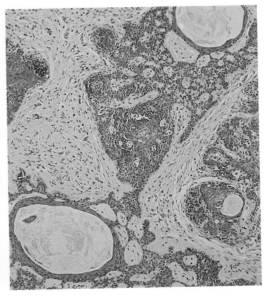

Fig. 6.75 Trichoepithelioma. In this very well-differentiated example, islands of small basaloid cells are present in the lower half of the field. Several abortive follicular structures are present in the upper half of the field.

Calcifying Epithelioma of Malherbe (Pilomatrixoma)

This not uncommon tumour occurs predominantly in children and has a predilection for the face (especially the cheeks), the neck and upper limbs. The lesion is small, solitary and painless. It has a characteristic firm to hard consistency, is often lobulated and may be slightly yellow in colour (Fig. 6.76). It is quite benign but usually requires excision for cosmetic reasons.

Histology

This tumour of follicular origin is siutated within the dermis and may sometimes involve the subcutaneous fat. It has a rather classical appearance, being composed of a dual but inter-related population of cells. In early lesions small, uniform cells consisting of regular, oval basophilic nuclei with scant cytoplasm predominate (Fig. 6.77). While these cells may focally undergo squamous differentiation, more typically they 'mature' into so-called ghost cells. These, which are much more conspicuous in older lesions, consist of eosinophilic sheets in which the faint out-line of pre-existent epithelial cells may be seen (Fig. 6.78). Giant cells are very common in this tumour and are often located about the edges of the islands of ghost cells. Despite the name, calcification is present in only a minority of cases (Fig. 6.79). These tumours are also associated with marked chronic inflammation and scarring.

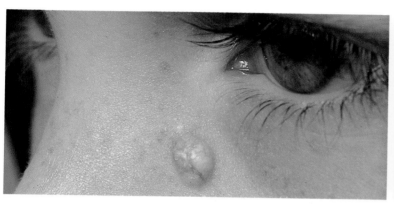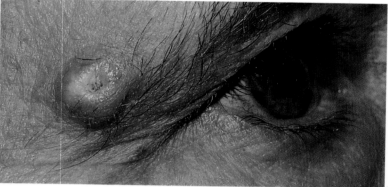

Fig. 6.76 Calcifying epithelioma of Malherbe (pilomatrixoma). The lesion is firm or hard in consistency. It may have a slightly yellow colour. Children are most prone to this lesion.

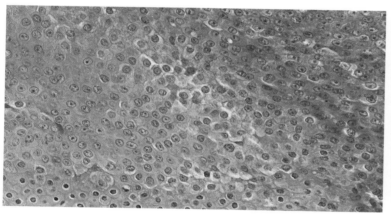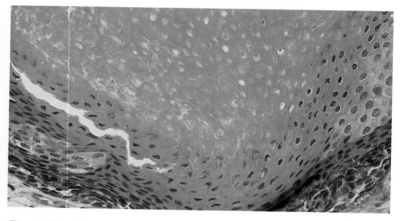

Fig. 6.77 Calcifying epithelioma. Small basaloid cells are present in the lower left of the field. With gradual maturation they appear longer and acquire paler-staining cytoplasm.

Fig. 6.78 Calcifying epithelioma. Abundant 'ghost cells' are present with intensely eosinophilic cytoplasm. Only the shadow cultures of nuclei are visible.

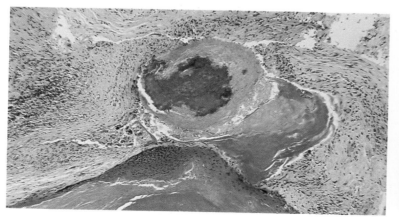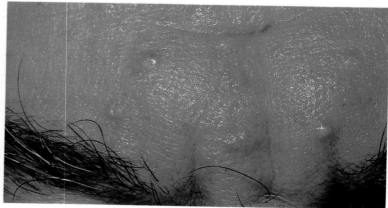

Fig. 6.79 Calcifying epithelioma. Calcification is seen in the lower part of the field, adjacent to the main fusion nodule. Note the scarring and chronic inflammatory changes surrounding the lesion.

Fig. 6.80 Senile sebaceous hyperplasia. Despite its name, this condition may occur quite early in adult life. Multiple lesions may occur. Confusion with a basal cell carcinoma is not uncommon as it occurs on the face.

SEBACEOUS GLAND TUMOURS
Senile Sebaceous Hyperplasia
This is very common and despite its name may occur in early middle-age. It occurs on the face, particularly the forehead and may be solitary or multiple (Fig. 6.80). The lesion is a small yellow papule with a central depression (Fig. 6.81) and is commonly mistaken for a basal cell carcinoma. It is, however, quite benign.

Histology
The papule is composed of a hyperplastic mature sebaceous gland which communicates with the surface by a dilated, debris-containing sebaceous duct (Fig. 6.82).

Steatocystoma Multiplex
This condition presents at puberty or thereafter and has an autosomal dominant mode of inheritance. The lesions are multiple (Fig. 6.83), measure 1–3 centimetres in diameter, have a smooth surface and are slightly yellow in colour. They are most commonly found on the neck, sternum, scrotum (Fig. 6.84) and in the axillae.

Histology
The lesions are variants of dermoid cysts. They are composed of a thin wall of stratified squamous epithelium from which conspicuous sebaceous glands can be seen to arise (Figs. 6.85 and 6.86). More rarely other adnexal structures e.g. hair follicles and glands may be found.

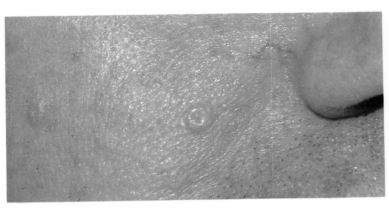

Fig. 6.81   Senile sebaceous hyperplasia. The lesion is a small yellow papule with a central depression.

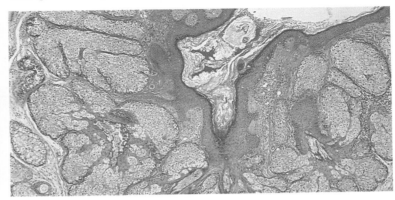

Fig. 6.82   Senile sebaceous hyperplasia. Numerous, mature hyperplastic sebaceous glands are seen.

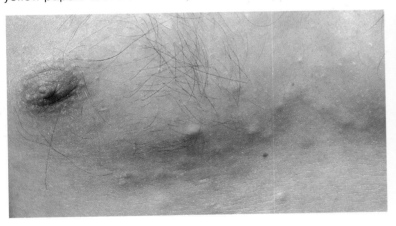

Fig. 6.83   Steatocystoma multiplex. These small cysts are multiple.

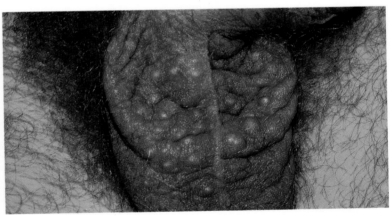

Fig. 6.84   Steatocystoma multiplex. The small intradermal cysts may occur on the scrotum. The condition is usually inherited as an autosomal dominant.

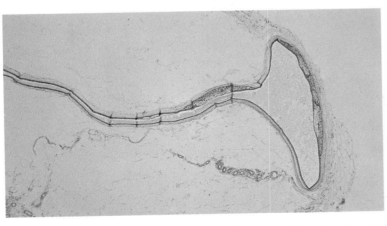

Fig. 6.85   Steatocystoma multiplex. Low power view showing the irregularity of the cyst.

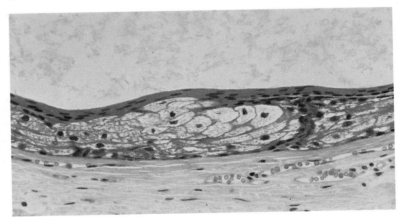

Fig. 6.86   Steatocystoma multiplex. Mature sebaceous cells are present in close apposition to the attenuated squamous epithelium.

SMOOTH MUSCLE TUMOURS
Leiomyoma

This is a benign tumour derived from the smooth muscle associated with hair follicles, the genitalia, nipples and blood vessels. The former often results in multiple nodules (Fig. 6.87) which are red, pink or brown in colour, less than 1.5 centimetres in size and subject to episodic pain especially precipitated by touch or low temperature. Some lesions may contract. Frequently this variant is familial. The other forms are solitary. The genital or nipple nodules are usually asymptomatic. Those associated with blood vessels are usually painful and most often are found on a limb.

Histology

Leiomyomas are composed of inter-lacing fascicles of smooth muscle cells characterized by their elongated, blunt-ended nuclei and abundant eosinophillic cytoplasm (Figs. 6.88 and 6.89).

Ganglion

This is a chronic painless cystic swelling which usually occurs over the dorsum of the wrist (Fig. 6.90) or ankle. It contains fluid which probably results from leakage of synovia through the sheath of tendon or capsule of a joint. The fluid becomes encapsulated by fibrous tissue and a cyst results.

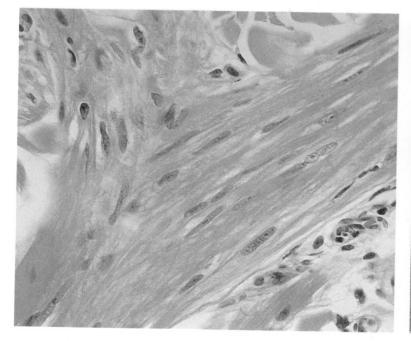

Fig. 6.87 Leiomyomata. Multiple lesions may occur in an individual. By courtesy of Dr. A.C. Pembroke.

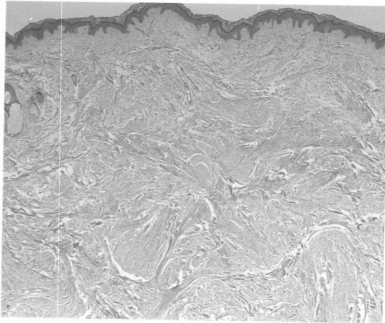

Fig. 6.88 Leiomyoma. Scanning view showing complete replacement of the dermis by broad, interlacing fascicles of eosinophilic spindle cells.

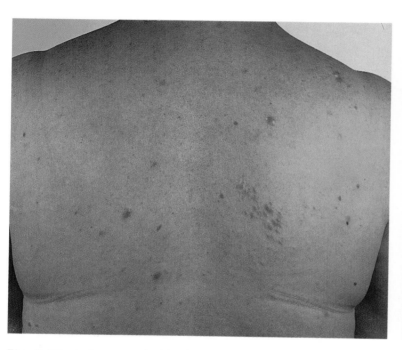

Fig. 6.89 Leiomyoma. The smooth muscle cells are elongated and characteristically have 'cigar'-shaped, blunt-ended nuclei.

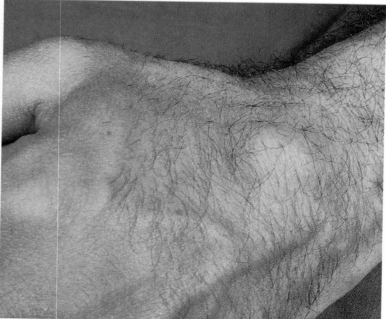

Fig. 6.90 Ganglion. A flesh-coloured swelling is present over the dorsum of the wrist. By courtesy of St. Mary's Hospital.

SALIVARY GLAND TUMOURS
Mucous Retention Cyst
This very common lesion is soft, fluctuant, spherical and sometimes red or blue in colour (Fig. 6.91). It is usually about 1 cm in size and occurs only on the lower lip.

NERVOUS TISSUE TUMOURS
Neurofibroma
Most commonly neurofibromata occur as part of von Recklinghausen's disease (qv) (Fig. 6.92) but occasionally solitary lesions occur (Fig. 6.93). These nodules are flesh-coloured, soft or firm, vary greatly in size and occur anywhere on the integument.

Histology
The neurofibroma (whether solitary or associated with von Recklinghausen's disease) is a discrete but unencapsulated tumour. It is composed of interlacing fascicles of Schwann cells, having irregular, wavy, elongated nuclei. Variable amounts of collagen and mucopolysaccharides are also present. A careful search of the tumour should reveal small nerve fibres coursing through its substance (Fig. 6.94).

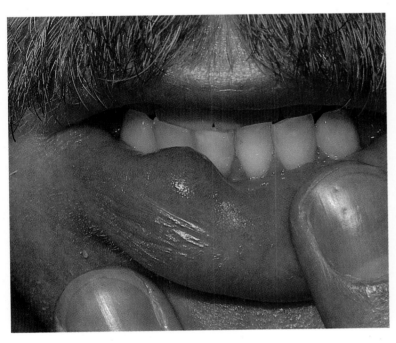

Fig. 6.91 Mucous retention cyst (mucocoele). This soft fluctuant spherical lesion occurs on the lower lip.

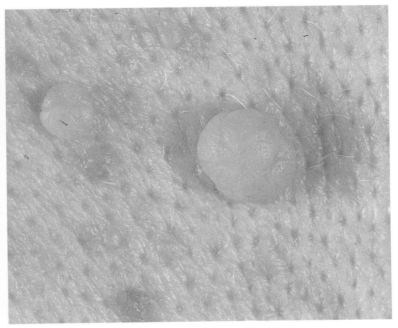

Fig. 6.92 Neurofibroma. The nodule is flesh-coloured and may be either soft or firm. A characteristic finding is that it can be invaginated with the tip of a finger.

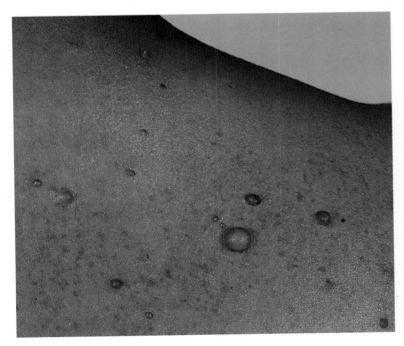

Fig 6.93 Neurofibromatosis. Neurofibroma may be multiple and vary greatly in size. They occur in von Recklinghausen's disease, in association with café au lait patches.

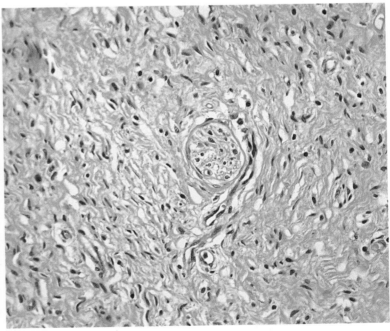

Fig. 6.94 Neurofibroma. A small nerve present in the centre of the field is surrounded by eosinophilic fibrillary connective tissue containing slender, wavy, spindle-shaped nuclei.

HISTIOCYTIC TUMOURS

Juvenile Xanthogranuloma (Naevoxanthoendothelioma)

This is an uncommon but easily recognized tumour of infancy. It presents as an orange or yellow nodule characteristically found on the face, scalp, trunk or limbs (Fig. 6.95). The tumour, which may be single or multiple, ultimately resolves. Presentation occurs before six months of age and most tumours achieve their full size by 18 months. Involution over the next year or two is usual. The lesion is quite benign and the child is otherwise perfectly healthy. Occasionally xanthogranulomata are found in association with von Recklinghausen's disease or histiocytosis X. The prognosis is then related to the associated lesion.

Histology

The juvenile xanthogranuloma consists of an irregular heterogeneous collection of inflammatory cells including lipid-laden histiocytes, eosinophils and giant cells (Fig. 6.96). Large numbers of Touton-type giant cells are characteristic (Fig. 6.97).

MISCELLANEOUS TUMOURS

Senile Comedo

This is a common consequence of chronic solar damage to the Caucasian skin (Fig. 6.98). The lesions are often multiple and are seen particularly on the face. They are colloquially known as blackheads.

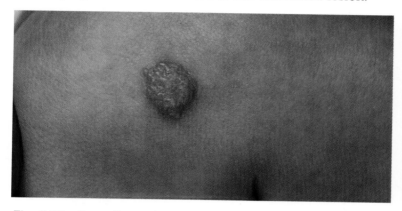

Fig. 6.95 Juvenile xanthogranuloma (Naevoxanthoendothelioma). The lesions may be solitary or multiple. They often have a yellow colour. They normally develop before the age of six months and subsequently involute spontaneously.

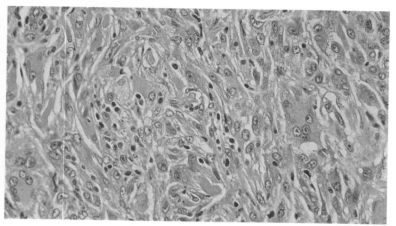

Fig. 6.96 Juvenile xanthogranuloma. This high power view shows a mixture of lymphocytes, xanthoma and giant cells.

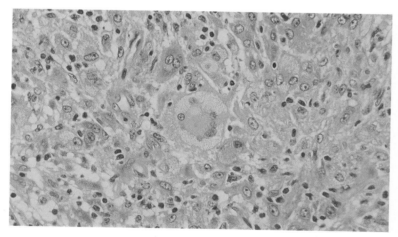

Fig. 6.97 Juvenile xanthogranuloma. In the centre is a typical Touton giant cell.

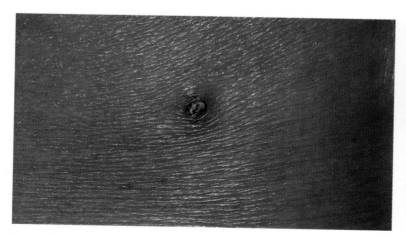

Fig. 6.98 Senile comedo. The lesion has a central keratinous core.

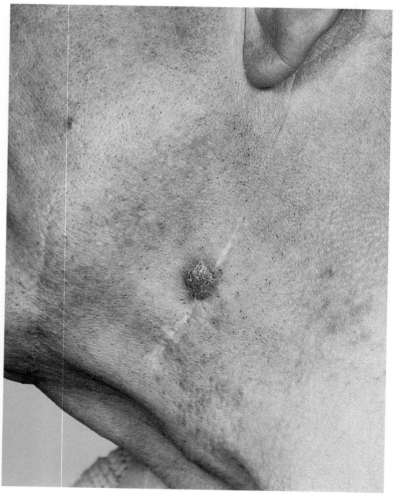

Fig. 6.99 Stitch abscess. The presence of a lesion which fails to heal within a scar should suggest the diagnosis.

Stitch Abscess

This iatrogenic lesion should not be difficult to recognize. The history of an operation and the presence of remnants of the suture material should make the diagnosis obvious (Fig. 6.99).

Histology

All suture material results in an intense inflammatory (granulomatous) reaction. Catgut is usually completely disposed of by the host, in contrast to silk or linen which, if not removed, will give rise to a persistent stitch granuloma/abscess. Histologically the lesion is easily diagnosed, consisting of suture fibres surrounded by numerous foreign body giant cells (Figs. 6.100 and 6.101).

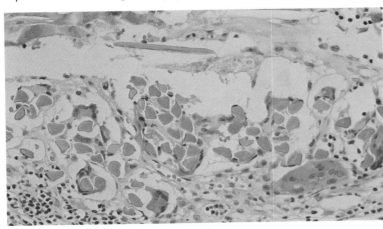

Fig. 6.100 Stitch abscess. Variably orientated suture particles are surrounded by foreign body giant cells.

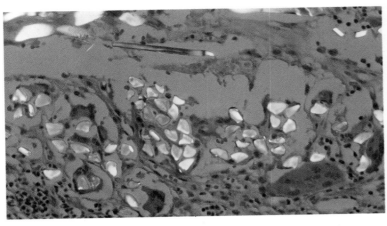

Fig. 6.101 Stitch abscess. The suture material shows positive birefringence when viewed under polarized light.

Accessory Nipple

This is occasionally mistaken for a pigmented naevus, but the appearance is that of a small nipple (Fig. 6.102). Multiple nipples may also be present. They occur along the course of embryological milk lines, that is from the anterior axillary fold to the inner thigh.

Histology

The accessory nipple typically has a rather papillomatous surface epithelium. The dermis contains lactiferous ducts and erectile smooth muscle bundles. In the deeper aspect secretory lobules may be identified (Figs. 6.103 and 6.104).

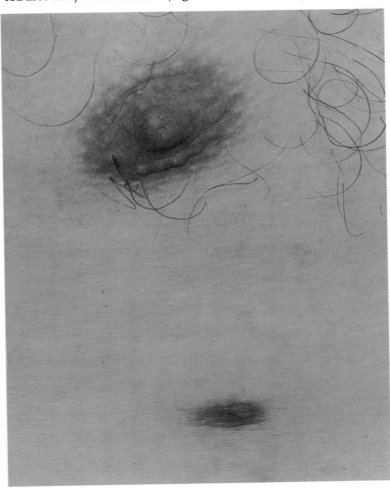

Fig. 6.102 Accessory nipple. In most cases the appearance is that of a very small nipple. They may be bilateral and multiple, occurring along the course of embryological milk lines.

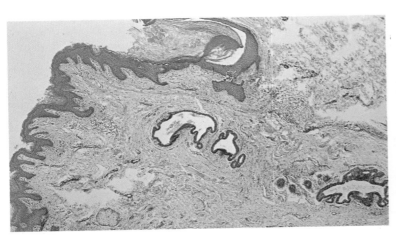

Fig. 6.103 Accessory nipple. The edge of an accessory nipple is shown with normal skin on the right. Several sections through a dilated lactiferous duct are visible.

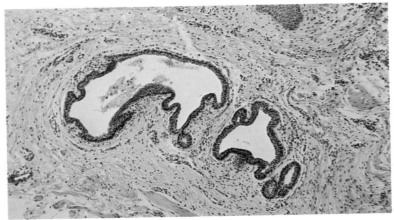

Fig. 6.104 Accessory nipple. A high power view of a lactiferous duct. Note the bundles of smooth muscle present in the lower field.

6.23

Subungual Exostosis (Osteochondroma)

This lesion is normally mistaken for a wart for it occurs most frequently below the toenail, particularly the big toenail (Fig. 6.105). It is an outgrowth of normal bone and the diagnosis can be confirmed by X-ray (Fig. 6.106).

Histology

The osteochondroma (cartilaginous exostosis) is the most common benign tumour of bone, although presentation as a subungual mass is very rare. The lesion, derived from ectopic epiphyseal cartilage, consists of a cartilagenous cap overlying bony trabeculae and accompanying marrow. Chondrosarcoma is a rare complication.

Dental Sinus

A chronic periapical dental abscess may eventually perforate bone and form a sinus which discharges either into the mouth or into the skin. The latter are found on the cheek, chin or just below the angle of the jaw (Fig. 6.107). An X-ray will confirm the diagnosis (Fig. 6.108). The offending tooth should be extracted.

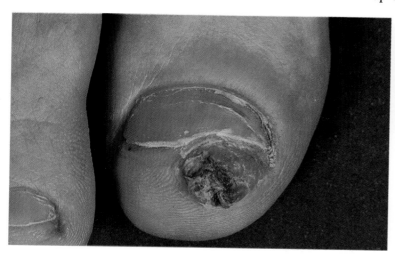

Fig. 6.105 Subungual exostosis. The lesion characteristically occurs on the big toenail. It is often mistaken for a wart.

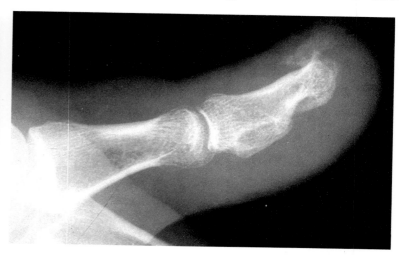

Fig. 6.106 Subungual exostosis. Calcification under the nail is seen on X-ray of the patient in Fig. 6.105.

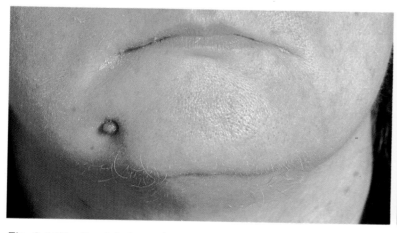

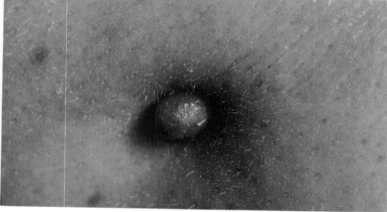

Fig. 6.107 Dental sinus. A chronic periapical abscess may perforate bone and form a sinus which discharges into the mouth or skin. The jaw is a common site.

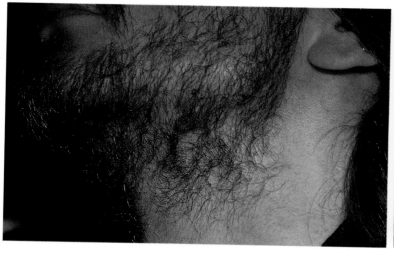

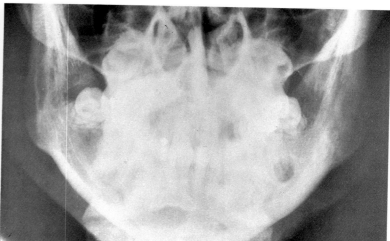

Fig. 6.108 Dental sinus. Here, the sinus has discharged under the jaw into the patient's beard. The X-ray reveals a translucency in the left mandible.

7 Malignant Tumours of the Skin

Anthony du Vivier MD, FRCP

Phillip H. McKee MB BCh, BaO, MRC Path

The great majority of primary malignant tumours of the skin are caused by excessive exposure to ultra-violet light. While the most susceptible individual is the ginger-haired, blue-eyed and fair-skinned Celt or Anglo-Saxon, some people with dark hair, brown eyes and olive skin tend to burn readily in the sun and are therefore also at risk. It would seem that a tendency to sunburn is probably of greater importance than skin and hair colouring in determining the risk factor. The various clinical sub-types of skin are summarized in Fig. 7.1.

Certain cutaneous neoplasms, particularly solar (senile) keratoses, are directly related to the duration of sun-exposure. Thus, solar keratoses may develop in the third decade in Anglo-Saxons living in sunny climates such as California, whereas in Great Britain where both the intensity and duration of sunlight is much less, such lesions tend to develop at a much greater age.

Malignant melanoma, in contradistinction, appears to be associated with the intensity rather than the duration of exposure and tends to be observed more often in white-collar office workers who holiday in the sun rather than in outdoor workers who suffer from chronic sun exposure.

Sunburn, which is caused by UVB (290–320nm), results in painful erythema (Fig. 7.2), oedema (Fig. 7.3) and sometimes blistering. Desquamation or peeling follows. UVA or long wave ultra-violet light (320–400nm) as delivered by so-called sunbeds results in tanning without sunburn and its role as a carcinogen is much less well-defined.

Freckles develop after sunburn. They are found predominantly on the face in childhood and increase in summer but disappear during the winter. A *freckle* (Fig. 7.4) is caused by an increase in melanin synthesis in the absence of melanocytic proliferation. Although often regarded as a sign of health, freckles are actually one of the earliest indications of sun damage. A further complication of excessive sun exposure is the development of fixed pigmentary lesions known as lentigines. A *lentigo* (Fig. 7.5) is a benign proliferation of melanocytes in which there is no evidence of junctional activity (Fig. 7.6) in contrast to that seen in a melanocytic naevus (c.f. Fig. 5.28). Several or many lesions are present, usually on those areas of skin which have been chronically exposed to sunlight (Fig. 7.7). A lentigo is an even-coloured macule varying from light tan to dark brown in appearance. It may be quite flat or just slightly raised with a matt surface and sometimes its distinction from an early seborrhoeic wart is impossible. All these changes are seen in an accelerated form in xeroderma pigmentosum (Fig. 7.8) where there is an enzymatic failure to repair ultra-violet light-damaged epidermal DNA.

Chronic solar exposure results in damage to the elastic fibres in the dermis (solar elastosis, Fig. 7.9), producing a yellow and wrinkled appearance (Fig. 7.10). On the face, comedones and milia may also be present (Fig. 7.11). *Cutis rhomboidalis nuchae*, an exaggerated form of solar elastosis, where the skin is thrown into coarse folds (Fig. 7.12) is seen particularly on the sides and

The clinical sub-types of skin
Type 1 Always burns, never tans.
Type 2 Always burns, sometimes tans.
Type 3 Sometimes burns, always tans.
Type 4 Never burns, always tans.
Type 5 Negro skin.

Fig. 7.1 The clinical sub-types of skin.

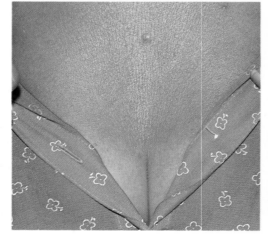

Fig. 7.2 Sunburn. This is ultimately responsible for premature ageing of the skin and the majority of cutaneous malignancies. Proper use of sunscreens should make it easily avoidable.

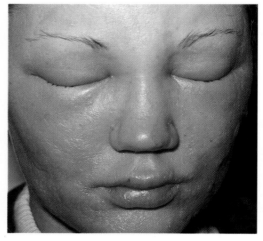

Fig. 7.3 Sunburn. Erythema and oedema are the acute changes caused by ultra-violet irradiation of the skin. This patient had exposed herself to a UVB lamp for several minutes.

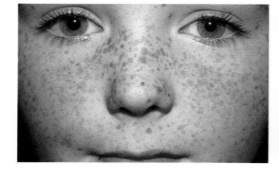

Fig. 7.4 Freckles (ephelides). These appear in the summer and fade in the winter. They indicate that damage is occurring in the skin.

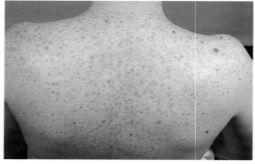

Fig. 7.5 Lentigines. These are permanent pigmentary changes in the skin. They represent a later stage of sun damage. This 27-year-old man also had a malignant melanoma on his chest.

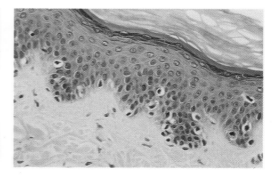

Fig. 7.6 Lentigo simplex. There is hyperkeratosis. The epidermis shows slight elongation of the ridges and increased numbers of basally located melanocytes are present. Note the absence of any junctional activity.

back of the neck (Fig. 7.13). On the dorsal aspects of the hands and forearms the skin loses its elasticity and becomes dry, wrinkled and atrophic. The blood vessels are prominent and vulnerable and purpura result from the least trauma (Fig. 7.14).

Many patients fail to equate ordinary sun exposure with ageing of the skin or cancer (Fig. 7.15), believing that sunbathing is necessary, not appreciating that the sun bathes their skin in such seemingly otherwise innocent pursuits as golfing or gardening. They attribute their cutaneous changes to ageing rather than to the effects of sunlight. However, a comparison of the extensor (exposed) with the flexor (shielded) aspects of the forearm will yield profoundly different cutaneous appearances.

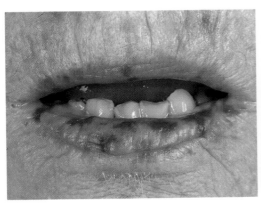

Fig. 7.7   Lentigines. These are not due to ageing, contrary to popular opinion, but to excess solar exposure.

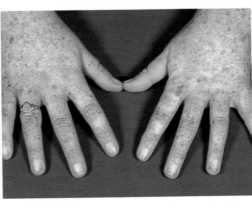

Fig. 7.8   Lentingines. This is the skin of a 12-year-old with xeroderma pigmentosum, a disorder of extreme photosensitivity. The lentigines appear very early in life.

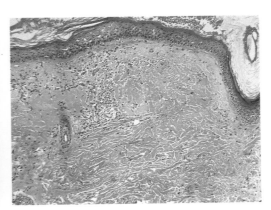

Fig. 7.9   Solar elastosis. Deep to a solar keratosis, the upper reticular dermis shows a diffuse homogenization of its connective tissue components. A focal chronic inflammatory infiltrate is also seen.

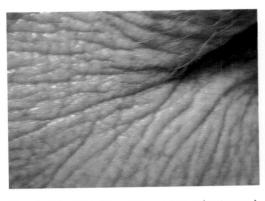

Fig. 7.10   Wrinkles. These are a feature of solar damage. This 40-year-old man was an ardent skier.

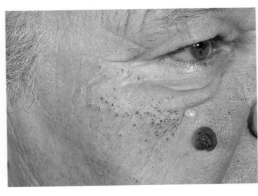

Fig. 7.11   Solar elastosis. Multiple comedones (blackheads) are features of chronic sun damage. This patient also has a seborrhoeic wart.

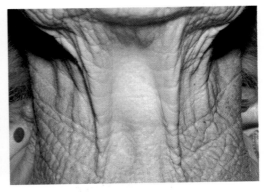

Fig. 7.12   Solar elastosis. Yellowing and furrowing of the skin result from chronic solar exposure. The area under the chin which is protected from the light is undamaged.

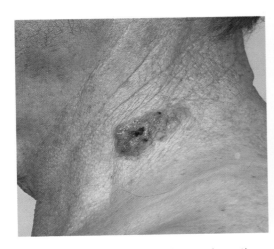

Fig. 7.13   Basal cell carcinoma in cutis rhomboidalis nuchae. A large cystic basal cell carcinoma is present in an area of chronic sun damage.

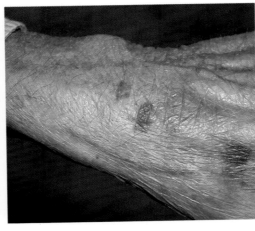

Fig. 7.14   Solar purpura. Chronic solar damage results in atrophy and purpura of the skin, especially on the backs of the hands and forearms.

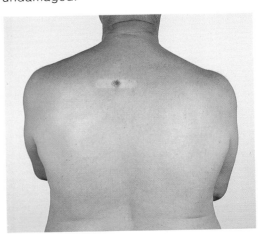

Fig. 7.15   Sunburn and a basal cell carcinoma. Many patients fail to appreciate the hazards of ultra-violet irradiation. In this case the basal cell carcinoma has been protected by a plaster and the rest of the skin has been exposed and burnt.

SOLAR KERATOSIS

A solar (senile) keratosis is a well-defined, raised, red papule (Fig. 7.16) or plaque (Fig. 7.17) with a roughened surface. The surface scale which varies in colour from yellow to brown may be removed to leave a raw, bleeding surface. Lesions may be single or multiple (Fig. 7.18) and are most commonly located on light-exposed surfaces such as the face or dorsal aspects of the hands (Fig. 7.19) and forearms but will obviously occur on any area of skin which has received excessive ultra-violet irradiation. Thus, a bald scalp (Fig. 7.20) is especially vulnerable. Solar keratoses are potentially malignant, in that very occasionally invasive squamous carcinoma may develop after a number of years (Fig. 7.21) although metastases are rare.

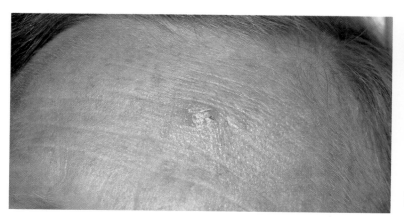

Fig. 7.16   Solar keratosis. The lesion is a well-defined, raised, red papule with a rough surface.

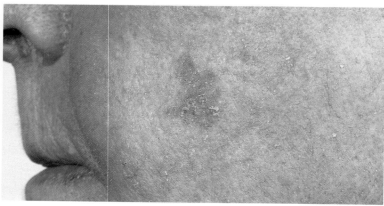

Fig. 7.17   Solar keratosis. A red, raised plaque with an adherent scale is present.

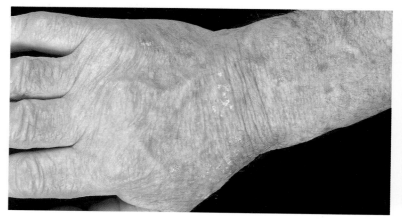

Fig. 7.18   Solar keratosis. Multiple lesions are common.

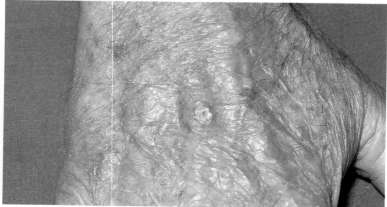

Fig. 7.19   Solar keratosis. The lesions commonly appear on the backs of the hands and forearms.

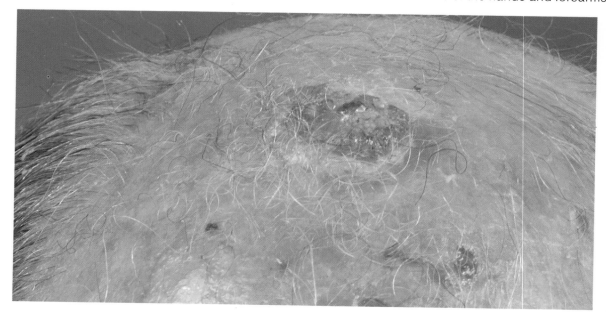

Fig. 7.20   Solar keratoses and squamous cell carcinoma. The scalp receives maximal solar irradiation but the hair provides protection. The bald scalp is, however, very vulnerable.

Applications of liquid nitrogen are commonly employed to treat solar keratoses, with excellent results. Curettage and cautery may also be used. 5-fluorouracil (Efudix), a cytostatic drug, is a useful topical therapy (Fig. 7.22) for multiple lesions, particularly on the face. It is less effective for keratoses on the backs of the hands and forearms, possibly because penetration is not as effective as it is on the face. It has, however, been used successfully in combination with retinoic acid. The application of 5-fluorouracil results in an intense inflammatory reaction (Fig. 7.23) and therefore requires experience in its use and careful explanation of its effects to the patient. Its major advantage is that it appears to select out early cutaneous lesions which may be difficult to discern macroscopically (Fig. 7.24).

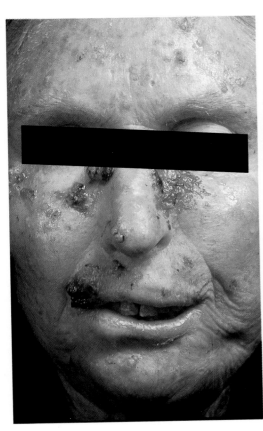

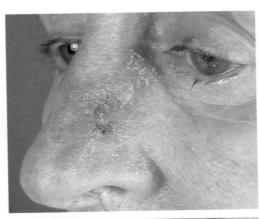

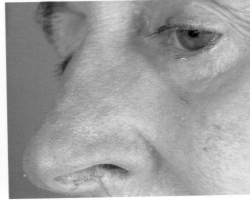

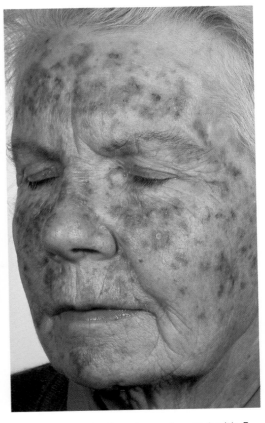

Fig. 7.21 Squamous cell carcinomata. Multiple squamous cell carcinomata arising from chronically solar-damaged skin and solar keratoses. By courtesy of St. John's Hospital for Diseases of the Skin.

Fig. 7.22 Solar keratosis treated with 5-fluorouracil cream. This plaque of solar keratosis was treated effectively. By courtesy of St. Mary's Hospital.

Fig. 7.23 Solar keratoses treated with 5-fluorouracil cream. 5-fluorouracil cream produces an intense inflammatory reaction of the skin so that its use should be restricted to an experienced physician. Excellent clinical results may be obtained.

Fig. 7.24 5-fluorouracil reaction. The drug appears to select out early abnormalities of the skin before they may be macroscopically obvious. As a result, the solar keratoses and surrounding skin react. By courtesy of St. John's Hospital for Diseases of the Skin.

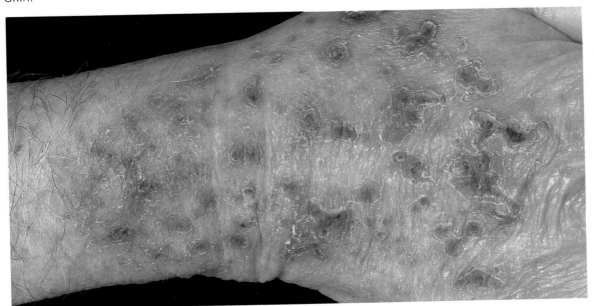

Histology

Solar keratoses are premalignant lesions which are characterized by variable degrees of dysplasia, ranging from mild changes through to carcinomata *in situ*. Obviously, examples of the latter should be carefully scrutinized for evidence of invasive tumour. A number of patterns of solar keratoses are recognized.

The most frequent type of solar keratosis is composed of variably acanthotic squamous epithelium covered by a thickened scale of alternating parakeratotic and hyperkeratotic horn (the former overlies the dysplastic epidermis and the latter is related to uninvolved intra-epidermal adnexal structures) (Fig. 7.25). The epidermis frequently buds down into the underlying dermis. Epithelial dysplasia is constant and manifests as loss of maturation, abnormalities of cellular polarity, nuclear and cytoplasmic pleomorphism, individual cell keratinization and abnormally located (and often abnormally structured) mitotic figures (Fig. 7.26). In contrast to Bowen's disease, the dysplasia tends not to involve the intra-epidermal components of the adnexal structures but may surround the latter giving a 'mantle-like' effect. Elastosis is a frequent manifestation in all solar keratoses.

The atrophic variant is characterized by hyperkeratosis and parakeratosis overlying a thinned epidermis showing pre-dominantly basal and suprabasal epithelial dysplasia (Fig. 7.27). Bowenoid solar keratoses show full thickness dysplasia and are histologically indistinguishable from Bowen's disease (Fig. 7.28). The acantholytic solar keratosis, in addition to epithelial dysplasia, is typified by suprabasal cleft formation due to tumour acantholysis (Figs. 7.29 and 7.30). In such instances it is important not to confuse the lesion with any of the acantholytic bullous dermatoses.

ACTINIC CHEILITIS

The lips, particularly the lower (Fig. 7.31), are vulnerable to the effects of chronic solar irradiation. Well-defined white patches, so-called leukoplakia, may develop (Fig. 7.32). Actinic cheilitis is of special importance because it may be complicated by an aggressive squamous cell carcinoma with significant metastatic potential. Prophylactic excision is therefore advisable.

Histology

The features of actinic cheilitis range from epidermal dysplasia to carcinoma *in situ* and not infrequently invasive squamous cell carcinoma (Fig. 7.33). At this site, it is particularly important to assess the surgical limits of excision, and the use of frozen section techniques to examine the latter is to be encouraged.

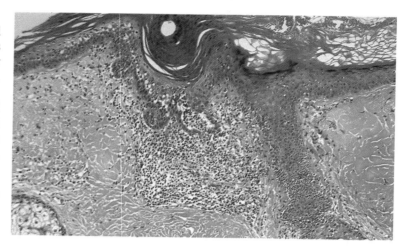

Fig. 7.25 Solar keratosis. Conspicuous parakeratosis overlies the dysplastic epithelium. In contrast, the stratum corneum related to the pilosebaceous follicle (right) is ortho-hyperkeratotic and associated with prominence of the granular cell layer. Acantholysis has resulted in the suprabasal cleft formation seen in the middle of the picture. Note the lichenoid distribution of the accompanying chronic inflammatory cell infiltrate.

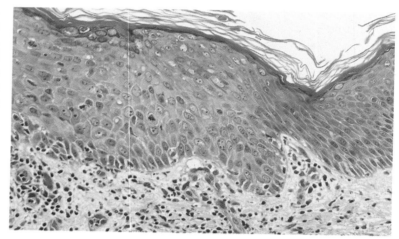

Fig. 7.26 Solar keratosis. Compare the normal epithelium on the right with the abnormal on the left. The latter shows severe dysplasia with lack of epidermal maturation, nuclear pleomorphism and increased numbers of abnormally located mitotic figures. In the superficial dermis there is a fairly heavy chronic inflammatory cell infiltrate surrounding the conspicuous vasculature.

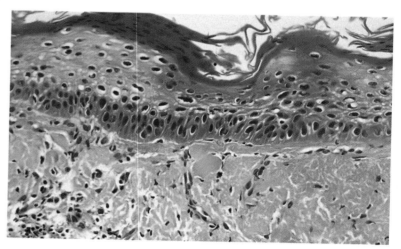

Fig. 7.27 Atrophic solar keratosis. There is focal parakeratosis. Basal and suprabasal dysplasia is manifest as nuclear enlargement, hyperchromatism and slight irregularity in shape and orientation. Note the conspicuous underlying solar elastosis.

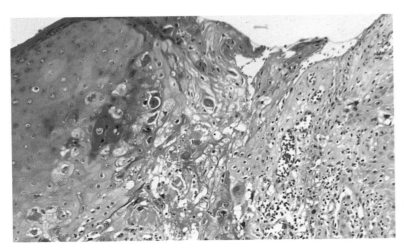

Fig. 7.28   Bowenoid solar keratosis. The epithelium is extremely dysplastic. Scattered, individually keratinized cells are present.

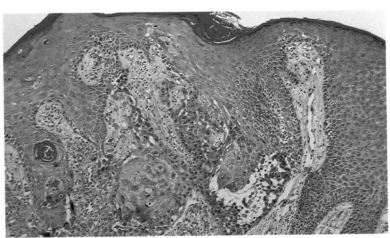

Fig. 7.29   Acantholytic solar keratosis. This example, which is also markedly dysplastic, shows conspicuous acantholysis with vesicle formation seen below and to the right of centre.

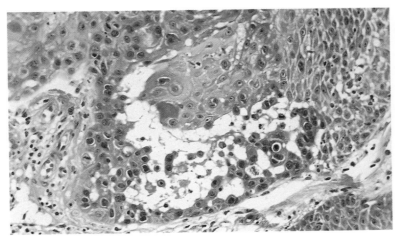

Fig. 7.30   Acantholytic solar keratosis. Note the hyperchromasia and nuclear pleomorphism of the basally located keratinocytes. A degenerate mitotic figure is seen below and to the right of centre.

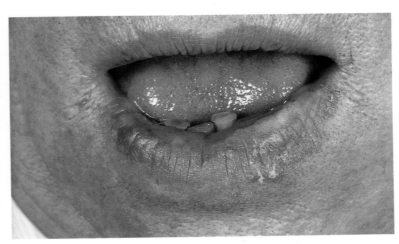

Fig. 7.31   Actinic cheilitis. The lower lips are vulnerable to solar irradiation. Well-defined premalignant white patches may result.

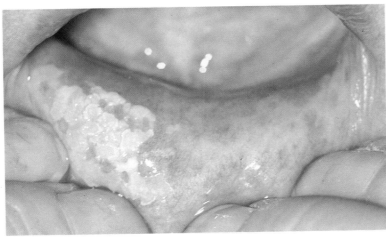

Fig. 7.32   Actinic cheilitis. White patches (so-called leukoplakia) may result from chronic solar exposure. Prophylactic excision is indicated. By courtesy of St. Mary's Hospital.

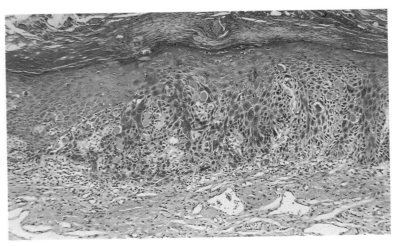

Fig. 7.33   Actinic cheilitis. There is marked hyperkeratosis and parakeratosis. Beneath the latter, the epithelium shows marked dysplasia with irregular stranding into the lamina propria. The features are those of early invasive squamous cell carcinoma.

7.7

CUTANEOUS HORN

This is a clinical descriptive term indicating marked keratin cohesion but without identifying its cause (Fig. 7.34). Lesions which may be complicated by keratin horn formation include seborrhoeic warts, solar keratoses, viral warts, basal cell carcinomata and squamous cell carcinomata. Excision and histological examination is the management of choice.

DISSEMINATED SUPERFICIAL ACTINIC POROKERATOSIS

This is a benign condition which presents predominantly on the legs of people who have had excessive exposure to sunlight (Fig. 7.35). Although not premalignant, it is discussed in this chapter because it may easily be mistaken for a solar keratosis, although it does have a characteristic clinical appearance. A typical lesion measures a few millimetres in diameter and has a very well-defined, slightly raised keratotic margin with a some-what atrophic red centre. Multiple lesions are usually present. No particularly effective treatment is as yet available.

Histology

Fundamental to the process of porokeratosis is the formation of the cornoid lamella. This consists of an angulated tier of keratin which is orientated at an obtuse angle to the epidermis. At its lower border the epithelium is vacuolated, while at its edges there is a well-formed granular cell layer (Fig. 7.36). Towards the centre of the lesion the epithelium is often atrophic.

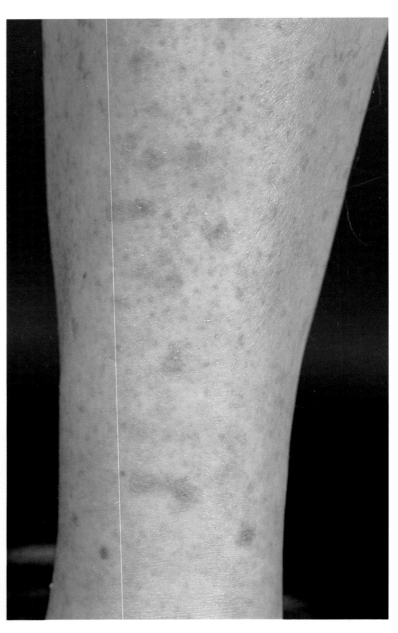

Fig. 7.35 Disseminated actinic porokeratosis. Multiple lesions occur on the legs. They have a well-defined, slightly raised, keratotic margin with an atrophic red centre. By courtesy of St. Mary's Hospital.

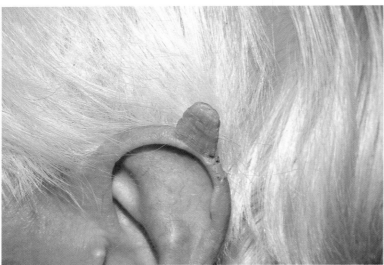

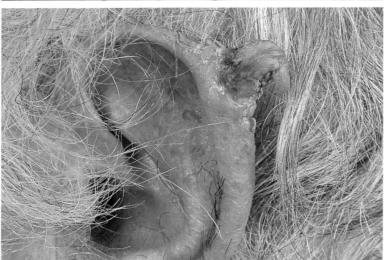

Fig. 7.34 Cutaneous horn. The keratin is unusually adhesive and a horn results. The underlying lesion may be a seborrhoeic wart (upper), solar keratosis or even squamous cell carcinoma (lower). By courtesy of St. Mary's Hospital.

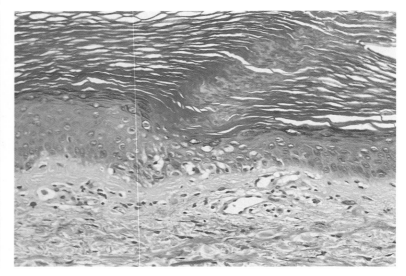

Fig. 7.36 Disseminated superficial actinic porokeratosis. Typical lesion showing cornoid lamella, absence of granular cell layer and conspicuous cytoplasmic vacuolation of the base of the tier. By courtesy of Dr. Neil Smith, Institute of Dermatology.

BOWEN'S DISEASE (Intra-epidermal Carcinoma)
Intra-epidermal Carcinoma of the Skin

This lesion which is usually solitary (Fig. 7.37) may appear anywhere on the integument, but occurs predominantly on the legs (Fig. 7.38), backs of the hands (Fig. 7.39) or fingers (Fig. 7.40) and face. The lesion is a well-defined, slightly raised red plaque with an adherent scale (Fig. 7.41) and may be misdiagnosed as eczema or psoriasis. However, solitary eczema or psoriasis is unusual and therefore a biopsy is wise.

Although the great majority of cases of Bowen's disease are due to excessive exposure to ultra-violet radiation, some cases, especially if lesions are multiple, are due to arsenical ingestion. Arsenic is used industrially and has been used therapeutically for a variety of disorders including psoriasis, epilepsy and syphilis and has been incorporated into many tonics and homeopathic preparations. The latent period between the time of ingestion of arsenic and the development of the cutaneous changes is lengthy, so that many patients will not be aware of, or will have forgotten, their exposure, particularly those who have been given tonics in childhood. Since arsenic may also be related to the development of internal malignancies, the latter should be excluded in any patient with arsenic-associated Bowen's disease. Although potentially malignant, invasive squamous cell carcinoma is an infrequent consequence of cutaneous Bowen's disease and usually takes many years to develop.

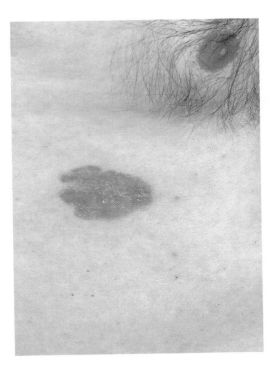

Fig. 7.37 Intra-epidermal carcinoma of the skin (Bowen's disease). The lesion is usually solitary. Although often mis-diagnosed as eczema or psoriasis, such lesions should be biopsied. By courtesy of St. Mary's Hospital.

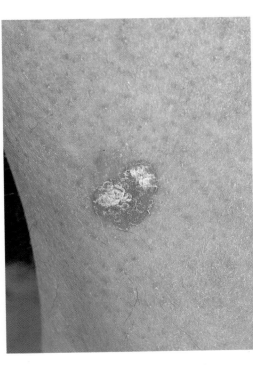

Fig. 7.38 Bowen's disease. A solitary patch on the lower leg, which may simulate psoriasis, is a common presentation.

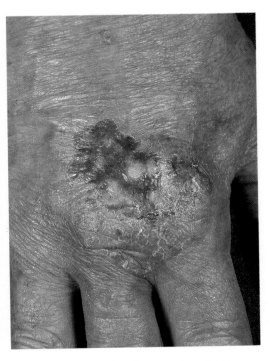

Fig. 7.39 Bowen's disease. A solitary, well-defined, slightly raised plaque with a raw surface and adherent scale is present. This lesion was mistaken for eczema. Biopsy is mandatory.

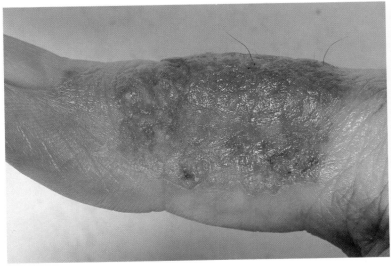

Fig. 7.40 Bowen's disease. The dorsum of a finger is a common site. The lesion has a very well-defined margin.

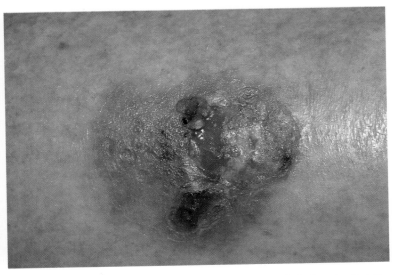

Fig. 7.41 Bowen's disease. The lesion is a well-defined, slightly raised red patch with an adherent scale. The surface may become eroded.

Histology

The histological features of Bowen's disease are those of carcinoma *in situ*. A typical lesion is characterized by parakeratosis, acanthosis and full-thickness dysplasia (Fig. 7.42). The epithelial architecture is completely disorganized; there is loss of cellular maturation and orientation, nuclear and cytoplasmic pleomorphism and increased mitotic activity, both normal and abnormal at varying levels within the epidermis (Fig. 7.43). Occasionally, individual cell keratinization may be a feature and sometimes cytoplasmic vacuolation is prominent (especially in arsenic-induced lesions).

Intra-epidermal Carcinoma of the Mucous Membranes

Bowen's disease may develop on the mucous membranes (Fig. 7.44) as well as on the skin. It presents as a well-defined, slightly raised red plaque which may have a velvety texture and is often sore or itchy. On the male genitalia it is sometimes known as erythroplasia of Queyrat (Fig. 7.45). It does not appear to occur in those circumcized in infancy. If Bowen's disease of the mucous membranes is neglected, squamous cell carcinoma frequently supervenes.

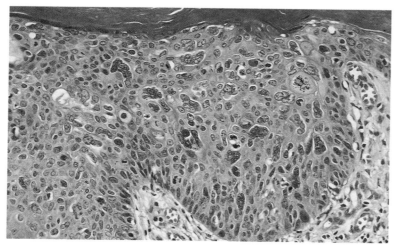

Fig. 7.42 Bowen's disease. There is massive hyperkeratosis. The epidermis, which is thickened, shows full thickness dysplasia with numerous pleomorphic and very enlarged nuclei. An enlarged degenerate mitotic figure is seen in the upper right quadrant.

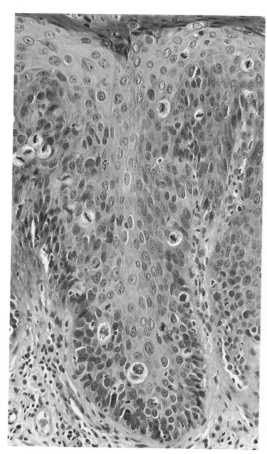

Fig. 7.43 Bowen's disease. Note the intense mitotic activity at varying levels within the epidermis.

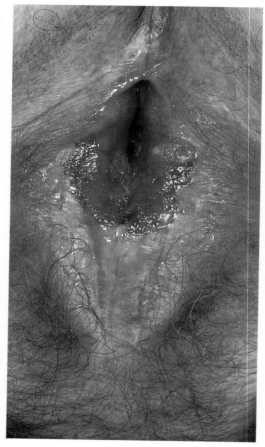

Fig. 7.44 Bowen's disease of the vulva. A raw, well-defined plaque of intra-epidermal carcinoma has occurred around the urethra and introitus. The surrounding skin is white (leukoplakia) and the patient had had lichen sclerosus et atrophicus for many years.

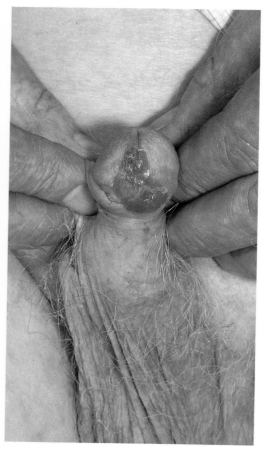

Fig. 7.45 Erythroplasia of Queyrat. Intra-epidermal carcinoma may occur on the glans penis. The lesion is a red, well-defined, slightly raised patch.

Bowenoid Papulosis

Bowenoid papulosis is something of an enigma representing an incompletely understood disorder characterized histologically by the features of epidermal dysplasia or carcinoma *in situ*, but apparently associated with a benign prognosis. The lesions are multiple, slightly raised, red-brown or pigmented papules or plaques (Figs. 7.46 and 7. 47). Lesions usually affect the glans or shaft of the penis or vulva but in some patients there is involvement of the peri-anal region. Occasionally in severely affected patients the papules may be numbered in hundreds and in females may involve the vagina and ectocervix. The exact nature of Bowenoid papulosis is unknown, but in some instances it is probably due to a viral infection. Human papilloma and herpes simplex viruses are probable aetiological candidates. The correct clinical management of Bowenoid papulosis is uncertain, but as there is some evidence that the multiple lesions may regress of their own accord, local conservative therapy e.g. curettage and cautery is more appropriate than any more radical surgical approach. Until its true nature is understood, the diagnosis of Bowenoid papulosis merits an exceedingly careful follow-up.

Histology

The papules are characterized by acanthosis associated with varying degrees of dysplasia ranging from mild changes through to carcinoma *in situ* (Fig. 7.48) and thus may be indistinguishable from those of Bowen's disease. Diagnosis depends upon careful clinico-pathological correlation. Bowen's disease is typified by a slowly enlarging, solitary lesion occurring in older age groups, while Bowenoid papulosis is characterized by multiple, rapidly growing, small papules occurring in younger people and often associated with a history of condylomata accuminata.

Management of Intra-epidermal Carcinoma of the Skin

Management depends upon the size of the lesion and upon the age of the patient. Excisional biopsy is the treatment of choice but if the lesion is too large, radiotherapy, curettage and cautery or cryotherapy may be satisfactory alternatives. 5-fluorouracil is an effective mode of therapy.

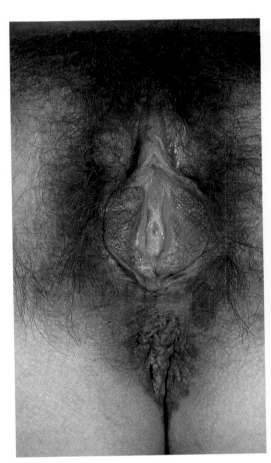

Fig. 7.46 Multicentric pigmented genital Bowen's disease. Well-defined, pigmented plaques surround the anus and involve the labia.

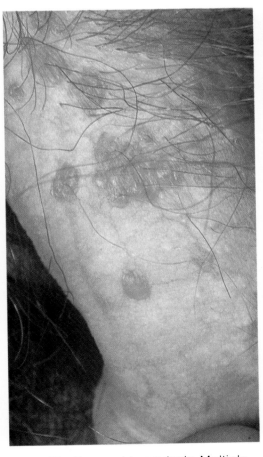

Fig. 7.47 Bowenoid papulosis. Multiple red-brown papules are present on the shaft of the penis. By courtesy of St. John's Hospital for Diseases of the Skin.

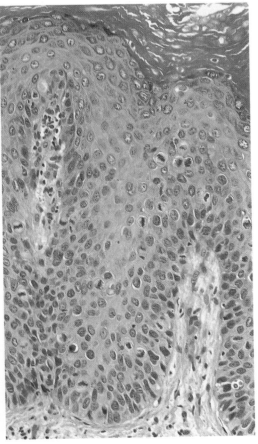

Fig. 7.48 Bowenoid papulosis. The epithelium is dysplastic. There are numerous mitotic figures. These features are *histologically* indistinguishable from Bowen's disease. Microscopic changes such as these in a young person should alert the pathologist to the possibility of Bowenoid papulosis. The biopsy came from the vulva of a young woman aged 23 years who clinically suffered from widespread genital condylomata.

7.11

PAGET'S DISEASE

This occurs as a solitary, red, slightly raised, well-defined plaque around one nipple and areola (Figs. 7.49–7.51) and is invariably associated with an underlying invasive or intraduct carcinoma of the breast. It may sometimes be mistaken for eczema (Fig. 7.52), or vice-versa, but a biopsy will distinguish the two. A much less common occurrence is extramammary Paget's disease (Figs. 7.53–7.55) which is found around the anus or genitalia and is usually, but not invariably, associated with carcinoma of the cutaneous adnexae or more distant sites such as malignant disease of the bowel or genitourinary tract. The diagnosis of extramammary Paget's disease should result in an intensive investigation of the patient for an underlying malignancy. The treatment is thus that of the underlying neoplastic disease. The affected skin should be managed surgically since radiotherapy and topical 5-fluorouracil are essentially ineffective.

Histology

The epidermis in both mammary and extramammary Paget's disease is infiltrated by variable numbers of large cells with abundant pale staining cytoplasm, and prominent oval vesicular nuclei with conspicuous eosinophilic nucleoli (Fig. 7.56). The cells which may be present singly, in clusters or sometimes totally replace the epithelium, classically show a diastase-resistant, periodic acid Schiff positive reaction (Fig. 7.57). The cytoplasm may also show a variably positive alcian blue staining reaction. The latter features may be of value in distinguishing Paget's disease from an atypical Bowen's disease or unusual *in situ* superficial spreading malignant melanoma. In some instances, scrutiny of the dermis may reveal infiltration by malignant cells from the underlying neoplasm.

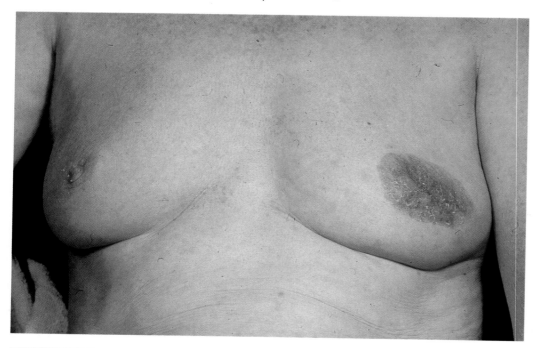

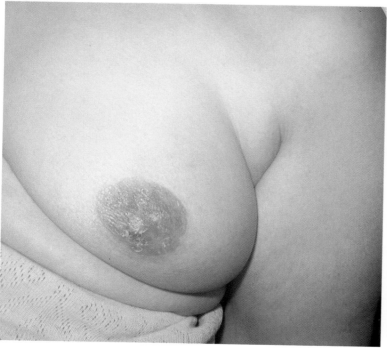

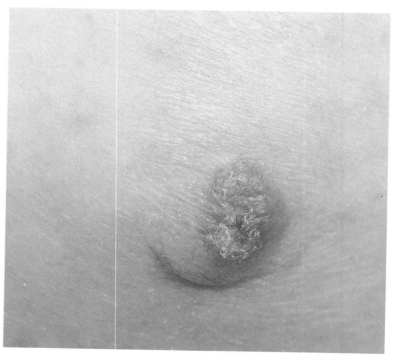

Fig. 7.49 Paget's disease of the breast. The lesion is unilateral and indicates an underlying intraduct carcinoma of the breast.

Fig. 7.50 Paget's disease of the breast. The whole of the nipple and areola has been replaced by a red, slightly raised, well-defined plaque.

Fig. 7.51 Paget's disease of the breast. This is an early example of the disease. Scaling is present on the surface of this well-defined red plaque. By courtesy of Dr. A.C. Pembroke.

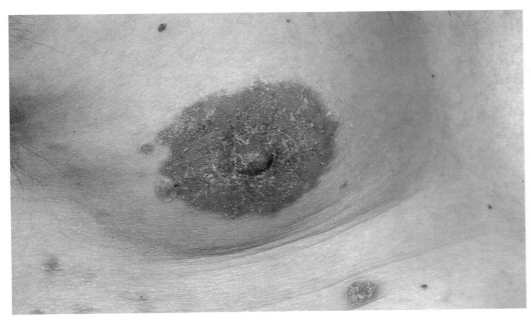

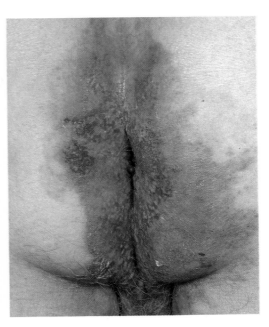

Fig. 7.52 Eczema of the nipple. The eruption is itchy, may weep and involve the surrounding skin. Eczema may be present elsewhere.

Fig. 7.53 Extramammary Paget's disease. The eruption is usually mistaken for eczema. However, note how well-defined the margin of the eruption is on the left. The patient may have underlying malignant disease. By courtesy of Dr. A.C. Pembroke.

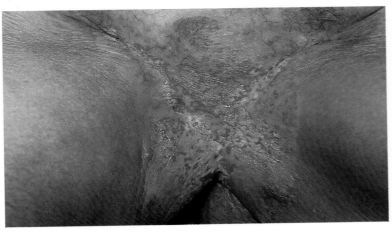

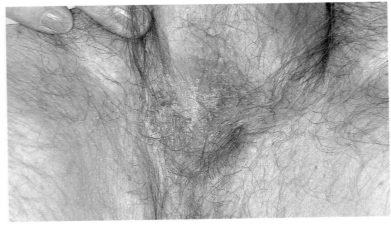

Fig. 7.54 Extramammary Paget's disease. The eruption is extremely extensive. The condition had recurred following an inadequate vulvectomy.

Fig. 7.55 Extramammary Paget's disease. A well-defined red, scaly plaque is present. The eruption had defied all attempts at treatment until a biopsy was performed and the correct diagnosis was made. By courtesy of St. Mary's Hospital.

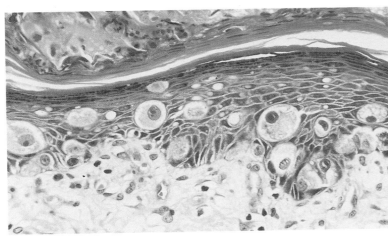

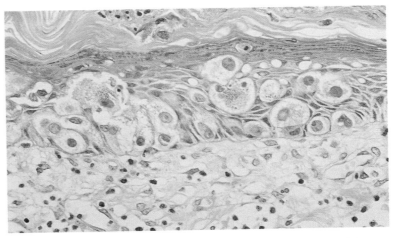

Fig. 7.56 Paget's disease of the nipple. There is superficial crusting. The irregular epidermis is infiltrated by characteristic cells with abundant pale-staining granular cytoplasm and large oval vesicular nuclei with prominent nucleoli.

Fig. 7.57 Paget's disease of the nipple. The cytoplasm of the tumour cells contains magenta-coloured, diastase-resistant, periodic acid-Schiff positive granules.

7.13

SQUAMOUS CELL CARCINOMA

Cutaneous squamous cell carcinoma is a potentially dangerous tumour which may occasionally infiltrate surrounding structures and metastasize to lymph nodes and subsequently be fatal. The aetiology is variable and includes the following:

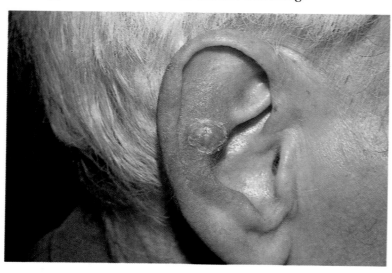

Fig. 7.58 Squamous cell carcinoma. The lesion starts as a firm, indurated nodule. The ear is a common site.

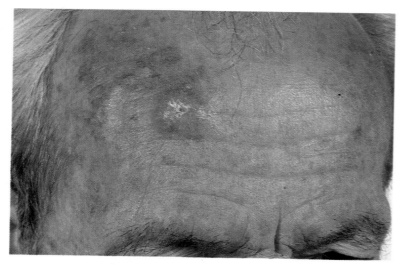

Fig. 7.59 Squamous cell carcinoma. The nodule enlarges and becomes fixed to surrounding structures.

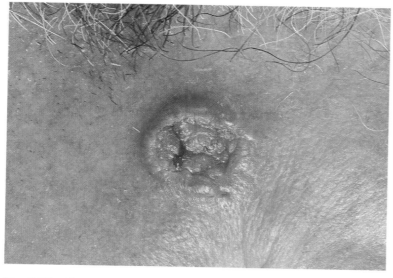

Fig. 7.60 Squamous cell carcinoma. The lesion is ulcerated with a raised, firm, indurated margin.

1. Ultra-violet Radiation
This is by far the commonest cause. Lesions may commence *de novo* or arise within a preceding solar keratosis (Fig. 7.58) or plaque of Bowen's disease.

2. X-rays
In the days before the dangers of X-rays were appreciated, radiologists were particularly at risk. X-ray treatment of certain diseases e.g. ankylosing spondylitis or tinea capitis is sometimes complicated many decades later by the development of squamous cell carcinoma.

3. Polycyclic Hydrocarbons
Tar, mineral oils, pitch and soot are also carcinogens. Indeed, soot was the first carcinogen to be discovered. Percival Pott in 1775 noted the development of scrotal tumours in men who had been chimney sweeps during childhood.

4. Mucosal Diseases
(a) Lichen planus affecting the lips or oral cavity and genital lichen sclerosus et atrophicus are very occasionally followed by malignant change.
(b) Mucosal Bowen's disease and oral and vulval hyperplastic epithelial dystrophy (leukoplakia) are premalignant.

5. Scars
Carcinoma may be a late complication of burns or of a skin disorder which results in scarring, e.g. dystrophic epidermolysis bullosa.

6. Chronic Skin Diseases
Squamous cell carcinoma may develop in chronic leg ulcers or untreated lupus vulgaris and leprosy.

7. Genetic Disorders
Squamous carcinoma may complicate genodermatoses such as albinism or xeroderma pigmentosum. In the former, there is a failure of melanization, i.e. the photoprotective mechanism. In the latter, there is a defect in the repair mechanism for DNA damaged by ultra-violet light.

8. Human Papilloma Virus
There is circumstantial evidence that cutaneous verrucous carcinoma (carcinoma cuniculatum) may be aetiologically related to a pre-existent wart virus infection.

Squamous cell carcinoma is an uncommon tumour. It may present either as a *nodule* or an *ulcer*. It starts as a nodule (Fig. 7.59) which grows laterally and vertically and gradually becomes fixed. The nodule is firm and thus feels indurated. It may have a crusted surface. The ulcer (Fig. 7.60) often has a purulent base surrounded by a firm and everted margin which is irregular in shape. The lesion grows more rapidly than a basal cell carcinoma.

Most lesions develop on sun-exposed areas. Thus, the face (Fig. 7.61) including the ears and lower lip (which are unusual sites for basal cell carcinomata), the backs of the hands and forearms are the more commonly involved sites. Lesions may occur on the lower leg (Fig. 7.62) and may be misdiagnosed as varicose ulcers (Fig. 7.63). The skin surrounding a squamous cell carcinoma often shows actinic damage (Fig. 7.64) although occasionally the tumour may arise from skin which appears normal (Fig. 7.65) or from solar-protected skin such as around the genitalia and anus (Figs. 7.66 and 7.67). A rare variant occurs on the sole of the foot (*epithelioma cuniculatum*, Fig. 7.68).

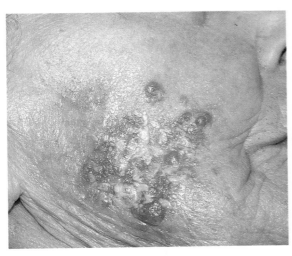

Fig. 7.61 Squamous cell carcinoma. Multiple nodules are present in a diffusely spreading variety on the face.

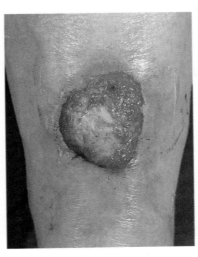

Fig. 7.62 Squamous cell carcinoma. It is important to include the margin of the lesion in a biopsy. Biopsy of the ulcerated area alone may fail to provide the diagnosis.

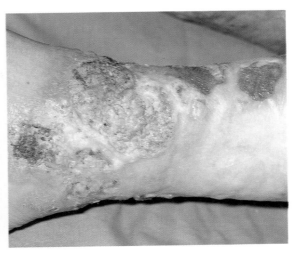

Fig. 7.63 Squamous cell carcinoma. This developed in a patient with a chronic blistering and scarring skin condition. By courtesy of Dr. A.C. Pembroke.

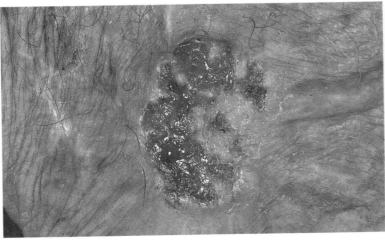

Fig. 7.64 Squamous cell carcinoma. The back of the hand is a common site for squamous cell carcinoma but an unusual one for basal cell carcinoma. Note the surrounding atrophic solar-damaged skin.

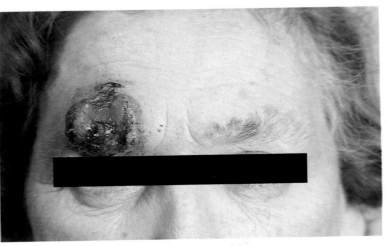

Fig. 7.65 Squamous cell carcinoma. A rapidly growing ulcerated nodule occasionally occurs on otherwise seemingly normal skin. By courtesy of St. Mary's Hospital.

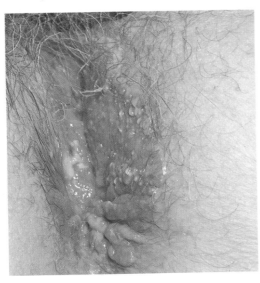

Fig. 7.66 Squamous cell carcinoma. A vegetating, well-defined, eroded plaque of tumour is present around the anus.

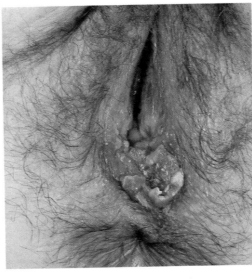

Fig. 7.67 Squamous cell carcinoma. Early invasion and metastasis occurs with perineal squamous cell carcinoma.

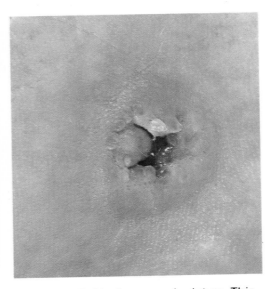

Fig. 7.68 Epithelioma cuniculatum. This is a squamous cell carcinoma of the sole of the foot. The lesion is frequently misdiagnosed clinically and even histologically, unless adequate material is provided by a deep surgical biopsy.

Squamous cell carcinomata have a variable natural history. Those arising within solar keratoses are much less aggressive than those arising *de novo* (Fig. 7.69) or from other causes such as mucosal Bowen's disease, irradiation, burns or chronic skin disorders. Lesions on the genitalia or lips (Figs. 7.70 and 7.71) tend to become invasive and metastasize early.

Squamous cell carcinoma should be managed jointly by a plastic surgeon and radiotherapist. Surgical excision is the treatment of choice, but radiotherapy is also effective in many cases and therefore the treatment will depend upon the age of the patient and the site and size of the lesion.

Histology

The histological appearances of cutaneous squamous carcinoma are variable and depend upon the degree of differentiation. Tumours are sub-divided into well differentiated, moderately differentiated and poorly differentiated variants. Rarely the tumour is so anaplastic that recognition of its precise nature is dependent upon detection of an epidermal origin.

Well differentiated squamous carcinoma is typified by infiltrating islands of tumour showing obvious squamous differentiation with well-formed desmosomes (Figs. 7.72 and 7.73) and usually conspicuous and frequently abundant keratinization. Mitotic activity is usually not markedly increased and pleomorphism is minimal.

Moderately differentiated tumours are characterized by a more pleomorphic appearance with architectural disorganization, increased (and often abnormal) mitotic activity and imperfect keratinization; the latter is manifest as individual cell keratinization and keratin pearl formation (Fig. 7.74).

In poorly differentiated variants there is marked pleomorphism, diagnosis being dependent upon detection of small foci of

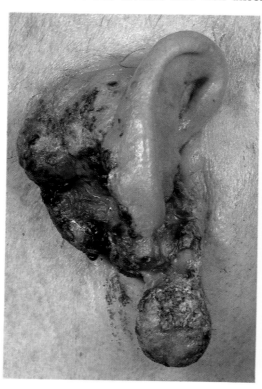

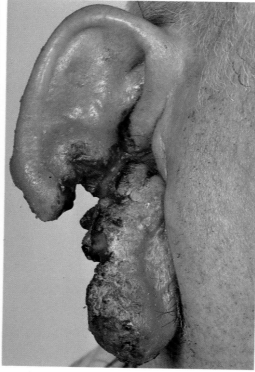

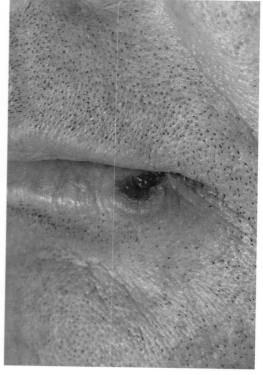

Fig. 7.69 Squamous cell carcinoma of the ear. This lesion was ignored until it had reached an advanced stage. It is nodular, ulcerated and destructive. The patient died two years later from involvement of the cervical lymph nodes, a mass in the chest and cervical vertebral bony destruction.

Fig. 7.70 Squamous cell carcinoma. An ulcer with an indurated margin is present on the lower lip. By courtesy of St. Mary's Hospital.

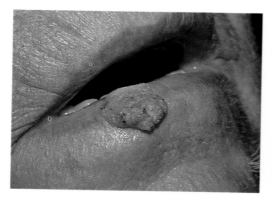

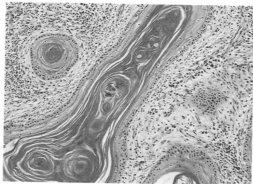

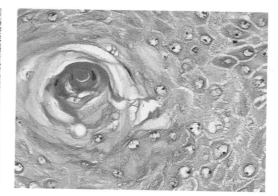

Fig. 7.71 Squamous cell carcinoma. This lesion has a warty, crusted surface but the base was firm and suspicious of malignant disease.

Fig. 7.72 Well differentiated squamous cell carcinoma. The dermis is infiltrated by islands of mature squamous epithelium showing obvious keratinization.

Fig. 7.73 Well differentiated squamous cell carcinoma. In this high power view, intercellular bridges (prickles) are conspicuous.

keratinization or occasional desmosomes (Fig. 7.75). A number of rare but important variants of squamous cell carcinoma are recognized.

Spindle cell squamous carcinoma, which is particularly associated with extreme solar damage, burns or radiotherapy may be a source of diagnostic confusion (Fig. 7.76). In tumours where a spindle cell pattern predominates, distinction from superficial sarcomatous conditions e.g. dermatofibrosarcoma protruberans or spindle cell amelanotic melanoma may be difficult and necessitate the study of numerous tumour sections in order to detect an epidermal origin or focus of tumour keratinization.

Clear cell squamous carcinoma is characterized by abundant intracytoplasmic glycogen resulting in distended, vacuolated cells (Fig. 7.77). Occasionally, the lesion may be confused with a clear cell metastasis from sites such as the lung or kidney.

Cutaneous verrucous carcinoma is a rare variant which occurs most often on the sole of the foot and is characterized by an exceedingly well differentiated histological appearance, a long clinical history and a usually favourable outcome. Some tumours, although not all, may arise in pre-existent viral warts. The tumour is typified by the development of deeply penetrating, keratinizing epithelial sinuses giving the tumour a characteristic clinical appearance. Its particular importance is that it may easily be misdiagnosed histologically if an adequate clinical history is not available. Diagnosis depends in part upon clinico-pathological correlation and also upon the typical histological features of deeply penetrating, bulbous processes of well-differentiated squamous epithelium showing marked keratinization (Figs. 7.78 and 7.79).

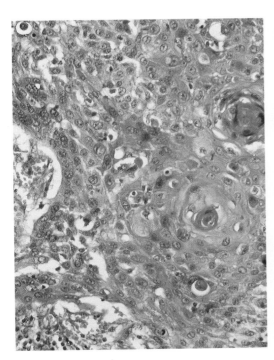

Fig. 7.74 Moderately differentiated squamous cell carcinoma. The tumour epithelium is obviously much more disorganized. Intercellular bridges, however, are still evident and scattered horn cysts are present.

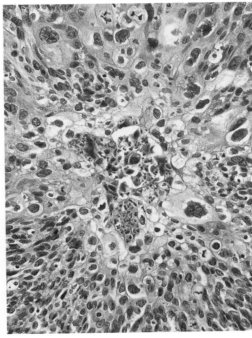

Fig. 7.75 Poorly differentiated squamous cell carcinoma. There is marked pleomorphism with hyperchromatic and sometimes bizarre nuclei and conspicuous mitotic figures. In the degenerate central region scattered dyskeratotic cells are present.

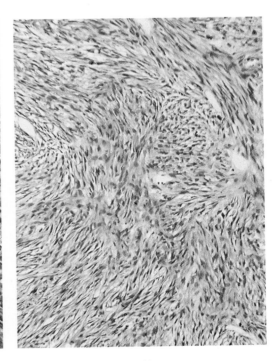

Fig. 7.76 Spindle cell squamous carcinoma. These histological appearances of a diffuse spindle cell tumour are only recognized as being of squamous derivation because of the detection of an epithelial origin in this actinically-derived variant.

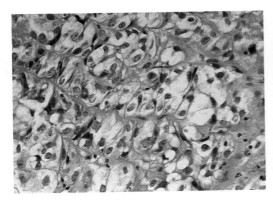

Fig. 7.77 Clear cell squamous carcinoma. In this field, abundant intracytoplasmic glycogen has resulted in a clear cell pattern.

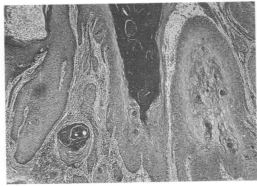

Fig. 7.78 Plantar verrucous carcinoma (carcinoma cuniculatum). This low power view shows extensive permeation of the reticular dermis by downgrowths of exceedingly well differentiated squamous epithelium. Note the extensive keratinization and characteristic blunt lower border of the tumour.

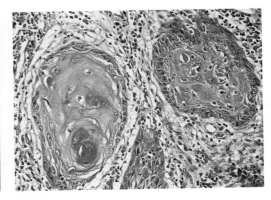

Fig. 7.79 Plantar verrucous carcinoma (carcinoma cuniculatum). The well differentiated epithelium has a typically watery appearance as seen on the left side of this picture.

KERATOACANTHOMA

This not uncommon tumour may be suspected clinically by a history of very rapid growth over a period of a few weeks. The tumour usually reaches its zenith within a couple of months and then involutes spontaneously to leave a pitted scar, the whole process taking three to four months (Figs. 7.80 and 7.81). It occurs largely on light-exposed areas and consists of a flesh-coloured nodule which stands up proud and elevated from the surrounding skin (Figs. 7.82 and 7.83). It is well-defined and has a central keratin plug (Figs. 7.84 and 7.85). Common sites are the central portions of the face and the backs of the hands so that sun exposure does appear to be the most important aetiological factor. However, these tumours also occur in those who work with pitch and tar and in immunosuppressed patients, particularly those who have been treated with immunosuppressive agents following renal transplantation. Curettage and cautery gives good cosmetic results, but often the lesion is seen late in its development and removal would be more destructive than leaving it to heal spontaneously. However, incisional biopsy is wise to confirm the diagnosis.

Histology

The diagnosis of keratoacanthoma calls for careful clinico-pathological correlation. Well-differentiated squamous carcinoma may mimic it and in such instances the diagnosis is totally dependent upon the typical clinical features and short natural history. In any cases where doubt exists (particularly if excision is incomplete), it is in the patient's best interests to regard the lesion as carcinomatous and to treat accordingly.

In its fully evolved state a keratoacanthoma is typified by a flask-shaped lesion with well-developed lateral borders – the so-called collarette, and a central keratin-filled epithelial invagination (Fig. 7.86). Although epithelial dysplasia may be present, more typically in keratoacanthoma the proliferating epithelium is well-differentiated, often has a ground glass appearance (Fig. 7.87) and shows marked keratinization. In contrast to squamous cell carcinoma where deep infiltration is a usual feature, in keratoacanthoma proliferation is more marked along the lateral aspects of the lesion.

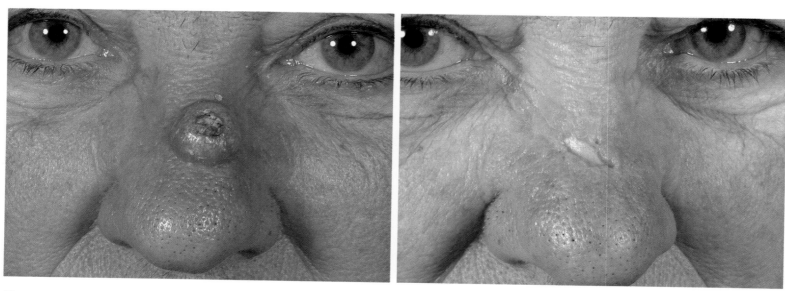

Fig. 7.80   Keratoacanthoma. Keratoacanthomata resolve spontaneously to leave a pitted scar.

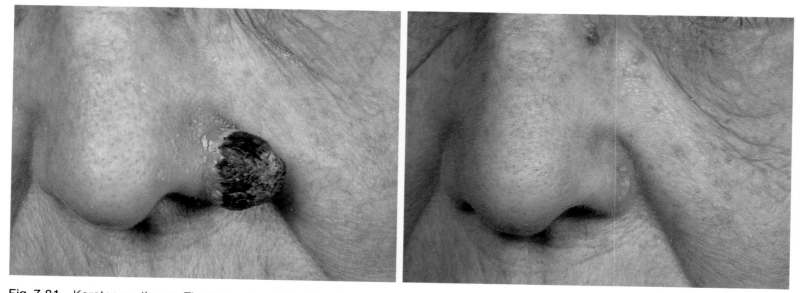

Fig. 7.81   Keratoacanthoma. The lesion is self-healing. Eleven weeks have elapsed between these two pictures.

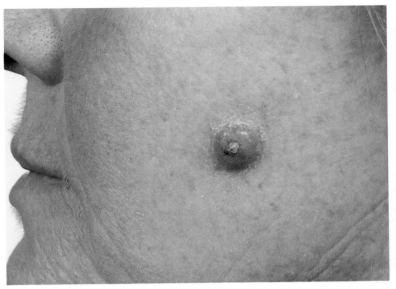

Fig. 7.82 Keratoacanthoma. The lesion is a well-defined nodule with a central keratin plug. It grows rapidly, reaching its maximum size within about six weeks.

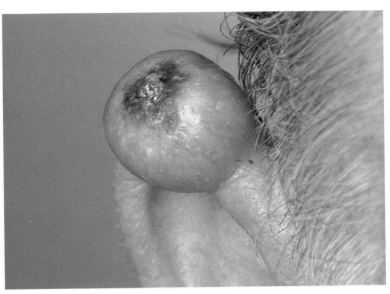

Fig. 7.83 Keratoacanthoma. This nodule is particularly well-circumscribed, stands up proud away from the skin and has a crusted centre.

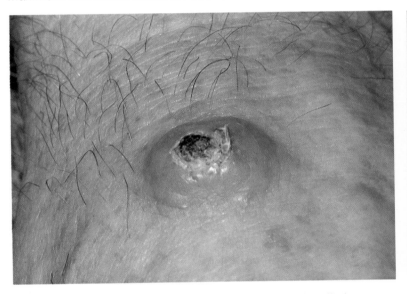

Fig. 7.84 Keratoacanthoma. The nodule is raised well above the surface. The back of the hand is a common site.

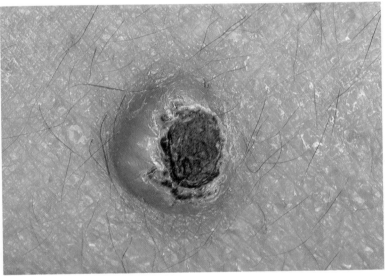

Fig. 7.85 Keratoacanthoma. The lesion has a crusted centre.

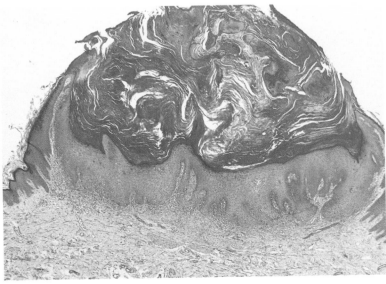

Fig. 7.86 Keratoacanthoma. Typical low power view showing the keratin plug fitting the central invagination and the well-formed lateral collarette.

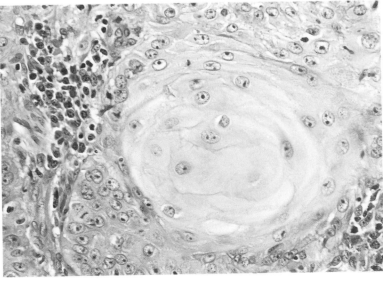

Fig. 7.87 Keratoacanthoma. Characteristically, in a well-developed lesion the epithelium adopts a 'ground glass' appearance. The dermis contains a heavy lymphocytic and plasma cell infiltrate.

7.19

BASAL CELL CARCINOMA

The basal cell carcinoma is the commonest cutaneous malignancy. Although sunlight is an important factor, it is curious that the lesion is almost always seen on the face and yet rarely on other sun-exposed sites. It is a slow-growing tumour in contrast to a squamous cell carcinoma or keratoacanthoma. While it very rarely metastasizes, it is locally invasive and this is of particular importance when situated near to the eye, nose and ear. If neglected it may infiltrate deeply through tissue planes into the cranial cavity. There are five clinical sub-types of basal cell carcinoma.

1. The Rodent Ulcer (Figs. 7.88–7.91)

This starts as a small papule which subsequently ulcerates. It is painless and therefore is frequently ignored by the patient. The ulcer margin is well-defined, slightly raised and rolled with a colour similar to that of a pearl. Tiny blood vessels (telangiectasia) may be seen coursing over the margin. Patients observe that the lesion tends to bleed, subsequently scabs, but never quite seems to heal.

2. Cystic Type (Figs. 7.92–7.96)

In this variant the central part of the tumour does not break down until quite late in the course of its evolution. The tumour may achieve quite a large size but is often neglected, being mistaken for a benign cyst. It is a slightly lobulated nodule, pearly in colour, with a smooth, telangiectatic surface.

3. Pigmented Basal Cell Carcinoma (Figs. 7.97 and 7.98)

This lesion has similar features to a rodent ulcer except that the margins of the tumour are heavily pigmented. The lesion is often misdiagnosed as malignant melanoma.

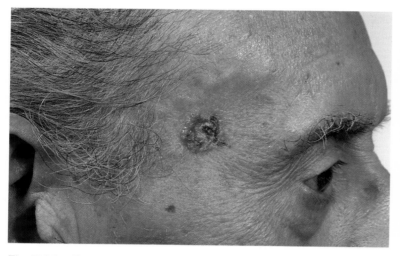

Fig. 7.88   Rodent ulcer. This usually appears on the face. It has a well-defined, rolled margin and an ulcerated centre.

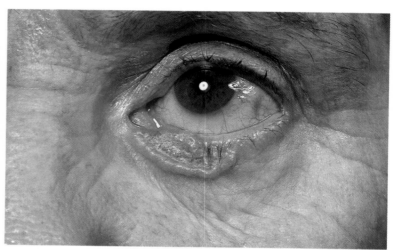

Fig. 7.89   Rodent ulcer. The rolled margin is particularly obvious. It has a pearly colour. Lesions close to the eye may be very destructive.

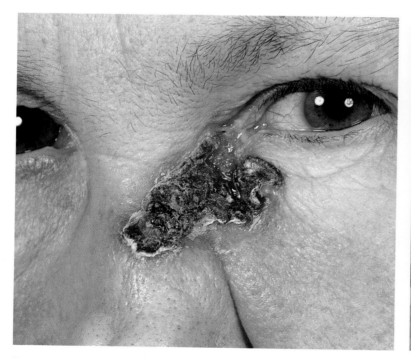

Fig. 7.90   Rodent ulcer. This lesion has penetrated widely and deeply. The erosive and gnawing nature of the tumour gives rise to its name.

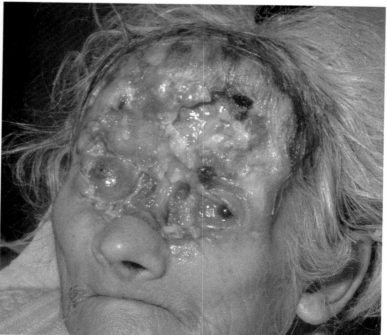

Fig. 7.91   Basal cell carcinoma. If neglected, the tumour grows inexorably causing fearful destruction. By courtesy of Dr. D.E. Sharvill.

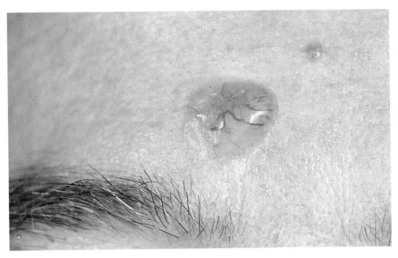

Fig. 7.92 Cystic basal cell carcinoma. The lesion is well-defined and somewhat lobulated.

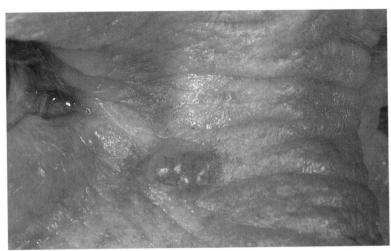

Fig. 7.93 Cystic basal cell carcinoma. The lesion has the colour of a pearl and is covered by tiny blood vessels (telangiectasia).

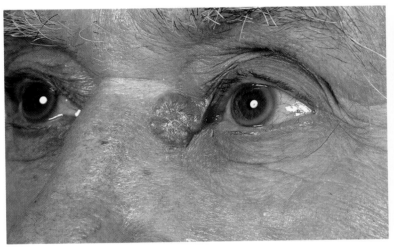

Fig. 7.94 Cystic basal cell carcinoma. The inner canthus of the eye is one of the commonest sites for basal cell carcinomata.

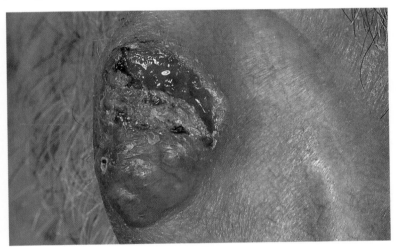

Fig. 7.95 Cystic basal cell carcinoma. This lobulated cystic lesion on the back of the ear has attained a large size before becoming ulcerated.

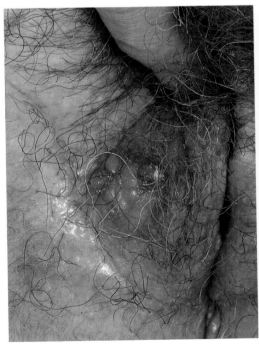

Fig. 7.96 Cystic basal cell carcinoma of the vulva. Basal cell carcinomata rarely occur at sites other than the face.

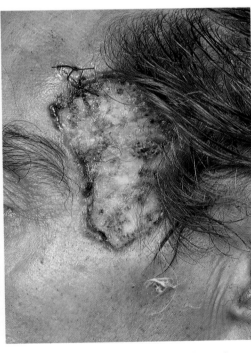

Fig. 7.97 Pigmented basal cell carcinoma. The rolled margin of the ulcerated lesion is strikingly pigmented.

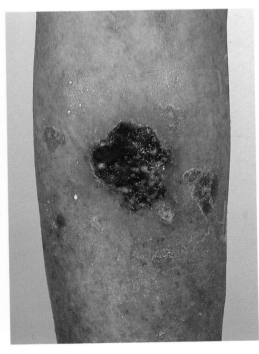

Fig. 7.98 Pigmented basal cell carcinoma. This lesion occurred on the leg: an unusual site. The margin of the ulcer is rolled and pigmented.

7.21

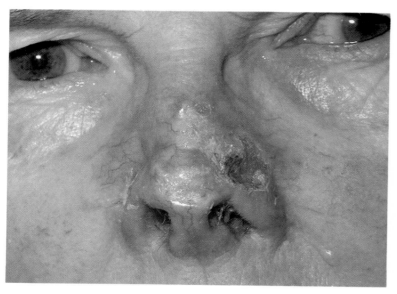

Fig. 7.99 Morphoeic basal cell carcinoma. The lesion is a pearly coloured plaque rather than a nodule and telangiectasia is present.

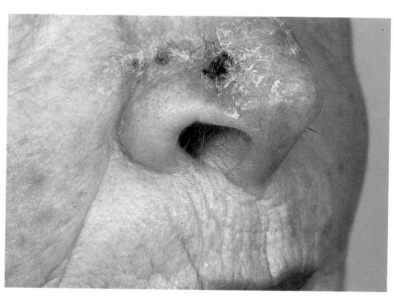

Fig. 7.100 Morphoeic basal cell carcinoma. These destructive lesions are often diagnosed late.

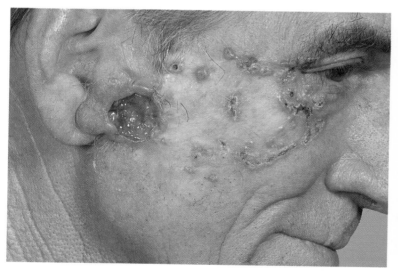

Fig. 7.101 Morphoeic basal cell carcinoma. The scarring sclerodermatous appearance is marked. The lesion has become extremely extensive.

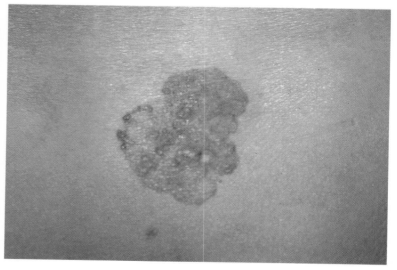

Fig. 7.102 Superficial basal cell carcinoma. The lesion is a plaque with a rolled pearly margin, which is a miniature version of that of the rodent ulcer.

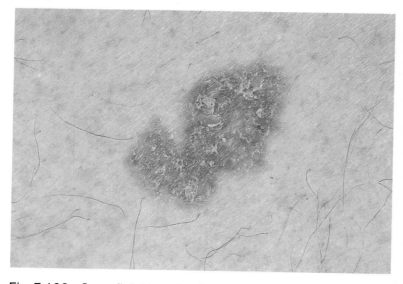

Fig. 7.103 Superficial basal cell carcinoma. A red, scaly plaque with indented margins is found on the trunk.

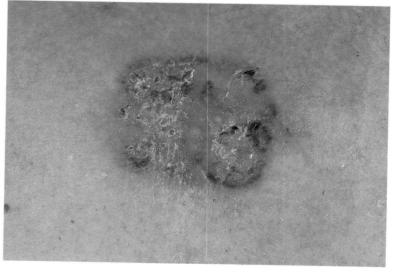

Fig. 7.104 Superficial basal cell carcinoma. The fine rolled margin is clearly delineated and in this case is pigmented.

4. Morphoeic Type (Figs. 7.99–7.101)

The morphoeic basal cell carcinoma is the type most likely to be misdiagnosed, because it does not appear as a tumour, but rather as a slightly elevated plaque. The term morphoea refers to the similarity to sclerodermatous skin. Thus, the plaque feels thickened and tethered. Telangiectasia and the pearly coloration are important diagnostic features. The lesion spreads insidiously. Nests of tumour cells infiltrate beyond the apparent clinical margins of the plaque as well as infiltrating deeply into the dermis. Thus, it can be extremely difficult to determine the limits of the tumour by visual inspection, so recurrences after surgery and radiotherapy by the unwary are commonplace.

5. Superficial Basal Cell Carcinoma (Figs. 7.102–7.104)

This lesion occurs almost invariably on the trunk. It is a red plaque with an adherent scale and is only slightly raised, although after a number of years it becomes invasive and a nodule or ulcer develops. The most important diagnostic feature is that there is a minute finely raised, well-delineated margin which is rolled, telangiectatic and pearly. Very careful inspection in a good light is often required to appreciate this. Sometimes multiple basal cell carcinomata (Fig. 7.105) occur on the trunk, often in patients who have previously received arsenic. Keratoses (Fig. 7.106) on the palmar surfaces may also be present. Superficial basal cell carcinomata are frequently mistaken for psoriasis, but their asymmetrical distribution and the fact that they do not respond to anti-psoriatic therapy should alert the practitioner to the diagnosis and suggest the need for biopsy to confirm it. Patients with psoriasis may have been treated with arsenic, so it is quite possible to see a patient with genuine psoriasis and superficial basal cell carcinoma.

Management

Basal cell carcinomata have the propensity for deep invasion and are potentially extremely destructive. Therefore they must be eradicated at the first attempt. There are a number of effective modalities but the choice depends on the size, site and nature of the lesion and the physical condition of the patient. The lesion may be excised and the defect closed primarily or repaired by a graft or rotation flap. Curettage and cautery are acceptable for small lesions away from dangerous sites on the face or larger lesions on the trunk. Radiotherapy is equally effective. Superficial basal cell carcinomata may be treated with topical 5-fluorouracil.

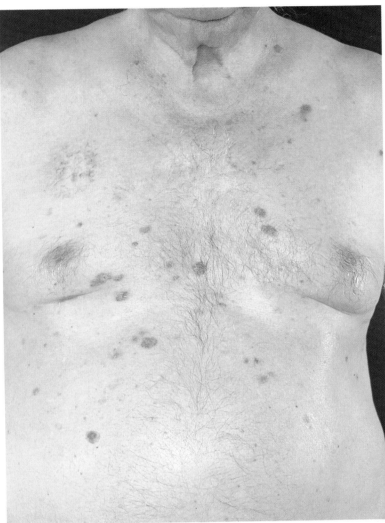

Fig. 7.105 Multiple basal cell carcinomata on the trunk. The occurrence of multiple basal cell carcinomata on the trunk suggests the previous ingestion of arsenic. This man had received arsenic for a severe dermatitis 30 years previously. By courtesy of St. Mary's Hospital.

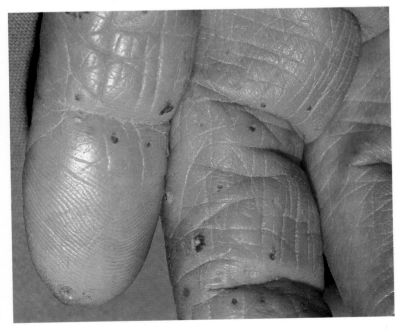

Fig. 7.106 Arsenical keratosis. Arsenic produces keratoses on the palms and fingers.

BASAL CELL NAEVUS SYNDROME (Gorlin's Syndrome)

In this dominantly inherited condition, multiple basal cell carcinomata develop from childhood onwards (Fig. 7.107). A characteristic feature is the presence of palmar and plantar pits (Fig. 7.108) which show the histology of mini-basal cell carcinomata. X-ray abnormalities such as mandibular cysts and bifid ribs are frequently found.

Histology

Basal cell carcinomata show a variety of histological appearances with variable differentiation thereby reflecting their probable derivation from undifferentiated epithelial germ cells.

In its prototype form the tumour is composed of discrete islands of small cells with darkly staining, uniform nuclei and scant ill-defined cytoplasm. Peripheral pallisading is a typical feature (Figs. 7.109 and 7.110). In most, but not all, instances an origin from the overlying epidermis may be detected (Fig. 7.111). The tumour islands are invariably accompanied by an actively proliferating connective tissue stroma. The latter appears to be an integral part of the tumour. Excessive connective tissue proliferation results in the morphoeic pattern (Fig. 7.112). Mitotic activity may be quite marked but this should *not* be interpreted as necessarily being associated with any sinister implication. It is important to recognize those tumours showing an aggressive infiltrating pattern with narrow tongues of epithelium extending deeply into the adjacent connective tissue.

A not infrequent finding in basal cell carcinoma is the presence of cystic foci (Fig. 7.113). In extreme examples this may give rise to a generalized lacy pattern – so-called adenoid basal cell carcinoma. Whether this phenomenon occurs as a result of degenerative changes or is in reality a manifestation of sweat duct differentiation is uncertain.

Pilar keratinization is also commonly found and in extreme examples may result in the formation of very numerous horn cysts so that differentiation from trichoepithelioma is impossible in the absence of adequate clinical history. Occasional foci of sebaceous differentiation may much less commonly be a feature (Fig. 7.114). Pigmented basal cell carcinoma depends upon a large inherent population of melanocytes for its typical dark coloration (Fig. 7.115).

Finally, superficial basal cell carcinoma is typified by multiple discrete foci of tiny basal cell carcinomata (Fig. 7.116). Although on examination of a single section, they appear separate, serial sectioning reveals an interconnected arborizing tumour. Superficial basal cell carcinoma is of particular importance in that due to difficulty in determining the precise lateral limits of the tumour, recurrences are to be particularly anticipated.

Although metastatic basal cell carcinoma does occur, it is exceptionally rare. The finding of apparent secondary deposits should stimulate an intensive investigative regime to exclude the much more likely possibility of an alternative source for the primary tumour.

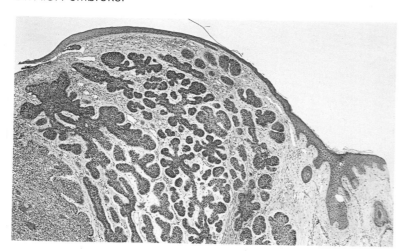

Fig. 7.107 Basal cell naevus (Gorlin's) syndrome. Multiple basal cell carcinomata develop from childhood onward. The condition is inherited as an autosomal dominant. By courtesy of Dr. A.C. Pembroke.

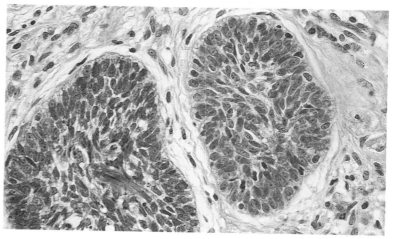

Fig. 7.108 Basal cell naevus syndrome. Tiny pits on the palms are characteristic additional features. By courtesy of Dr. Eugene van Scott, Skin and Cancer Hospital, Philadelphia.

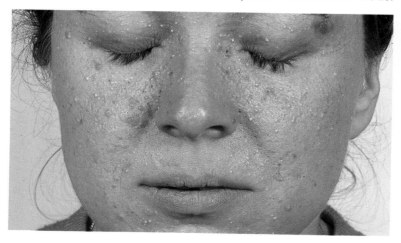

Fig. 7.109 Basal cell carcinoma. This low power view shows the characteristic appearances of a nodular basal cell carcinoma. The dermis is extensively invaded by discrete islands of small, darkly-staining uniform cells.

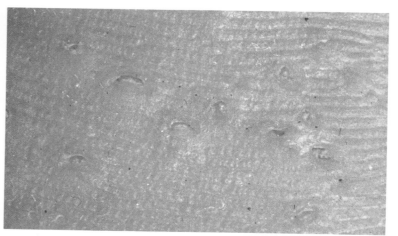

Fig. 7.110 Basal cell carcinoma. Peripheral pallisading of the tumour nucleus is characteristic. The retraction of the connective tissue component around the tumour islands is a fixation artefact typically seen in this neoplasm.

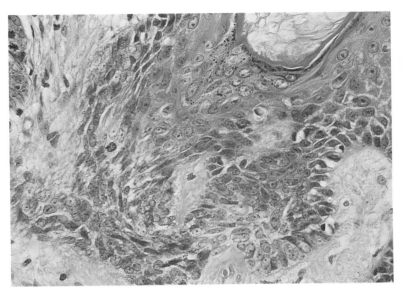

Fig. 7.111 Basal cell carcinoma. The tumour origin. Note the presence of scattered mitotic figures.

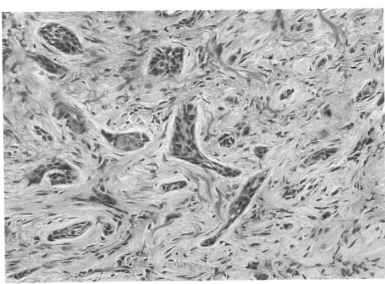

Fig. 7.112 Morphoeic basal cell carcinoma. In this tumour the epithelial component is compressed into narrow strands by the intense fibroblastic stroma.

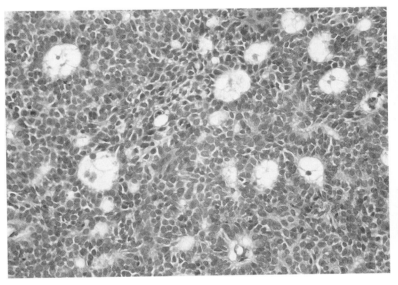

Fig. 7.113 Adenoid basal cell carcinoma. This lace-like pattern may be a focal change in an otherwise typical lesion or represent the bulk of the tumour.

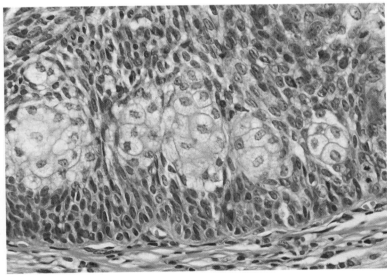

Fig. 7.114 Basal cell carcinoma. Sebaceous differentiation with the appearance of large cells with bubbly cytoplasm and vesicular nuclei is a rather uncommon finding.

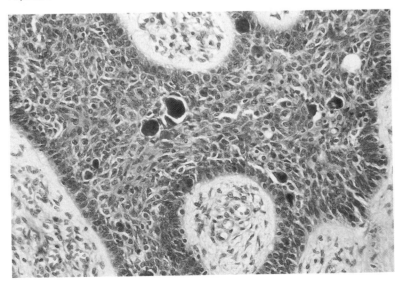

Fig. 7.115 Pigmented basal cell carcinoma. Dense deposits of melanin are present both within the tumour cells and as larger extracellular aggregates.

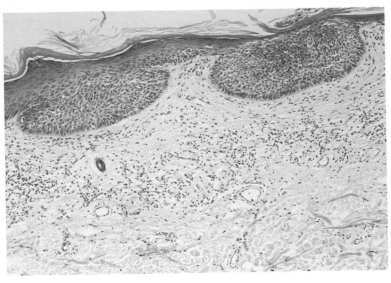

Fig. 7.116 Multifocal superficial basal cell carcinoma. Two discrete foci of basaloid proliferative change are present in this arsenic-induced lesion.

MALIGNANT MELANOMA

Malignant melanoma is the commonest serious cutaneous malignancy seen by dermatologists. The incidence of the tumour has risen disproportionately, for example doubling in Scandinavia and Australia over a period of one decade. At present, there are five new cases per 100,000 population per annum in the United Kingdom. Comparable figures for Scandinavia and Australia are 12 and 32 respectively. Females appear to be affected twice as often as males.

Ultra-violet light is the most important cause. Its incidence is increased in those with red hair, blue eyes, freckles and poor tanning ability, living in those parts of the world where solar exposure is high. However, malignant melanoma develops more commonly in white collar office workers than in outdoor workers and it is probable that intense but infrequent exposure on vacation is more important than chronic and continual irradiation.

The malignant melanoma metastasizes via the lymphatics to the lymph nodes and via the blood stream principally to the brain, lungs, bones and skin and is ultimately fatal. Previously, the prognosis was thought to be very poor indeed, but it has become clear that the growth characteristics and therefore the prognosis of the different types of malignant melanoma vary. Essentially, the more superficial the lesion at the time of excision, the better the prognosis. Thus, lentigo maligna (Hutchinson's freckle) and superficial spreading malignant melanoma have a prolonged horizontal growth phase before vertical invasion occurs and thus the prognosis is usually favourable. In contrast, nodular malignant melanoma has no horizontal growth phase. It grows vertically from the start and consequently has a much worse outlook. Prognosis is also determined by the site of the lesion, e.g. it is worse on the trunk than on the limb. Females fare better than males.

Most malignant melanomata develop *de novo* on skin which was previously normal. However, about one-third of malignant melanomata develop in close association with a pre-existant junctional naevus. As most Caucasians have twenty or more moles, prophylactic removal is neither warranted nor practicable. There are, however, certain exceptions.

The Bathing Trunk Naevus Syndrome

Malignant transformation is frequent in this rare condition. Unfortunately, prophylactic excision is not possible in many of these patients because of the extent of the naevi (Fig. 7.117).

Congenital Melanocytic Naevi

Malignant change (Fig. 7.118) in large congenital naevi occurs very rarely. There is no agreed policy for their management and technically prophylactic excision is often difficult without skin grafting. The vast majority are therefore left alone with generally no ill effects. Solar irradiation of the lesions should be avoided.

Dysplastic Naevus Syndrome
(Family Atypical Mole Malignant Melanoma)

The dysplastic naevus syndrome is a recently recognized condition in which patients develop large numbers of atypical naevi and are at an increased risk of developing malignant melanomata. Cases may be sporadic or familial. Examples of the latter are sometimes referred to as the B-K mole syndrome (named after two of the families in the original series). Patients develop naevi in the first and second decades which gradually enlarge (often over 1.0cm in diameter) and acquire atypical clinical appearances, with irregular margins and variable pigmentation (Fig. 7.121). Most individuals give a history of intense solar irradiation.

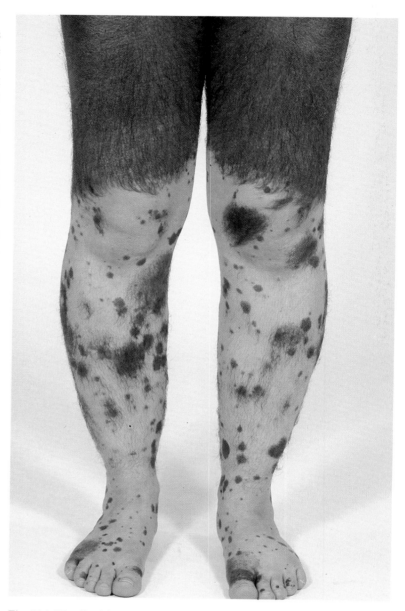

Fig. 7.117 Bathing trunk naevus syndrome. Extensive pigmented naevi are present from birth. There is a significant malignant change in the condition.

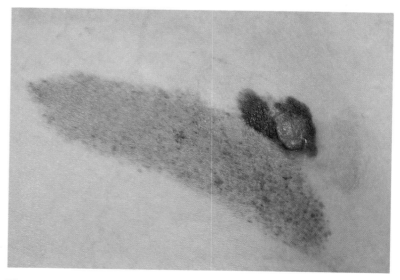

Fig. 7.118 Malignant melanoma. Exceptionally, malignant melanoma develop in large melanocytic naevi which have been present from birth.

Histology

While some lesions from a patient with the B-K mole syndrome may histologically only show the features of melanocytic naevi, others will be characterized by varying degrees of atypia and therefore fall into the dysplastic category. Dysplastic naevi may be subdivided into lentiginous and epithelioid variants. The former, the more common, is typified by basally located melanocytes showing nuclear pleomorphism, hyperchromatism and a conspicuous peri-cellular retraction halo (Fig. 7.119). The epidermal ridge pattern is accentuated as in a lentigo. A characteristic finding is desmoplasia within the papillary dermis following the lower borders of the epidermal ridges. Epithelioid dysplastic naevi are composed of larger cells with eosinophilic cytoplasm containing fine granular melanin pigment, vesicular nuclei and sometimes prominent nucleoli (Fig. 7.120). In both variants, a lymphocytic response is present in the superficial dermis. All dysplastic naevi should be carefully sectioned to exclude focal development of invasive (superficial spreading) malignant melanoma.

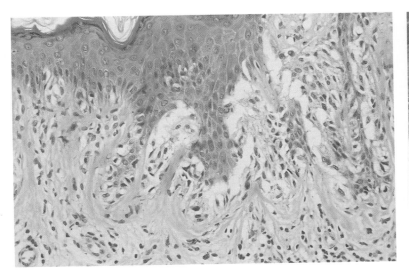

Fig. 7.119 Dysplastic naevus. The left side of the picture shows a lentiginous pattern with abundant pallisaded melanocytes showing conspicuous retraction artefact. This merges with marked junctional acitivity on the right. Note the presence of marked desmoplasia (lamellar fibroplasia), pigmentary incontinence and a lymphocytic infiltrate in the dermis.

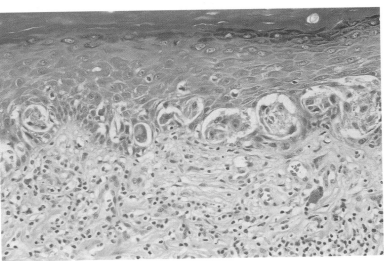

Fig. 7.120 Dysplastic naevus. The lesion is characterized by nests of basally localized melanocytes with abundant eosinophilic cytoplasm, vesicular nuclei and prominent nucleoli. There is dermal fibrosis, quite marked pigmentary incontinence and a lymphocytic infiltrate is evident.

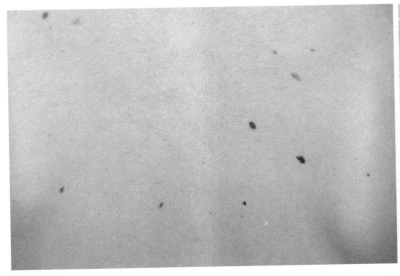

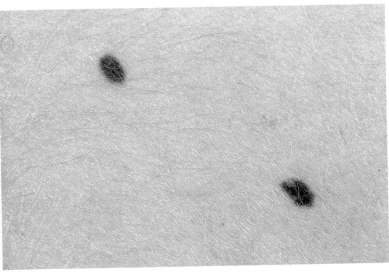

Fig. 7.121 Dysplastic naevus. This 15-year-old girl had a family history of malignant melanoma. These two moles were atypical with irregular margins. The one on the far right was malignant.

There are four clinical types of cutaneous malignant melanoma: lentigo maligna, superficial spreading malignant melanoma, acral lentiginous malignant melanoma and nodular malignant melanoma.

1. Lentigo Maligna (Hutchinson's Freckle)

This commences as a malignant melanoma *in situ* which grows very slowly, but after a number of years may become invasive (lentigo maligna melanoma). It is seen in the elderly, most commonly on the face (Fig. 7.122), and chronic solar exposure would appear to be the most important factor in the aetiology of this particular lesion (Fig. 7.123). It first appears as a flat pigmented lesion which gradually enlarges. The pigment varies from light tan to brown or black. Red, blue, grey and white areas may also be present (Fig. 7.124). The margin of the lesion is also irregular, being notched and indented (Fig. 7.125). Eventually, when invasion occurs nodules develop (Fig. 7.126). The lesion is often quite sizable by the time the patient presents for diagnosis and therefore surgical excision and repair of the defect is technically difficult. Since the malignant potential of these lesions is low, and they often occur in elderly and infirm patients in whom operation under general anaesthesia might be hazard-ous, many physicians observe them at regular intervals and intervene only if the lesion becomes raised and thus invasive. Others, however, advocate cryotherapy or radiotherapy at an early stage if surgery is contra-indicated.

Histology

Lentigo maligna is invariably accompanied by the features of actinic damage, i.e. epidermal atrophy and solar elastosis. An established lesion is characterized by proliferation of atypical melanocytes. The latter are situated predominantly along the basal layer of the epidermis, have irregular hyperchromatic nuclei and characteristically show marked cytoplasmic vacuo-lation (Fig. 7.127). Pigmentation is variable but in most instances is markedly increased and many involve adjacent keratinocytes, dermal macrophages (melanophages) and may sometimes be found within the keratin lamellae of the stratum corneum. Characteristically in lentigo maligna the atypical melanocytes involve the basal layers of hair follicles (Fig. 7.128). With progression of the lesion, clusters of atypical cells gather at the epidermo-dermal junction often adopting a spindle-cell form. Invasion is typically multifocal and the resultant tumour, lentigo maligna melanoma, most often has a spindle cell pattern.

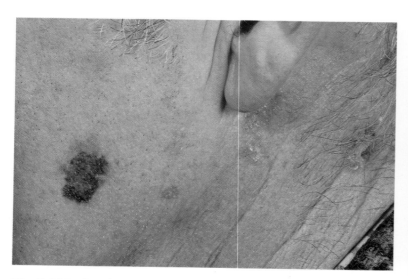

Fig. 7.122 Lentigo maligna. This patient had two basal cell carcinomata behind his ear in addition to the lentigo. Chronic solar irradiation is an important cause of this condition.

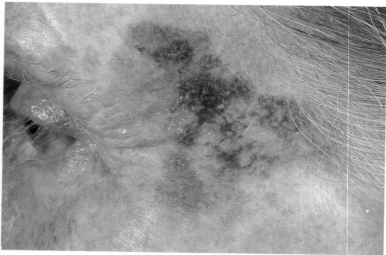

Fig. 7.123 Lentigo maligna. The lesion is made up of various colours and has an irregular indented margin. It grows slowly and may attain a large size before presentation.

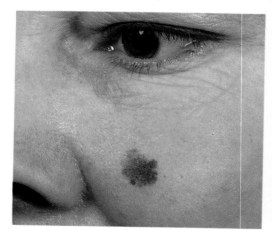

Fig. 7.124 Lentigo maligna. Although known as a condition of the elderly, this is now occurring more frequently in younger individuals. Note the irregular indented outline of the lesion.

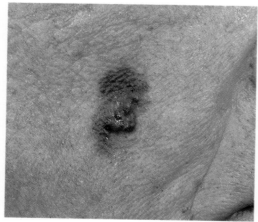

Fig. 7.125 Lentigo maligna melanoma. This lesion has become nodular.

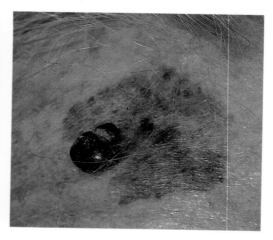

Fig. 7.126 Lentigo maligna melanoma. Eventually the lesion begins to grow vertically and invade the dermis. The lesion thickens and becomes nodular.

2. Superficial Spreading Malignant Melanoma

This is most probably the commonest sub-type of malignant melanoma (Figs. 7.129–132). If it is diagnosed early the prognosis is excellent with a 5 year survival in the order of 95%. It may be found anywhere on the integument but the torso and lower limbs are most frequently involved. It is a tumour predominantly

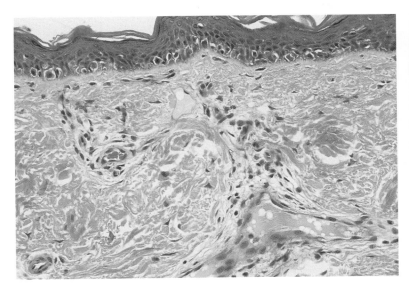

Fig. 7.127 Lentigo maligna. The epidermis is atrophic. Situated within the basal layer of the epithelium are atypical melanocytes having enlarged, irregular hyperchromatic nuclei and showing characteristic peri-nuclear vacuolation (a fixation artefact). Pigmentation which is variably increased also involves the adjacent keratinocytes. Solar elastosis is present.

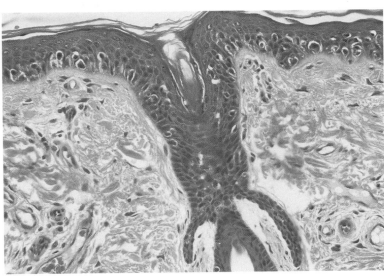

Fig. 7.128 Lentigo maligna. The atypical melanocytes are present in the basal layers of the superficial component of this hair follicle.

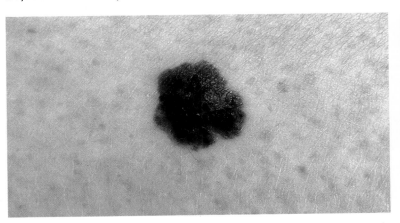

Fig. 7.129 Superficial malignant melanoma. The lesion is a slightly raised plaque with an irregular outline. It is black and brown in colour.

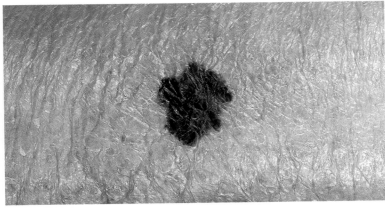

Fig. 7.130 Superficial malignant melanoma. The irregular indented and notched margin is clear.

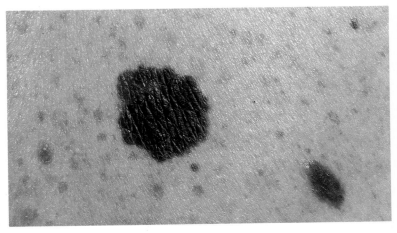

Fig. 7.131 Superficial malignant melanoma. The lesion is almost totally black except for a brown area at one edge. Note the surrounding lentigines from sun damage. The other mole was benign.

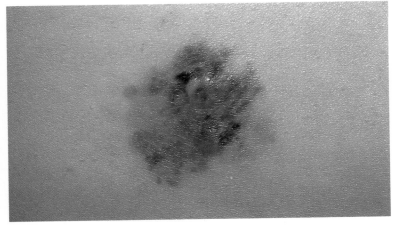

Fig. 7.132 Superficial malignant melanoma. The lesion is irregular in outline and colour. There are several pigmentary shades of which black is barely evident. Malignant melanomata are by no means always black.

of young adults. The tumour, which is raised just above the surface has an irregular outline and variable unevenly distributed pigmentation. Admixed with various shades of brown and black are foci of red, blue and purple coloration probably related to underlying vascular changes. As with lentigo maligna, areas of white and grey probably indicate sites of partial regression of the lesion. Ultimately the lesion grows vertically and a nodule (Fig. 7.133) develops. The lesion may then metastasize (Figs. 7.134–7.136).

The management of superficial spreading malignant melanoma is surgical. In most instances it is possible to make the diagnosis clinically but in any doubtful cases the lesion should be completely excised rather than biopsied. It has been the practice to excise these lesions widely and close the defect with a skin graft. However, primary excision with direct closure is now practised much more frequently by many plastic surgeons.

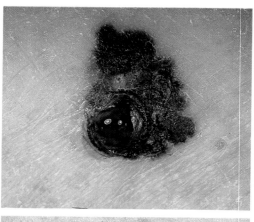

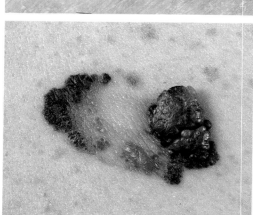

Fig. 7.133 Malignant melanoma. Vertical growth and deep invasion follows the horizontal spreading phase of superficial malignant melanoma.

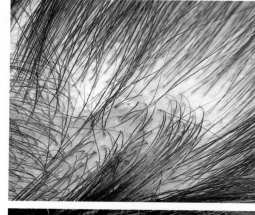

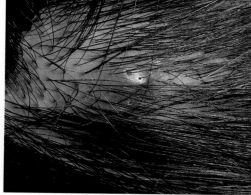

Fig. 7.134 Metastatic malignant melanoma. Grey-black nodules are present. The scalp is a common site. The primary was on the face.

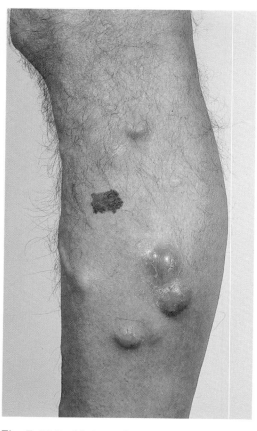

Fig. 7.135 Metastatic malignant melanoma. Hard, flesh and plum-coloured tumours have evolved from this man's neglected malignant melanoma. The leg is a common site for malignant melanomata.

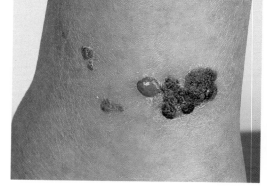

Fig. 7.136 Metastatic malignant melanoma. Local spread from this invading superficial malignant melanoma has produced a plum-coloured nodule as well as pigmented papules.

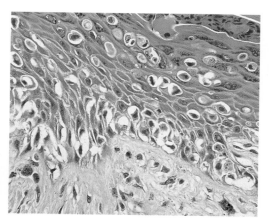

Fig. 7.137 Superficial spreading malignant melanoma (in situ). The appearances are quite dramatic. Scattered throughout all levels of the epidermis are large dysplastic melanocytes. Marked pigmentary incontinence is seen in the papillary dermis.

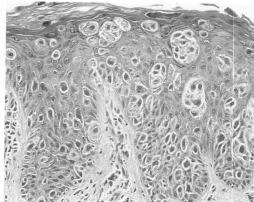

Fig. 7.138 Superficial spreading malignant melanoma. Clusters of 'pagetoid' melanocytes are present at all layers of the epidermis. Note the widely distributed melanin pigment (so-called 'buckshot scatter').

Histology

In contrast to lentigo maligna melanoma, superficial spreading malignant melanoma is not usually associated with features of severe actinic damage. Individual cells and clusters are irregularly distributed throughout the epidermis, often involving the upper layers in a pattern reminiscent of Paget's disease, hence its alternative designation of *Pagetoid melanoma* (Figs. 7.137 and 7.138). The cells are large with abundant cytoplasm and pleomorphic vesicular nuclei with prominent eosinophilic nucleoli. Pigmentation is variable but often it is marked. Tumour cells are found characteristically spreading from one epidermal ridge over a dermal papillae to the adjacent ridge. In cases of doubt this is a useful feature as benign lesions are typified by involvement of the epidermal ridges only. Invasive tumour is very common in the lesions of superficial spreading type and thus many sections should be examined before accepting a diagnosis of *in situ* melanoma. The infiltrating tumour is usually of the epithelioid cell type.

3. Acral Lentiginous Malignant Melanoma (Palmar-plantar-mucosal Melanoma)

This lesion begins in a manner similar to that of lentigo maligna (Fig. 7.139). However, it has a much more aggressive biological behaviour and vertical growth and metastases occur early on. It is an uncommon lesion that is initially flat with irregular margins and pigmentation, but soon becomes raised and subsequently nodular (Fig. 7.140). It occurs on the palms (Fig. 7.141) and soles (Fig. 7.142) and is the type of malignant melanoma to which orientals and negroes are prone. The lesion also occurs on the mucosa and extremities and, in particular, under the nail.

The clinical features of malignant melanoma arising from the nailbed are similar to those described for other sites (Fig. 7.143) but the nailplate becomes disrupted and split (Fig. 7.144) because of the growth of the tumour underneath. Acral lentiginous malignant melanoma is best managed surgically and in the case of malignant melanoma of the nailbed, amputation of the digit is the treatment of choice.

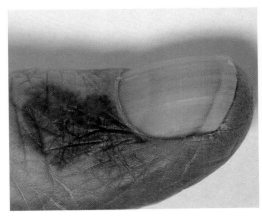

Fig. 7.139 Acral malignant melanoma. The clinical appearances are similar to those of Hutchinson's lentigo but this lesion grows much more quickly. By courtesy of Dr. A.C. Pembroke.

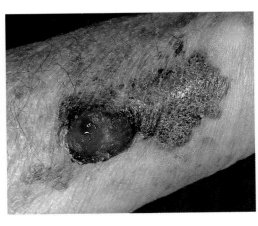

Fig. 7.140 Acral malignant melanoma. This nodule on the forearm has developed in an area of skin of similar appearance to lentigo maligna. However, they have a much more aggressive biological behaviour.

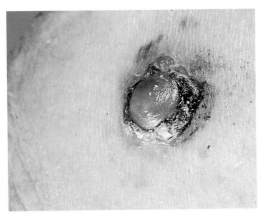

Fig. 7.141 Nodular acral malignant melanoma. These lesions bleed easily. The nodule has various colours including red which indicates vascular tissues. By courtesy of St. Mary's Hospital.

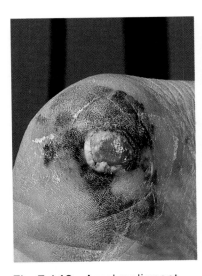

Fig. 7.142 Acral malignant melanoma. A nodule has occurred within a flat area of pigmentary variation and irregular outline. The sole of the foot is the classical site for this tumour.

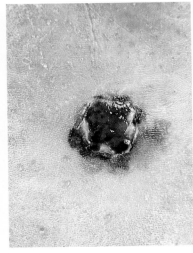

Fig. 7.143 Nodular acral malignant melanoma. These lesions also ulcerate. Note the irregularity of the outline and the shades of grey accompanying the overall sinister black appearance. By courtesy of St. Mary's Hospital.

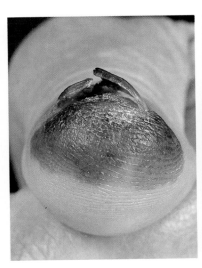
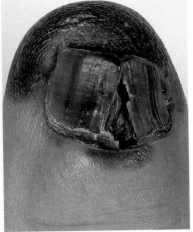

Fig. 7.144 Malignant melanoma of the nailbed. The lesion has an irregular outline and its colours vary from black to grey and blue. As it invades, the lesion distorts and splits the nailplate. By courtesy of Dr. A.C. Pembroke.

Histology

The features are similar to those of lentigo maligna except that the epidermis is hyperplastic. The most common variant is typified by atypical melanocytes situated predominantly along the basal aspect of the epidermis, although the higher reaches including stratum corneum may also be involved. Individual cells are pleomorphic with hyperchromatic nuclei and conspicuous nucleoli (Fig. 7.145). Mitotic figures are frequent. Nest formation with both epithelioid and spindle cell forms is common but a true Pagetoid variant is much less common than the lentiginous form. Similarly nodular melanoma may rarely be the mode of presentation of the acral lentiginous variant.

4. Nodular Malignant Melanoma

This lesion does not appear to have a horizontal growth phase but grows quickly and vertically from its inception (Figs. 7.146 and 7.147). The lesion is raised, nodular and sometimes ulcerated. The outline of the lesion may be irregular and its colour varied as described for the other varieties of malignant melanoma. Occasionally the tumour has no apparent visible pigmentation – so-called *amelanotic malignant melanoma* (Fig. 7.148). In such instances, however, careful inspection may reveal a minute focus of pigmentation at the edge of the nodule. Malignant nodular melanoma may occur on any area of the body and usually diagnosis is not difficult. It has a much worse prognosis than the superficial spreading type because of the speed at which it evolves and the depth of penetration so often reached.

Nodular melanoma should be widely excised and grafted. If adjacent lymph nodes are palpable they should be cleared. There is no accepted successful treatment for metastatic disease at the present time. In such instances, the patient should be referred to centres specializing in its management. Various regimens of combined chemotherapeutic agents are used as well as local perfusion of affected regions with cytotoxic drugs.

Histology

Nodular melanoma is by definition a lesion in which there is no evidence of an adjacent intra-epidermal lesion of either lentigo maligna, acral lentiginous or superficial spreading sub-types (Figs. 7.149 and 7.150). As nodular melanoma has such a poor prognosis it is essential that numerous sections are examined before such a diagnosis is accepted. The histological features of invasive melanoma arising within any of the above sub-types are similar and are thus considered together in the following section.

Invasive malignant melanoma is associated with junctional activity (Fig. 7.151) and varying proportions of epidermal and dermal infiltration. Although traditionally the tumour cells are classified into epithelioid and spindle cell types, with the former

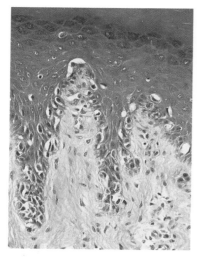

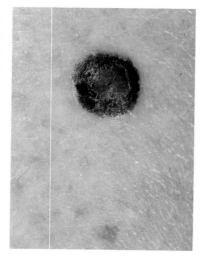

Fig. 7.145 Acral lentiginous malignant melanoma. Note the prominent epidermal ridge pattern with basally located atypical melanocytes showing conspicuous vacuolation. There is dermal fibrosis (lesion from sole of foot).

Fig. 7.146 Nodular malignant melanoma. This lesion grows vertically from the beginning and invasion produces a nodule. Note the surrounding lentigines.

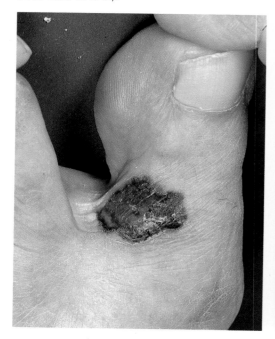

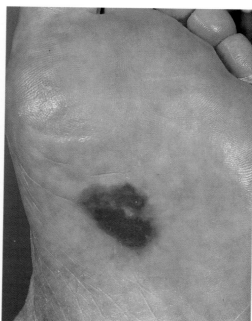

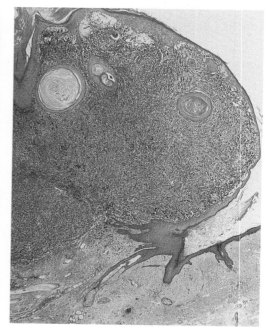

Fig. 7.147 Nodular malignant melanoma. This black nodule represents the classic conception of a malignant melanoma and could hardly fail to be diagnosed. The prognosis for these lesions is grim and yet diagnosis of the less obvious lesions at an earlier stage may be life-saving.

Fig. 7.148 Amelanotic malignant melanoma. This is a rare occurrence. The lesion is a plum-coloured nodule and although the tumorous nature of the lesion may suggest malignant disease, its precise nature may not be suspected.

Fig. 7.149 Nodular melanoma. The epidermis is elevated into a pedunculated nodule by this heavily pigmented tumour. Note the presence of accompanying squamous epithelial proliferation with the formation of superficial horn cysts.

most often being associated with superficial spreading and nodular variants and the latter being particularly seen with lentigo maligna melanoma and acral lentiginous melanoma, many tumours are composed of a mixture of the two cell types.

A typical melanoma is characterized by pleomorphic tumour cells infiltrating the epidermis (which may often be ulcerated) and extending to a varying degree into the dermis. The cells may have abundant cytoplasm and large nuclei with eosinophilic nucleoli (epithelioid type) or adopt a spindle cell form (Figs. 7.152 and 7.153). Examples of the latter, particularly amelanotic variants may be confused with other spindle cell tumours if an origin from the epidermis is not recognized. In such instances the use of a Masson-Fontana reaction may reveal small traces of pigment not detected with routine haematoxylin and eosin stained preparations. Tumours may sometimes show marked pleomorphism with giant cell forms and abundant, often atypical mitotic figures (Fig. 7.154). In cases where the diagnosis of malignancy versus benignancy is uncertain the finding of mitoses in the dermal component of a melanocytic lesion (excepting juvenile melanoma) is an absolute diagnostic indicator of malignant melanoma. This feature may be of particular value in those lesions that appear to have arisen in a previously benign melanocytic naevus. Pigmentation is variable but in many examples it is very heavy, being present both within malignant melanocytes and melanophages. An important feature which must be carefully recorded in each case is the presence or absence of a lymphocytic infiltrate along the lower border of the lesion. Its presence may be associated with a better prognosis.

In all cases of invasive melanoma both the tumour thickness (Breslow) and depth of invasion should be assessed. The depth of invasion should be recorded according to Clark's levels viz.

Level 1 *in situ* malignant melanoma
Level 2 infiltration of papillary dermis
Level 3 infiltration to the level of the papillary/reticular dermis interface
Level 4 infiltration of the reticular dermis
Level 5 infiltration of the subcutaneous fat

Tumour thickness should be measured from the most superficial aspect of the granular cell layer to the point of maximum depth of invasion or in those instances where ulceration is present, from the surface of the ulcerated area to the deepest extent of infiltration. In general those tumours with a thickness of less than 0.76mm have a very good outcome, those greater than 1.5mm being associated with a much poorer prognosis.

A complete report on a malignant melanoma should therefore include the histogenetic sub-type, the level of invasion, the tumour thickness, the presence or absence of a lymphocytic infiltrate and an assessment of the mitotic activity of the tumour (mitotic rate recorded as the number of mitotic figures identified per five high power fields using a x 300, wide field objective).

Patients with malignant melanoma should be monitored for the rest of their lives and examined for local recurrence, metastasis and fresh malignant disease (Fig. 7.155). They should be advised regarding photoprotection.

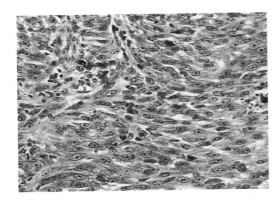

Fig. 7.150 Nodular melanoma. The adjacent epithelium is characteristically free from any *in situ* melanocytic lesion. Note the presence of solar elastosis on the right side of the picture.

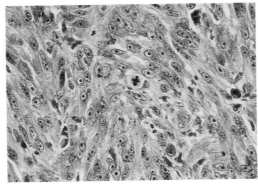

Fig. 7.151 Nodular melanoma. Conspicuous junctional activity is present.

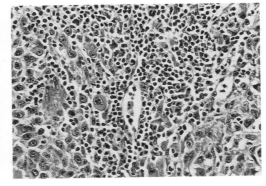

Fig. 7.152 Nodular melanoma. Epithelioid cells predominate in this field. They are large with abundant pink cytoplasm and vesicular nuclei, often with conspicuous darkly staining nucleoli. Note the presence of a lymphocytic infiltrate.

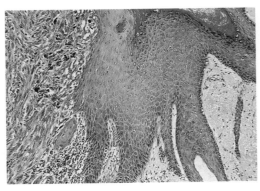

Fig. 7.153 Nodular melanoma. In this field a predominantly spindle cell pattern is evident. Pigmentation is marked.

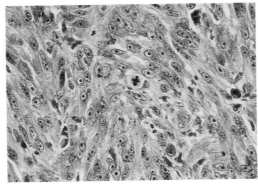

Fig. 7.154 Nodular melanoma. Note the quadri-polar mitotic figure in the centre of the picture.

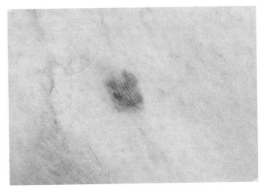

Fig. 7.155 A second malignant melanoma. During follow-up of the patient in Fig. 7.133 (upper), a second very early malignant melanoma developed. Histologically it was confined to the epidermis.

XERODERMA PIGMENTOSUM

This extremely rare disorder is of particular importance because it sheds some light on the mechanisms involved in the induction of cutaneous malignant tumours. It has an autosomal recessive mode of inheritance and is characterized by extreme photosensitivity and a tendency to develop malignant skin tumours at an early age. Neurological abnormalities may also occur in some patients. The disease is due to an inability to repair damage which normally occurs to epidermal DNA following ultra-violet light irradiation. There is failure of enzymatic excision of thymine dimers which result from irradiation of thymidine base pairs in DNA.

Xeroderma pigmentosum presents as severe sunburn (Fig. 7.156) on the exposed parts on the first occasion that the infant is outside on a sunny day. This photosensitivity is followed by the development of masses of freckles on the exposed areas of the skin (Fig. 7.157). Subsequently solar keratoses, basal cell carcinomata, squamous cell carcinomata, keratoacanthomata (Fig. 7.158) and malignant melanomata supervene. Death before the end of adolescence was considered the norm. However, with obsessional avoidance of ultra-violet light combined with the application of sun-blocking agents and close supervision of the skin with a view to early diagnosis and treatment of malignant tumours, the prognosis of this otherwise grim disease has somewhat improved.

X-IRRADIATION OF THE SKIN

Cutaneous X-irradiation results in atrophy, scarring, telangi-ectasia and pigmentary abnormalities (Fig. 7.159); so-called *radiodermatitis*. Over-irradiation of the skin may result in ulceration (Fig. 7.160) and exposure of deep structures. Basal or squamous cell carcinomata may ensue after several decades. Thus, irradiation was a procedure commonly used for the treatment of scalp ringworm in children until 1959 when griseofulvin became available. Over-irradiation caused permanent alopecia due to scarring, and several decades later malignancy sometimes ensued (Fig. 7.161). Irradiation is now very rarely used for the treatment of benign conditions of the skin. Careless use of X-ray equipment may result in radiodermatitis (Fig. 7.162).

Histology

The effects of chronic radiation damage to the integument include most importantly the development of cutaneous neoplasia. The epidermis is hyperkeratotic and variably acanthotic and atrophic (Fig. 7.163). It may show the features of solar (radiation) keratoses and be the site of origin of basal cell and squamous cell carcinomata. The latter may cause particular diagnostic difficulties as it is often of a poorly differentiated anaplastic type (Fig. 7.164). The dermis is typically fibrosed and homogenized (Fig. 7.165) and while superficially telangiectatic vessels are the rule, in its deeper aspects endarteritis obliterans is a common feature (Fig. 7.166). Although spindle cell sarcomatous conditions have been reported as a feature of chronic radiation dermatitis it is more likely that most, if not all, represent spindle cell squamous carcinomata.

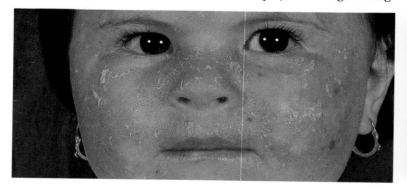

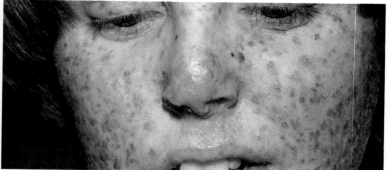

Fig. 7.156 Xeroderma pigmentosum. Extreme photosensitivity is the key feature of this condition. Persistent erythema occurs after seemingly innocent solar exposure.

Fig. 7.157 Xeroderma pigmentosum. Permanent freckling of exposed skin quickly ensues. This patient developed her first squamous cell carcinoma at the age of two.

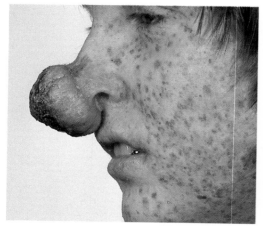

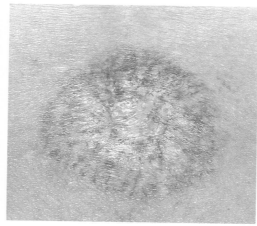

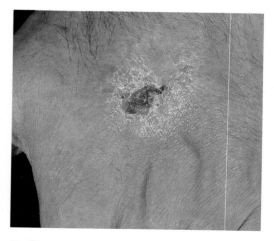

Fig. 7.158 Xeroderma pigmentosum. Malignant change occurs early in life. This keratoacanthoma developed in a 12-year-old girl. The lesion did, however, resolve spontaneously.

Fig. 7.159 Radiodermatitis. Irradiation of the skin results in atrophy, scarring and telangiectasia.

Fig. 7.160 Radionecrosis. Ulceration has occurred secondary to inappropriate irradiation of Bowen's disease on the back of the hand.

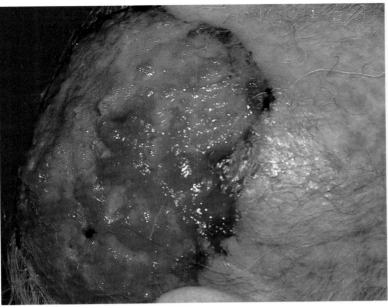

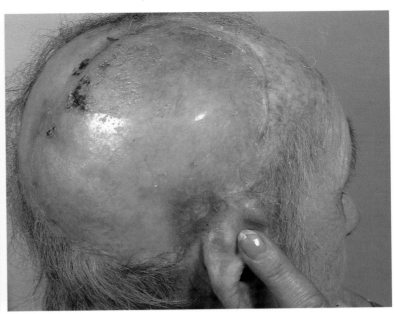

Fig. 7.161 Radiation-induced malignant disease. A basal cell carcinoma developed on this lady's scalp 60 years after irradiation of tinea capitis as a child. She has always had alopecia following the overirradiation. The lesion was successfully excised (right). By courtesy of Mr.J.P. Bennett.

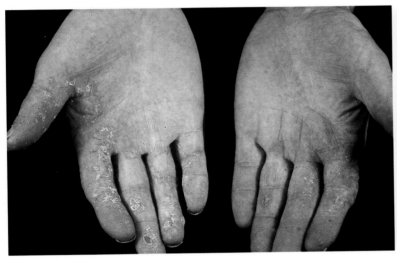

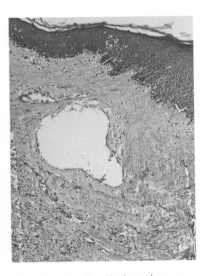

Fig. 7.162 Radiodermatitis in a dentist. Careless use of X-ray equipment resulted in radiodermatitis of the skin of the hands, a common occurrence in radiologists before the hazards of X-rays were appreciated. By courtesy of Dr. A. Warin, St. John's Hospital for Diseases of the Skin.

Fig. 7.163 Radiation dermatitis. There is acanthosis. The dermis is fibrosed and contains telangiectatic blood vessels.

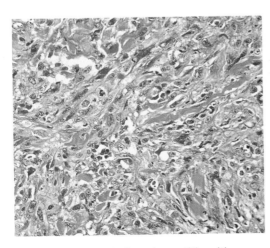

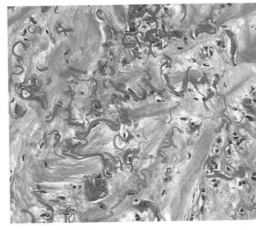

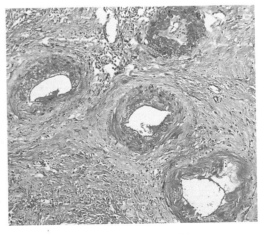

Fig. 7.164 Radiation dermatitis with anaplastic carcinoma. The dermis is infiltrated by a highly undifferentiated malignant tumour composed of pleomorphic cells with irregular nuclei.

Fig. 7.165 Radiation dermatitis. This field shows dermal fibrosis, elastosis and occasional bizarre post-irradiation fibroblasts. The latter may be a cause of diagnostic confusion for the unwary.

Fig. 7.166 Radiation dermatitis. Conspicuous vascular changes are evident.

7.35

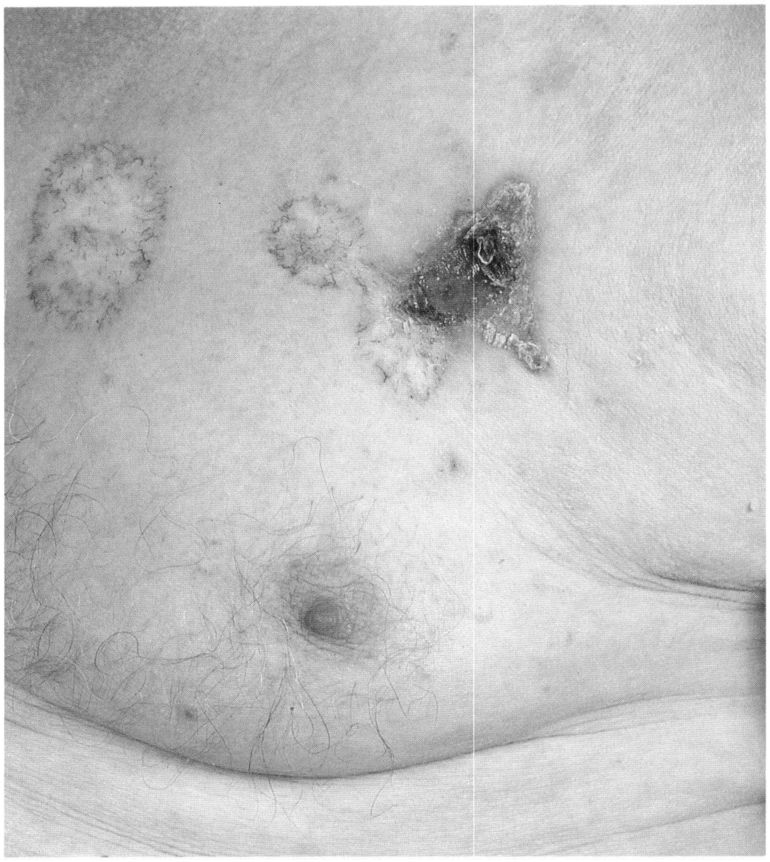

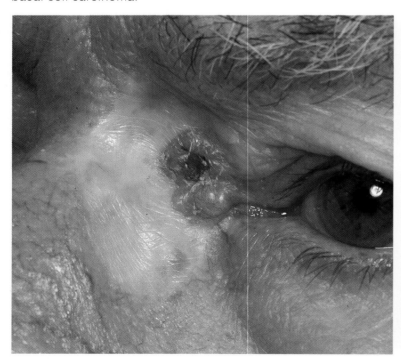

Fig. 7.167 Management of cutaneous malignant disease. Recurrence of superficial basal cell carcinoma after irradiation. Cutaneous malignant disease should be managed in a joint clinic. Irradiation is not the treatment of choice for superficial basal cell carcinoma.

MANAGEMENT OF CUTANEOUS MALIGNANT DISEASE

Diagnosis is often the initial problem so that it is appropriate to refer the patient to a dermatologist. Morphoeic basal cell carcinomata, superficial basal cell carcinomata, Bowen's disease and superficial spreading malignant melanomata are the most frequently misdiagnosed lesions. Seborrhoeic warts, especially those which have bled, are those most commonly suspected as malignant melanomata by the general practitioner. The dermatologist has facilities for immediate biopsy or exfoliative cytology, has liquid nitrogen available for the treatment of solar keratoses, and is experienced in the use of 5-fluorouracil. Equally, the dermatologist usually has a joint clinic with a radiotherapist (Fig. 7.167) and a plastic surgeon where a decision may be made as to the appropriate therapy for the individual patient concerned. Specific referral to a general surgeon or radiotherapist by a general practitioner is an implied decision to treat accordingly. Complete irradication of the disease is mandatory. The plastic surgeon has the special skills to excise completely and either close primarily or repair the defect with an appropriate graft or flap. These skills are not usually possessed by the general surgeon (Figs. 7.168 and 7.169). Radiotherapy is often more appropriate in the elderly and may produce better cosmetic results in certain sites than surgery. Equally, the radiotherapist has the oncological skills to deal with metastatic disease. Thus, a combined approach to the management of cutaneous malignant disease is appropriate.

Patients who have had a malignancy of the skin should be followed for life. This is probably best done by the dermatologist. New lesions are common and can therefore be diagnosed and treated early if the skin is adequately supervised. In addition, advice regarding photoprotection and the appropriate use of sunscreens with a high protection factor may prevent further damage.

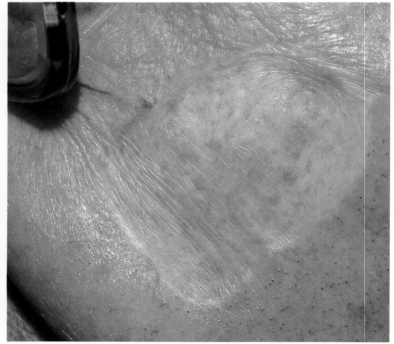

Fig. 7.168 Recurrence of basal cell carcinoma in a skin graft. Cutaneous malignant disease should be managed in a combined clinic of dermatologist, plastic surgeon and radiotherapist. The average general surgeon does not have the skills of a plastic surgeon and serious recurrences may occur.

Fig. 7.169 Management of cutaneous malignant disease. The specialized surgery of cutaneous malignant disease should be managed by a plastic surgeon, otherwise poor cosmetic results may occur.

8 Mycosis Fungoides and Allied Conditions

Anthony du Vivier MD, FRCP

Phillip H. McKee MB BCh, BaO, MRC Path

The important lymphomas which present primarily in the skin are mycosis fungoides and the Sézary syndrome. In the majority of patients mycosis fungoides remains in the skin such that some authorities regard it as a reactive process which only occasionally becomes malignant and spreads to the lymphoreticular system. Others believe it to be a malignant process throughout its course. The Sézary syndrome is an erythroderma with so many features in common with mycosis fungoides that it is believed to be a leukaemic overspill of this condition. Because of abnormalities in thymus-derived lymphocytes found in these and other related disorders, the conditions are sometimes grouped together and called cutaneous T-cell lymphomas. However, this term does not convey anything concerning the natural history of a particular process, so the old terminology is retained here.

Non-Hodgkin's lymphoma usually affects the skin only incidentally, long after it is well-established in lymph nodes and other organs. However, occasionally it may present and remain in the skin for a limited period before becoming systematized. Leukaemia, equally, may occasionally deposit in the skin but the primary disease is active elsewhere. Hodgkin's disease very rarely presents in the skin although cutaneous complications are frequent.

There are some rare conditions which, very occasionally, are associated with either mycosis fungoides or lymphoma. These, viz. actinic reticuloid, follicular mucinosis and lymphomatoid papulosis are mentioned because they are distinctive and serve to illustrate the complexity of the clinical picture. Finally, Jessner's lymphocytic infiltrate and lymphocytoma cutis are described. These conditions present as purple nodules, papules or plaques in the skin, that is, in a manner simulating the clinical appearances of lymphoma and yet, although having a pronounced lymphocytic infiltrate of the skin, are entirely benign.

LYMPHOMAS PRESENTING PRIMARILY IN THE SKIN
Mycosis Fungoides

Mycosis fungoides is a rare condition in either sex, which can present at any age. It shows great variation in behaviour, ranging from a very slowly progressive disorder, which is not life-threatening, to an aggressive disease resulting in tumours on the skin and involvement of the liver, spleen, lymph nodes and other organs, resulting in death. It was given the name mycosis fungoides in 1835 by Alibert because of the mushroom-like tumours which arose in the late stages of the disease (Fig 8.1).

The *pre-mycotic stage* begins as barely palpable patches on the trunk and limbs. The patches are pink or red and may easily be mistaken for eczema or psoriasis (Fig. 8.2). However, the lesions do not respond to the standard treatment for these diseases and it is this lack of response which may, in itself, suggest the diagnosis. The lesions become widespread (Fig. 8.3) on the trunk and limbs. The patches tend to be asymmetrical and vary in colour and in shape (Fig. 8.4). Thus, they may be pink or various shades of red, which become darker as the condition progresses. The shapes of the lesions may be quite angulated (Fig. 8.5) and bizarre (Fig. 8.6), rather than just round or oval (Fig. 8.7). In addition, their surface may be scaly and sometimes wrinkled and atrophic (Fig. 8.8). The term *'parapsoriasis en plaque'* is sometimes

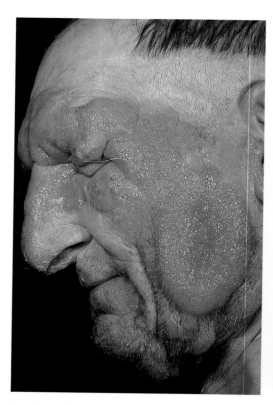

Fig. 8.1 Mycosis fungoides. Alibert gave the name of mycosis fungoides to a disease which may eventuate in mushroom-like tumours on the skin.

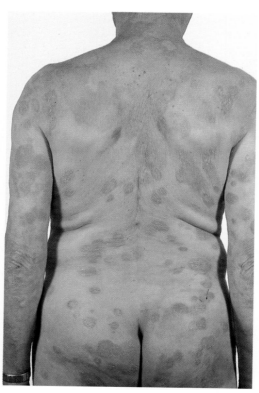

Fig. 8.2 Mycosis fungoides. Widespread lesions simulating psoriasis are present. However, the lesions are asymmetrical which is unusual for psoriasis. Skin biopsy confirmed the diagnosis. By courtesy of Dr. A.C. Pembroke.

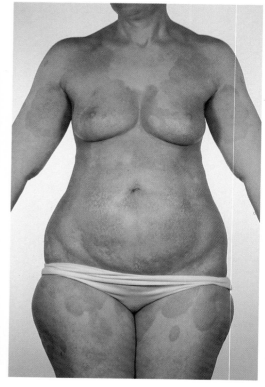

Fig. 8.3 Mycosis fungoides. Widespread patches occur on the trunk and limbs. The lesions are asymmetrical.

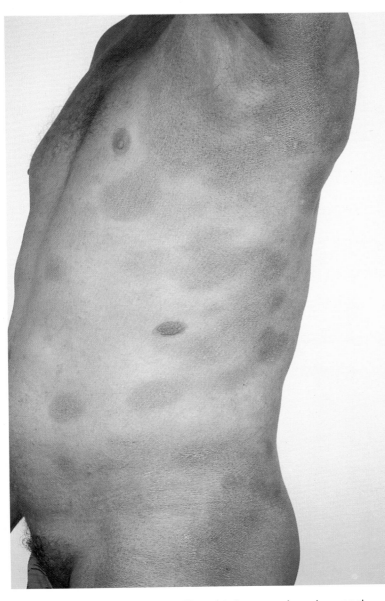

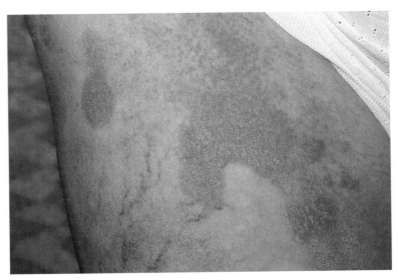

Fig. 8.5 Mycosis fungoides. Some lesions are strangely indented and angulated.

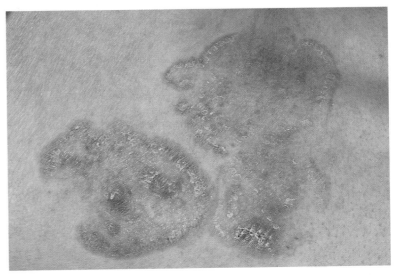

Fig. 8.4 Mycosis fungoides. The patches vary in colour and shape. There is considerable post-inflammatory hyperpigmentation in all the lesions because the patient was partly of Indian origin.

Fig. 8.6 Mycosis fungoides. The eruption may have quite bizarre shapes.

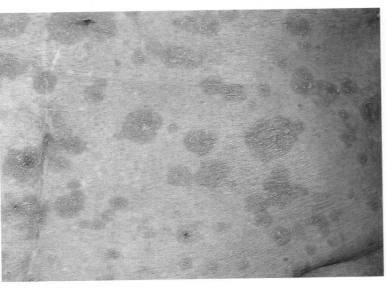

Fig. 8.7 Mycosis fungoides. The lesions are various shapes and sizes. This early stage is sometimes known as parapsoriasis en plaque.

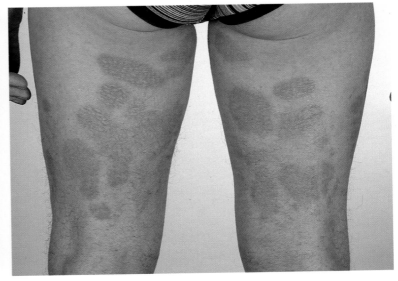

Fig. 8.8 Mycosis fungoides. Several skin biopsies may be necessary to establish the diagnosis of this early stage of parapsoriasis en plaque. The variety of shapes, of sizes and asymmetry of the lesions suggest the mycotic stage clinically. The lesions have an atrophic, wrinkled appearance.

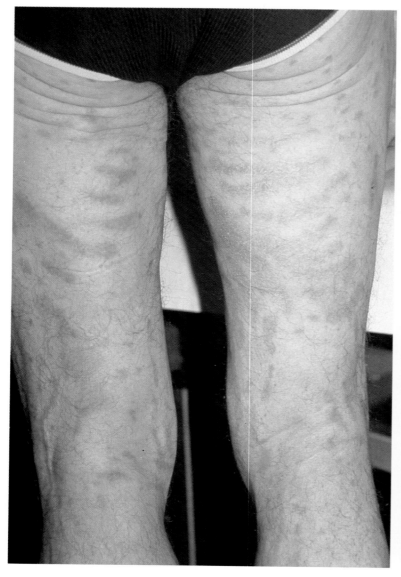

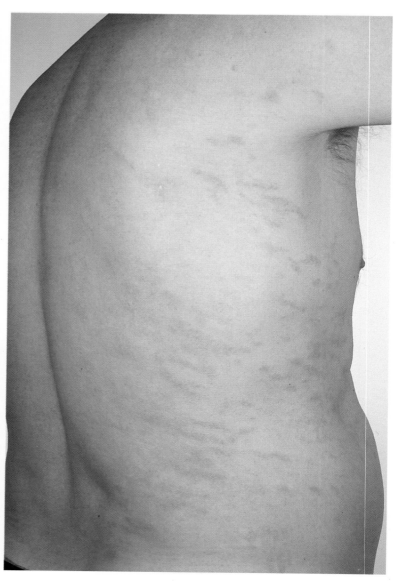

Fig. 8.9 Digitate dermatosis. Finger-like processes of constant colour and size occur. The lesions are symmetrical. This variety of parapsoriasis is benign and usually never progresses to mycosis fungoides.

Fig. 8.10 Digitate dermatosis (chronic superficial scaly dermatosis). This condition is also known as parapsoriasis en plaque benign (or small) type. Symmetrical finger-like processes occur on the trunk and limbs.

Fig. 8.11 Poikiloderma. This is a pre-mycotic sign. Atrophy and telangiectasia occur in a network pattern. The breast is a common site.

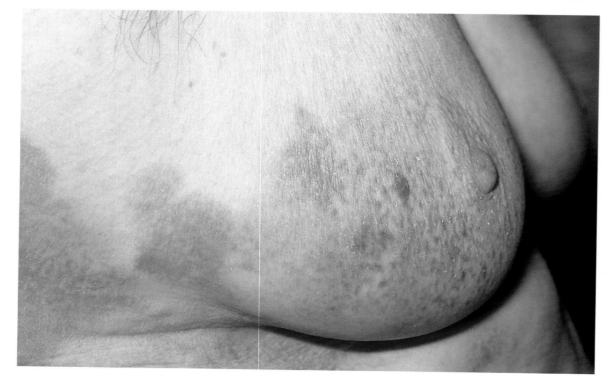

used interchangeably with this appearance of the skin. The matter is complicated because of a condition of the same name which very rarely ever progresses to true mycosis fungoides and which has a non-specific histology. It is known as 'parapsoriasis en plaque benign (or small) type' or 'digitate dermatosis' or 'chronic superficial scaly dermatosis'. It has a distinctive clinical pattern of symmetrical (Fig. 8.9), well circumscribed, oval or finger-like (Fig. 8.10) (hence digitate) processes on the skin of the trunk and limbs. The lesions are flat or just palpable and have a red, pink or yellow-orange hue. The eruption begins in middle-age and is persistent but responds temporarily to ultra-violet light, both natural and artificial, including PUVA.

A readily identifiable pre-mycotic appearance of the skin is poikiloderma. This is characterized by telangiectasia, atrophy and a combination of hyper- and hypopigmentation of the skin. One or a limited number of patches may occur, particularly over the breasts (Fig. 8.11) or buttocks (Fig. 8.12) within a framework of pre-mycotic lesions, as previously described or, alternatively, the whole eruption is made up of these poikilodermatous patches and the condition is known as poikiloderma atrophicans et vasculare (Figs. 8.13 and 8.14).

Very occasionally, solitary patches of mycosis fungoides occur (Fig. 8.15). A skin biopsy is necessary for confirmation of the diagnosis.

As the condition progresses, the lesions become more infiltrated. This 'infiltrative' stage is relatively easy to diagnose. The lesions are palpable and thickened and deeper in colour (Fig. 8.16). They often become intolerably pruritic.

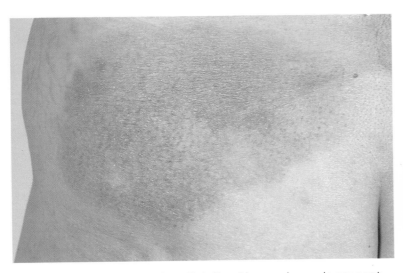

Fig. 8.12 Poikiloderma. A well-defined large plaque is present over the buttock, a common site. There is pronounced telangiectasia. By courtesy of St. Mary's Hospital.

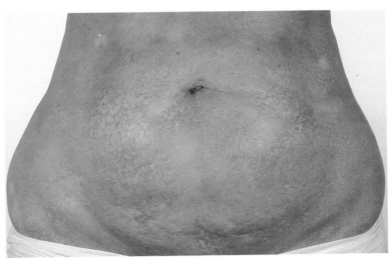

Fig. 8.13 Poikiloderma. Stippled telangiectatic patches occur in addition to conventional patches of mycosis fungoides.

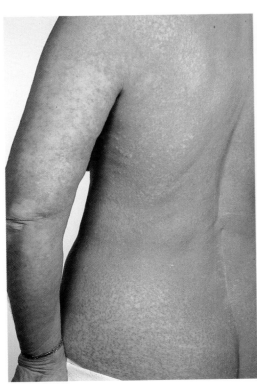

Fig. 8.14 Poikiloderma atrophicans et vasculare. Very occasionally the whole eruption has the features of poikiloderma.

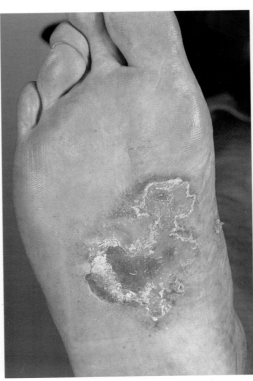

Fig. 8.15 Mycosis fungoides. Solitary patches very rarely occur. Skin biopsy is required for the correct diagnosis of mycosis fungoides.

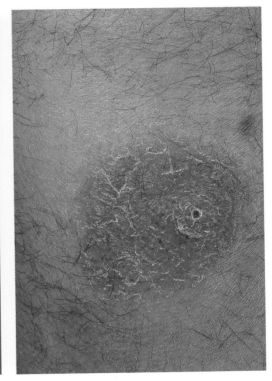

Fig. 8.16 Mycosis fungoides. A deep red colour results as the lesions become more infiltrated.

Ultimately, the 'tumorous' stage develops. The lesions are of a red-brown or purple colour (Fig. 8.17) and consist of nodules (Figs. 8.18 and 8.19) or thickened plaques or ulcers (Fig. 8.20).

The progress from minimally infiltrative plaques to the tumour stage may take a lifetime or may never occur at all. On the other hand, it may take only a few years. The development of tumours is an ominous sign and the likelihood of involvement of lymph nodes (Fig. 8.21), liver, spleen and other organs is increased. Patients then succumb to the consequences of obstruction or overwhelming infection.

Histology

Mycosis fungoides is a malignant tumour of T-lymphocytes of lymph node derivation (Fig. 8.22). The cells show a remarkable tendency to colonize the epidermis (epidermotrophism). In earlier stages of the disease they are recognized as medium sized (<12μm) cells with an irregular hyperchromatic nucleus (Lutzner cells). They may be present in both the dermis and epidermis: in the latter situation they may be distributed singly or in clumps. To a lesser extent in early lesions and much more obviously so in later stages, much larger cells (15–30μm) with highly convoluted (cerebriform), hyperchromatic nuclei become apparent (mycosis Sézary cells). While such cells are present in abundance in the peripheral blood in Sézary syndrome (Fig. 8.23), they may also be similarly detected (although in smaller numbers) in a minority of patients with mycosis fungoides. It must be stressed, however, that small numbers of these cells may sometimes be present in both the lesions and bloodstream of patients with a number of quite benign dermatoses including lichen planus and lupus erythematosus. Electron-microscopically they are characterized by multi-lobed, convoluted nuclei with peripheral chromatin margination (Figs. 8.24 and 8.25).

Recent studies have shown that most of the malignant cells in the infiltrate bear OKT4 (helper-inducer) markers. A much smaller proportion of cells bear OKT8 (suppressor-cytotoxic) markers. Langerhan's cells are almost invariably present within the infiltrate. Recent concepts of the pathogenesis of mycosis fungoides suggest that the condition may develop as a consequence of antigen persistence, resulting in increased nodal production of OKT4 lymphocytes, which return to the epidermis with eventual malignant transformation. There is some evidence to suggest that persistent infection of Langerhan's cells by Human T-cell leukaemia/lymphoma virus with resultant OKT4 lymphocyte proliferation may be responsible.

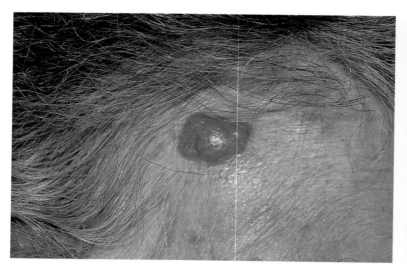

Fig. 8.17 Tumour stage mycosis fungoides. Red-coloured nodules occur as the disease progresses. The prognosis becomes guarded at this stage.

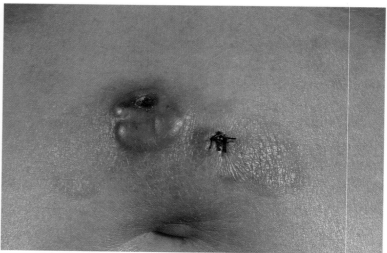

Fig. 8.18 Tumour stage mycosis fungoides. A tumour has arisen on a background of plaque mycosis fungoides. The lesion is plum-coloured.

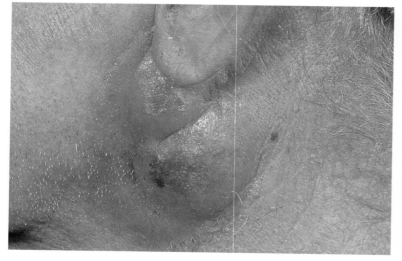

Fig. 8.19 Tumour stage mycosis fungoides. A large tumorous mass is present. The patient had widespread infiltrated plaques elsewhere (see Fig. 8.2). By courtesy of Dr. A.C. Pembroke.

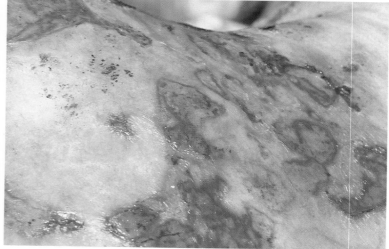

Fig. 8.20 Ulcerative mycosis fungoides. Very occasionally ulcerative lesions occur. The lesions responded to PUVA but ultimately the patient succumbed.

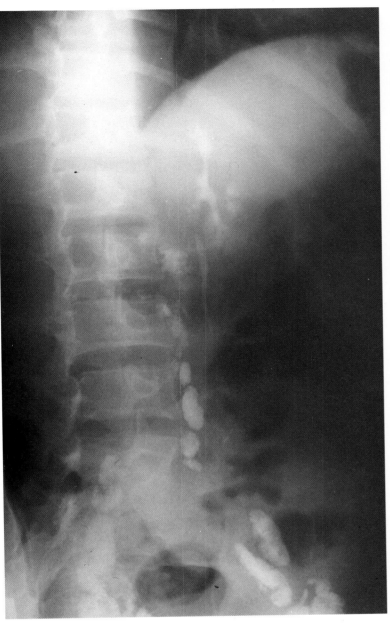

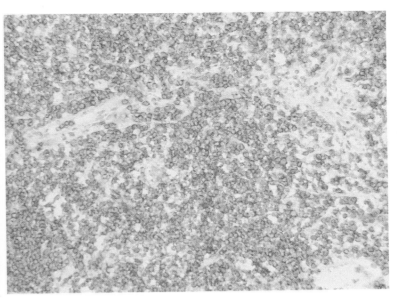

Fig. 8.22 Tumour stage mycosis fungoides. The infiltrate is positively labelled with anti leu 4 (a pan T cell marker).

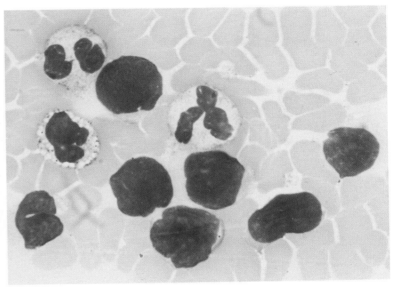

Fig. 8.21 Lymph node involvement. Ultimately lymph node involvement occurs and the patient may develop obstructive features. This man had massive lymphoedema of his leg, before he died of overwhelming infection.

Fig. 8.23 Mycosis/Sézary cells. Cerebriform, hyperchromatic nuclei are present in this peripheral blood smear (Giemsa stain).

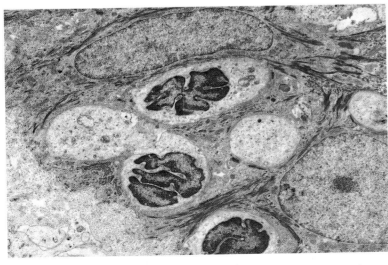

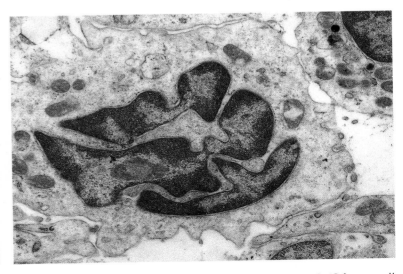

Fig. 8.24 Mycosis fungoides. This electronphotomicrograph shows epidermis (upper) and superficial papillary dermis. The squamous epithelium is infiltrated by three typical mycosis/Sézary cells.

Fig. 8.25 Mycosis fungoides. Characteristic mycosis/Sézary cell with abundant cytoplasm and a centrally located, irregular, highly convoluted nucleus with a peripheral chromatin distribution.

8.7

Biopsies (particularly of the punch-type) of the early, pre-mycotic (patch) stage may not necessarily always be diagnostic and therefore it is recommended that for these lesions an adequate surgical specimen is submitted to the laboratory. The epidermis may be normal or slightly thickened and show ortho-

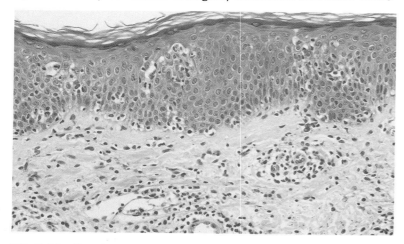

Fig. 8.26 Patch stage mycosis fungoides. There is mild hyperkeratosis overlying a slightly thickened epidermis. The latter is diffusely infiltrated by mononuclear cells with irregular, hyperchromatic nuclei and surrounded by a clear vacuole. A chronic inflammatory cell infiltrate is present around the superficial blood vessels.

hyperkeratosis. Scattered singly or in clusters are collections of mononuclear lymphoid cells, often surrounded by a clear halo (Fig. 8.26). While classical mycosis cells may be apparent (Fig. 8.27), more often than not they are either very few in number or not detectable. In the dermis, pigmentary incontinence may be a feature and a lympho-histiocytic infiltrate surrounds the blood vessels of the superficial plexus. In areas the infiltrate may adopt a lichenoid distribution. As with the epidermal component, mycosis cells may be sparse or absent. By way of contrast, chronic superficial dermatitis is characterized by a spongiotic process (Fig. 8.28) and therefore should *not* be mistaken histologically for the patch stage.

The features of plaque stage mycosis fungoides are merely an exaggeration of those described above. The epidermis is often acanthotic, sometimes adopting a psoriasiform appearance (Fig. 8.29), and there may be marked superficial crusting. The infiltrate is much more intense and large numbers of mononuclears are present in the epidermis (Fig. 8.30). While many of these cells do not show obvious atypicality, invariably numbers of large, hyperchromatic and irregular nuclei will be identified. These may be present singly or accompanied by collections of smaller lymphocytes to form the intra-epithelial Pautrier micro-abscesses (Fig. 8.31). In addition to the epidermis, adnexal, particularly hair-follicle, epithelium may be involved. The dermis, which is sometimes fibrosed, contains a dense, sometimes lichenoid infiltrate which, in addition to lymphoid cells, may

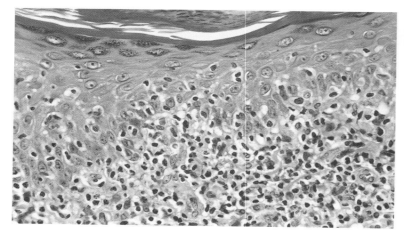

Fig. 8.27 Patch stage mycosis fungoides – a rather more advanced lesion. There is parakeratosis, hyper-orthokeratosis and acanthosis. The epidermis and dermis are diffusely infiltrated by large numbers of cells with highly irregular, darkly staining nuclei (mycosis cells).

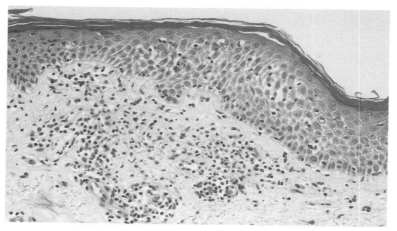

Fig. 8.28 Chronic superficial dermatitis. The epidermis is focally infiltrated by lymphocytes with associated intercellular oedema (spongiosis). A perivascular lympho-histiocytic infiltrate is present in the superficial dermis.

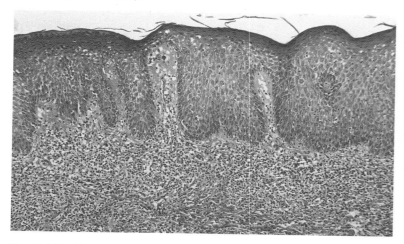

Fig. 8.29 Plaque stage mycosis fungoides. The epidermis shows psoriasiform hyperplasia. In addition to epithelial involvement, a dense cellular infiltrate occupies both papillary and reticular dermis.

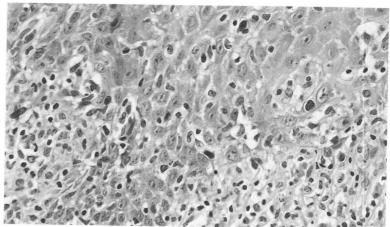

Fig. 8.30 Plaque stage mycosis fungoides. This high power view shows atypical mononuclear cells and several pleomorphic mycosis cells in the epidermis.

also contain eosinophils, histiocytes etc. (Figs. 8.32 and 8.33).

In tumorous mycosis fungoides, dense infiltrates occupy both the dermis and subcutaneous fat. Typically, pleomorphism is much more marked so that confusion with other lymphomatous processes, especially Hodgkin's disease, becomes a distinct possibility (Fig. 8.34).

Poikiloderma atrophicans vasculare is an important pre-reticulotic condition. Histologically it is characterized by hyperkeratosis, epidermal atrophy, basal cell liquefactive degeneration and a lichenoid or perivascular superficial dermal inflammatory cell infiltrate (Fig. 8.35). Variable numbers of small, hyperchromatic, irregular lymphocytes are to be found in the epithelium and dermis. Pigmentary incontinence may be a feature and telangiectatic vessels are commonly found (Fig. 8.36).

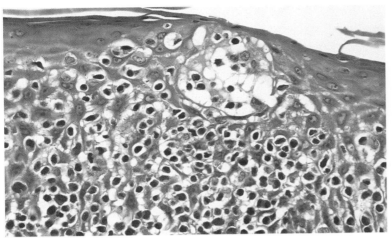

Fig. 8.31 Plaque stage mycosis fungoides. A characteristic Pautrier micro-abscess is situated just below the stratum corneum.

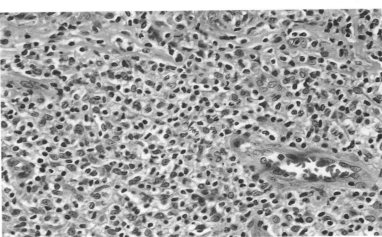

Fig. 8.32 Plaque stage mycosis fungoides. The dermis is diffusely infiltrated by large numbers of mycosis cells. Note the mitotic figure in the centre of the field.

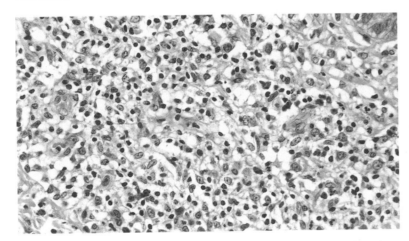

Fig. 8.33 Plaque stage mycosis fungoides. This view shows the infiltrate to contain many eosinophils and more primitive lymphoid cells with irregular vesicular nuclei.

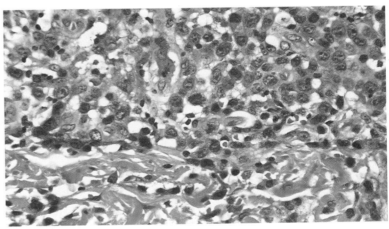

Fig. 8.34 Tumour stage mycosis fungoides. The infiltrate is composed of rather monomorphic large cells with irregular vesicular nuclei and abundant cytoplasm. Several mitotic figures are evident. In the absence of clinical information it would be difficult to classify precisely this high grade malignant tumour.

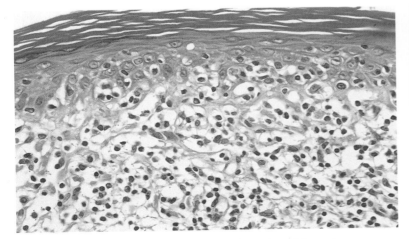

Fig. 8.35 Poikiloderma atrophicans vasculare. There is hyperkeratosis, epidermal atrophy and a very indistinct lower border to the squamous epithelium. Atypical mononuclear cells are conspicuous both within the epidermis and dermis.

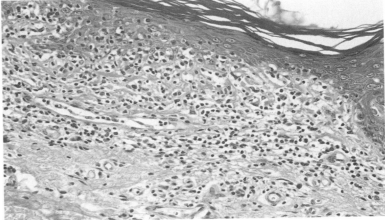

Fig. 8.36 Poikiloderma atrophicans vasculare. In addition to the features described for Fig. 8.35, note the presence of ectatic blood vessels within the dermis.

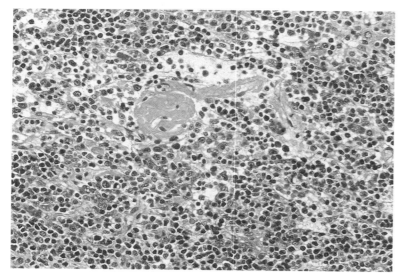

At an early stage of both mycosis fungoides and Sézary syndrome (see later), lymph nodes may show only reactive hyperplasia or dermatopathic lymphadenopathy (Figs. 8.37 and 8.38) but with progression, destruction of the nodal architecture by typical mycosis cells becomes evident (Fig. 8.39). While the infiltrate may become very pleomorphic and difficult to differentiate on histological grounds from other 'end-stage' lymphomas, it must be stressed that mycosis fungoides remains a T-cell lymphoma and does *not* transform into other lymphoproliferative disorders, in particular Hodgkin's disease. Autopsy examination of internal viscera in patients with both mycosis fungoides and Sézary syndrome may disclose surprisingly widespread internal involvement in the absence of frank symptomatology.

Fig. 8.37 Dermatopathic lymphadenopathy. This is a reactive condition in which the para-cortical zone of the lymph node becomes infiltrated by histiocytes containing lipid, haemosiderin or melanin pigment. Here, abundant melanin is present.

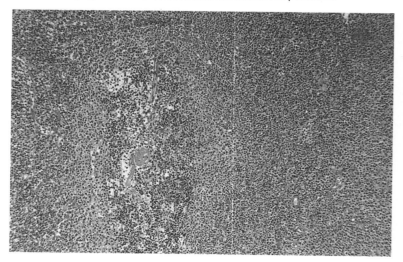

Fig. 8.38 Mycosis fungoides. The lymph node architecture is disturbed by a heavy cellular infiltrate (right).

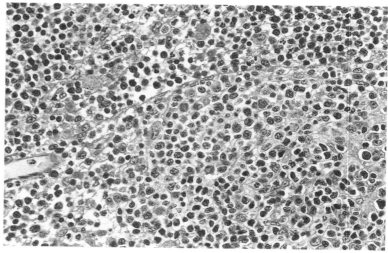

Fig. 8.39 Lymph node – mycosis fungoides. The infiltrate contains numerous cells with highly convoluted nuclei.

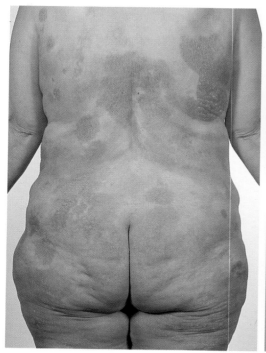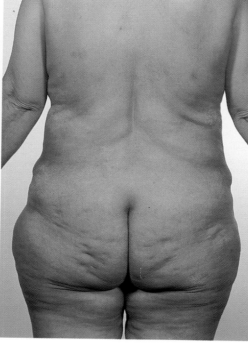

Fig. 8.40 PUVA and nitrogen mustard treatment of early stage mycosis fungoides. Early stages of disease respond well to topical applications of dilute solutions of nitrogen mustard. The eruption (left) was initially cleared with PUVA and then remission was ultimately maintained with topical application of mustard every 10 days (right).

Treatment

Mycosis fungoides was largely untreatable until recently. Now, topical applications of dilute solutions of nitrogen mustard (Fig. 8.40) and photochemotherapy (Fig. 8.41) using oral psoralens combined with long-wave ultra-violet light (PUVA) are used to clear early stage disease. Both treatments are suppressive but gratifying long-term remissions may be obtained with persistent therapy. Topical nitrogen mustard does cause contact dermatitis (Fig. 8.42) in the majority of patients, but most can easily be desensitized. Nitrogen mustard can be applied at home and can be used to treat areas of skin which may be sheltered from ultra-violet irradiation (Fig. 8.43). Both treatments have the disadvantage that ultimately they are cutaneous carcinogens (Fig. 8.44) although the resultant lesions reported so far have been treatable. Tumour stage mycosis fungoides is usually treated with localized radiotherapy or, if lesions are widespread, with electron beam irradiation. Some centres have advocated radical therapy from the start, following the major advances that have been made in the aggressive treatment of Hodgkin's disease. They have suggested whole-body electron beam therapy and treatment with cytotoxic drugs systemically. However, the condition is so variable in its behaviour, probably being relatively benign in the majority of patients, that it is difficult to assess the results and it is questionable whether whole-body irradiation is justifiable in every case. Presently available systemic cytotoxic drugs do not seem to be effective against this T-cell lymphoma of the skin.

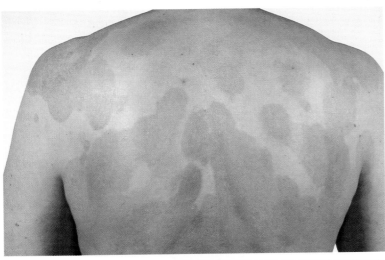

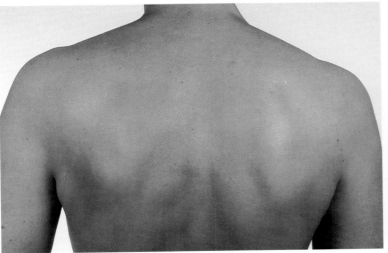

Fig. 8.41 PUVA treatment of early stage mycosis fungoides. Early stages of the disease respond well to PUVA. This patient subsequently maintained remission with PUVA once a month.

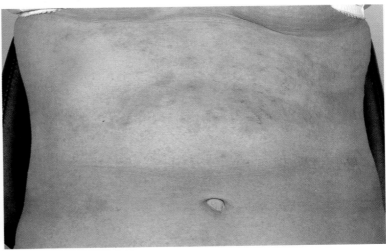

Fig. 8.42 Contact dermatitis to topical nitrogen mustard. Contact dermatitis develops after a few weeks of therapy in the majority of patients. Desensitization, however, is possible in most.

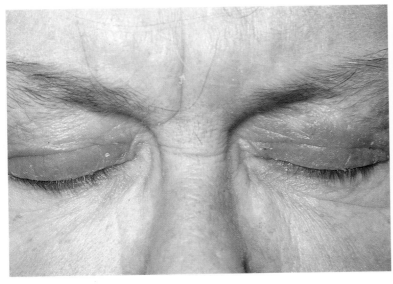

Fig. 8.43 Sanctuary site disease. During treatment with PUVA, mycosis fungoides may occur in shielded sites such as the groin or axillae or, as in this case, the eyelids due to shielding by the protective glasses. These areas may be cleared with topical nitrogen mustard.

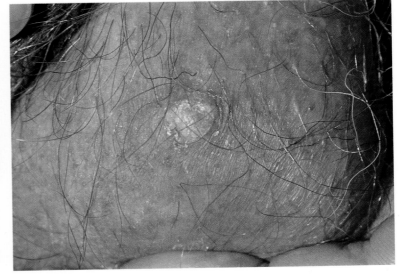

Fig. 8.44 Treatment-induced carcinogenesis. Topical nitrogen mustard and PUVA are known carcinogens. This early squamous cell carcinoma of the scrotum developed after a decade of nitrogen mustard therapy. By courtesy of Dr. Eugene van Scott, Skin and Cancer Hospital, Philadelphia.

Sézary Syndrome

This uncommon disorder is thought by some authorities to be a variant of mycosis fungoides because similar pathological changes may be found in the skin, peripheral blood and lymph nodes in both conditions. However, it does present an entirely different clinical picture. It was first described by Hallopeau, a distinguished French dermatologist, in 1891; he referred to his patient as 'the red man' (l'homme rouge). This description is apposite for, although it can occur in both sexes, the patients are universally red (Fig. 8.45) and usually have associated scaling (Fig. 8.46). The condition is therefore an erythroderma or exfoliative dermatitis. These conditions are synonymous and simply reflect whether scaling is present to a marked degree or not. Other causes of erythroderma must be considered such as psoriasis, eczema, drug reactions and, very occasionally, a cutaneous reaction to Hodgkin's disease, but the diagnosis of Sézary's syndrome may be confirmed by a skin biopsy. The histology is essentially the same as that of mycosis fungoides often with large numbers of atypical lymphocytes showing marked epidermotropism (Fig. 8.47). Large, abnormal cells with convoluted cerebriform nuclei (described by Sézary as 'cellules monstreuses') are found in the peripheral blood and bone marrow so that the condition is considered as a T-lymphocyte leukaemic version of mycosis fungoides. There is frequently generalized lymphadenopathy (Fig. 8.48) and node biopsy may show infiltration with these cells.

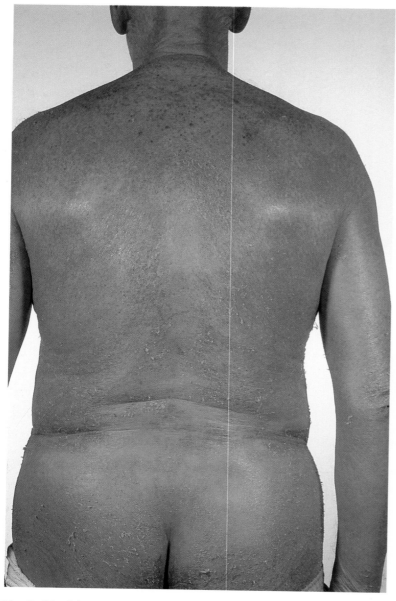

Fig. 8.45 Sézary syndrome. The condition results in a universal redness of the skin (erythroderma).

Fig. 8.46 Sézary syndrome. A close-up of the patient in Fig. 8.45 shows the scaling of the skin.

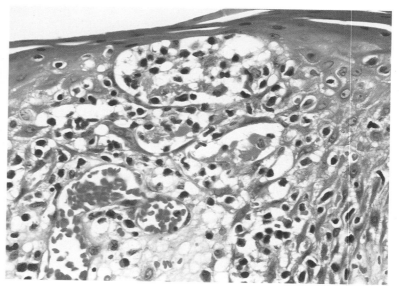

Fig. 8.47 Sézary syndrome. There is epidermal infiltration by large numbers of Sézary cells resulting in almost confluent Pautrier abscess formation. A congested dilated blood vessel is situated just below the epithelium on the left side of the picture.

The condition begins insidiously and is usually diagnosed as a drug eruption, psoriasis or eczema, but it fails to respond to therapy and it spreads, resulting in universal involvement of the skin. Once the erythroderma is established, there is oedema and thickening of the skin and it has a tendency to hang in folds. Ectropion may be a marked feature as in any erythroderma. There is a characteristic hyperkeratosis of the palms and soles. Pruritus may become an extremely distressing symptom of the disease. As the disease progresses, tumours may develop on the skin, particularly on the face and scalp (Figs. 8.49 and 8.50).

The prognosis of the disease is variable. Some patients may enjoy tolerable health for a number of years before generalized involvement of the reticulo-endothelial system and skin tumour

formation occurs. Indeed, some patients, although erythrodermic, never, or only latterly, develop obvious Sézary cells in the peripheral blood and marrow and the disease is referred to as either pre-Sézary syndrome or *erythrodermic mycosis fungoides*. Patients usually eventually die secondary to overwhelming infections. The treatment of Sézary syndrome is unsatisfactory at the present time and it differs from mycosis fungoides in showing a limited or no response to photochemotherapy or topical nitrogen mustard. A combination of various cytotoxic drugs and, in particular, chlorambucil and steroids have been used with variable success, as has cyclosporin A, an anti-T-cell agent. Retinoids may be helpful. Radiotherapy, particularly whole-body electron beam therapy, may produce temporary relief.

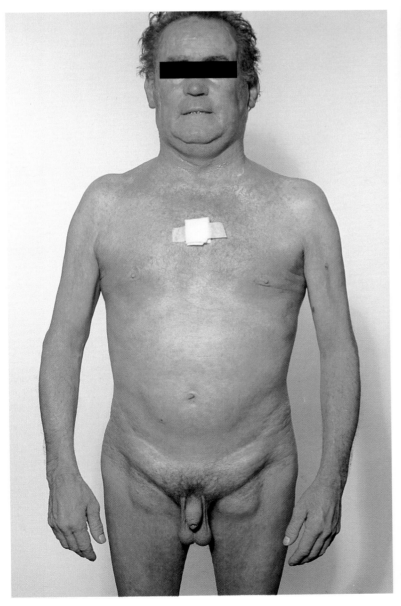

Fig. 8.48 Sézary syndrome. Lymph nodes and the bone marrow are infiltrated with Sézary cells as well as the skin. The cells may be demonstrable in the peripheral blood. Note the inguinal lymphadenopathy. By courtesy of St. Mary's Hospital.

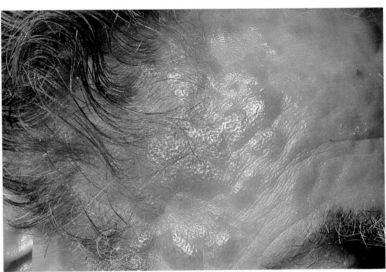

Fig. 8.49 Sézary syndrome. As the disease progresses tumours may occur on the face. This is an ominous sign. By courtesy of St. Mary's Hospital.

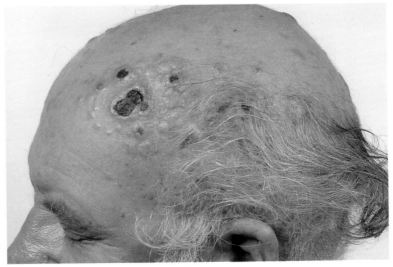

Fig. 8.50 Sézary syndrome. The tumours may ulcerate. The scalp is a common site.

LYMPHOMAS OCCASIONALLY PRESENTING IN THE SKIN

Hodgkin's Disease

Specific involvement of the skin is rare in Hodgkin's disease. However, generalized pruritus secondary to the disease is quite common although it is usually well-established by the time itching develops and it is a rare presenting feature of the disease. Very occasionally the disease may present as the recent development of a dry skin (Fig. 8.51). A tendency to xeroderma and ichthyosis is normally present from birth, so an acquired xeroderma should be viewed with suspicion. Hyperpigmentation and erythroderma sometimes occur as part of Hodgkin's disease. Patients are, however, particularly prone to infections of the skin since they are immunosuppressed and also treated with immunosuppressive drugs. Herpes zoster, particularly, the disseminated form, is a common cutaneous complication of the disease (see Fig. 10.21).

Non-Hodgkin's Lymphoma

Specific lesions of the skin do occur quite commonly in the course of non-Hodgkin's lymphoma but usually the diagnosis has already been established. However, occasionally a patient may present with skin lesions (Fig. 8.52). They are papules (Figs. 8.53 and 8.54), plaques (Fig. 8.55), nodules (Fig. 8.56) or tumours which may or may not break down and ulcerate (Fig. 8.57). The lesions are frequently purple or plum-coloured. It is probable that this presentation was formerly given the name 'tumeur d'emblée' and mistakenly thought to be a variety of mycosis fungoides.

The diagnosis is easily established by performing a skin biopsy. There is an infiltrate in the dermis consisting of malignant-appearing lymphocytes which extend deep down into the subcutaneous fat. There is usually a characteristic sparing of

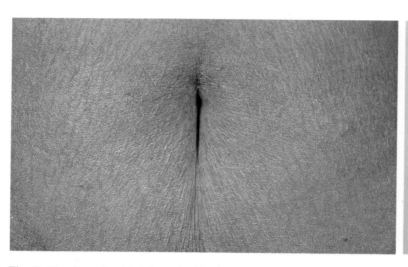
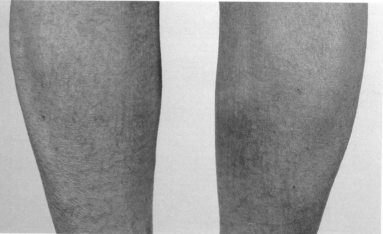

Fig. 8.51 Acquired ichthyosis. Hodgkin's disease occasionally presents as acquired dry skin. By courtesy of Dr. R.H. Marten.

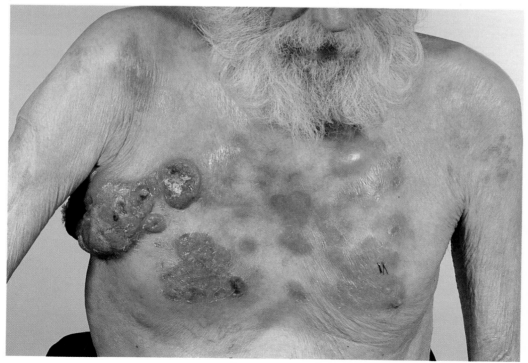
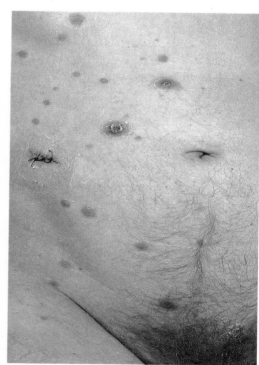

Fig. 8.52 Non-Hodgkin's lymphoma. Large nodules and fungating tumours may occur. They are often a deep red or plum colour. This patient had a tumour excised and grafted on his right arm three years before this recurrence. There was no lymphadenopathy or marrow involvement.

Fig. 8.53 Non-Hodgkin's lymphoma. Scattered, small, firm purple papules and nodules are present. Skin biopsy is simple and essential for diagnosis.

the uppermost portion of the dermis; the so-called grenz zone (Fig. 8.58). This is in marked contrast to the histology of mycosis fungoides where the infiltrate tends to be in the upper part of the dermis and to actually infiltrate the epidermis. The lymphocytes of non-Hodgkin's lymphoma are usually derived from bone marrow (B-cells) as opposed to the thymus-derived lymphocytes (T-cells) of mycosis fungoides.

The management and course of non-Hodgkin's lymphoma is outside the scope of this book, but in those cases where the lymphoma appears to be confined to the skin, the prognosis is quite variable. In some there is a fairly swift involvement of other organs, but in others it may remain confined only to the skin for a number of years.

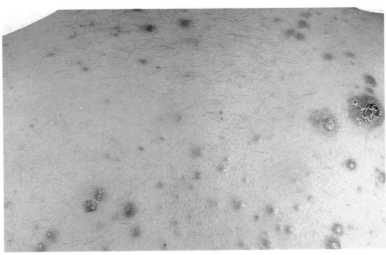

Fig. 8.54 Non-Hodgkin's lymphoma. Multiple purple papules or nodules occur, some of which are crusted.

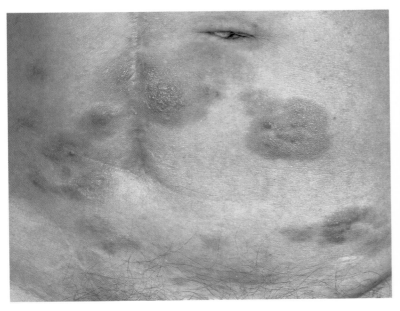

Fig. 8.55 Non-Hodgkin's lymphoma. Infiltrated plum-coloured plaques are present. Skin biopsy is essential for diagnosis and distinction from mycosis fungoides.

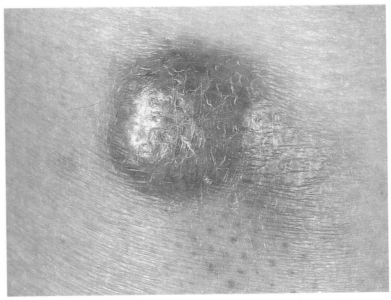

Fig. 8.56 Non-Hodgkin's lymphoma. The nodules have a deep red or purple colour.

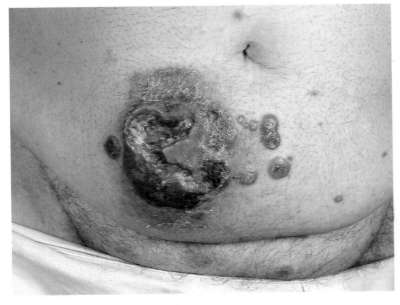

Fig. 8.57 Non-Hodgkin's lymphoma. Purple papules, nodules and a large ulcerating nodule are present. This man presented with these lesions but disease was found in other organs.

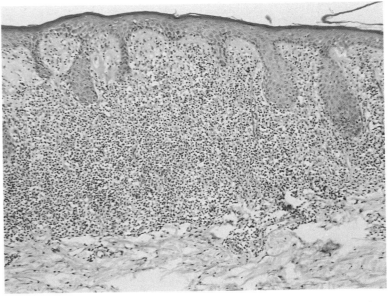

Fig. 8.58 B-cell lymphoma. The epidermis is not involved and a grenz zone is present. A dense band-like infiltrate occupies the upper and mid dermis.

Leukaemic Deposits

Leukaemic deposits in the skin are rare, particularly as a presenting feature. However, papules (Fig. 8.59), nodules or thick plaques may occasionally occur, especially on the face (Fig. 8.60). The lesions are often a deep red colour. Skin biopsy, a full blood count and bone marrow biopsy will help to establish the diagnosis. Very occasionally, erythroderma may be a presenting feature of leukaemia.

Non-specific presentations of leukaemia are much more common, particularly widespread purpura (Fig. 8.61). Generalized pruritus and infections of the skin consequent to immunosuppression, such as sepsis or viral disorders, are common.

DISORDERS OCCASIONALLY ASSOCIATED WITH LYMPHOMA

Included in this section are three disorders which seemingly have little in common. Actinic reticuloid is an abnormal reaction of the skin to ultra-violet light irradiation. Lymphomatoid papulosis is a variant of pityriasis lichenoides where the pathology centres around blood vessels while the pathology of follicular mucinosis centres around the hair follicles. However, all three conditions have occasionally been associated with mycosis fungoides or lymphoma and it is convenient to describe them here.

Actinic Reticuloid (Chronic Actinic Dermatitis)

Originally, actinic reticuloid was the name given to a condition affecting exclusively males with extreme photosensitivity and with a malignant 'reticuloid' histology. The spectrum of the condition has now widened and the name has been modified to chronic actinic dermatitis. It commences insidiously on solar-exposed sites such as the face and backs of the hands (Fig. 8.62) as a persistent eczema and gradually acquires a 'reticuloid'

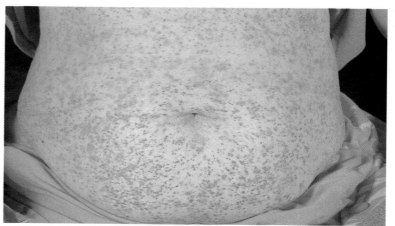

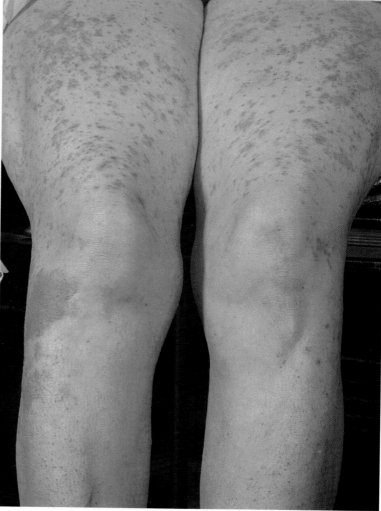

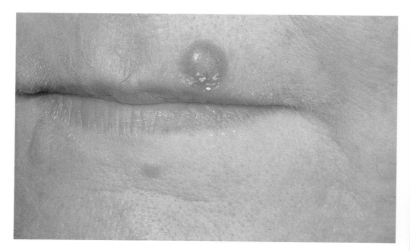

Fig. 8.59 Leukaemia cutis. Firm purple papules or nodules may occasionally occur in leukaemia, especially on the face.

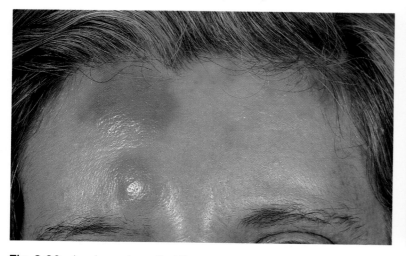

Fig. 8.60 Leukaemia cutis. Plum-coloured plaques may be found on skin biopsy to be deposits of leukaemia. By courtesy of Dr. A.C. Pembroke.

Fig. 8.61 Leukaemia. The most common cutaneous presentation of leukaemia is purpura.

histology in advanced cases. The skin is red, scaling and thickened and thrown into folds such that the face almost has a leonine appearance (Fig. 8.63). The eruption gradually spreads to covered sites. Patients frequently have positive patch tests (including photo-patch tests) to a number of allergens but avoidance of the allergen may not effect much improvement. Light testing indicates a photo-sensitivity ranging throughout the UBV and the UVA ranges. In severe cases, a nocturnal existence is sometimes necessary to diminish the intensity of the affliction. The condition very occasionally progresses to lymphoma.

Histology
The features vary from those of a mild non-specific chronic dermatitis to a histology virtually indistinguishable from that of mycosis fungoides (Fig. 8.64).

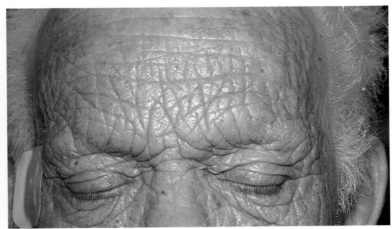

Fig. 8.63 Chronic actinic dermatitis. This condition was originally reported to occur only in men. In this case the eruption was lichenified secondary to rubbing. Skin biopsy and light testing are necessary to establish the diagnosis.

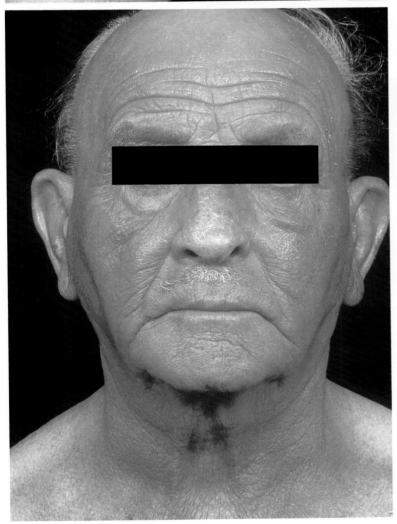

Fig. 8.62 Chronic actinic dermatitis. The light-exposed areas of the backs of the hands, face and 'V' of the neck are involved. The lesions are deep red, scaling and thickened. Skin biopsy and monochromatic light tests established the diagnosis.

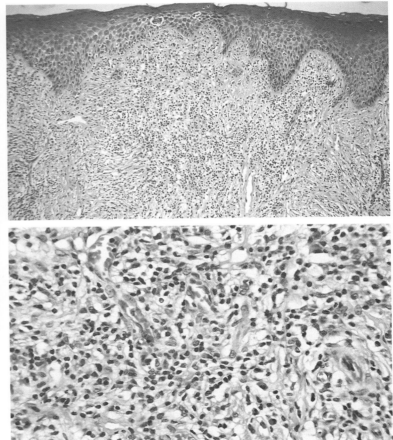

Fig. 8.64 Actinic reticuloid. The low power view shows patchy hyperkeratosis, marked but irregular acanthosis and two small collections of lymphoid cells resembling the Pautrier microabscesses of mycosis fungoides (top). There is a fairly dense chronic inflammatory cell infiltrate occupying the dermis, which consists of lymphocytes, plasma cells, eosinophils and histiocytes (bottom). Some of the lymphocytic nuclei are irregular and hyperchromatic, increasing the resemblance to mycosis fungoides.

Lymphomatoid Papulosis

The precise nosological position of this entity is uncertain. Most authors consider it to be an atypical variant of pityriasis lichenoides et varioliformis acuta (PLVA) but some regard it as a distinct clinico-pathological entity. Others have viewed it as a pityriasis lichenoides-like lymphoma or even a cutaneous T-cell lymphoma. This, however, only adds to the confusion, so it is probably best to regard lymphomatoid papulosis as being, in general, a variant of PLVA while recognizing that in some instances it does appear to have its own independent identity. This is of some importance in that a small proportion of patients appear to eventually succumb to a cutaneous lymphoma, but in the great majority the disease has a benign outcome.

Clinically, while the disease may become manifest at either extreme of life, most cases develop around the fifth decade. It presents as recurrent erythematous papules (Fig. 8.65) or nodules which soon become haemorrhagic and necrotic, with subsequent healing often resulting in scarring. Lesions occur predominantly on the trunk and extremities. Despite its worrying histology, the results of extensive clinical investigations for systemic involvement are usually negative. Unfortunately neither clinical nor pathological studies have enabled one to predict which patients will transform into a truly malignant process.

Histology
The fully established lesion has a rather characteristic morpho-

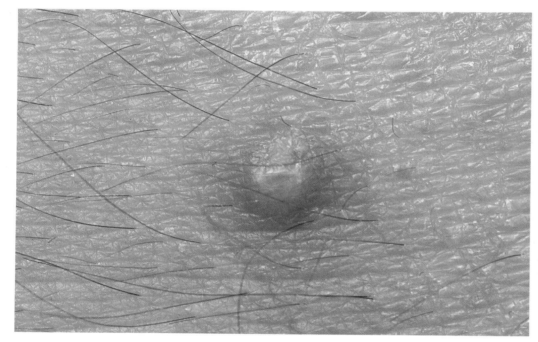

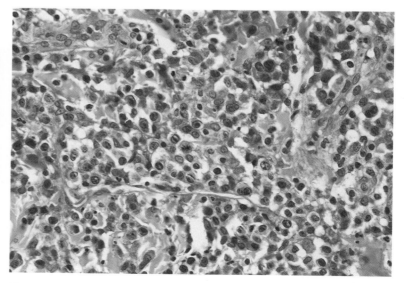

Fig. 8.65 Lymphomatoid papulosis. Indurated papules occur especially on the limbs. By courtesy of St. John's Hospital for Diseases of the Skin.

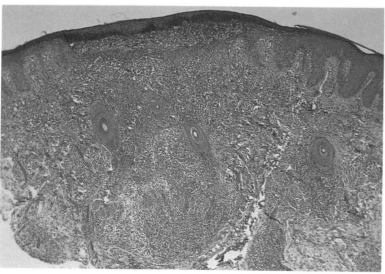

Fig. 8.66 Lymphomatoid papulosis. Low power view showing an ulcerated papule with typical wedge-shaped cellular infiltrate.

Fig. 8.67 Lymphomatoid papulosis. High power view of the infiltrate. Note the polymorphism: lymphocytes and plasma cells admixed with larger cells with abundant cytoplasm and irregular vesicular nuclei and prominent nucleoli. Mitotic figures are conspicuous.

logy (Fig. 8.66). A dense, wedge-shaped infiltrate (with its broad base uppermost) extends from the epidermis often into the superficial aspects of the subcutaneous fat. The infiltrate is typically polymorphous consisting of an admixture of polymorphs, eosinophils, plasma cells and variably differentiated lymphoid cells; the latter including many bizarre forms including immunoblasts. Variable numbers of Langerhan's cells are also present. Characteristic of lymphomatoid papulosis is the pleomorphism of the infiltrate and its often high mitotic activity (Figs. 8.67 and 8.68). The infiltrate typically involves the epidermis which is acanthotic and parakeratotic. Endothelial swelling, diapedesis of red blood cells both in the dermis and epidermis is the rule (Fig. 8.69).

Follicular Mucinosis

This is a rare disorder of unknown aetiology, which is characterized by the finding of acid mucopolysaccharides, which stain positively with Alcian blue, in the sebaceous glands and the outer root sheath of the hair follicle.

There appear to be three variants of this condition. The first is confined to the head and neck region and consists of infiltrative plaques affecting the hair-bearing areas (Fig. 8.70) such as the beard, eyebrows or scalp, so that hair-loss occurs. The lesions are well-defined, infiltrated and red (Fig. 8.71). Occasionally, a mucinous material may be expressed from the hair follicles which are usually prominent and patulous. This is the most common variety and is ordinarily followed by remission after a couple of years.

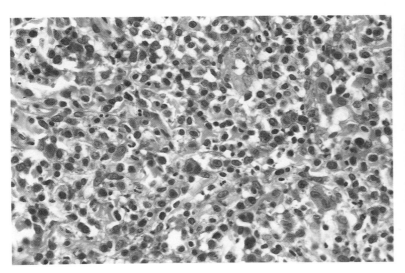

Fig. 8.68 Lymphomatoid papulosis. In addition to the features described in Fig. 8.67, note the presence of two binucleate cells.

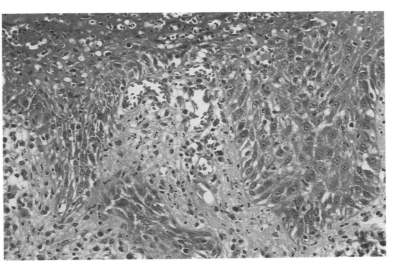

Fig. 8.69 Lymphomatoid papulosis. The epidermis overlying the lateral border of the lesion is acanthotic, oedematous and infiltrated by large numbers of red blood cells.

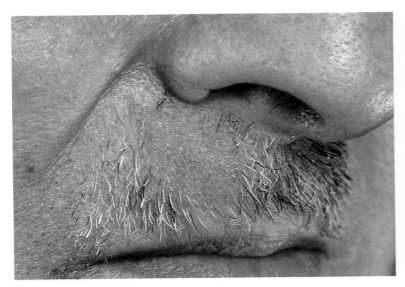

Fig. 8.70 Follicular mucinosis. A red infiltrated plaque in the moustache area has caused loss of hair. By courtesy of St. John's Hospital for Diseases of the Skin.

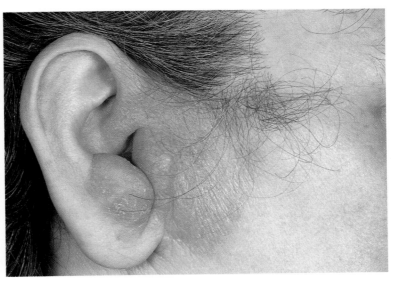

Fig. 8.71 Follicular mucinosis. A thickened, well-defined, oedematous plaque is present in and around the ear. The head and neck are the usual sites for limited forms of the disease. Biopsy is necessary to establish the diagnosis. By courtesy of Dr. Dorothy Vollum.

There is a second variety which is much more extensive and occurs in an older age group and is not confined to the head and neck. The clinical features are the same as those described previously. This variety may also resolve but the process takes longer.

The third variety appears to be a variant of mycosis fungoides and the diagnosis is suspected because there may be typical patches of mycosis fungoides or poikiloderma interspersed with the extensive follicular mucinosis lesions. The eruption is more widespread than in the preceding two varieties and usually occurs in an older age group (Fig. 8.72). Skin biopsy is mandatory to confirm the diagnosis of mycosis fungoides.

Histology

The appearances are those of mucinous degeneration involving the sebaceous glands and the external root sheath of the hair follicles (Figs. 8.73 and 8.74). In the third variant, the changes of mycosis fungoides are superimposed.

BENIGN LYMPHOCYTIC INFILTRATIONS OF THE SKIN

These are considered here because the clinical presentation and the histological appearances of the nodules or plaques may be mistaken for lymphoma.

Lymphocytoma Cutis (Spiegler-Fendt Pseudolymphoma)

This rare, benign condition may occur at any age but particularly affects adolescents or young adults. It is of unknown aetiology.

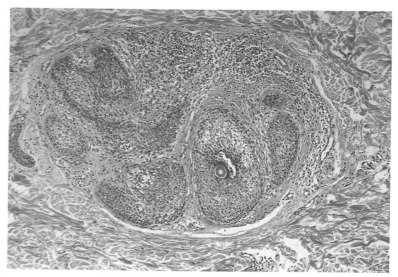

Fig. 8.73 Follicular mucinosis. Intercellular deposition of mucin has resulted in the vacuolated appearance of the follicular epithelium. A non-specific chronic inflammatory cell infiltrate is present.

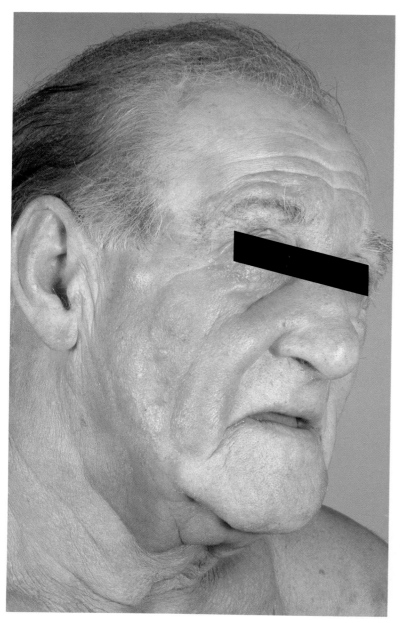

Fig. 8.72 Follicular mucinosis. Indurated plaques are present and typical patches of mycosis fungoides occurred on the limbs and trunk. Skin biopsy was necessary to establish the diagnosis.

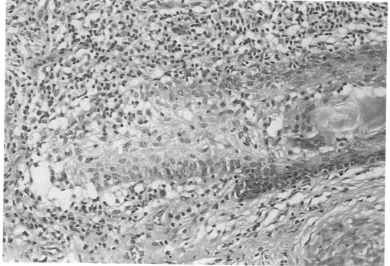

Fig. 8.74 Follicular mucinosis. The outer root sheath shows gross mucinous degeneration and a mild infiltrate of chronic inflammatory cells. The dermis contains large numbers of lymphocytes with occasional plasma cells and eosinophils.

Persistent purple or brown papules or nodules (which may be clinically indistinguishable from true lymphomatous deposits) arise on the head and neck (Fig. 8.75). The lesions may be circumscribed or diffusely dispersed throughout the skin. Biopsy is mandatory for diagnosis. The condition responds well to small doses of radiotherapy. Its major importance is its recognition as a *pseudo*-lymphoma.

Histology
The appearances are those of an over-exuberant reactive B-cell hyperplasia. The epidermis is uninvolved and a papillary dermal grenz zone is usual. Occupying the dermis and often subcutaneous fat is a dense nodular, polymorphic inflammatory cell infiltrate. Lymphoid follicle with germinal centre formation is characteristic (Fig. 8.76). The cellular infiltrate consists of mature lymphocytes, plasma cells, eosinophils and occasional giant cells (Fig. 8.77). The polymorphic nature of the infiltrate accompanied by lymphoid follicle formation enables one to distinguish lymphocytoma cutis from a true lymphoma.

Jessner's Lymphocytic Infiltrate of the Skin
This relatively common disease is characterized by multiple purple or red-brown papules, nodules or plaques which occur on the face and trunk (Fig. 8.78). They tend to come and go randomly, unlike the infiltrations of lymphocytoma cutis. The course of the condition is quite benign. The cause is unknown.

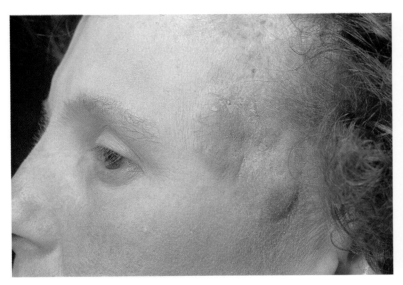

Fig. 8.75 Lymphocytoma cutis. A diffused infiltrated purple nodular lesion is present on the face. A skin biopsy is necessary for precise diagnosis. By courtesy of St. John's Hospital for Diseases of the Skin.

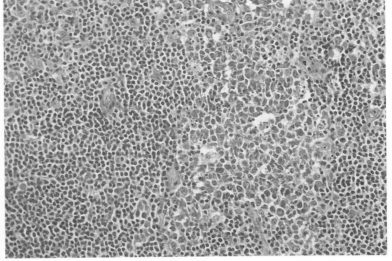

Fig. 8.76 Lymphocytoma cutis. A dense dermal infiltrate is present. The right side of the picture contains a large reactive follicle with characteristic scattered nuclear dust.

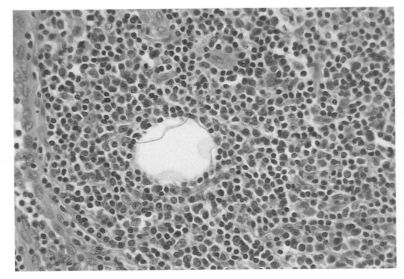

Fig. 8.77 Lymphocytoma cutis. The infiltrate is polymorphic, being composed of lymphocytes, plasma cells and scattered eosinophils. Note the absence of primitive cell forms and mitoses.

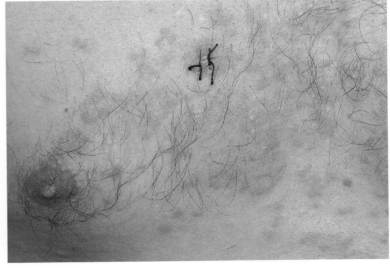

Fig. 8.78 Jessner's lymphocytic infiltration of the skin. Purple infiltrated plaques are present on the chest. The lesions tend to relapse and remit spontaneously.

8.21

Histology

The epidermis is unaffected. Within the dermis is a monomorphic lymphocytic infiltrate surrounding blood vessels and sometimes cutaneous adnexae (Figs. 8.79 and 8.80). It is thus indistinguishable from chronic lymphatic leukaemia. The absence of hyperkeratosis, epidermal atrophy and basal cell liquefactive degeneration distinguishes it from discoid lupus erythematosus. In addition, the epidermo-dermal junction shows negative immunofluorescence.

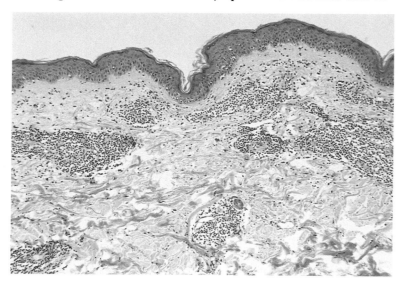

Fig. 8.79 Lymphocytic infiltrate of Jessner. This typical example shows discrete collections of mononuclear cells around the blood vessels and sweat ducts in the dermis.

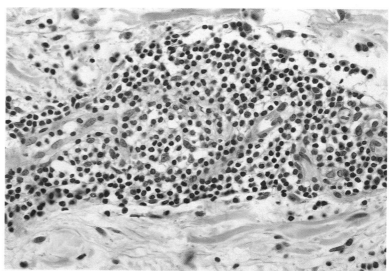

Fig. 8.80 Lymphocytic infiltrate of Jessner. The infiltrate consists of uniform, mature lymphocytes.

9 Bacterial Infections of the Skin and Syphilis

IMPETIGO

This is a superficial cutaneous infection caused by either *Staphylococcus aureus* or a β-haemolytic streptococcus or both. It is particularly common in children and adolescents. The condition is highly contagious and will spread rapidly in any institution such as a boarding school or a nursery. The primary lesion is a vesicle or blister (Fig. 9.1) containing yellow pus (Fig. 9.2). It extends, becoming circinate or polycyclic (Fig. 9.3) before rupturing, and produces a yellow, honey-coloured crust (Fig. 9.4). The lesions occur most often on the face (Fig. 9.5), but may be found anywhere on the skin. The condition is an acute one and autoinoculation causes it to spread to other sites. It most frequently arises *de novo* although predisposing causes, such as infestation and, in particular, pediculosis capitis or eczema (Fig. 9.6) may be present. Treatment with the appropriate antibiotic either topically or, more often, systemically will result in resolution of the condition within a day or so. Many staphylococcal infections are resistant to penicillin so erythromycin is the usual choice of antibiotic. The streptococcal infections are sensitive to penicillin but also to erythromycin.

FOLLICULITIS

When correctly used, this term implies a superficial bacterial infection of the hair follicle. However, it is also used to describe sterile, follicular pustules from which pathogenic bacteria can not be recovered and which probably would be better classified as pseudofolliculitis.

Bockhart's Impetigo

This is an acute, staphylococcal or streptococcal infection of the skin, seen particularly on the lower limbs of hirsute individuals (Fig. 9.7). It is also fairly common in patients using topical glucocorticosteroids for eczema and psoriasis (Fig. 9.8). Small, discrete, painful, yellow, follicular pustules are evident. The condition responds rapidly to appropriate systemic antibiotics.

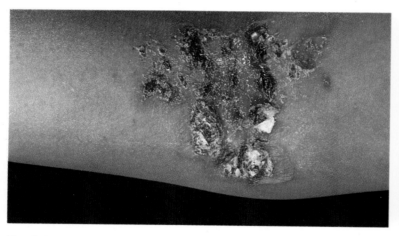

Fig. 9.1   Impetigo. The lesions start as blisters which contain pus and subsequently become eroded and crusted.

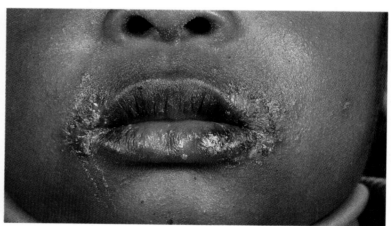

Fig. 9.2   Impetigo. The lesions ooze pus.

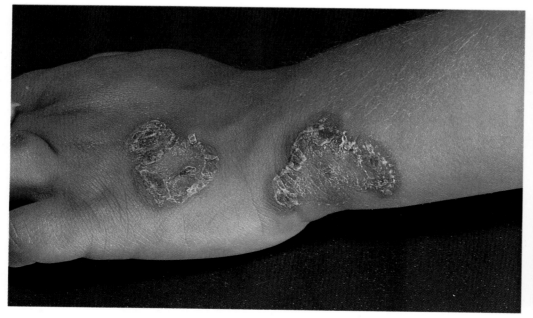

Fig. 9.3   Impetigo. The lesions may be polycyclic and heal centrally.

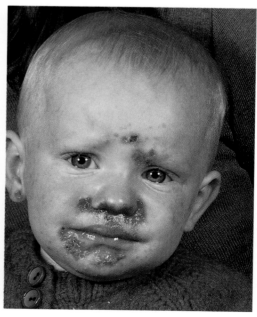

Fig. 9.4   Impetigo. The face is a common site. Golden crusts are present. Infants and children are particularly at risk.

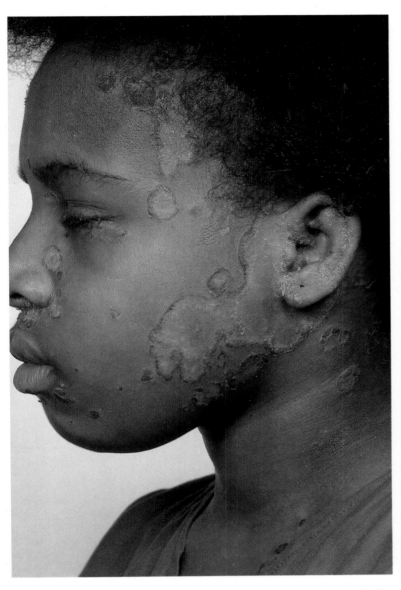

Fig. 9.5 Impetigo. The lesions may spread rapidly especially if topical steroids are inappropriately prescribed.

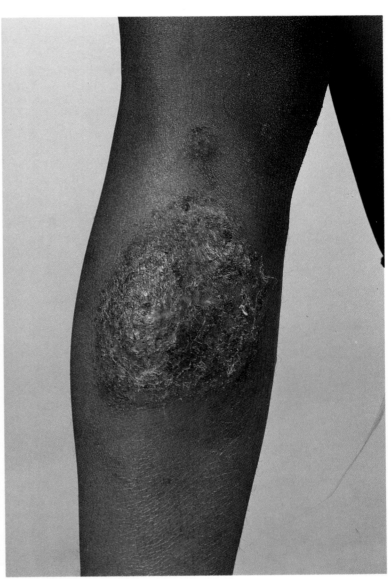

Fig. 9.6 Impetiginized eczema. Impetigo may occur as a secondary event. Eczema often becomes infected and yellow brown crusting results.

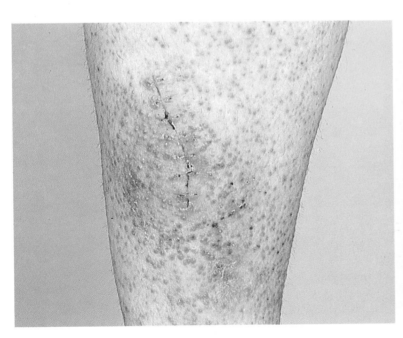

Fig. 9.7 Folliculitis. Septic pustules have occurred under an occlusive dressing following a leg operation.

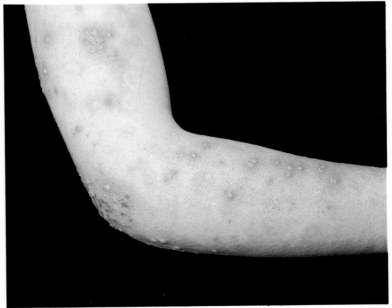

Fig. 9.8 Folliculitis. Discrete yellow pustules surrounded by erythema are a common complication of topical glucorticosteroid treatment of skin disorders. By courtesy of St. John's Hospital for Diseases of the Skin.

Sycosis Barbae

This is a chronic deep-seated staphylococcal infection of the beard area (Fig. 9.9). It is only seen in men and is now very rare in Western societies, probably as a result of better hygienic conditions and the widespread availability and early use of antibiotics. There is, however, a common condition caused by ingrowing hairs which is frequently misnamed sycosis barbae.

Folliculitis Secondary to Ingrowing Hairs

This condition is found commonly, but not exclusively, in negroes. The hairs in the beard area, particularly under the jaw, tend to grow back into the skin resulting in an acneiform, follicular, pustular eruption (Fig. 9.10). In negroes, this may result in keloid formation (Figs. 9.11 and 9.12). The disorder responds poorly to antibiotics although there may be a marginal response to long-term, low-dose antibiotics given in a similar manner as in the treatment of acne vulgaris. The condition can,

however, be resolved by growing a beard, although this is not always acceptable.

Folliculitis of the Scalp

This is relatively common in negroes where yellow pustules are seen surrounding the hairs. Although *Staphylococcus aureus* is readily cultured from the lesions, the condition is not eradicated by treating with the appropriate antibiotic. It tends to be recalcitrant and chronic with fresh lesions developing all the time and may well result in considerable keloid formation, particularly at the back of the neck (Fig. 9.13).

Pseudomonas Folliculitis

Outbreaks of folliculitis have been reported in the United States since 1975, secondary to the use of contaminated whirlpools. Pustules develop on the torso and limbs (Fig. 9.14) within 24—48 hours of exposure. *Pseudomonas aeruginosa* may be cultured from

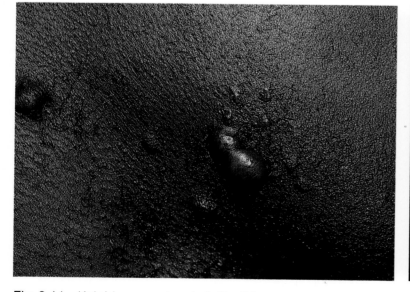

Fig. 9.9   Sycosis barbae. Staphylococcal infection of the beard area is uncommon in Western societies probably because of improved hygiene and early use of antibiotics.

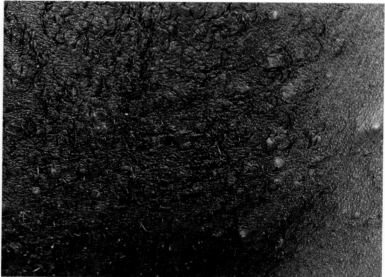

Fig. 9.10   Folliculitis secondary to ingrowing hairs. A sterile acneiform eruption develops secondary to ingrowing hairs. It is particularly common in negroes.

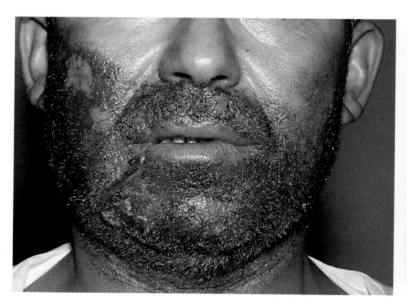

Fig. 9.11   Keloids secondary to folliculitis. Keloids may result from the pseudofolliculitis associated with ingrowing hairs.

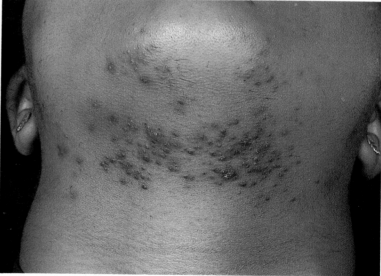

Fig. 9.12   Keloids secondary to ingrowing hairs in a hirsute female.

the pustules. The patient may be unwell with malaise and low-grade fever and lympadenopathy. Otitis externa, mastitis, ocular and urinary tract infections may also occur. Whirlpools are much more prone to contamination than swimming pools, partly because of difficulties in maintaining adequate chlorination of the water. The chlorine evaporates easily due to the high temperatures and continual agitation of the water by the pressurized jets of the jacuzzi. There is usually a high concentration of organic matter which encourages the growth of the bacteria and tends to reduce the chlorine to less-active forms. The heat of the water also dilates the follicular openings and facilitates the entry of the bacteria. The condition is self-limiting and the patient recovers in a week or ten days without treatment.

Folliculitis due to Acne and Oils
Sterile follicular pustules are common on the limbs, particularly the thighs, of individuals who have a tendency to acne and are hirsute. Those who wear tight, occlusive clothing or have an occupation where their clothes become contaminated with oil (Figs. 9.15 and 9.16) are particularly prone to this kind of folliculitis.

FURUNCULOSIS (Boils)
This is an acute staphyloccal infection of the hair follicles (Fig. 9.17). It differs from folliculitis in that there is a greater degree of inflammation and the infection spreads away from the hair follicle into the surrounding dermis. Pus may become

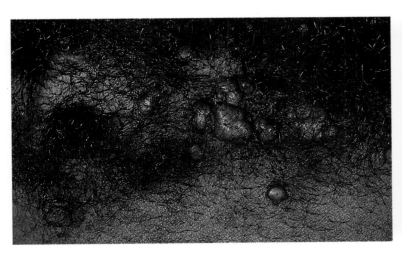

Fig. 9.13 Nuchal keloids. Folliculitis of the scalp often results in keloids especially at the back of the neck.

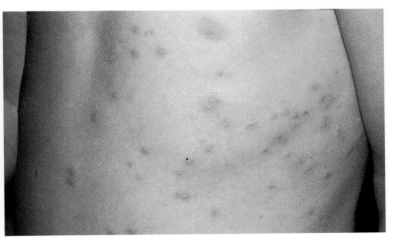

Fig. 9.14 Pseudomonas folliculitis. Widespread pustules surrounded by erythema may develop from the use of jacuzzis contaminated with *Pseudomonas aeruginosa*.

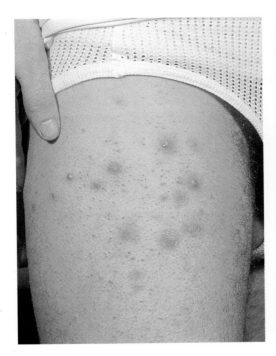

Fig. 9.15 Folliculitis due to oils. Sterile acneiform papules and pustules develop secondary to follicular occlusion due to oils.

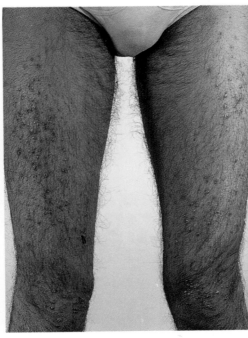

Fig. 9.16 Folliculits due to oils. Hirsutism predisposes to this condition. The thighs are a common site particularly if oily tight-fitting trousers are worn. By courtesy of Dr. A.C. Pembroke.

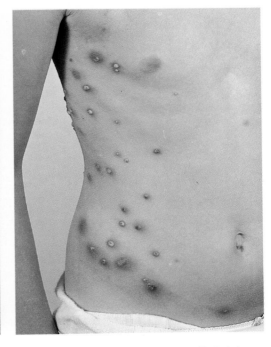

Fig. 9.17 Furunculosis (boils). Painful red nodules are present in various stages of development.

9.5

visible on the surface of the lesion as it evolves (Fig. 9.18) and will discharge either spontaneously or as a result of lancing. A deep abscess may leave scarring (Fig. 9.19). A carbuncle is a collection of boils such that multiple draining sites occur. The patient is usually unwell and has a fever. The condition responds rapidly to appropriate antibiotics. Occasionally, however, boils may become recurrent. In these cases the patient is usually a chronic carrier of staphylococci, either in the anterior nares, perineum or axillae, often acquired after a period of hospitalization. Swabs should be taken from these sites and the carrier sites treated with topical antibiotics for several weeks. It may be necessary to take an additional prolonged course of antibiotics, and also it is useful to sterilize the skin by adding hexachlorophane to the daily bath.

Although always recorded in textbooks, it is rare that a patient presenting with boils proves to have previously unsuspected diabetes mellitus, but it is routine practice to test the urine for glycosuria. Occasionally, immunosuppressed patients may present with boils.

STYES (Hordeoli)

A stye is a staphylococcal infection of an eyelash (Fig. 9.20) and has the same clinical features as a boil although it is much smaller in size. Many affected patients also carry the staphylococcus in their anterior nares, which should also be treated. Chronic staphylococcal infections of the eyelashes occasionally occur (Fig. 9.21).

ECTHYMA

This is a bacterial infection of the skin caused by either *Staphylococcus aureus* or streptococci. It begins in a similar way to impetigo (as a superficial vesicle containing pus) but extends more deeply and enters the dermis. The condition presents as crusted ulcers, particularly on the lower legs (Fig. 9.22). It is a common consequence of insect bites and particularly occurs in hot countries. It presented particular problems to American troops in Vietnam.

TOXIC EPIDERMAL NECROLYSIS ('Scalded Skin' Syndrome)

This is an uncommon condition of children, particularly of the very young. Early recognition of the disease and treatment with appropriate antibiotics may be life-saving. It is caused by an epidermolytic toxin, usually produced by a Group 2 staphylococcus, phage type 71. It appears to be an individual idiosyncratic response since other members of the same family may

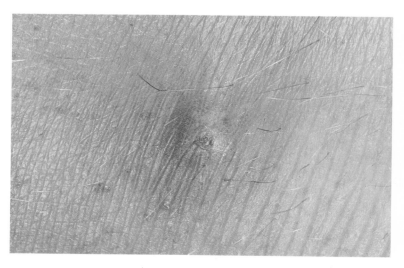

Fig. 9.18 Furunculosis. The pus is pointing on the surface of this red tender nodule.

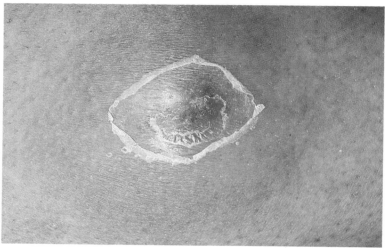

Fig. 9.19 Furunculosis. As the boil expands there is a peeling of the overlying skin.

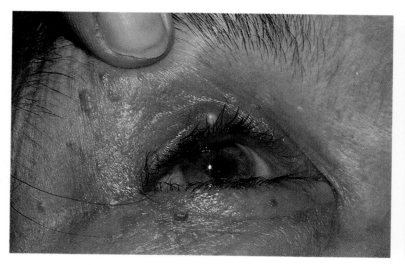

Fig. 9.20 Stye. This is an acute staphylococcal infection of an eyelash. The pus is pointing.

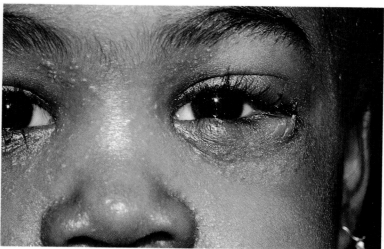

Fig. 9.21 Chronic sepsis of the eyelashes. Chronic staphylococcal infections may be associated with carriage of the bacteria in the nose.

have staphylococcal infection which is manifest only as impetigo. A most characteristic symptom is extreme tenderness of the skin followed shortly by redness and widespread desquamation of the epidermis in sheets (Fig. 9.23). This reveals red, raw and eroded skin resembling a superficial burn (Fig. 9.24). Most, or all, of the body surface may be involved with the desquamation.

A similar eruption occurs in adults, but this is drug-induced and not caused by a staphylococcus and does not respond to antibiotics. The histopathology of the staphylococcal 'scalded skin' syndrome reveals the damage to be superficial, in the granular cell layer, whereas in drug-induced disease the damage is in the region of the dermo-epidermal junction.

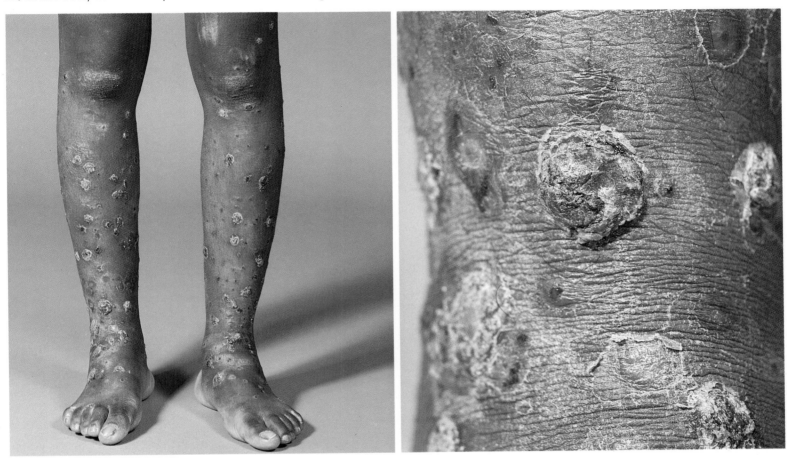

Fig. 9.22 Ecthyma. Crusted and eroded lesions are present mainly on the lower legs. Insect bites are the most common cause and sepsis results. By courtesy of St. Mary's Hospital.

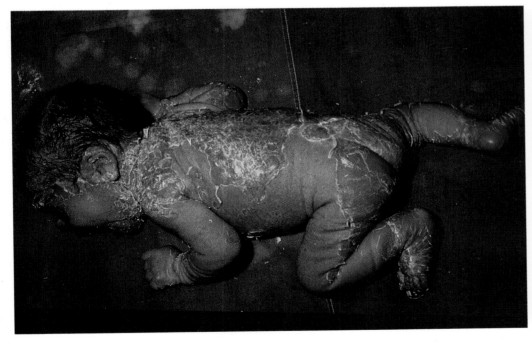

Fig. 9.23 Scalded skin syndrome (Lyell's syndrome). Epidermal necrolysis occurs secondary to staphylococcal toxin. The skin may be universally red and desquamating resembling a burn.

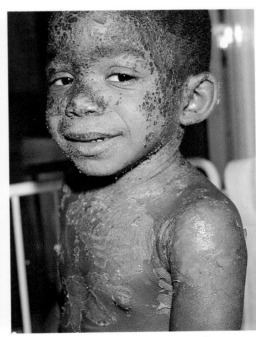

Fig. 9.24 Scalded skin syndrome. The skin becomes raw and eroded. The similarity to impetigo is clear. The condition responds rapidly to antibiotics.

ERYSIPELAS

This is an acute, superficial infection of the skin, normally caused by a streptococcus. The condition is sometimes known as 'St. Anthony's fire'. The clinical distinction of erysipelas from cellulitis is often difficult; erysipelas is more superficial and usually affects the face (Fig. 9.25), while cellulitis also affects the subcutaneous tissue. Cellulitis may also be caused by staphylococcus, usually involving the lower leg.

The onset of the condition is sudden. The patient is ill, has a high fever and rigors, may vomit and become quite delirious. Examination reveals a unilateral eruption, occurring either on one leg or on one side of the face or scalp. The area involved is sharply delineated, red and tender (Fig. 9.26) and there is associated oedema and sometimes blistering (Fig. 9.27) and erosions (Fig. 9.28). The condition responds dramatically to appropriate antibiotic therapy although the patient may be left with a persistent oedema of the lower leg.

It is thought that the organism penetrates the skin via a breach in the epidermis. On the face, this may be difficult to identify but on the leg there is often associated tinea pedis. The condition may become recurrent, probably due to a relative deficiency of lymphatics. This lymphatic hypoplasia may be present primarily or result from the erysipelas. Recurrent attacks should be treated with long-term antibiotics. Small doses of penicillin or erythromycin taken daily are often very effective. Associated predisposing causes such as otitis externa or tinea pedis should be treated.

LYMPHANGIITIS

This is an inflammation of the subcutaneous lymphatic channels secondary to infection, usually by a steptococcus. It presents as linear red streaks on the skin (Fig. 9.29) associated with tender regional lymphadenopathy. It responds to treatment of the source of the infection.

ERYSIPELOID

This is an uncommon infection with the Gram-positive bacteria *Erysipelothrix rhusiopathiae.* It occurs in those whose occupation includes handling contaminated raw fish or meat. The organism enters the skin through an abrasion and is most likely to be seen on the hand. Erysipeloid involves a slowly evolving process lasting a few weeks and consisting of a purple to red, slightly oedematous eruption (Fig. 9.30) with a well-defined, raised edge which spreads over the fingers, with a tendency to heal at its original site. Unlike erysipelas, there is no systemic disturbance. It responds to treatment with penicillin.

ERYTHRASMA

This is a bacterial infection of the skin caused by *Corynebacterium minutissimum.* The disease causes an intertrigo and is most common in the groins (Fig. 9.31), axillae (Fig. 9.32) or under the breasts. It causes a well-defined brown discoloration (Figs. 9.33 and 9.34) with a fine wrinkled, slightly scaly surface. It fluoresces a coral-pink colour under Wood's light and this aids the diagnosis (Fig. 9.35). It is often present as maceration of the skin between the toes, and is more common in those who live in hot countries. It responds to topical imidazoles or oral erythromycin.

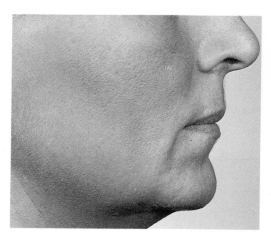

Fig. 9.25 Erysipelas. There is erythema and oedema usually unilaterally. The onset is sudden. The patient feels ill and may have a rigor.

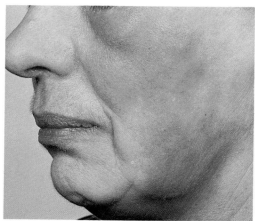

Fig. 9.26 Erysipelas. Recurrent attacks are common probably due to lymphatic deficiency. Continual low dose antibiotic therapy usually prevents further episodes.

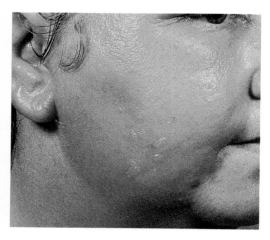

Fig. 9.27 Erysipelas. There may be blistering in addition to the erythema and oedema.

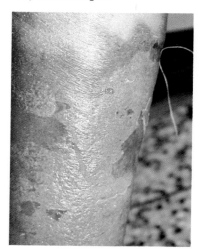

Fig. 9.28 Erysipelas. Erosions may follow erythema, oedema and blistering. The lower leg is a common site.

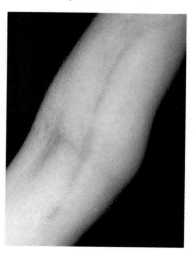

Fig. 9.29 Lymphangiitis. A linear red streak has resulted from an infected condition of the hand. Lymphadenopathy is usually present.

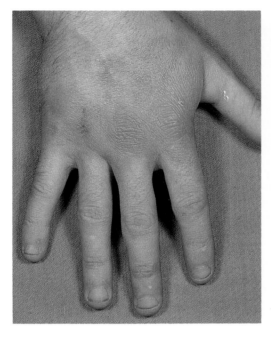

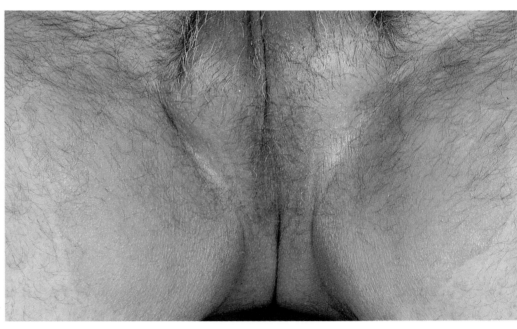

Fig. 9.30 Erysipeloid. Erythema and oedema are present on the back of the hand. By courtesy of St. Mary's Hospital.

Fig. 9.31 Erythrasma. A brown discoloration occurs in intertriginous areas. The groin is a common site.

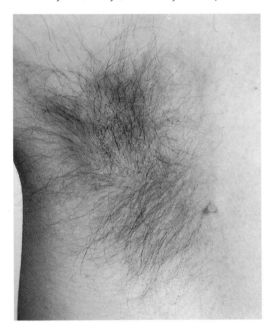

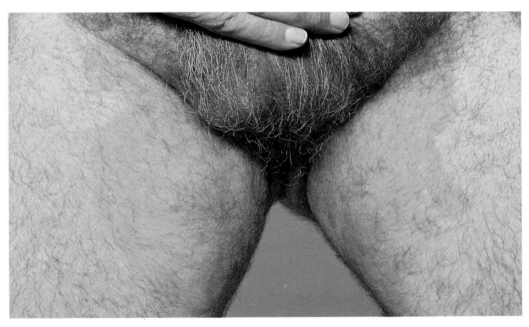

Fig. 9.32 Erythrasma. The axillae are commonly involved. The condition is more common in hot climates.

Fig. 9.33 Erythrasma. The discoloration is caused by *Corynebacterium minutissimum*. By courtesy of St. Mary's Hospital.

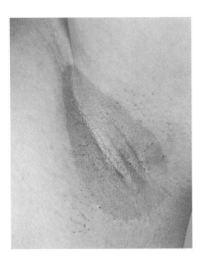

Fig. 9.34 Erythrasma. A brown discoloration is present in the axillae.

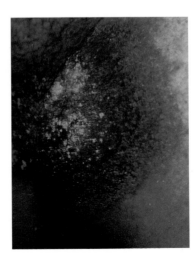

Fig. 9.35 Erythrasma. The organism fluoresces a coral-pink colour under a Wood's light. By courtesy of Dr. Y.M. Clayton, St. John's Hospital for Diseases of the Skin.

TUBERCULOSIS OF THE SKIN

Cutaneous tuberculosis is becoming increasingly uncommon in Western countries following the advent of drugs which can successfully combat the disease and reduce the foci of infection and also as a result of improvements in the nutritional and economic state of the community. The type of lesion produced in the skin depends on whether or not the patient has acquired any immunity to the disease in the past. There is thus both primary tuberculosis of the skin and so-called 'post-primary' disease. In addition, there are cutaneous reactions to the presence of tuberculosis elsewhere in the body which are known as tuberculides.

Primary Tuberculosis of the Skin

Susceptible individuals are those who have never had a previous infection with *Mycobacterium tuberculosis*. The Mantoux test is negative. Direct inoculation of the bacilli into the skin produces a chancre with associated lymphadenitis. The chancre starts as a brown papule which frequently ulcerates and persists as a sore. The edge of the ulcer may be undermined with an adherent crust on the surface. It may occur anywhere on the body but since the bacilli are thought to be introduced via traumatized skin it is usually seen on exposed parts such as the face or limbs, particularly in children.

Post-primary Tuberculosis

BCG Granuloma

A similar lesion to the above may occur after BCG vaccination of an already immune individual (Figs. 9.36 and 9.37). Biopsy of the lesion reveals a granulomatous histology and acid-fast bacilli are demonstrable on Ziehl-Neelsen staining of the section.

Lupus Vulgaris

This variety of cutaneous tuberculosis results from lymphatic or

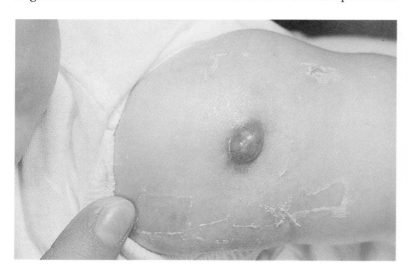

Fig. 9.36 BCG vaccination. A solitary brown nodule is present at the site of BCG vaccination against tuberculosis. The child had had no previous exposure to the disease.

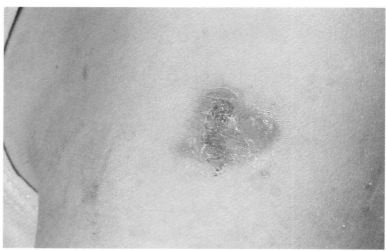

Fig. 9.37 BCG granuloma. The lesion ulcerates and persists as a sore.

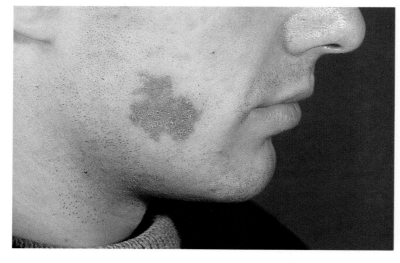

Fig. 9.38 Lupus vulgaris. There is a solitary plaque on the face. The cheek is the commonest site.

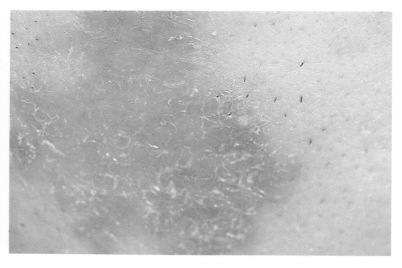

Fig. 9.39 Lupus vulgaris. The plaque has an 'apple jelly' colour and scaling is present.

haematogenous spread from a focus in a bone, joint or lymph node. There is usually a solitary lesion on the face (Fig. 9.38), neck or on a limb. It is a red-brown, somewhat raised, well-demarcated plaque (Fig. 9.39). By pressing the lesion with a glass slide (a procedure known as diascopy) small nodules within the plaque appear as a translucent brown colour, somewhat reminiscent of apple jelly. Subsequently the epidermis overlying the dermal granuloma becomes scaly and atrophic (Fig. 9.40). Superficial ulceration and scarring may result. Similar lesions may occur on a limb (Figs. 9.41 and 9.42). Biopsy of the skin confirms the diagnosis (Fig. 9.43). The condition should clear with appropriate anti-tuberculosis therapy but occasionally the disorder is chronic. After many decades there is a risk of squamous cell carcinoma developing in the lesion.

Tuberculosis Verrucosa Cutis

This is a rare condition secondary to direct inoculation of tubercle bacilli into the skin (Fig. 9.44), usually through an abrasion in a person whose occupation might involve handling material contaminated with the bacilli. Thus, butchers can contract the disease from animals ('butchers' warts') and pathologists from humans during post-mortem examinations. The lesion is usually single and consists of a hyperkeratotic warty plaque on a hand or limb. The red-brown colour of the lesion is suggestive of the diagnosis but a skin biopsy is mandatory. This should confirm the diagnosis.

Scrofuloderma

This term refers to direct infection of tubercle bacilli from an underlying infected lymph node (Fig. 9.45) or bone to the skin. The side of the neck, supraclavicular fossa or axillae are common sites. There is a fluctuant swelling which suppurates and ulcerates. The condition heals on treatment but leaves considerable scarring.

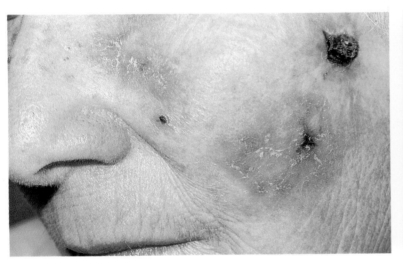

Fig. 9.40   Lupus vulgaris. The skin becomes atrophic and scarred.

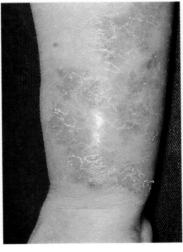

Fig. 9.41   Lupus vulgaris. The brown colour is very typical of lupus on this woman's arm.

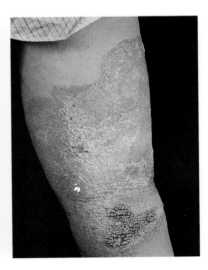

Fig. 9.42   Lupus vulgaris. The lesion is raised, well-demarcated and warty. Skin biopsy for culture and histology can easily be performed.

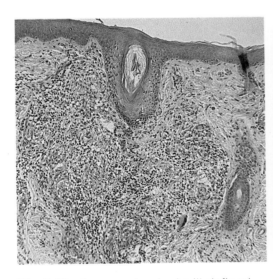

Fig. 9.43   Lupus vulgaris. An ill-defined granulomatous infiltrate containing giant cells is situated in the upper dermis, in close proximity to a hair follicle. There is a heavy admixture of lymphocytes and caseation necrosis is absent. Such features although not absolutely diagnostic are highly suggestive of lupus vulgaris. As is often the case, a Ziehl-Neelsen stain for tubercle bacilli was negative.

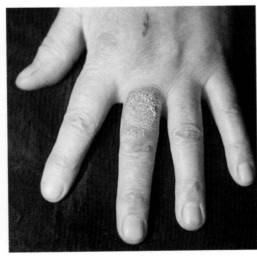

Fig. 9.44   Tuberculosis verrucosa cutis. This condition results from direct inoculation of tubercle bacilli into the skin. It usually occurs as a solitary lesion in a person whose occupation could entail handling contaminated material. By courtesy of St. John's Hospital for Diseases of the Skin.

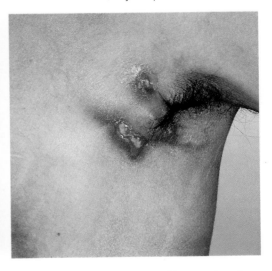

Fig. 9.45   Scrofuloderma. Direct extension to the skin has resulted from infected lymph nodes in the axillae.

Tuberculides

These are cutaneous immunological reactions to tuberculosis elsewhere in the individual, but no tubercle bacilli are demonstrable in the skin lesions.

Erythema Induratum (Bazin's Disease)

These skin lesions are essentially similar to those of erythema nodosum but they may ulcerate, unlike erythema nodosum, and they particularly affect the calves (Fig. 9.46) rather than the shins. The condition is probably the result of circulating immune complexes. The patient complains of painful swellings on the legs. There may be a concomitant fever and joint pains.

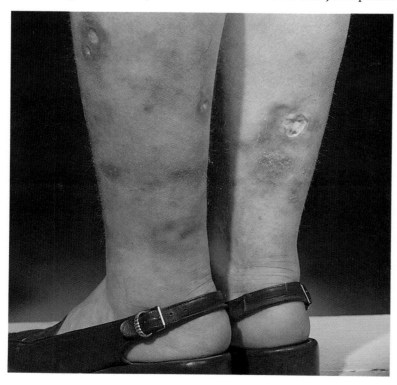

Fig. 9.46 Bazin's disease. Ulcerated tender nodules on the calves are suggestive of tuberculosis.

On examination, red, tender, warm swellings are seen. Nodules can also occur on the fronts of the shins, ankles and feet and occasionally even on the upper limbs. Erythema nodosum or erythema induratum are indications to search for evidence of tuberculosis elsewhere. The eruptions will respond to anti-tuberculous therapy. Occasionally no focus of tuberculosis is found in erythema induratum and yet the Mantoux test may be strongly positive. This particular variety does, however, respond to anti-tuberculous treatment.

Papulonecrotic Tuberculide

This is a rare condition occurring predominantly in young individuals who have active tuberculosis elsewhere. There is an eruption of necrotic, inflammatory, indolent papules which occur in crops on the extremities (Fig. 9.47). This is thought to be an immunological reaction. The histopathology is suggestive of a granuloma but no bacilli can be demonstrated in the lesions. The condition responds to the treatment of the tuberculosis elsewhere.

FISH-TANK AND SWIMMING POOL GRANULOMA

This infection is caused by *Mycobacterium marinum*. It is contracted from contaminated water via a skin abrasion. Fish-tanks or swimming pools are the usual sources. The patient may give a history of having cut the skin whilst cleaning out a fish-tank that previously housed diseased fish (Fig. 9.48). Alternatively, the patient may have abraded the skin of the face or a limb in a contaminated swimming pool. Purple-red nodules (Fig. 9.49) develop at the site of the injury and may subsequently appear along the line of lymphatic drainage from the inoculation site. Healing usually occurs spontaneously after a number of weeks or months.

The diagnosis is made by skin biopsy which shows a granulomatous histopathology. *Mycobacterium marinum* (syn. *balnei*) causes tuberculosis in fish. It is an acid-fast bacillus which can be grown on culture but must be incubated at 31°C and not the usual 37°C required for human tuberculosis.

There is no really specific effective treatment but success has been reported with rifampicin, septrin and minocycline.

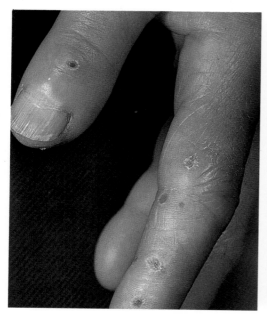

Fig. 9.47 Papulonecrotic tuberculide. Crops of necrotic indolent papules occur particularly on the extremities.

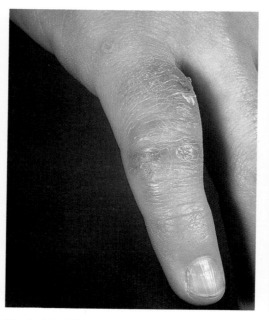

Fig. 9.48 Fish-tank granuloma. This young man had cut his skin on a fish-tank which he was cleaning. The tank had previously housed fish which had died of *Mycobacterium marinum*. By courtesy of St. Bartholomew's Hospital.

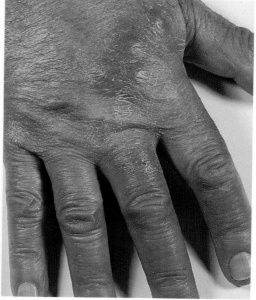

Fig. 9.49 Fish-tank granuloma. This man has developed purple nodules at the site of abrasions acquired whilst cleaning a fish-tank.

GONOCOCCAEMIA

Disseminated gonococcal infections may occur in untreated patients with gonorrhoea. They occur more commonly in females. The organism appears to be slightly different from that causing gonococcal urethritis, which remains limited to the mucous membranes.

The condition essentially affects the skin and the joints,

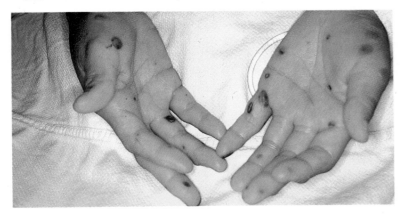

Fig. 9.50 Gonococcaemia. The lesions are haemorrhagic pustules on an erythematous base. By courtesy of Dr. Frank Dann, Honolulu.

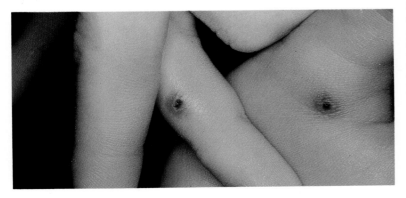

Fig. 9.51 Gonococcaemia. The extremities, particularly the hands are affected. By courtesy of Dr. Frank Dann, Honolulu.

although occasionally a pericarditis or meningitis occurs. The patient is unwell and feverish. The skin lesions are vesicles or pustules on an erythematous base (Fig. 9.50) and are found on the extremities, particularly the fingers (Fig. 9.51). They are sparse. The knees, wrists and ankles are the joints most commonly involved and often only one joint is affected.

SYPHILIS

Syphilis is an infection with the spirochaete *Treponema pallidum*. Spirochaetes are thin-walled, flexible, helical rods. They have some features in common with bacteria but are unusual in that their mobility is due to an internal axial filament rather than the external flagella used by other mobile bacteria. Syphilis is usually transmitted sexually, particularly among homosexual men but may be acquired from maternal disease *in utero* or from infected blood products or instruments. The disease is divided into stages known as primary, secondary, latent and tertiary. The former two stages are infectious. If the disease is untreated, it may progress through all four stages or remit.

Primary Syphilis

The primary lesion or chancre occurs at the site of inoculation between ten days and three months after infection. It is thus usually on the genitalia or around the anus, but may occur anywhere on the body, particularly on the lips, inside the mouth or rectum or on a finger. The chancre is a painless ulcer with an indurated edge (Fig. 9.52). The base is yellow and harbours a large number of spirochaetes which may be demonstrated by dark ground microscopy. The local lymph nodes are enlarged but are quite painless. The chancre heals spontaneously, often without trace, within one to three months.

Secondary Syphilis

Most patients are diagnosed during the primary stage. However, if the chancre is not visible to the patient, either around the anus or in the rectum, the disease may evolve to the secondary stage. This occurs about two months after the chancre.

The patient usually has a fever and presents because of a rash. The eruption is widespread (Figs. 9.53 and 9.54) and particularly

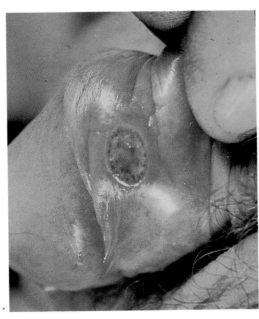

Fig. 9.52 Primary syphilis. The lesion is a painless ulcer with an indurated edge. The base is yellow and harbours large numbers of spirochaetes. By courtesy of Dr. F. Lim, King's College Hospital.

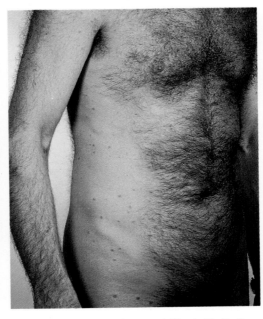

Fig. 9.53 Secondary syphilis. Initially the rash is macular and pink and is most obvious on the trunk. It does not itch. The serology is positive at this stage.

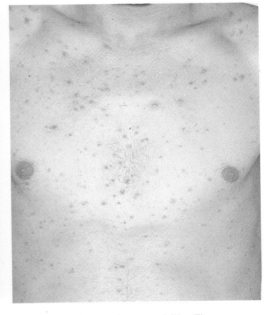

Fig. 9.54 Secondary syphilis. The lesions become papular and more widespread. There is a tendency towards cropping of the lesions. By courtesy of St. Mary's Hospital.

involves the genitalia (Figs. 9.55 and 9.56), palms and soles (Fig. 9.57) and face (Fig. 9.58). It does not itch although clearly if there is some complicating factor such as hepatitis or a second sexually acquired disease such as scabies, the skin will be pruritic. There is a generalized lymphadenopathy. The primary lesion may still be visible.

Initially the rash is macular and pink (roseolar) and is most obvious on the trunk. It becomes papular and more widespread. There is a tendency to cropping of lesions. The papules become brown and may resemble pityriasis rosea or psoriasis. Later lesions may become more infiltrated (Fig. 9.59). The lesions may be more profuse around the frontal hair margin (crown of Venus) and sides of the neck (collar of Venus). Genital and palmar/plantar involvement are constant features. In the intertriginous areas the papules may be eroded (condylomata lata). Condylomata usually occur around the anus or in the groin but may occur under the axillae or breasts, in the umbilicus or between the toes. These lesions are usually moist and exude treponemes in the serum; they are therefore highly infectious.

Slightly raised oval patches occur on the mucous membranes (Fig. 9.60). The tongue, buccal mucous membranes, soft palate and fauces are most usually involved. The lesions have an off-white surface membrane. Several contiguous lesions are known as 'snail-track' ulcers.

Hair loss is common, either as part of the cutaneous eruption (Fig. 9.61) or subsequently as a telogen effluvium response to the systemic upset.

The patient may not be ill at all, but most have some degree of malaise. Headache, sore throat, hoarseness, deafness, photophobia, neck stiffness, polyarthritis and noctural bone pains may all occur. There may also be hepatitis and renal involvement. Anaemia, leucocytosis and a raised ESR are common. At this stage, the serological tests are positive.

Secondary Relapse and Latent Syphilis
If untreated, the patient recovers with a variety of possible sequelae. There may be a secondary relapse of a mucocutaneous nature within two years. The eruption particularly affects the

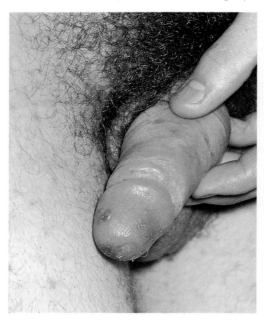

Fig. 9.55 Secondary syphilis. The genitalia are usually involved. By courtesy of St. Mary's Hospital.

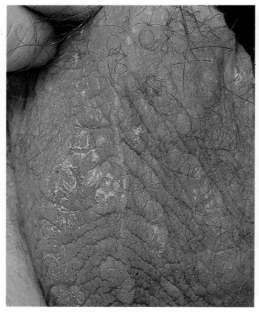

Fig. 9.56 Secondary syphilis. Scaly, red, firm patches are present on the scrotum.

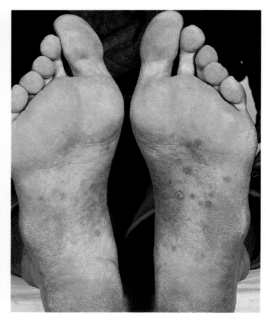

Fig. 9.57 Secondary syphilis. The soles (and palms) are invariably affected with papules.

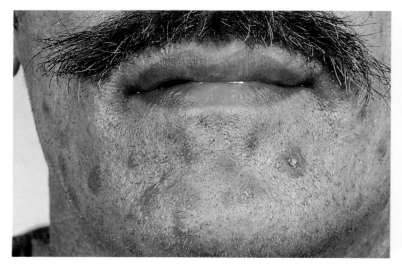

Fig. 9.58 Secondary syphilis. The face is usually involved. The papules may become scaly and resemble pityriasis rosea or psoriasis. Indeed, syphilis tends to mimic other diseases. This is the same patient as in Fig. 9.53.

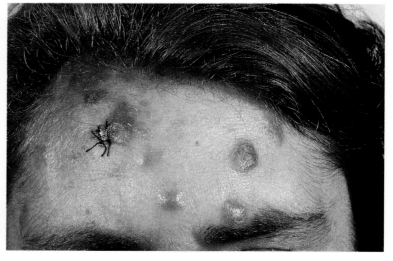

Fig. 9.59 Secondary syphilis. In the later stages, infiltrated plaques may develop. The brown colour of the lesions is characteristic. A skin biopsy was necessary and the histology suggested the diagnosis. Syphilis is uncommon in women; this woman's husband was bisexual.

genitalia and palms and soles. This condition is still infectious. The disease then passes into a latent asymptomatic phase but with positive serology. Even during this phase, sero-negative conversion and spontaneous cure may occur. If it does not, the disease may proceed to cardiovascular or neurosyphilis or other organ involvement. This is known as tertiary syphilis.

Tertiary Syphilis

The gumma is the hallmark of tertiary syphilis. It is a chronic granuloma. It develops a number of years after the primary inoculation and is non-infectious. Only the mucocutaneous manifestations will be dealt with here.

The dermal gummata are firm brownish-red papules or nodules which are usually arranged in an annular pattern as raised plaques (Fig. 9.62). The lesions are asymmetrical and sparse or solitary, with a smooth or scaly surface, resembling psoriasis. They heal with scarring. Subcutaneous lesions may break down and ulcerate. The ulcer is several centimetres in diameter and has a vertical punched-out wall (Figs. 9.63 and 9.64). The base

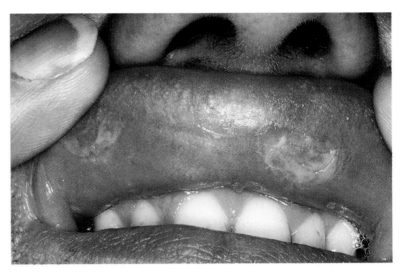

Fig. 9.60 Secondary syphilis. White, slightly eroded patches are present inside the upper lip. By courtesy of Dr. B. Monk.

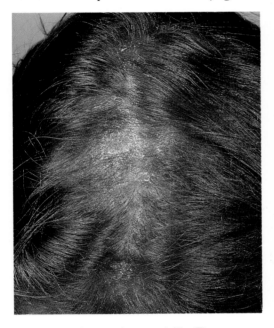

Fig. 9.61 Secondary syphilis. There are patches of erythema, scaling and alopecia in the scalp.

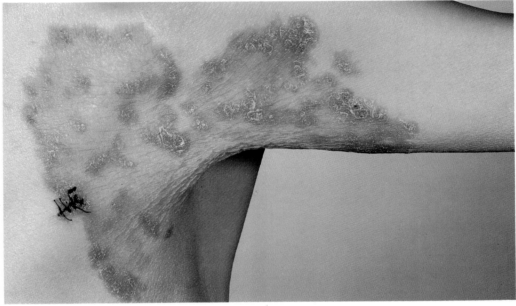

Fig. 9.62 Tertiary syphilis. The lesions are annular and consist of red-brown papules and infiltrated scaling plaques within the lesion. The diagnosis was suggested after a skin biopsy.

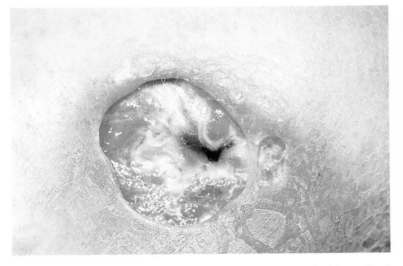

Fig. 9.63 Tertiary syphilis. The ulcer is well-defined with vertical edges and appears 'punched-out'. The base has a yellow slough. By courtesy of St. Mary's Hospital.

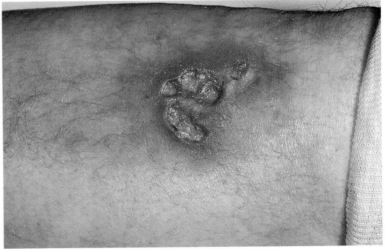

Fig. 9.64 Tertiary syphilis. The ulcers are well-defined with vertical edges. A skin biopsy is necessary to establish the diagnosis.

has a yellow slough rather like a chamois leather. These lesions occur particularly over the upper shins, the chest, face and scalp. Mucosal gummata may occur and the tongue may be diffusely infiltrated, producing white patches, erosions and fissuring. These may be premalignant.

Congenital Syphilis

This disorder is extremely rare where routine ante-natal care demands serological examination of all expectant mothers. The result of transplacental infection depends on the immunological maturity of the fetus and the degree of the infection. Early in pregnancy, abortion or still-birth is the rule and the fetus is covered in blisters. If pregnancy progresses to a later stage, the child may be born with papules and blisters on the palms and soles, or born healthy with subsequent failure to thrive and an eruption similar to secondary syphilis with hepatosplenomegaly and pulmonary and bone involvement. Late congenital syphilis presents with tertiary-like manifestations in childhood. The stigmata include perforation of the palate and collapse of the nose due to gummata and frontal bossing and bowing of the tibia due to periostitis. Nerve deafness, abnormal teeth and interstitial keratitis (Hutchinson's triad) and joint effusions occur. Neurosyphilis may result.

10 Viral Infections
of the Skin

Many human viral disorders have cutaneous manifestations as part of a more general disturbance, for example measles and smallpox, but their description classically lies within the speciality of infectious diseases. The viral disorders which are referred to a dermatologist are described here and in the main they have little or no constitutional disturbance.

HERPES SIMPLEX

Herpes simplex is a double-stranded DNA virus which causes an acute self-limiting eruption on the skin or mucous membranes. When it occurs on the face, it is temporarily disfiguring but produces little morbidity. When it occurs on the genitalia, it can give rise to enormous distress and anxiety.

The disease is contagious and results in an initial primary infection (Figs. 10.1 and 10.2) which may be followed by recurrent attacks without further reinfection. During primary infection, the virus reaches the dorsal root ganglion via peripheral nerves, and it lies dormant there until it is subsequently reactivated. Primary infection often occurs in childhood and is acquired from a parent (Fig. 10.3); a gingivostomatitis may result. The severity of the infection varies but there is an incubation period of three to ten days followed by a fever and sore throat. Painful, grouped vesicles develop on the lips (Fig. 10.4), tongue, gums, buccal mucosae and palate. Erosion and crusting follow and regional lymphadenopathy is present.

Primary infections may occur at other sites, particularly on the genitalia, in adults. Most individuals, however, have no personal or parental recollection of a primary infection and would appear to have had a subclinical primary infection as judged by the presence of antibodies and the tendency to recurrent attacks.

The herpes simplex virus is classified into Type I and Type II. Differentiation could originally be made on a clinical basis because type II infections were limited to ano-genital sites, but this no longer pertains and laboratory tests are required to distinguish the two. Recurrent attacks occur within the area of the initial primary inoculation. The reason for recurrences may be obscure, but the most frequent causes are menstruation, sunlight, fever, stress, trauma and general illness. It is of note that lobar pneumonia is almost invariably accompanied by 'fever blisters', even in those who do not recall having had herpes simplex infections previously. The regularity of the recurrences varies greatly between individuals. Most have one or two a year but some seem to be rarely without attacks, especially in the case of genital lesions.

The eruption begins with tingling or discomfort in the skin and a cluster of lesions develops (Fig. 10.5). These evolve rapidly from a macule to a papule to a vesicle surounded by erythema. The vesicles may coalesce. They dry and scab and, in the majority, heal without scarring. In some, however, they become eroded and necrotic and scarring may result. Secondary bacterial

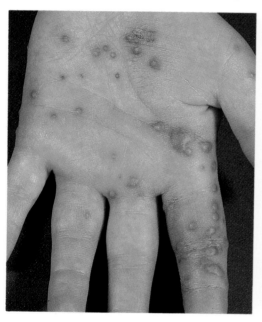

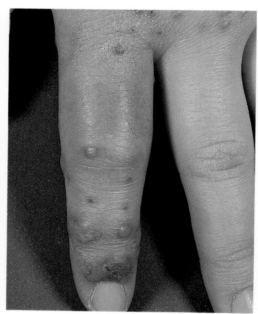

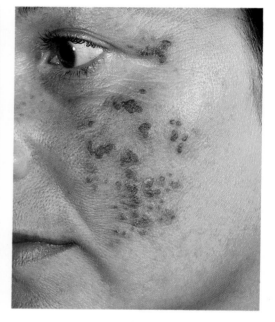

Fig. 10.1 Primary herpes simplex. Widespread vesicles surrounded by erythema are present on the back and front of the hand. Type II herpes simplex was recovered. By courtesy of Dr. Michèle Clement.

Fig. 10.2 Primary herpes simplex. Grouped crusted vesicles surrounded by erythema are present.

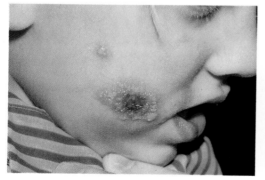

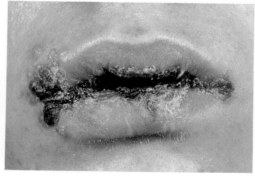

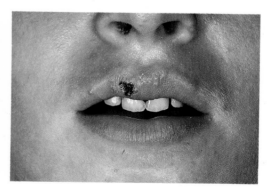

Fig. 10.3 Herpes simplex. The virus is often acquired when an infant or child is kissed by an infected parent. Grouped vesicles, crusting and erythema occur

Fig. 10.4 Primary herpes simplex. A few vesicles are present but most of the lesions have become crusted. This was a primary attack of herpes simplex.

Fig. 10.5 Recurrent herpes simplex. The 'cold sore' occurs most commonly on the lips. Vesicles and crusting are present.

infection occasionally occurs (Fig. 10.6). The length of the attack varies from five to fourteen days.

Infection with herpes simplex may occur anywhere on the mucocutaneous surface but the commonest sites are the lips or face. The genital form (Fig. 10.7) has become increasingly frequent since the late 1960s. Part of the problem is that a woman may have an infection limited to the cervix and therefore experience no symptoms, so the disease is unwittingly transmitted. The virus is active during the vesicular stage and may be a hazard to medical and dental personnel. This may result in inoculation of the skin of an examining finger and result in a so-called 'herpetic whitlow' (Fig. 10.8).

In the main, the cold sore is an innocuous inconvenience but there are certain complications. The eye may become infected, with resultant keratitis and, occasionally, blindness. The early use of the anti-viral agents has, however, been gratifyingly effective.

Sufferers from atopic eczema are particularly susceptible to the virus. The eczema becomes superimposed by the virus and a severe, potentially life-threatening illness known as 'eczema herpeticum' may result (Figs. 10.9 and 10.10). This, fortunately, now responds dramatically to the new anti-viral agent Acyclovir.

Herpes simplex infections are occasionally followed by erythema multiforme or Stevens-Johnson syndrome. The virus causes meningitis and encephalitis. The immunosuppressed are at risk, as are infants born to mothers with active herpes simplex cervicitis or vulvitis. This may result in disseminated cutaneous infection with severe neurological and other organ involvement. Maternal genital infection at the time of parturition is an indication for Caesarean section. Patients with advanced malignant disease, particularly those being treated with immunosuppressive drugs, are similarly at risk from the disseminated disease. There is evidence that the herpes simplex Type II virus could be implicated in the aetiology of carcinoma of the cervix. These women have a higher incidence of herpes simplex antibodies and the virus has been recovered from cell cultures of cervical carcinoma.

The specific treatment of viral disorders is still unsatisfactory. Undoubtedly, however, more progress has been made with the herpes simplex virus than most other viruses. Idoxuridine in dimethyl sulphoxide is gradually being replaced by Acyclovir. This drug reduces the length and the morbidity of recurrent attacks when applied topically, but does not prevent recurrences. Taken orally and continuously it does prevent recurrences. However, the attacks return on stopping the drug and the long-term hazards of continuous therapy are unknown. Oral and intravenous Acyclovir have dramatically improved the treatment of eczema herpeticum and primary and disseminated infections.

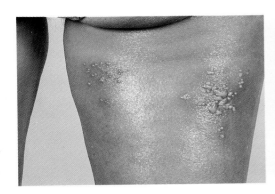

Fig. 10.6   Herpes simplex. The vesicles may become purulent with secondary bacterial infection.

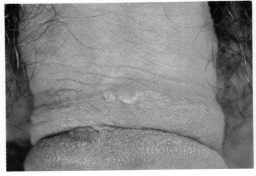

Fig. 10.7   Genital herpes simplex. This disorder is becoming common and causes considerable distress. By courtesy of St. John's Hospital for Diseases of the Skin.

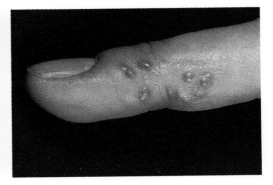

Fig. 10.8   Herpes simplex. Medical personnel and dentists may unwittingly contract the virus on a finger from tending an infected patient.

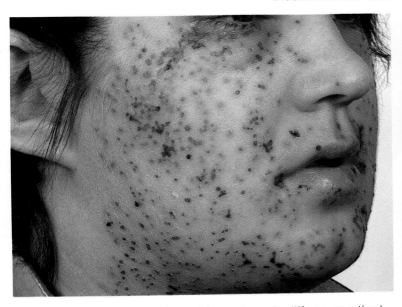

Fig. 10.9   Eczema herpeticum (Kaposi's varicelliform eruption). Eczematous subjects are prone to widespread herpes simplex infections.

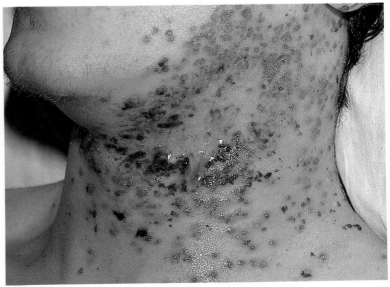

Fig. 10.10   Eczema herpeticum. A myriad of vesicles are present, surrounded by erythema with erosions centrally. Acyclovir has dramatically improved the treatment of this condition.

HERPES ZOSTER (Shingles)

Herpes zoster is an infection caused by the same virus as that which causes varicella (chickenpox) (Fig. 10.11). The disease represents a reactivation of the chickenpox virus which lies dormant in the dorsal root or cranial nerve ganglion after the initial attack. There may be an interval of several decades of latency before the virus spreads along the cutaneous nerves. Shingles cannot be caught from another individual; it occurs only in those carrying the dormant virus. The reactivation of the latent virus is a purely personal event. However, since live varicella virus is present in the lesions of shingles, chickenpox can be contracted by an individual who has never had chickenpox from a patient who is suffering from shingles.

The first symptom is the fairly acute onset of pain or discomfort. By the time of presentation there is usually a vesicular eruption on one side of the body corresponding to a dermatome (Figs. 10.12–10.15). Each individual lesion commences as a macule which rapidly becomes a vesicle surrounded by erythema (Fig. 10.16). The lesions evolve over the next two or three weeks, becoming pustular, haemorrhagic (Fig. 10.17) and finally scabbed (Fig. 10.18). As the scabs fall off, a scar may result (Fig. 10.19). The lesions are to be found at various stages of development. Many become confluent. There are usually satellite lesions to be found elsewhere on the body away from the originally involved dermatome. Secondary bacterial sepsis is common. There may be associated local lymphadenopathy.

For most individuals, an attack of shingles represents a tiresome interlude of two to three weeks during which they feel unwell and uncomfortable but make a full recovery with no sequelae. However, involvement of certain dermatomes may have important complications. Thus, the eye may be involved (Fig. 10.20) if the ophthalmic branch of the trigeminal nerve is attacked. This requires urgent treatment with acyclovir to prevent permanent damage. In these cases, the ciliary ganglion is usually involved and there are vesicles on the side and the tip of the nose. Involvement of the geniculate ganglion gives rise to Ramsay Hunt's syndrome. This is a facial nerve palsy with involvement of the external ear, or tympanic membrane. There may be tinnitus, vertigo and deafness. Involvement of the sacral nerves may be extremely debilitating and may lead to difficulties with micturition and defaecation. Paralysis of an upper or lower limb (usually temporary) may occur secondary to disruption of motor nerves involved by the dermatome. The elderly are particularly at risk from herpes zoster, for there is a significant incidence of post-herpetic neuralgia which may be intractable and very disheartening.

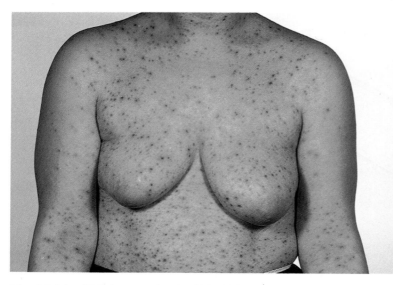

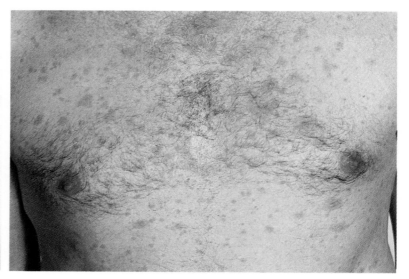

Fig. 10.11 Chickenpox (varicella). Chickenpox and shingles (herpes zoster) are caused by the same virus. Chickenpox may be contracted from a patient with herpes zoster but not vice-versa.

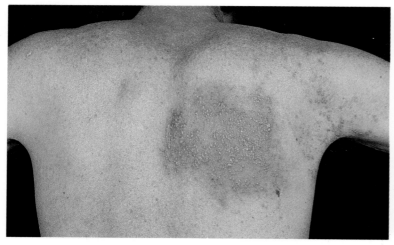

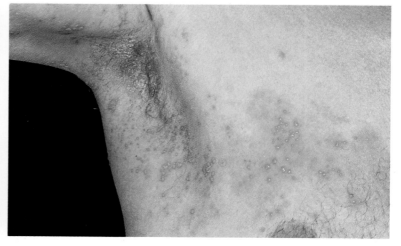

Fig. 10.12 Herpes zoster. The eruption occurs in a unilateral distribution, corresponding to the limits of a dermatome. By courtesy of St. John's Hospital for Diseases of the Skin.

Fig. 10.13 Herpes zoster. Front view of the patient depicted in Fig. 10.12. By courtesy of St. John's Hospital for Diseases of the Skin.

The factors governing the reactivation of the dormant chicken-pox virus are unknown, but clearly, immunosuppressed individuals are at risk. Patients with lymphoma, particularly those undergoing therapy with immunosuppressive drugs, may develop widespread disease such that in addition to the initial single dermatome involvement, there are lesions all over the cutaneous surface, as in chickenpox (Fig. 10.21). In such individuals, the disorder may be life-threatening with visceral, pulmonary, hepatic and neurological involvement.

Treatment is still unsatisfactory. For the majority, adequate analgesia is enough. Some authorities have advocated high doses of systemic steroids as anti-inflammatory agents in an attempt to prevent post-herpetic neuralgia in the elderly. Forty percent Idoxuridine in DMSO has been used topically with some degree of success. Systemic acyclovir is now the treatment of choice for herpes zoster in the immunosuppressed.

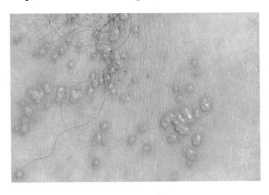

Fig. 10.14 Herpes zoster. Vesicles surrounded by erythema are the hallmark of shingles. This is a close-up of lesions in Fig. 10.13. By courtesy of St. John's Hospital for Diseases of the Skin.

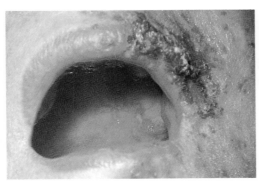

Fig. 10.15 Oral herpes zoster. Vesicles are present in the mucous membranes and on the skin in trigeminal nerve involvement. The eruption is unilateral. By courtesy of St. Mary's Hospital.

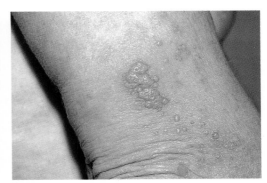

Fig. 10.16 Herpes zoster. Vesicles are surrounded by erythema and subsequently become confluent.

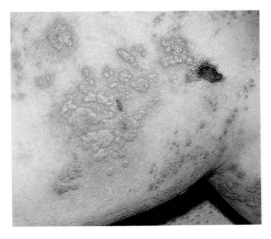

Fig. 10.17 Herpes zoster. The lesions become more haemorrhagic and turbid as they progress.

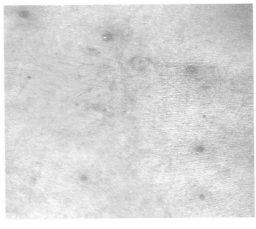

Fig. 10.18 Satellite zoster. Satellite vesicles are usually found away from the involved dermatome in most patients.

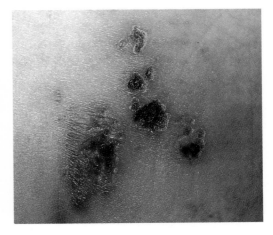

Fig. 10.19 Herpes zoster. Necrotic lesions result and scarring is common following the disorder. By courtesy of St. Mary's Hospital.

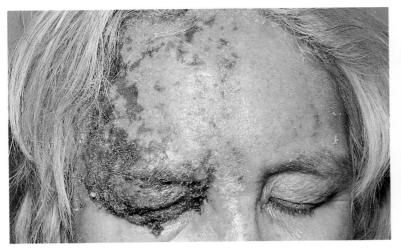

Fig. 10.20 Ophthalmic zoster. Crusting and erosion are present. The ophthalmic branch of the right trigeminal nerve is affected. It is essential to treat the eye if it is involved. By courtesy of St. Mary's Hospital.

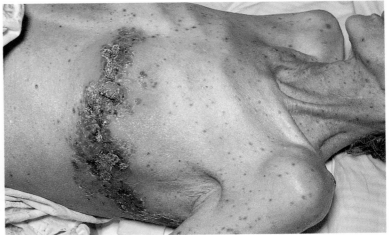

Fig. 10.21 Disseminated zoster. In the immunosuppressed, the virus may be disseminated to involve most of the cutaneous surface as in chickenpox. By courtesy of St. Bartholomew's Hospital.

VACCINIA

Vaccination against smallpox with the vaccinia virus is no longer routine since the virtual eradication of the disease worldwide, so complications of the technique are no longer likely to be encountered. Bacterial sepsis of the vaccination site is the most common complication, but toxic eruptions such as erythema multiforme may also occur. *In utero*, in infants, in the immunosuppressed and in eczema, generalized or progressive vaccinia may occur. Encephalitis is a rare complication. Accidental autoinoculation from the vaccination site occasionally results in an eruption of umbilicated vesicles identical to those of the initial vaccination (Fig. 10.22).

WARTS

These are an extremely common, self-limiting condition of the skin or mucous membranes, particularly in the young. The causative papilloma virus can infect many sites and is serologically different in each area. Warts are harmless but give rise to symptoms because they are unsightly, embarrassing and painful, particularly on the feet. They are infectious and may be contracted from other individuals or from swimming pools and public changing facilities.

Common Warts

Common warts are seen most often on the hands and fingers (Fig. 10.23) and around the nails. However, they may occur anywhere of the body. Clinically, they are firm, discrete papules with a rough, 'warty' surface. They vary in size from one millimetre to well over a centimetre. They may be single or multiple and occasionally, they coalesce and may produce larger masses.

Plane Warts

Plane warts are very small lesions which are just slightly raised with a smooth, flat, skin-coloured or slightly pigmented surface (Figs. 10.24 and 10.25). They occur particularly on the face and the backs of the hands. They are often misdiagnosed, probably because they are quite small and do not have a rough, 'warty' surface and are erroneously treated with topical glucocorticosteroids, in which case they spread. Frequently, they occur in lines corresponding to a scratch or some other such trauma. This is known as the Koebner phenomenon. Plane warts may be peculiarly persistent.

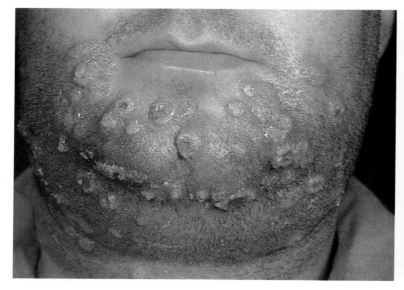

Fig. 10.22 Vaccinia. Accidental autoinoculation of the virus from a vaccination site results in umbilicated vesicles identical to those of the original vaccination.

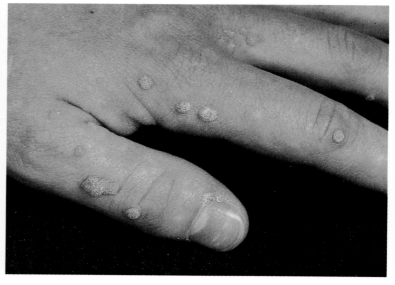

Fig. 10.23 Common warts. The hands and fingers are the most common sites. The lesions are discrete, firm papules with a rough surface.

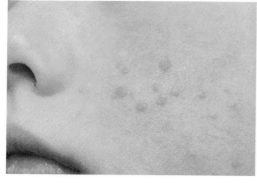

Fig. 10.24 Plane warts. Discrete slightly raised small lesions occur on the face. They are often mistaken for acne or, worse, for eczema and mistreated with topical steroids, in which case they spread.

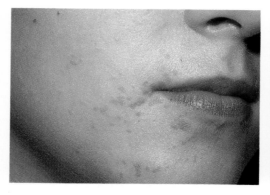

Fig. 10.25 Plane warts. The lesions may be quite pigmented. They are often persistent.

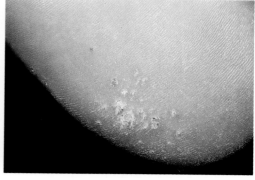

Fig. 10.26 Plantar warts (verrucae). The lesions are frequently multiple and coalesce to produce a mosaic pattern. They are well-defined and have a rough surface. They bleed on paring.

Plantar Warts

Plantar warts are often known colloquially as 'verrucae'. Single lesions may occur but frequently they coalesce and then are known as 'mosaic' warts (Fig. 10.26). If they occur on the direct pressure-bearing areas of the feet they can be painful and interfere with walking. Because direct pressure forces them deep into the dermis they are flat, almost circular lesions, with a rough surface. Pin-point black spots may be seen on the surface due to thrombosed capillaries. The capillaries will bleed on paring the wart and serve to differentiate them from corns (callosities). A corn (Figs. 10.27 and 10.28) represents a thickening of the skin overlying a bony prominence, resulting from friction between the skin, the bony prominence and tight-fitting shoes. The skin becomes more and more normal-looking on paring in contrast to a wart. Plantar warts can be extremely persistent.

Filiform or Digitate Warts

Filiform or digitate warts are often found on the face, neck or anogenital area (Figs. 10.29–10.32). In the latter site they are known as 'condylomata accuminata'. They may invade the vagina, urethra or rectum. Certain serological types may be implicated in cervical carcinoma.

The treatment of warts is unsatisfactory. There are no suitable anti-viral agents available. All warts ultimately resolve so that conservative measures are usually preferred, especially since recurrences are common. Salycilic acid, podophyllin and formalin are the mainstays of conservative therapy. Applications of liquid nitrogen are effective for warts in most sites but may be painful, especially on the feet. Surgery is useful for single lesions.

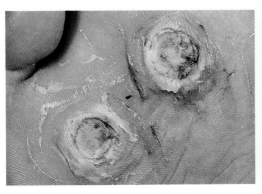

Fig. 10.27 Corns. A corn is a thickening of the skin resulting from friction. On the sole they occur over bony prominences and are distinguished from verrucae because the skin appears more normal on paring and does not bleed.

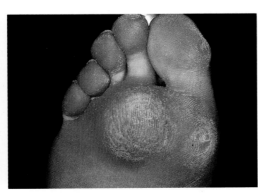

Fig. 10.28 Callosities. The hyperkeratotic skin has occurred over the metatarsal phalangeal joints and the medial side of the big toe, areas which are easily compressed by ill-fitting shoes.

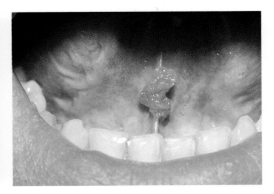

Fig. 10.29 Digitate (filiform) warts. Warts may occur on mucous membranes. This wart was probably contracted sexually.

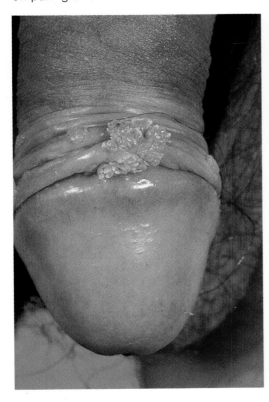

Fig. 10.30 Penile warts. Filiform warts on the genitalia are usually sexually transmitted and the patient should be screened for other sexually transmissible disorders.

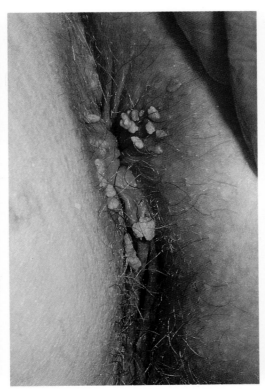

Fig. 10.31 Perianal warts. Discrete raised pedunculated warty lesions are present. They may be treated with podophyllin applied by an experienced operator (or else a perilesional dermatitis may occur), liquid nitrogen or surgery.

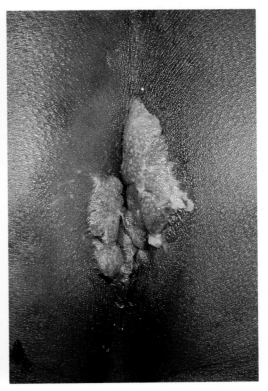

Fig. 10.32 Perianal warts. Large accumulations of warts may occur especially if they are initially treated with topical steroids. The source of these warts in this ten-year-old was not established.

MOLLUSCUM CONTAGIOSUM

This is a common eruption affecting the skin and mucous membranes and is caused by a large DNA virus which is a member of the pox group. The lesions are flesh-coloured, dome-shaped papules (Fig. 10.33) which vary in size from minute lesions to a centimetre or so in diameter. A central depression is visible in the surface of the lesion (Fig. 10.34). This 'umbilication' is a most important diagnostic sign. The lesions occur anywhere on the body but particularly on the face and trunk in children and around the genitalia in adults (Fig. 10.35). The lesions are fairly infectious. Children acquire them from one another at school, and swimming pools are common sources of infection. Genital lesions in adults (Fig. 10.36) are usually acquired sexually. The lesions disappear spontaneously after several months.

As they disappear they often develop a surrounding patch of eczema (Fig. 10.37). They can vary in number from a single lesion (Figs. 10.38 and 10.39), which may be difficult to diagnose prior to histological examination, to multiple lesions. Patients with eczema are prone to this infection. The lesions are then commonly mistaken for the eczema and are inappropriately treated with topical steroids and therefore spread extensively.

The lesions respond well to treatment by destructive methods such as liquid nitrogen therapy, curettage and cautery, or piercing the lesions with an orange-stick dipped in aqueous phenol or iodine. Once they have gone they rarely recur.

ORF

This condition is also due to a pox virus and is contracted from infected sheep. The condition causes vesicles around the mouth of the animals and is sometimes known as 'scabby mouth'. The virus survives on fences and feeding troughs from which the infection may be acquired. The disease occurs in butchers (Fig. 10.40), meat porters and farmers and others who have occasion to encounter contaminated material. There is usually a solitary lesion on a finger, which lasts just over a month. It is a papule with the characteristic appearance of a red centre surrounded by a white ring, with red in the periphery (Figs. 10.41 and 10.42). It weeps and then crusts over before separating away from the underlying healing skin. There is frequently regional lymphadenopathy and a fever. Occasionally, a toxic eruption, such as erythema multiforme, occurs in addition. There is no specific treatment.

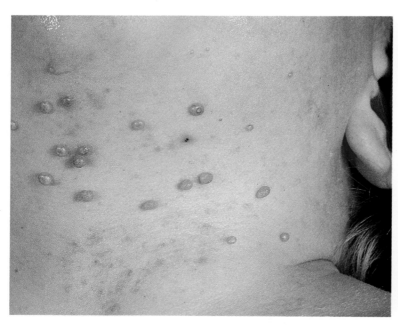

Fig. 10.33 Molluscum contagiosum. Several discrete dome-shaped papules are present on the neck of this two-year-old.

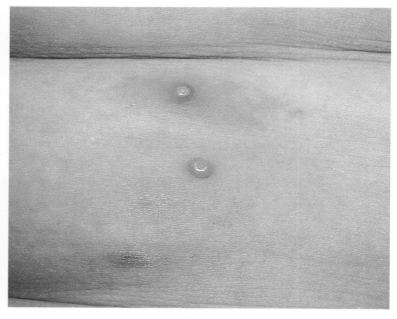

Fig. 10.34 Molluscum contagiosum. A central depression ('umbilication') is visible on the surface of the lesions.

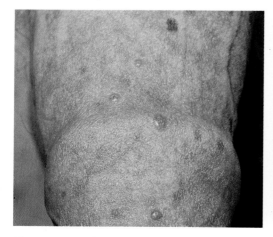

Fig. 10.35 Genital molluscum contagiosum. These lesions are contracted sexually.

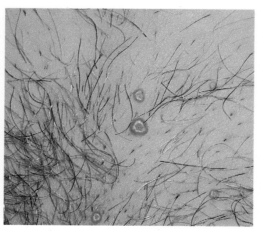

Fig. 10.36 Pubic molluscum contagiosum. It is wise to screen for other sexually transmissable disease in adults with genital lesions.

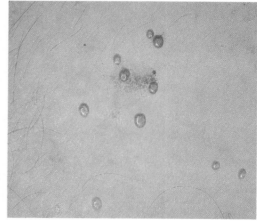

Fig. 10.37 Molluscum contagiosum. Eczema frequently develops around the lesions as they resolve.

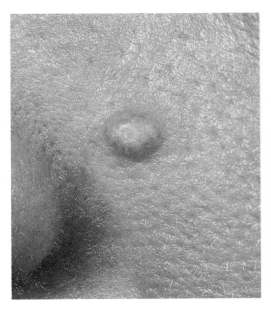

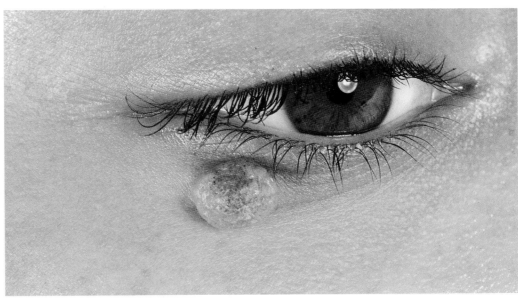

Fig. 10.38 Solitary molluscum contagiosum. The central depression in the surface of the lesion is a helpful diagnostic physical sign.

Fig. 10.39 Solitary molluscum contagiosum. Solitary lesions may be difficult to diagnose clinically. They are often quite large ('giant molluscum'). This lesion is well-defined, raised and dome-shaped and there is central change.

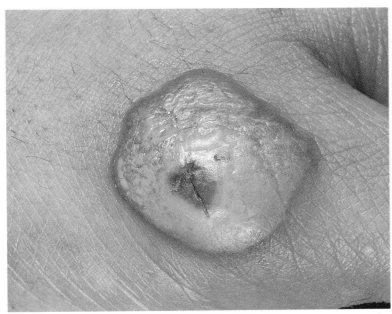

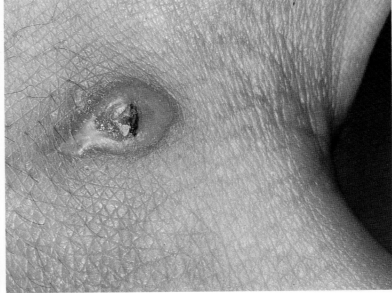

Fig. 10.40 Orf. The lesion is vesicular and weeps. These two Arab brothers were amateur butchers preparing halal meat for Ramadan. They had not recognized the sheep's 'scabby mouth'.

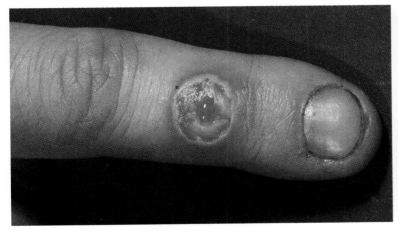

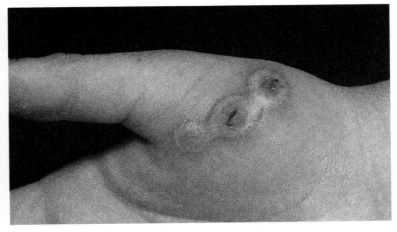

Fig. 10.41 Orf. The lesion often has a red centre, surrounded by white with red at the periphery.

Fig. 10.42 Orf. The fingers or hand are the most common sites. It is contracted from sheep infected with the virus. Three lesions are present.

10.9

HAND, FOOT AND MOUTH DISEASE

This is a disorder of children and young adults. It is caused by a Coxsackievirus, usually of the A16 strain. This is an Enterovirus of the picorna family. There is a three-day incubation period during which the virus enters via the buccal mucosa and the small intestine. It travels to the regional lymph nodes and there is then a generalized viraemia with localizing of the virus to the mouth, hands and feet. The condition lasts above seven days. The clinical picture is distinctive. There are a limited number of oval, slightly yellow, vesicles surrounded by erythema on the hands and feet (Fig. 10.43). In the mouth, erosions (Fig. 10.44) are more common since the roof of the vesicle is quickly removed by the tongue. There is a mild systemic disturbance and the condition does not usually recur.

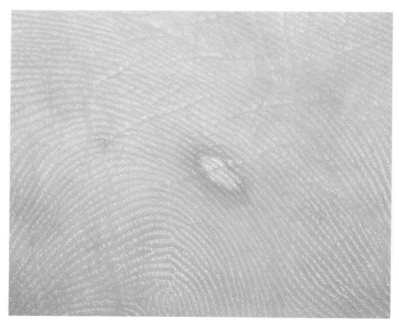

Fig. 10.43 Hand, foot and mouth disease. The lesion is an oval white vesicle surrounded by erythema on the palm. There are usually only a few lesions. By courtesy of St. Bartholomew's Hospital.

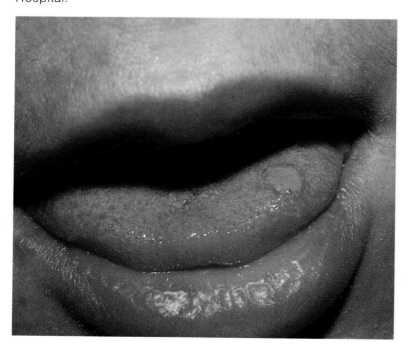

Fig. 10.44 Hand, foot and mouth disease. Discrete, small oval or round erosions occur in the mouth. The disorder is self-limiting and caused by Coxsackievirus.

11 Fungal Infections of the Skin

Superficial fungal disorders of the skin are very common and usually respond admirably to treatment. If misdiagnosed, however, they are almost invariably treated with topical glucocorticosteroids and since these drugs are immuno-suppressives, the fungi will flourish and the disease process worsen.

PITYRIASIS VERSICOLOR

This is a common, insidious condition of young, healthy adults caused by *Pityrosporum orbiculare*, a lipophilic yeast. It occurs after puberty and the development of mature sebaceous glands. The yeast is a unicellular commensal of normal skin but in the pathogenic state it reproduces by budding and produces filaments known as pseudohyphae. In this form the organism is known as *Malassezia furfur*. The yeast is an opportunist. Pathogenicity is encouraged by an increase in environmental temperature and humidity, such that many individuals notice its presence after a summer vacation. It is also a common cutaneous complication in individuals who are immuno-suppressed, either through disease, for example lymphoma, or through drugs, for example systemic steroids.

The physical signs are small macules which coalesce as they increase in size, so that lesions of various shapes and sizes occur (Fig. 11.1). They tend to surround the orifices of hair follicles. The fungus is keratinophilic and thus occurs in the stratum corneum and produces scaling (Fig. 11.2). This scaling may not be immediately obvious on examination but can be demonstrated by gentle scraping of a lesion with a blunt scalpel. The colour of the lesions varies (hence 'versicolor') but is distinctive. In the pale, non-suntanned Caucasian the lesions are brown or fawn-coloured (Fig. 11.3). In the suntanned individual the lesions appear pale in comparison with the surrounding normal skin (Fig. 11.4). This was originally thought to be caused by the fungus shielding the melanocytes from ultra-violet light irradiation. However, it is now clear that dicarboxylic acids produced by the fungus temporarily impair melanocytic function and thus cause hypopigmentation. In any one individual, including dark-skinned people, both hyper- (Fig. 11.5) and hypopigmented lesions (Fig. 11.6) may occur.

The eruption is asymmetrical and occurs on the back, chest (Fig. 11.7) and neck. It is most unusual to see the disease on the face, despite the fact that it is well supplied by sebaceous glands. The explanation for this is not clear, but possibly covered areas of the body produce the occlusive environment which favours pathogenicity. In widespread cases, especially those mistreated with topical steroids (Fig. 11.8), lesions may also occur on the limbs.

The diagnosis can be confirmed by taking scrapings of the skin with a blunt scalpel. The scales are put on a microscope slide and 30% potassium hydroxide solution is added. The thick-walled, spherical yeasts with pseudohyphae may then be seen. Certain ink stains are taken up by the organism, giving a better microscopic preparation (Fig. 11.9). This fungus is not readily grown on culture media and therefore culture methods are not routinely performed.

The fungus is easily treated. Half-strength Whitfield's ointment, selenium sulphide shampoo or topical applications of imidazoles are all effective. Systemic ketoconazole, 200mg daily for five days, is also curative but should only be used rarely because it is a potentially hepatotoxic agent. The condition often recurs either because of inadequate therapy or because of a resurgence

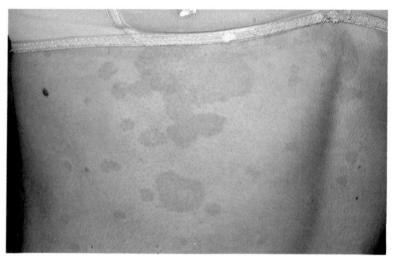

Fig. 11.1 Pityriasis versicolor. The lesions commence as small macules which coalesce resulting in lesions of different shapes and sizes.

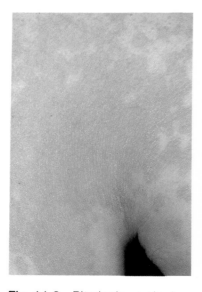

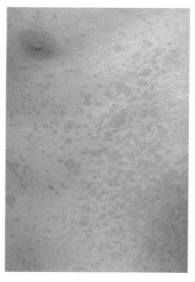

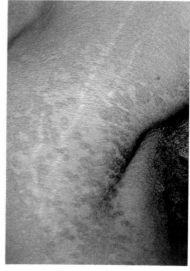

Fig. 11.2 Pityriasis versicolor. Slight scaling is just visible. Gentle scraping of the lesions with a blunt scalpel will enhance the scaling.

Fig. 11.3 Pityriasis versicolor. Fawn-coloured or brown macules coalesce to produce confluent patches.

Fig. 11.4 Pityriasis versicolor. The fungus produces dicarboxylic acids which temporarily impair melanocytic function resulting in hypopigmented macules.

Fig. 11.5 Pityriasis versicolor. Hyperpigmented macules are present in this West Indian.

of the original precipitating factors. It should be noted that pityriasis versicolor does not respond to oral griseofulvin unlike tinea infections. In order to avoid confusion, the condition's alternative name, tinea versicolor, is better abandoned.

Complete resolution of the rash occurs within three or four weeks of treatment. However, in those who have pronounced hypopigmentation, although the scaling (the sign of active pityriasis versicolor) disappears, white areas remain (Fig. 11.10) simulating vitiligo. It is usually several months before the melanocytes recover and start producing pigment again.

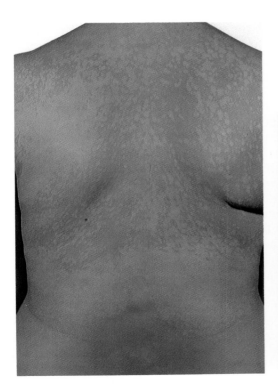

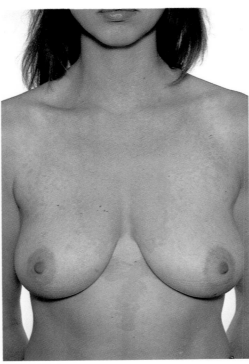

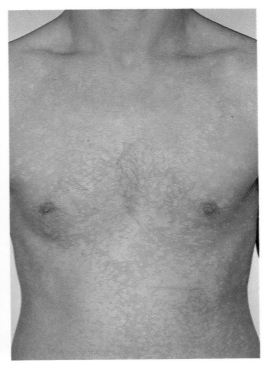

Fig. 11.6 Pityriasis versicolor. Both hypo- and hyperpigmented lesions may occur in one individual.

Fig. 11.7 Pityriasis versicolor. The eruption occurs mainly on the torso.

Fig. 11.8 Pityriasis versicolor. Hypo- and hyperpigmented macules are present. The eruption becomes wide-spread if mistreated with topical steroids.

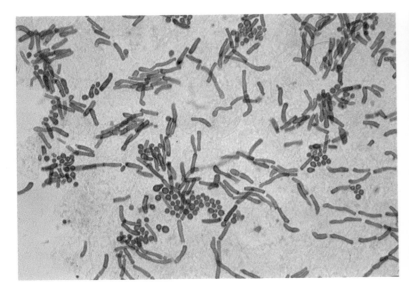

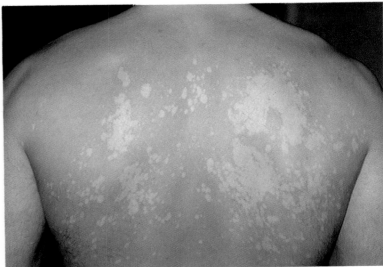

Fig. 11.9 Pityriasis versicolor. *Malassezia furfur* is found in the skin. Parker's stain (equal parts 30% potassium hydroxide and Parker's blue-black ink) (x 128). By courtesy of Miss G. Midgley, St. John's Hospital for Diseases of the Skin.

Fig. 11.10 Pityriasis versicolor. The hypopigmentation may be mistaken for vitiligo, especially after treatment, but the lesions are asymmetrical, of various shapes and sizes and confined to the torso unlike vitiligo.

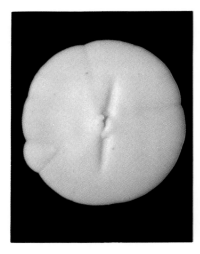
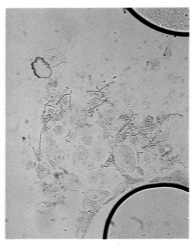

Fig. 11.11 *Candida albicans.*
Candida albicans is a yeast. It
has a pasty appearance on
culture. By courtesy of Dr. Y.M.
Clayton, St. John's Hospital for
Diseases of the Skin.

Fig. 11.12 *Candida albicans.*
Candida albicans in 30%
potassium hydroxide (x 128).
By courtesy of Miss G.
Midgley, St. John's Hospital for
Diseases of the Skin.

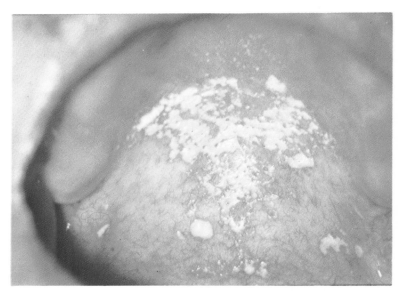

Fig. 11.13 Oral candidosis. White and yellow pustules are
present on the palate. By courtesy of St. Mary's Hospital.

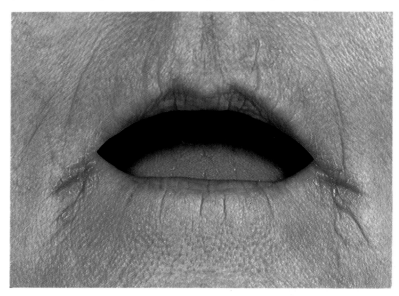

Fig. 11.14 Angular cheilitis. The condition occurs in the
edentulous, especially those whose dentures are ill-fitting such
that the conformation of the mouth is altered.

CANDIDA ALBICANS

Candida albicans is a yeast (Figs. 11.11 and 11.12). It is a
commensal of the gastrointestinal, upper respiratory and
genital tracts and also of warm and moist skinfolds. It becomes
pathogenic quite readily and particularly favours a warm,
occluded, wet environment. The disease states that result are
oral and genital candidosis (mucous membrane candidosis,
commonly known as thrush), candida intertrigo and chronic
paronychia.

Oral Candidosis

Certain groups of individuals are at risk. The condition is
common in infancy where immunological defence mechanisms
are poorly-developed and the infection is frequently contracted
from the genital tract of the mother. Ill and debilitated patients
are particularly susceptible. These patients are usually immunosuppressed, either because of their underlying condition or
because they are being treated with immunosuppressive drugs
(particularly systemic steroids). Alternatively, broad spectrum
antibiotics alter the normal bacterial flora permitting *Candida* to
take their place. Otherwise healthy individuals who are edentulous, wear dentures and have poor dental hygiene are at risk. The
denture provides occlusion which in turn implies increased
moisture and warmth: the ideal environmental conditions for
the overgrowth of *Candida albicans.*

The diagnosis of oral candidosis is not difficult. Well-defined
white or yellow pustules (Fig. 11.13) or plaques are visible on the
palate, tongue, buccal mucous membranes or gums. The lesions
are easily scraped away with a spatula leaving a red, raw,
bleeding base.

The condition responds to treatment of the predisposing
conditions and the use of nystatin or one of the imidazoles. Oral
ketoconazole is also effective but rarely required.

Angular Cheilitis (Perlèche)

Although a disorder classically associated with the under-
nourished, this is most commonly seen in patients who wear
dentures which do not fit properly. The conformation of the
mouth becomes distorted and sags, such that the upper lip tends
to overhang the lower and a groove is formed at the angles of the
mouth (Fig. 11.14). Saliva trickles imperceptibly down the fold
providing a perfect habitat for *Candida albicans* to flourish. The
area is sore, red, scaling and often fissured. Swabs taken from
the cheilitis will confirm the condition. Sometimes, *Staphylococcus
aureus* colonizes the area in addition to *Candida* or it may occur
on its own. Swabs from the denture and mouth may also be
positive for *Candida.* The condition responds to correcting the
dentures and also to improvement in oral hygiene. It is
important that the patients do not sleep in their dentures and are
also taught to sterilize the dentures properly.

Genital Candidosis
Candida Vulvo-vaginitis

Candida vaginitis is very common in young women. It may be
precipitated by oral contraceptive therapy, pregnancy or
systemic broad-spectrum antibiotics, all of which may alter the
local flora. Fashionable, tight-fitting clothing produces an
occluded, warm and moist environment which exacerbates the
problem. Severe pruritus and soreness result, with a thick,
abundant cream-coloured discharge. There is associated
erythema and oedema. This is a common presentation of diabetes
mellitus in middle-aged, often overweight women and it is
mandatory to test the urine of any female presenting with
candida vaginitis. If the vaginitis is neglected, the adjoining skin
becomes involved. The appearances are of red, raw, glazed,

oedematous skin (Fig. 11.15). The margin of the eruption is macerated and pustules seen away from the main body of the eruption are typical.

Predisposing causes should be attended to and the condition is treated with nystatin or imidazole pessaries. Recurrent attacks may be particularly troublesome. It may be necessary to sterilize the bowel with oral nystatin and occasionally, specific oral anti-candida treatment such as ketoconazole is necessary.

Candida Balanitis

Balanitis is usually contracted from a sexual partner with active disease. It is much more common in the uncircumcized since the prepuce provides an ideal occluded environment for the yeast to flourish. The glans may be red and swollen and studded with yellow pustules (Fig. 11.16). The condition responds to topical anti-candida agents.

Candida Intertrigo

Intertrigo is a dermatological term used to indicate a skin eruption occurring in an area between two opposing surfaces of the skin (Fig. 11.17). The axillae (Fig. 11.18), the groin (Fig. 11.19) and under the breasts are the major intertriginous areas. However, the interdigital, umbilical and other folds (particularly those occurring in the obese) and the posterior nailfolds are also intertriginous sites. There are various skin diseases which have a predilection for these areas, which include psoriasis, seborrhoeic eczema, erythrasma and tinea. An intertriginous site is ideal for candidosis because it is warm, moist and subject to friction and thus damage to the stratum corneum. Occlusive dressings or clothing, including napkins in infants, compound the problem.

The initial lesions are pustules on an erythematous base which become confluent. These break leaving red and raw skin. The outer margins of the eruption are often macerated. Maceration is a term used to describe excessive hydration of the stratum corneum. The skin appears thickened, white and sodden. Satellite lesions are characteristic and consist of fresh pustules away from the central core of the rash.

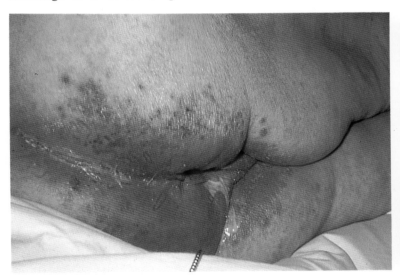

Fig. 11.15 Perineal candidosis. The skin becomes red and raw with discrete satellite pustules.

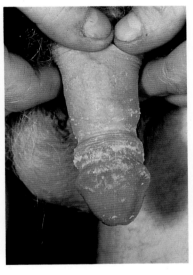

Fig. 11.16 Candida balanitis. The glans is studded with yellow pustules. It is more common in the uncircumcized. By courtesy of Dr. F. Lim.

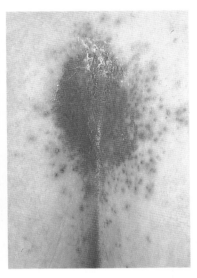

Fig. 11.17 Candida intertrigo. A raw erythema is present in the natal cleft with satellite pustules away from the central eruption. This lady was found to have glycosuria.

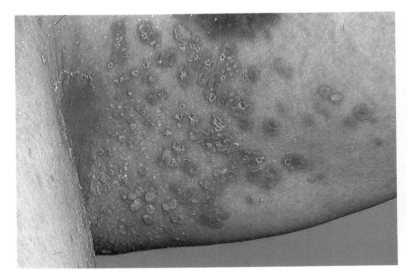

Fig. 11.18 Candida intertrigo. This lady had injured her arm in a fall; the bruising is evident. An eruption occurred between the two apposing skin surfaces because she was unwilling to move the arm. An erythema is present in the axilla and pustules are radiating out from it. By courtesy of St. Mary's Hospital.

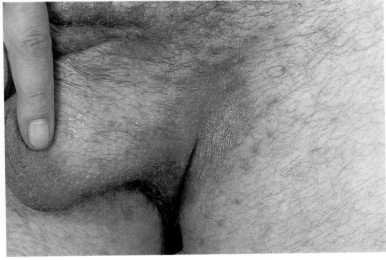

Fig. 11.19 Candida intertrigo. There is maceration in the fold with satellite pustules on the thighs and scrotum.

Erosio Interdigitale

The apposing folds of skin between the fingers are not usually colonized by *Candida* but if the skin becomes damp and macerated because of too much immersion in water it becomes an ideal environment. There is a central red, raw and eroded area surrounded by maceration of the skin (Figs. 11.20 and 11.21).

Candida Paronychia

This common condition of the nail and posterior nailfold is described in Chapter 21.

Chronic Mucocutaneous Candidosis

This is an extremely rare disorder. A detailed description is not appropriate here, suffice to say that chronic mucocutaneous changes occur as a result of various immunological defects, particularly of cell-mediated immunity, in association with multiple endocrine defects or thymoma. Their delineation is the province of the immunologist but the clinical features are those of persistent oral thrush, often producing chronic hypertrophic changes, vulvo-vaginitis and destructive nail changes from chronic paronychia (Fig. 11.22). There are often widespread cutaneous hypertrophic plaques over the face, hands and elsewhere. Advances in immunotherapy and the availability of ketoconazole have vastly improved the treatment of this distressing condition.

TINEA (Ringworm)

Ringworm is a superficial fungal disorder of the skin. The fungus lives in dead keratin, that is, in the hair, nails or stratum corneum. It does not, ordinarily, penetrate deeper into the living cells. The fungus is a dermatophyte, a multicellular organism characterized by hyphae, which mat together to form mycelia. The hyphae can be seen on direct microscopy of the affected hair, nails or skin scales treated with potassium hydroxide (Fig. 11.23). The dermatophytes reproduce by spore formation. Vegetative arthrospores may be visible on direct microscopy but asexual spores are only produced after culture of material on Sabouraud's medium. This takes about three weeks. The asexual spores are known as macroconidia. There are three genera of dermatophytes which are identified by their macroconidia. They are known as *Microsporum, Epidermophyton* and *Trichophyton*. Thus, the individual genus and its species cannot be identified prior to culture but certain clinical characteristics of the infection may suggest the presence of one dermatophyte rather than another.

Ringworm infections may be described under their causative genera but it is customary to describe the infections in relation to their site on the skin.

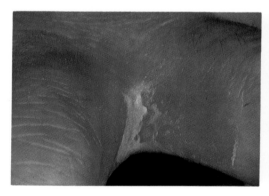

Fig. 11.20 Erosio interdigitale. There is maceration and erosion in the web between the fingers. This woman was a domestic and always had her hands in and out of water. Wet, occluded skin is ideal for colonization by *Candida albicans*.

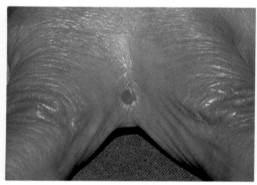

Fig. 11.21 Erosio interdigitale. This is a very early lesion. There is a central erosion surrounded by maceration. This occurred in a gynaecologist who was continually washing her hands after each consultation but not drying them carefully enough.

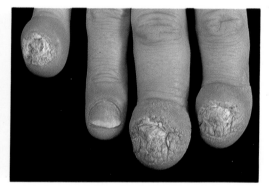

Fig. 11.22 Chronic mucocutaneous candidosis. Persistent nailfold erythema and oedema and severe dystrophic changes in the nails occur as a result of colonization by *Candida* due to immunoparesis. By courtesy of St. John's Hospital for Diseases of the Skin.

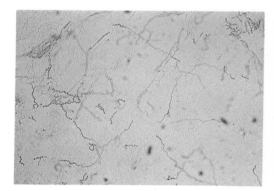

Fig. 11.23 Dermatophyte hyphae. Hyphae are present in scrapings of skin treated with potassium hydroxide (x 32). By courtesy of Miss G. Midgley, St. John's Hospital for Diseases of the Skin.

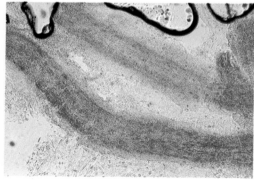

Fig. 11.24 Small-spored ectothrix. Infection of the outer hair root sheath is caused by *Microsporum* species. 30% potassium hydroxide preparation (x 32). By courtesy of Miss G. Midgely, St John's Hospital for Diseases of the Skin.

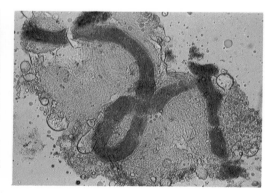

Fig. 11.25 Endothrix infection. The fungus invades the inner hair shaft. 30% potassium hydroxide preparation (x 96). By courtesy of Miss G. Midgley.

Tinea Capitis

Ringworm of the scalp presents as one or several patches of hair loss coupled with various degrees of inflammation of the skin. There may, in addition, be lesions elsewhere. The pattern of hair loss depends on the amount of damage done by the fungus. Certain fungi invade the outer root sheath of the hair (ectothrix, Fig. 11.24). The affected hairs are broken off above the surface of the scalp and the coating of spores gives the hair a rather dull appearance. Other fungi invade the inner hair shaft itself (endothrix, Fig. 11.25). The damage done by the hyphae and the spores is considerable such that the hairs are broken off close to the surface. The inflammatory changes depend on whether the fungus is of human (anthropophilic) or animal (zoophilic) origin. With a human ringworm infection, the inflammatory changes may be quite minor (Fig. 11.26) but with an animal infection, host resistance is high and considerable inflammation (Fig. 11.27) may result in a boggy mass known as kerion. The patterns of tinea capitis are traditionally typed into ectothrix and endothrix infections, kerion and a fourth category known as favus.

Ectothrix Infections

SMALL-SPORED ECTOTHRIX FUNGI. These all belong to the *Microsporum* genus. They are the most common ringworm infections of the scalp. They are virtually never seen after puberty, probably because growth is inhibited by fatty acids produced by the mature sebaceous glands. Thus, a child with the disorder would recover spontaneously at puberty. There are two common species – *M. canis* (Fig. 11.28) and *M. audouinii*. The former is zoophilic (originating in either a cat or dog) and the latter is anthropophilic. The fungi invade the outer hair shaft and deposit their spores. These spores can be seen on direct microscopy. Hairs infected with either of these fungi fluoresce a brilliant green colour (Fig. 11.29) under an ultra-violet lamp emitting radiation at 360nm (Wood's light). Infections with human ringworm are highly contagious and will spread from one child to another at school. Examination with a Wood's lamp can be extremely helpful in identifying those affected in an epidemic. *M. canis* is usually limited to the handlers of the affected animal and usually does not spread from human to human. The physical signs are patches of redness and scaling of the scalp with loss of hair (Fig. 11.30). The degree of inflammation with *M. audouinii* may be quite small but can be considerable with *M. canis*, even amounting to kerion formation on occasion.

LARGE-SPORED ECTOTHRIX FUNGI. The zoophilic species of the *Trichophyton* genus are responsible for large-spored ectothrix fungi. *T. verrucosum* is contracted from cattle or horses and *T. mentagrophytes* var. *granulare* from cattle, horses or rodents. The inflammatory response is considerable (Fig. 11.31). There is loss of hair in patches, redness and thick scaling. Kerion formation may occur. These species do not fluoresce with Wood's lamp. The anthropophilic species of the *Trichophyton* genus rarely cause tinea capitis.

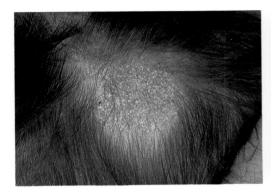

Fig. 11.26 Tinea capitis. In anthropophilic infections there is minimal scaling with loss of hair.

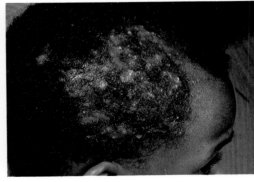

Fig. 11.27 Tinea capitis. There is pronounced weeping and crusting coupled with hair loss in this case of ringworm caught from an infected cat.

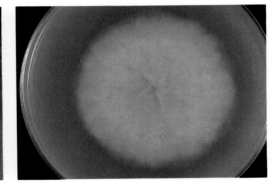

Fig. 11.28 *M. canis*. On culture, the underside of the plate is yellow. By courtesy of Dr. Y.M. Clayton, St. John's Hospital for Diseases of the Skin.

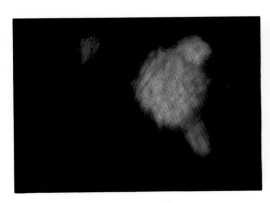

Fig. 11.29 Wood's light fluorescence. Microsporum hair infections fluoresce under Wood's light. This is helpful in identifying affected children in epidemics. By courtesy of Dr. Y.M. Clayton, St. John's Hospital for Diseases of the Skin.

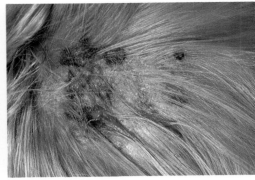

Fig. 11.30 Tinea capitis. In zoophilic infections there is considerable in-flammation (kerion) with loss of hair An infected kitten was the cause in this case,

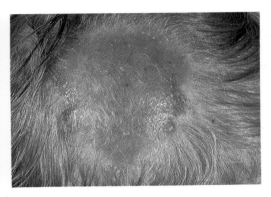

Fig. 11.31 Tinea capitis. Ringworm of the scalp due to animal fungi is characterized by severe inflammation which may result in kerion formation. This adult was infected by a cattle ringworm. Scalp ringworm in adults is very unusual.

Endothrix Infections

The hyphae and spores invade the hair shaft and the outer sheath is spared. The hair is completely destroyed down to its base and black dots are left behind. The degree of inflammation is not great and a patchy baldness without much scaling may be all that is to be found on examination. *T. tonsurans (T. sulphureum), T. soudanense* (Fig. 11.32) and *T. violaceum* are the fungi responsible. They are rarely seen in the United Kingdom.

Kerion

This is a severe inflammatory scalp reaction to a ringworm infection, usually of animal origin and particularly *T. verrucosum* or *T. mentagrophytes* var. *granulare*. The scalp is a red, warm, painful, pustular mass. There is crusting and the hairs become matted (Fig. 11.33) and fall out. The condition is self-limiting because of the host rejection but permanent scarring and alopecia may ensue if the condition is not treated.

Favus

This is very rare in Western Europe but common in the Middle East. It is important to diagnose this fungal infection immediately because neglect may lead to permanent scarring and thus alopecia (Fig. 11.34). This rarely happens with the other fungi covered here. Favus is caused by *T. schoenleinii*. It is an endothrix infection but the hyphae are not as abundant as in the other endothrix infections so the hair is less damaged and may grow quite long. Classically, small crusts occur around the hairs (Fig. 11.35). These are known as scutulae but they may not always be present. There is a characteristic mousy odour associated with this condition. It is imperative to examine and culture the hairs in any case of patchy alopecia.

Treatment

Tinea capitis responds well to griseofulvin or ketoconazole. The former has a long, safe track record and is the treatment of choice. Prior to 1958 when griseofulvin became available, treatment of this condition could be far from satisfactory. It was often treated with radiotherapy in order to induce epilation of the affected hairs. Occasionally, particularly in the earlier part of the century when radiation dosages were not very accurate, overdose occurred and permanent alopecia resulted (Fig. 11.36). In some cases, tumours of the head, neck and skin of the scalp have developed fifty or sixty years later (Fig. 11.37).

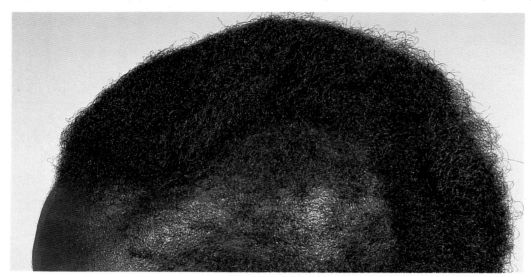

Fig. 11.32 Tinea capitis. *T. soudanense*, an anthropophilic fungus, was responsible for this boy's scalp ringworm. He came from West Africa where he had acquired this endothrix infection.

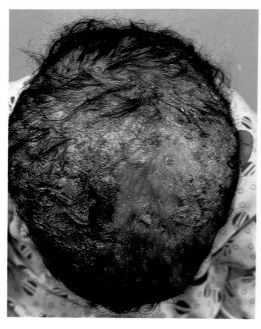

Fig. 11.33 Kerion. There is crusting and the hair is matted secondary to the severe inflammatory reaction. By courtesy of St. John's Hospital for Diseases of the Skin.

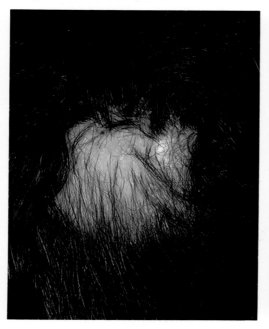

Fig. 11.34 Favus. Scarring alopecia often results from this infection with *T. schoenleinii*.

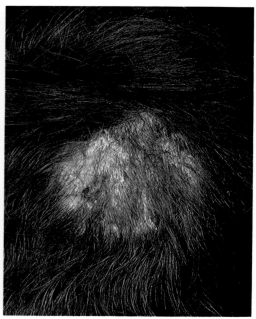

Fig. 11.35 Favus. Crusting occurs around the hairs. By courtesy of St. John's Hospital for Diseases of the Skin.

Tinea Corporis

This is the form of dermatophyte infection which is best described as ringworm (Fig. 11.38). However, the term 'ringworm' is still confusing because many common skin disorders, for example discoid eczema (Figs. 11.39 and 11.40) and the herald patch of pityriasis rosea (Fig. 11.41) are ring-shaped whereas dermatophyte infections may not be ring-shaped.

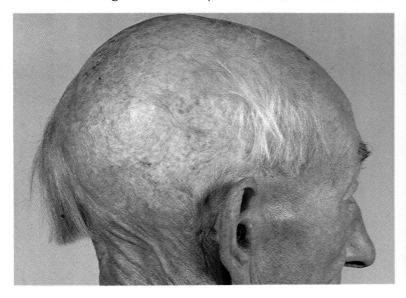

Fig. 11.36 Alopecia secondary to irradiation of scalp ringworm. Scalp ringworm was treated with irradiation before griseofulvin was available. Over-irradiation resulted in life-long alopecia.

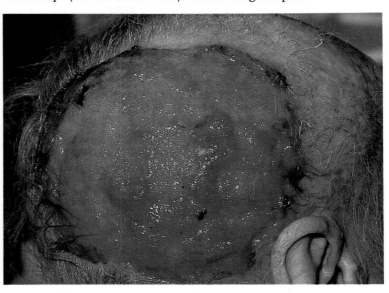

Fig. 11.37 Basal cell carcinoma secondary to irradiation of scalp ringworm. Over-irradiation of scalp ringworm may result in neoplastic change many decades later.

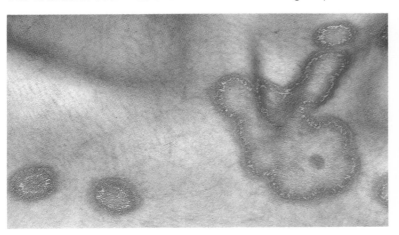

Fig. 11.38 Tinea corporis. The activity of ringworm occurs at the margins of the lesions which have a tendency to heal centrally. Scrapings should be taken from the red scaly margin for the identification of hyphae. By courtesy of Dr. A.C. Pembroke.

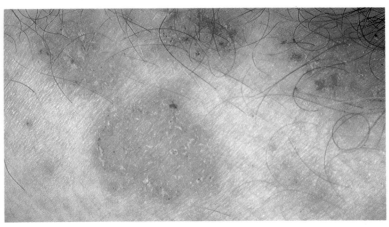

Fig. 11.39 Discoid eczema. The lesions do not show central healing or post-inflammatory pigmentation and are red and scaling across the lesion.

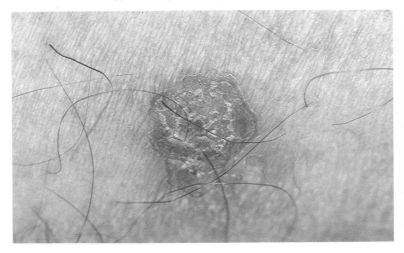

Fig. 11.40 Discoid eczema. The lesions may be crusted in discoid eczema. The activity of the eruption is even across the surface. By courtesy of St. John's Hospital for Diseases of the Skin.

Fig. 11.41 The herald patch of pityriasis rosea. This is often misdiagnosed as tinea but the erythema remains constant throughout the lesion. A few days later other small oval pink lesions develop.

The features which suggest tinea corporis are an annular eruption, with a tendency to active margins and a healing central area which is often hyperpigmented (Fig. 11.42). The fungus tends to migrate outwards for fresh nutrient material. The lesions are red and scaly and asymmetrically placed (Fig. 11.43). The degree of erythema and scaling depends on the type of fungus. Animal ringworm is much more inflammatory than human ringworm (Fig. 11.44).

Tinea Faciei

Tinea of the face has much the same characteristics as tinea corporis. The lesions are asymmetrical, annular red patches. There is scaling and redness at the periphery of each lesion (Fig. 11.45) and a tendency towards central healing and pigmentation (Fig. 11.46).

Tinea Cruris

Ringworm in the groin is a common pruritic eruption in young men but is unusual in women. It is caused by the anthropophilic fungi only, particularly *Trichophyton rubrum*, *Epidermophyton floccosum* and *T. mentagrophytes* var. *interdigitale*. It spreads outwards asymmetrically from the genito-crural folds and down the thigh, leaving post-inflammatory pigmentation (Fig. 11.47). The advancing border is well-defined, slightly raised, red and scaly (Fig. 11.48). It is frequently misdiagnosed and treated with topical glucocorticosteroids which permit the condition to spread (Figs. 11.49 and 11.50). It is, therefore, always wise to examine scrapings from any skin condition in the groin for the presence of fungi. There may well be evidence of tinea elsewhere, especially in the toe webs and toenails which may lead to recurrent attacks unless treated. The eruption may spread onto the buttocks (Figs. 11.51 and 11.52) and lower abdomen (Fig. 11.53).

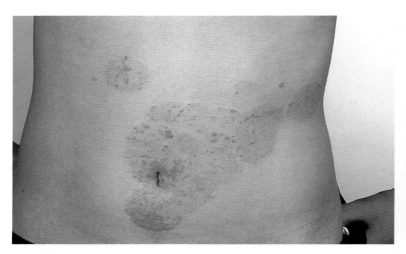

Fig. 11.42 Tinea corporis. Post-inflammatory hyperpigmentation is a feature of healing tinea. This eruption had been mis-diagnosed and treated with topical steroids which reduce the inflammatory response.

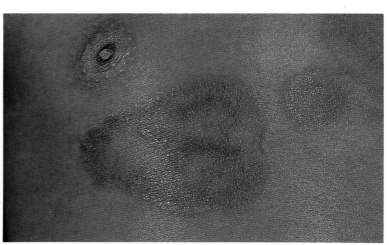

Fig. 11.43 Tinea corporis. The margin of the annular lesions is most active. The lesions are asymmetrically distributed.

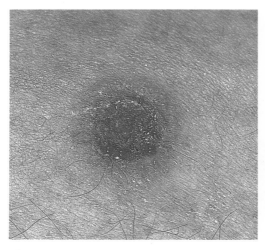

Fig. 11.44 Tinea corporis. Animal ringworm infections are more inflammatory than human. *Microsporum canis* was grown on culturing scales from this lesion.

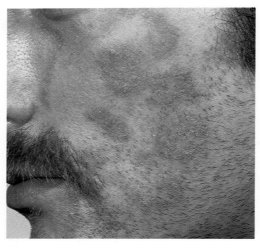

Fig. 11.45 Tinea of the face. Annular, red, scaly patches are present on the cheek. The condition had been misdiagnosed and treated with topical steroids which caused the eruption to spread.

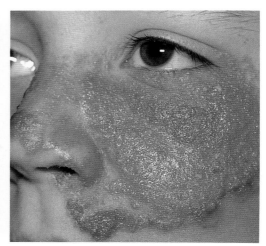

Fig. 11.46 Tinea of the face. The margin of the eruption is most active. Many pustules are present (kerion) as a result of mistreatment with topical steroids.

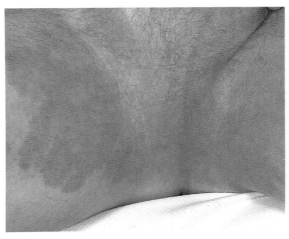

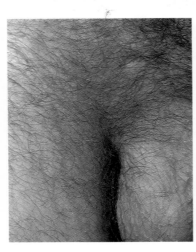

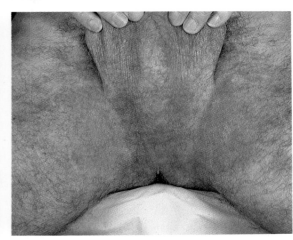

Fig. 11.47 Tinea cruris. The margins of the eruption on the thighs are red and there is post-inflammatory pigmentation in areas which have been invaded by the fungus.

Fig. 11.48 Tinea cruris. The margin of the eruption is red and scaling and tends to advance away from the genito-crural fold down the inner thigh. By courtesy of St. John's Hospital for Diseases of the Skin.

Fig. 11.49 Tinea cruris (tinea incognito). The eruption is frequently misdiagnosed and treated with topical steroids which suppress the physical signs of inflammation so that the linear border is not visible. Scrapings were, however, full of hyphae.

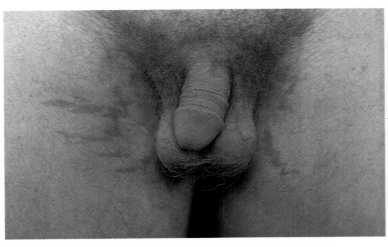

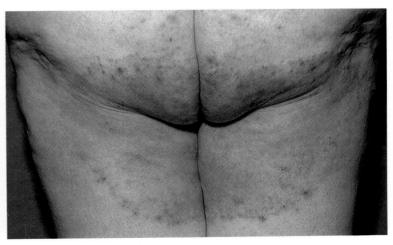

Fig. 11.50 Tinea cruris (tinea incognito). This had been treated with powerful topical steroids. Gross striae have resulted but the inflammatory physical signs are suppressed except for an active red and scaling edge in the lower part of the right inner thigh, where the patient had failed to apply the steroid. By courtesy of St. John's Hospital for Diseases of the Skin.

Fig. 11.51 Tinea of the buttocks. Tinea may spread from the groin onto the buttocks, especially if treated with topical steroids. The active edge is pronounced with central hyperpigmentation. There is considerable excoriation because tinea may be very pruritic in this area.

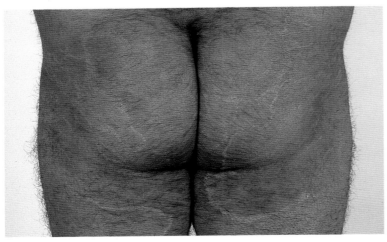

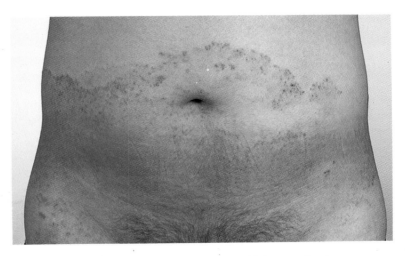

Fig. 11.52 Tinea of the buttocks. This man also had sarcoidosis and the accompanying immunosuppression permitted the rash to become extensive. *E. floccosum* was grown on cultures of his skin.

Fig. 11.53 Tinea of the lower abdomen. This man had a *T. rubrum* infection of the groin which had been treated with topical steroids and had become extensive.

Tinea Pedis

This is colloquially known as 'athlete's foot'. It is more common in men and is usually acquired from communal changing rooms in institutions or sports facilities. Only the anthropophilic fungi are responsible. *T. mentagrophytes* var. *interdigitale* and *E. floccosum* produce similar clinical appearances but *T. rubrum* is described separately because of its special characteristics.

The eruption is found in the toe webs. There is peeling, scaling and erythema. The skin is macerated (Fig. 11.54). The condition is itchy but may become sore if it is fissured (Fig. 11.55). The eruption is usually asymmetrical, one foot being more involved than the other. Many individuals have this condition between the webs of their fourth and fifth toes but only about a quarter of these cases are due to tinea. Most cases are due to compression of the fourth toe against the fifth by tight-fitting shoes, thus producing a macerated intertrigo but, no fungi will be recovered on culture of the skin scales. This condition may respond to toe spacers and better fitting footwear. Equally, soft corns (Figs. 11.56 and 11.57) caused by the rubbing of the fourth toe against the fifth secondary to ill-fitting shoes are regularly mistaken for tinea. However, infection of other toe webs is almost certainly due to tinea.

The condition spreads onto the sole of the foot and presents as an itchy, vesicular eruption (Figs. 11.58 and 11.59), usually unilaterally. The vesicles often coalesce and large confluent blisters result. In these acute, vesiculo-bullous eruptions, secondary bacterial infection may be superimposed and a lymphangiitis results. Occasionally, a vesicular eruption identical to that of an acute hand eczema (pompholyx) may result along the sides of the fingers (Fig. 11.60) and hands. This is referred to as an 'id' phenomenon. No fungi are recovered from these vesicles but the eruption does respond to treatment of the tinea pedis.

If tinea is untreated or mistreated with topical steroids it may spread onto the dorsa of the feet. The eruption is asymmetrical (Figs. 11.61 and 11.62) and tends to have an active red scaling margin (Fig. 11.63).

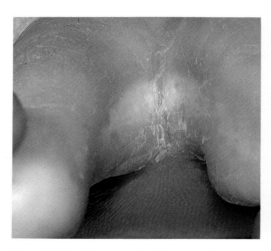

Fig. 11.54 Tinea pedis. The eruption starts as maceration between the toes.

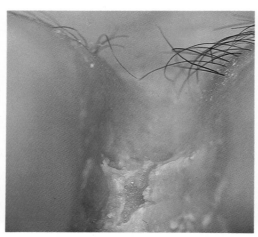

Fig. 11.55 Tinea pedis. Painful fissuring may occur in addition to the maceration. By courtesy of St. John's Hospital for Diseases of the Skin.

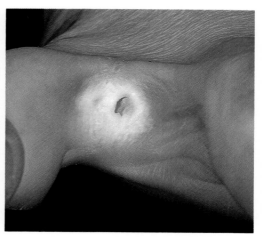

Fig. 11.56 Soft corn. Corns due to friction between the skin of the fourth and fifth toes due to ill-fitting shoes are sometimes misdiagnosed as tinea pedis.

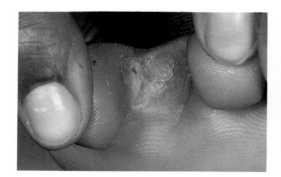

Fig. 11.57 Soft corn. The skin is thickened and hyperkeratotic. Only the lateral side of the web is involved.

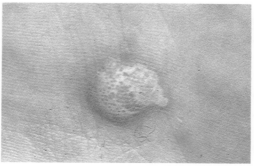

Fig. 11.58 Tinea pedis. Tinea may present as vesicles on the sole of the foot. The eruption is usually unilateral.

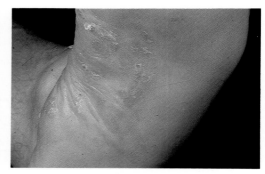

Fig. 11.59 Tinea pedis. Vesicles and scaling are present on the sole of the foot. This is often colloquially known as 'athlete's foot'.

Trichophyton Rubrum Infections

This is now the commonest dermatophyte infection in the United Kingdom (Fig. 11.64). It was rare before World War II but was imported by British troops who acquired it in the Far East. It commences, as do the other fungi, between the toes, causing macerated, fissured and scaling skin, but does not cause a vesicular response on the soles. The host's response is minimal so the degree of inflammatory change is correspondingly small.

Thus, the changes on the skin may be quite subtle (Fig. 11.65). The skin is dry and rather powdery, particularly in the skin creases and there is a peeling of the skin. Nail involvement is frequent and the fungus may subsequently spread to the hands and fingernails. Tinea cruris is very common. *T. rubrum* lesions may spread to the lower legs and produce a papular or nodular eruption on the calf or shin. The condition is known as Majocchi's granuloma (Fig. 11.66).

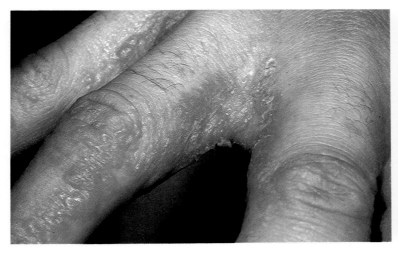

Fig. 11.60 Pompholyx. Acute eczema of the hand may occasionally result as a reaction to an acute tinea pedis (an 'id' phenomenon).

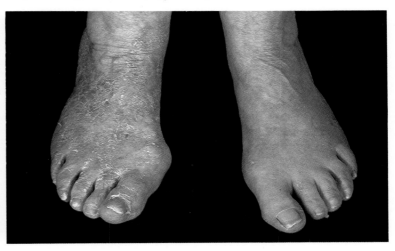

Fig. 11.61 Tinea pedis. The eruption is often unilateral. The toenails are also involved. Topical steroids were responsible for the spread of the rash.

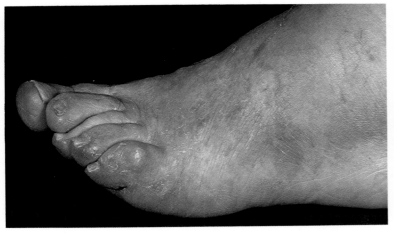

Fig. 11.62 Tinea pedis. The tendency to red rings is visible. The toenails are involved.

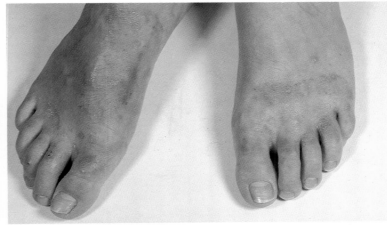

Fig. 11.63 Tinea pedis. This man had been prescribed a powerful topical glucocorticosteroid. The condition had spread considerably. The asymmetry of the eruption is suggestive of tinea.

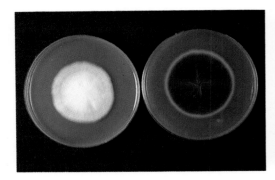

Fig. 11.64 *Trichophyton rubrum*. The underside of the plate is a red colour, hence the adjective rubrum. It is the most common cause of dermatophyte infections in the United Kingdom. By courtesy of Dr. Y.M. Clayton, St. John's Hospital for Diseases of the Skin.

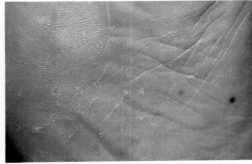

Fig. 11.65 *T. rubrum* infection of the feet. The condition presents as peeling of the skin.

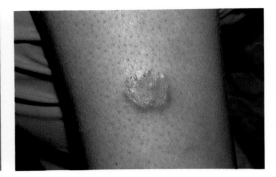

Fig. 11.66 Majocchi's granuloma. This is a nodular annular eruption on the back of the calf due to *T. rubrum*.

Tinea Manuum

Ringworm of the dorsum of the hand or wrist (Figs. 11.67 and 11.68) should be regarded as a form of tinea corporis, but ringworm of the palm presents special characteristics. It is almost invariably caused by *T. rubrum*. It is unilateral and may remain this way for decades, a situation for which there is no satisfactory explanation at the present time. There are crescentic, peeling scales (Fig. 11.69) to be seen and a powdery filling-in of the skin creases (Fig. 11.70). The palmar skin feels dry. Sooner or later the fingernails become involved.

Tinea Incognito

This is an artificial term to describe ringworm infections that have been misdiagnosed and treated with topical glucocorticosteroids. The use of topical steroids somewhat modifies the clinical picture of the eruption because there is a damping down of the usual inflammatory responses which indicate the presence of the disorder. Thus the margin of the eruption, which is usually slightly raised, red and scaly, may be barely perceptible. There may, however, be an untreated area which will suggest the correct diagnosis. It is imperative to take scrapings from any eruption with scales, particularly those which do not conform to the correct pattern of a skin disorder.

Tinea Unguium

The nails are often invaded by the anthropophilic fungi, especially *T. rubrum* (see Fig. 21.13). They are discussed fully in the chapter on nail disorders.

MANAGEMENT OF DERMATOPHYTE INFECTIONS

Griseofulvin was a major advance in the management of dermatophyte infections. It is a very safe drug and patients only occasionally experience side-effects, nausea and headaches being the most common. It is the only effective treatment for ringworm of the scalp and nails and for *T. rubrum* infections. Tinea corporis, tinea pedis and tinea cruris will show some response to topical anti-fungal agents such as the imidazoles and half-strength Whitfield's ointment but they are not as efficient as griseofulvin. Most cases will clear within four weeks of treatment with griseofulvin but nail involvement represents a special case (see Chapter 21). Ketoconazole is also effective but in view of its hepatotoxicity, it is a second line drug.

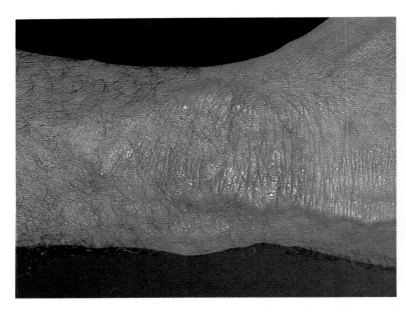

Fig. 11.67 Tinea of the wrist. The eruption is annular with central healing.

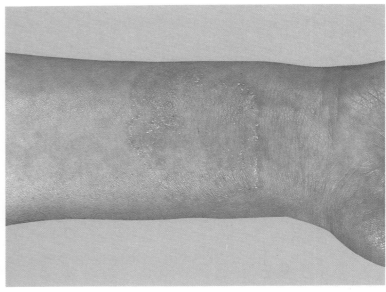

Fig. 11.68 Tinea of the wrist. This is frequently misdiagnosed as contact dermatitis to a wrist-watch but the red scaly margin and central healing suggest tinea.

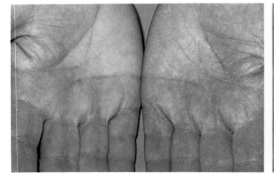
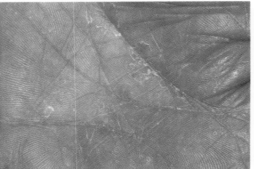

Fig. 11.69 *T. rubrum* infection of the hand. The eruption is invariably unilateral. Closer examination reveals crescentic peeling scales.

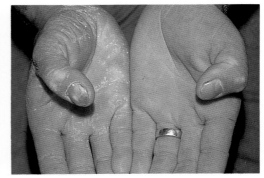

Fig. 11.70 Tinea of the hands. The eruption is unilateral and often remains so indefinitely. Note the involvement of the thumbnail.

12 Infestations of the Skin

SCABIES

Scabies is a common, intensely itchy disorder of the skin caused by an acarus or mite, *Sarcoptes scabei* var. *hominis* (Fig. 12.1). It is simple to diagnose and eminently treatable.

The mite is capable of crawling from one human skin to another but it does require relatively prolonged contact between the two. The condition is caught from a bedfellow where intimate contact is likely, but not from momentary contact between adults, such as shaking hands. However, the infection is readily transmitted between children where protracted physical contact is commonplace. Children, particularly infants, are constantly handled by adults and infection may easily be transmitted.

The pregnant female mite, having established herself on the skin of a new victim, will burrow into the horny layer of the skin and lay her eggs. The preferred sites for this are areas where the stratum corneum (horny layer) is at its thickest — for example, the palms and soles. Once infection has taken place it may be a month or two before the symptoms of pruritus commence. Although the burrows will be visible, they will not be noticed by the patients in the absence of symptoms; indeed, it is rare for a patient to note their rather distinctive morphology. This incubation period is important, as it enables a time to be calculated when the patient may have contracted the infection, so that contacts may be identified and treated.

The cardinal symptom is of itching all over the body, which is particularly intense at night or after a warm bath. It begins slowly at first but gradually becomes intense and often unbearable, driving the patient to distraction and inability to sleep at nights.

The diagnostic physical sign is the burrow (Figs. 12.2 and 12.3). This is a serpiginous track which is just palpable and about 10mm long. The mite is only just visible to the human eye as a minute white dot at the end of the track. It can be extracted with a needle and demonstrated under the microscope. The most common sites for the burrows are the hands, particularly along the sides of the fingers, in the web between the thumb and the first finger (Fig. 12.4), and at the wrist overlying the hypo- and hyperthenar eminences. The plantar surfaces are particularly involved in children (Fig. 12.5). These lesions are diagnostic because they appear in no other disease. The burrow may develop into an inflammatory papule or nodule in the anterior axillary folds (Fig. 12.6), the points of the elbows (Fig. 12.7) and the genitalia. Indeed, papules on the penis or the scrotum in an itching patient are highly suspicious of scabies (Figs. 12.8–12.10).

Once sensitization to the presence of the mite has occurred, a papular and urticarial eruption (Fig. 12.11) occurs on the trunk (Figs. 12.12–12.13), buttocks, inner thighs and forearms. Lesions are not seen on the face. Excoriations and bruising are commonplace as a result of scratching.

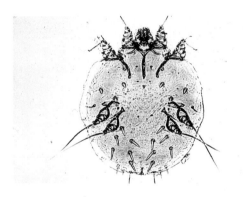

Fig. 12.1   Scabies. Scabies is caused by an acarus or mite, *Sarcoptes scabei* var. *hominis*. It burrows into the skin but may be extracted with a needle and identified under a light microscope.

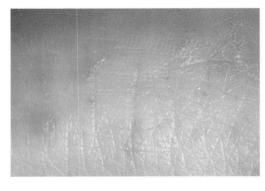

Fig. 12.2   Scabies. Linear, slightly raised serpiginous lesions (burrows) are diagnostic of scabies. By courtesy of St. Mary's Hospital.

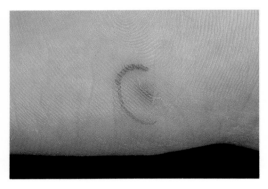

Fig. 12.3   Scabies. Linear burrows occur most often on the palmar surfaces.

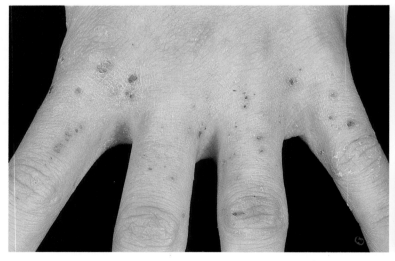

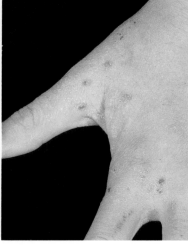

Fig. 12.4   Scabies. Papules and burrows occur between the fingers, especially in the web between the thumb and the index finger

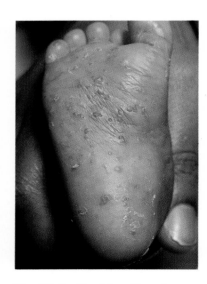

Fig. 12.5   Scabies. Papules and burrows occur on the soles and sides of the feet. Children are particularly affected in this manner.

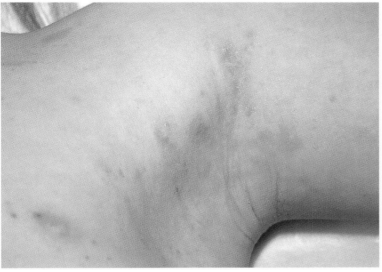

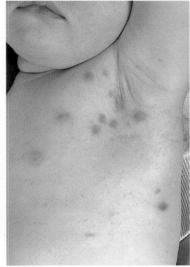

Fig. 12.6 Scabies. Papules commonly occur in the axillae (left) and nodules may develop (right).

Fig. 12.7 Scabies. Nodules around the elbows are characteristic.

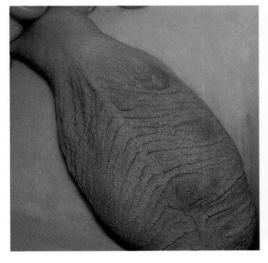

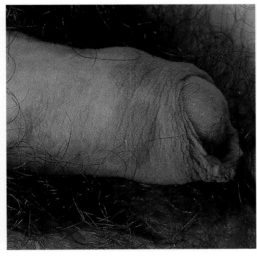

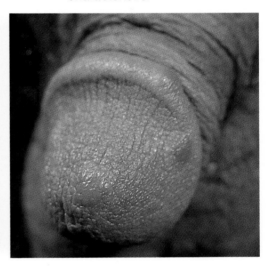

Fig. 12.8 Scabies. Genital papules are almost diagnostic of scabies.

Fig. 12.9 Scabies. Nodules may persist on the genitalia for many weeks after the disease has been treated.

Fig. 12.10 Scabies. Papules on the scrotum or penis are an almost universal finding in males with scabies. By courtesy of St. Mary's Hospital.

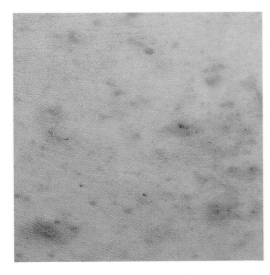

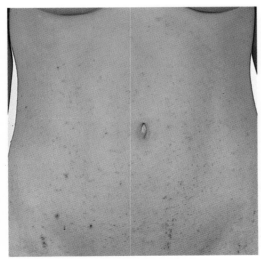

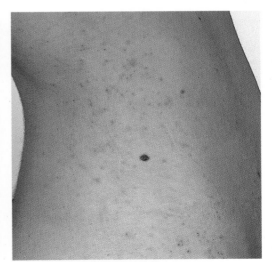

Fig. 12.11 Scabies. An excoriated papular eruption occurs in addition to the burrows.

Fig. 12.12 Scabies. This is an intensely pruritic condition. After an incubation period of approximately one month, generalized itching occurs, with a fine papular eruption on the trunk.

Fig. 12.13 Scabies. Widespread excoriations and bruising of the skin occur.

The extent of physical signs depends to a large extent on the personal hygiene of the patient, so that in the well-washed only one or two burrows may be found, although the pruritus will be just as intense. The scabies mite has no respect of status, so the condition is found in all social classes, contrary to popular belief. Sometimes the condition becomes secondarily infected, particularly in childhood, but this is not the rule – a surprising fact in view of the intensity of the scratching of the skin.

Very occasionally, extremely extensive infestation with acari occurs, so-called Norwegian or crusted scabies. This condition occurs in immunosuppressed patients. Institutionalized individuals with Down's syndrome are also prone to this, perhaps because they have disordered immunological function or possibly because they may not scratch and therefore eliminate a certain proportion of the mites mechanically. In recent years, patients have been misdiagnosed as having eczema (Fig. 12.14) and treated with powerful topical steroids (Figs. 12.15). These are immunosuppressive and allow easy dissemination of the mites. The diagnosis of Norwegian scabies is usually made after members of staff of an institution develop scabies in an epidemic form, as this variety of scabies is highly infectious requiring the minimum of contact. A myriad of burrows will be found on close examination of the skin, particularly on the hands, but the most striking feature is the degree of crusting and scaling of the skin. This may be virtually universal, including the face, but will predominate in those areas where the eruption of ordinary scabies is usually found, for example between the fingers (Fig. 12.16).

Scabies is easily treated, but the treatment must be done thoroughly and conscientiously, and some time must be spent in explaining this to the patient; otherwise treatment failures will occur. Gamma benzene hexachloride should be applied from the neck downwards to all parts of the body and this should be emphasized so that the soles of the feet, the hands, between the fingers, the genitalia and the natal cleft are all included. The treatment should be applied by the patient or a parent after a hot bath and allowed to dry for five minutes. Twenty-four hours later a second application is made after another bath. All members of the family and contacts should be treated, whether or not they have begun to itch.

It should be explained to the patient that the itching will not go away immediately, although it will usually diminish in intensity. This is important because the patient may be tempted to use the acaricidal lotion repeatedly. These lotions, especially benzyl benzoate, are primary irritants of the skin and will frequently lead to an eczematous eruption. The patient will itch as a consequence of this eczema; re-application of the lotions will only make the situation worse. Benzyl benzoate should probably no longer be used to treat scabies. It is important to follow the patient's progress because it may be necessary to prescribe a topical steroid to overcome the eczema resulting from the treatment. It is not uncommon for a patient to have pruritus for up to four weeks after successful treatment. Once a patient has had an attack of scabies it is most unlikely that it will occur again. On subsequent contact with the scabies mite the body mounts an immediate immune response to the acarus which is then unable to get a foothold. It is a myth that scabies can be contracted from infected clothing since the mite lives in the skin and not on the clothing. There is therefore no need to take any special measures regarding clothing or bedding

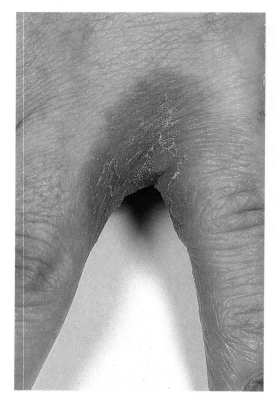

Fig. 12.14 Eczema. Eczema between the fingers is sometimes misdiagnosed as scabies or vice-versa.

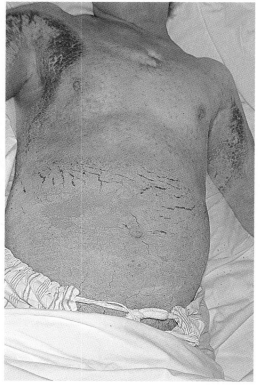

Fig. 12.15 Crusted (Norwegian) scabies. This man was misdiagnosed as having eczema and was admitted to hospital where he was treated with powerful topical and eventually systemic steroids. The correct diagnosis was made when several other patients, nurses and doctors developed irritation of the skin. This man was located as the source. By courtesy of St Mary's Hospital.

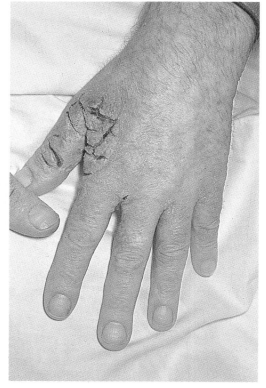

Fig. 12.16 Crusted scabies. Crusting is present between the finger webs. The lesions were teeming with acari and were therefore highly infectious. The condition responded rapidly to routine treatment with quellada. By courtesy of St. Mary's Hospital.

PEDICULOSIS

There are three varieties of louse which can be distinguished morphologically and which have a predilection for certain sites on the body. The head louse is elongated in shape, as is the body louse, but the latter is larger. The crab louse is shorter and is as broad as it is long; its name derives from the crab-like claws on the rear legs with which it grasps hair. Lice have six legs, are wingless and give rise to symptoms of irritation of the skin. Unlike the acarus, no immunity is developed to the louse and repeated infections may occur.

Pediculosis Capitis

Infestation of the scalp, particularly in children of school age, is still remarkably common. The lice are obvious to the naked eye on examination and may be seen to move. The eggs, which are known as nits, are seen attached to the hairs (Fig. 12.17). These can be distinguished from dandruff by the fact that nits cannot be shaken off the hair although they can be slid up the shaft and then pulled off. Secondary infection and lymphadenopathy often occur as a result of scratching. Because resistance to gamma benzene hexachloride has been reported, 0.5% malathion lotion is applied to the scalp and left on for 24 hours. The nits should be removed with a fine tooth comb and the treatment repeated after ten days. It is important that other members of the family and the rest of the children at the school are examined, otherwise infection can obviously recur. The condition is far more common in children because they are more likely to be in fairly close physical contact, although adults can also be affected.

Pediculosis Pubis

The crab louse (*Phthirus pubis*) is found primarily in the pubic area but also, especially in a hirsute individual, on the limbs, chest, in the axillae and even on the eyebrows or eyelashes but not on the scalp. The infection is usually transmitted sexually. The condition gives rise to intense pruritus. The crab louse can easily be identified with the naked eye and can often be seen to be moving. The nits are attached to the hairs and can be confirmed under a microscope. Treatment is with gamma benzene hexachloride applied thoroughly to all the affected areas. The application should be repeated ten days later to deal with any eggs which may have hatched out since the first application. Although *Phthirus pubis* lives primarily on the skin, it may be found on the underclothing and it is wise to examine this for evidence of lice and disinfect with DDT if necessary.

Pediculosis Corporis

Body lice are rarely seen in normal individuals, except under disaster conditions when there is chaos, overcrowding and a breakdown in hygiene. Vagrants, however, are frequently infested. These pediculi differ from the others in that although they feed off the skin, they breed and live in the clothing, including the bed clothing of the infested individual. They are found in the seams of the underclothing and cause extremely intense pruritus in the skin closest to the clothes such as the shoulders, neck, breasts, and around the buttocks. Secondary sepsis is common. Since repeated infection is commonplace in the lodging houses which vagrants frequent, chronic infestation ensues because there is no natural immunity. As a result of continual scratching, the skin becomes pigmented, thickened, dry and scaly; a situation known colloquially as 'vagabond's disease'. Under certain conditions the body louse may carry Rickettsia and result in typhus, trench or relapsing fevers.

The diagnosis of body lice is remarkably easy, provided the condition is considered and a search is made of the clothing. Treatment with gamma benzene hexachloride alone will not cure the patient: he must be separated from the infested clothing and have a fresh set provided. The infested clothing should be fumigated. DDT is effective.

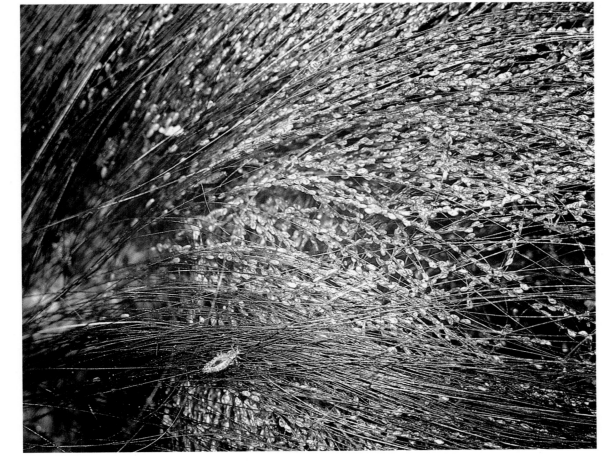

Fig. 12.17 Pediculosis capitis. A mass of nits and pediculi are present in this man's hair. A louse is clearly visible. By courtesy of St. Bartholomew's Hospital.

INSECT BITES

These are extremely common and must be considered in the differential diagnosis of any patient complaining of itching. Urticarial wheals (Fig. 12.18), often with a central punctum (Fig. 12.19), papules, vesicles and less commonly blisters (Fig. 12.20) amid excoriations may suggest the diagnosis. The lesions are usually scattered asymmetrically over the body, or concentrated on the lower legs (Fig. 12.21). The source requires detection and careful consideration of the personal habits of the

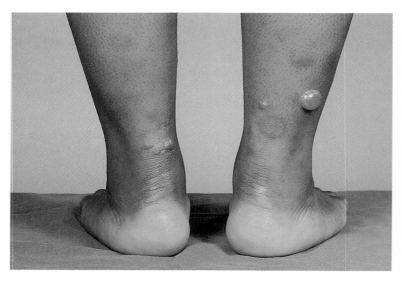

Fig. 12.18   Insect bites. Urticarial papular, bullous and post-inflammatory pigmented lesions are present in this West Indian child.

Fig. 12.19   Insect bites. A central punctum is sometimes visible within an urticarial lesion. By courtesy of St. John's Hospital for Diseases of the Skin.

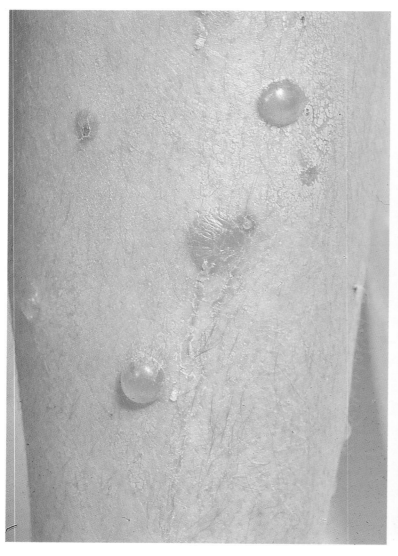

Fig. 12.20   Insect bites. Bullae sometimes develop, especially on the lower legs. By courtesy of St. Mary's Hospital.

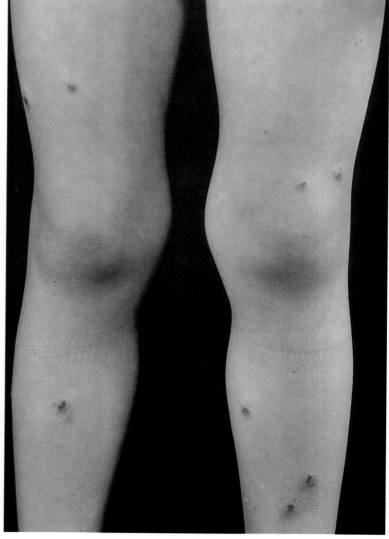

Fig. 12.21   Insect bites. The lower legs are a very common site. Bites are intensely pruritic and therefore excoriated. By courtesy of St. John's Hospital for Diseases of the Skin.

patient. Thus, pets may house fleas or mites, as may homes previously occupied by pets. Recently acquired old furniture may be the residence of bugs. Trips abroad or to the country, or work in the garden may bring the patient into contact with a host of insects including mosquitoes, caterpillars (Fig. 12.22), ticks and sandflies. These, in addition to causing bites, may harbour disease; for example, malaria (mosquitoes), Rocky Mountain spotted fever (ticks), and leishmaniasis (sandflies). The fact that only certain individuals seem to be attractive to insects and other members of the household or party may be spared, may incline the patient to discount insects when considering the diagnosis.

Domestic animals, especially cats and dogs, are responsible for many cases of unsuspected insect bites. The owners find it hard to believe that their pet could acquire an infestation. Fleas constitute the majority of ectoparasites living on pets. They breed in cracks and crevices in floorboards, amongst soft furnishings, in dust and dirt and they particularly enjoy centrally-heated, and fitted-carpet environments. The lesions seen on humans are usually grouped, often three at a time in a linear arrangement (Fig. 12.23) on the trunk or limbs. The eruption may become extremely widespread. It causes intense irritation.

Cheyletiella are mites which particularly favour cats and dogs as carriers, but cause them no symptoms. They attack man causing urticarial or papulo-vesicular eruptions. The distribution usually occurs when the animal is held in contact with the human, that is, in the lap area or the lower chest and abdomen, the forearms and thighs.

Animals may acquire scabies (sarcoptic mange). There is no incubation period and burrows are not usually found as in human scabies. The eruption occurs on the parts of the body which have been in contact with the infested animal, usually the arms. It has a red papular morphology and is very itchy.

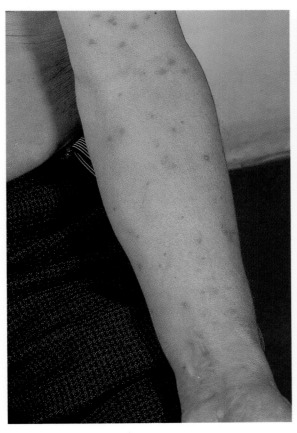
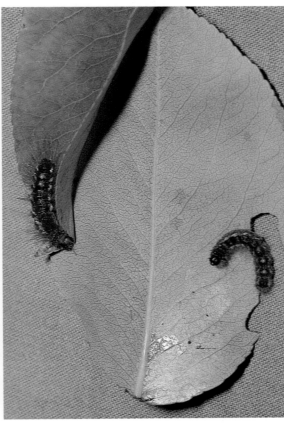

Fig. 12.22 Insect bites. These bites were found to be caused by caterpillars of the brown tail moth.

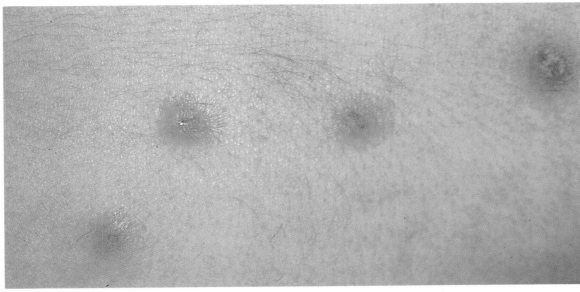

Fig. 12.23 Insect bites. Excoriated papules occurring in linear groups of three or four are characteristic. By courtesy of St. John's Hospital for Diseases of the Skin.

Bedbugs live in crevices in furniture and walls, and usually produce more inflammation than fleas. They must be suspected if the patient has acquired furniture, particularly a bed, or has moved into new lodgings prior to the appearance of the bite. The bugs shun the light and come out at night feeding particularly on exposed areas, such as the arms and face, i.e. parts not covered by night attire or bedclothing. The lesions may be quite substantial (Fig. 12.24) and blood may be found on the clothing the following morning. Many patients will sleep through an attack. The patient may feel quite unwell with a fever, secondary infection (Fig. 12.25) and sometimes lymphadenopathy, especially with recurrent attacks. It is wise to contact public health officials to eradicate the problem.

Management of Insect Bites
It is helpful to collect brushings from suspect animals onto the shiny surface of brown paper and have these examined by a parasitologist. The finding of evidence of ectoparasites helps to convince the patient of the diagnosis. The animal should be treated by a veterinary surgeon. It is often necessary to fumigate the rooms used by the animal. Occasionally it is necessary to contact public health departments for further investigation.

The patient may be helped by calamine or topical steroids. Secondary infection should be treated with antibiotics.

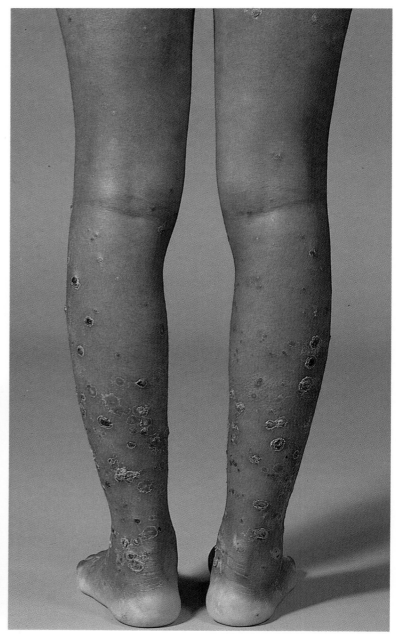

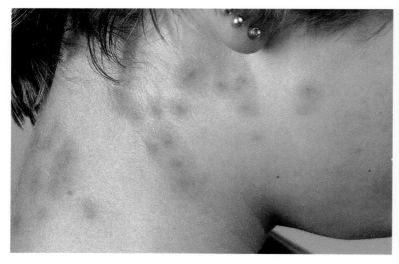

Fig. 12.24   Insect bites. Large urticarial wheals with a central punctum are present on the neck and face. Bed bugs frequently attack exposed areas at night.

Fig. 12.25   Insect bites. Secondary infection is common.

13 Tropical Infections of the Skin

LEPROSY (HANSEN'S DISEASE)

This is a chronic infection due to *Mycobacterium leprae* which produces physical signs principally in the skin and nervous tissue. The degree of involvement in either site depends largely on the immunological status of the patient and the bacteriological load. The socio-economic conditions and racial background of the patient are important contributory factors. The disease is transmitted by inhalation or ingestion of infected nasal droplets. The organism invades the Schwann cells which surround the cutaneous nerves. The various types of leprosy are arbitrarily divided into tuberculoid, borderline and lepromatous, based on the immunological status of the patient. These types are known as TT, BB and LL and the intermediate types between these are designated BT and BL. This immunological classification is determined on the basis of the clinical signs and the lepromin test (Fig. 13.1). This is the reaction to an intradermal injection of a standard extract of leprosy tissue. It is positive in tuberculoid leprosy and negative in lepromatous leprosy.

Leprosy is a disorder of tropical countries, particularly India, Africa, South-east Asia and South America. It is uncommon in Western societies. Clearly, it presents most frequently in the skin and only the cutaneous physical signs are described here. However, it is a complex disorder in immunological terms and its management requires considerable skill if nervous tissue function is to be preserved. It is thus usually treated by leprologists.

Tuberculoid Leprosy

The immunological resistance to the leprosy bacillus is high at this end of the spectrum. The skin lesions are few and asymmetrically distributed. The patches are well-defined and often annular in shape (Fig. 13.2). They are red with central hypopigmentation (Fig. 13.3). The surface is dry and scaly, does not sweat and is anaesthetic. The sites of predilection are the cool, peripheral parts of the body such as the face, buttocks, the elbows and knees (Fig. 13.4) and extensor surfaces of the limbs (Fig. 13.5). The peripheral nerves particularly the great auricular, ulnar and peroneal become involved in addition to nervous tissue within the skin lesion. These nerves are thickened and therefore palpable. Involvement leads to a peripheral neuropathy with sensory changes resulting in ulceration of the digits and motor changes in palsies such as footdrop or ulnar nerve

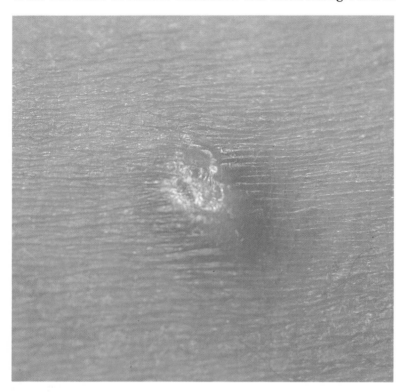

Fig. 13.1 Mitsuda (lepromin) test. This is a reaction to an intradermal injection of a standard extract of leprosy tissue. It is positive in tuberculoid leprosy but negative in lepromatous leprosy. By courtesy of St. John's Hospital for Diseases of the Skin.

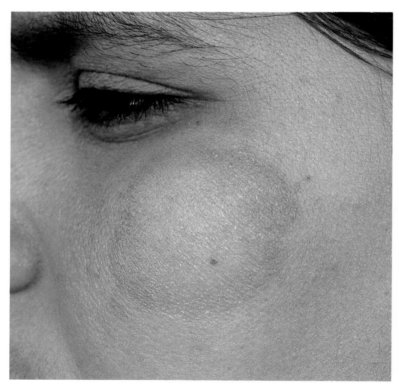

Fig. 13.2 Tuberculoid leprosy. There is a dry, annular, anaesthetic patch on the cheek. Skin biopsy established the diagnosis. By courtesy of St. John's Hospital for Diseases of the Skin.

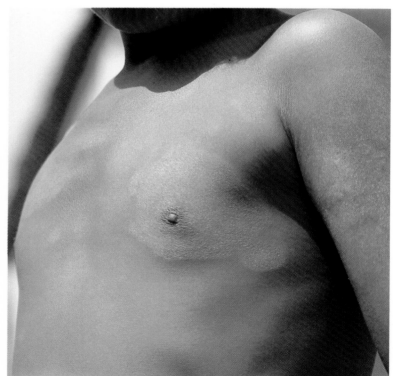

Fig. 13.3 Tuberculoid leprosy. Annular, anaesthetic, hypopigmented patches occur.

13.2

paralysis. Skin biopsy will confirm the diagnosis (Fig. 13.6). Non-caseating granulomata are found but bacilli are conspicuously few or likely to be absent.

Borderline Leprosy

This disorder is a mixture of both tuberculoid and lepromatous leprosy. It is, however, immunologically unstable and can downgrade to lepromatous leprosy or can reverse to tuberculoid leprosy. Neurological signs are often present.

Lepromatous Leprosy

In this variety of leprosy the immunological response of the host is minimal. It is a widespread, progressive disease with bacilli invading not only the skin and nerves but also the reticulo-endothelial system. The skin lesions are symmetrical and extensive, in contrast to those of tuberculoid leprosy. Neurological involvement occurs late in the disease, probably because the immunological response to the presence of the bacilli in the nervous tissue is minor and therefore little damage is done. The disease is highly infectious from nasal discharges, unlike tuberculoid leprosy which is not infectious at all.

The early cutaneous changes are often too subtle to be noticed by the patient. The first symptoms are usually nasal such as stuffiness, discharge and epistaxis. Swelling of the ankles and lower legs is common. The skin changes commence as symmetrical, small, red or slightly hypopigmented macules which are multiple and subsequently become extensive. They have vague and ill-defined borders. Anaesthetic papules,

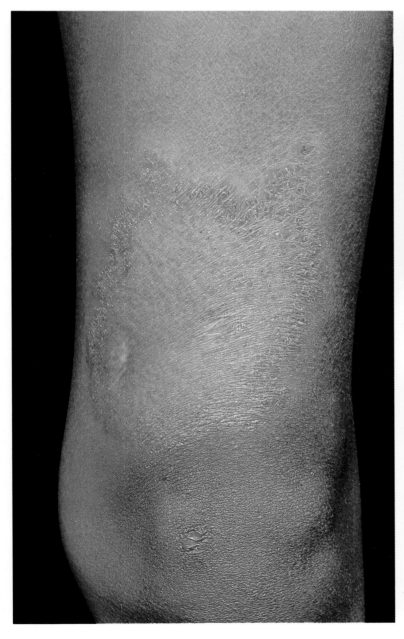

Fig. 13.4 Tuberculoid leprosy. Annular, dry, slightly scaly patches are characteristic. The extensor surface of the knee is a common site. By courtesy of St. John's Hospital for Diseases of the Skin.

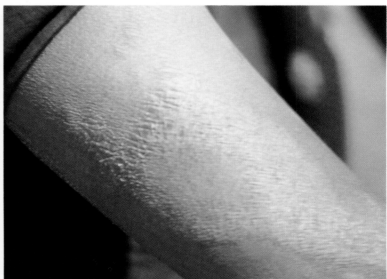

Fig. 13.5 Tuberculoid leprosy. The skin is dry, anaesthetic and hairless due to involvement of the sweat glands, nerves and hair follicles.

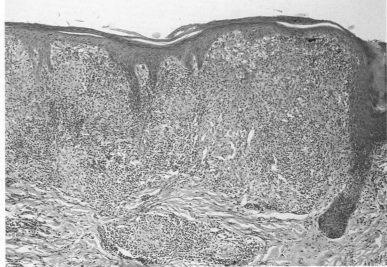

Fig. 13.6 Tuberculoid (TT) leprosy. Granulomata are eroding into the epidermis. No acid-fast bacilli are seen on Wade-Fite staining. By courtesy of Dr. S. Lucas, University College Hospital.

plaques and nodules (lepromata) develop later (Fig. 13.7). The face (Fig. 13.8), arms, legs and buttocks are characteristically affected but any area of the skin, other than warm sites such as the axillae and groin, may be involved. The cooler areas of the face, such as the lips, nose (Fig. 13.9) and earlobes (Figs. 13.10 and 13.11) are particularly involved. Diffuse infiltration of the skin of the forehead causes a leonine appearance (Fig. 13.12) and the eyebrows and eyelashes disappear. The nose, eyes,

testes and bone become involved. Glove and stocking anaesthesia develops from polyneuritis (Fig. 13.13) and destruction and shortening of the digits result from frequent unappreciated trauma (Fig. 13.14). The course of the disease is punctuated by frequent febrile exacerbations and erythema nodosum leprosum is a characteristic feature. The untreated patient ultimately succumbs from renal failure or concomitant tuberculosis.

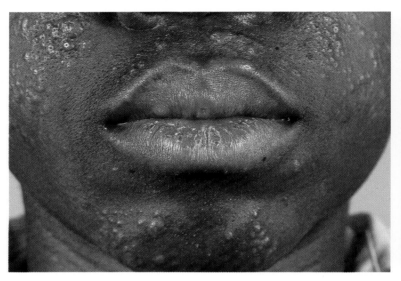

Fig. 13.7 Lepromatous leprosy. Extensive papules and nodules are present in this African. The lips are also involved.

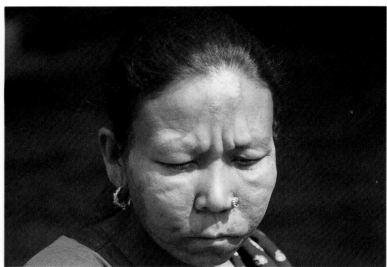

Fig. 13.8 Lepromatous leprosy. Diffuse infiltration of the face occurs.

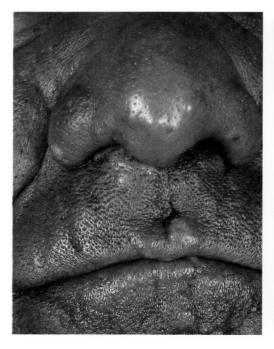

Fig. 13.9 Lepromatous leprosy. The nose and lips are characteristic sites.

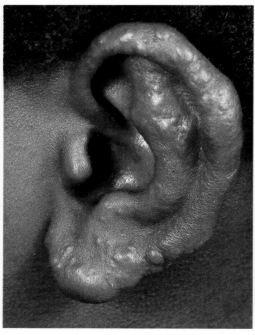

Fig. 13.10 Lepromatous leprosy. Papules and nodules around the ears are characteristic. Leprosy favours the peripheral areas of skin.

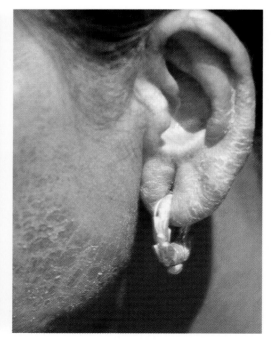

Fig. 13.11 Lepromatous leprosy. There is diffuse pink infiltration of the cheeks and ears.

The diagnosis can be made by biopsy of the skin (Figs. 13.15 and 13.16). There are relatively few lymphocytes, but a large number of acid-fast bacilli are demonstrable in foamy, so-called 'lepra' cells. The diagnosis can also be made by making a superficial slit into involved skin and smearing the tissue thus gained onto a slide. This can be stained for acid-fast bacilli and the organisms demonstrated.

The treatment of leprosy is the province of experts who have made the disease a life-long study. However, drugs such as dapsone, rifampicin and clofazimine have now turned this scourge of a disease into a treatable one.

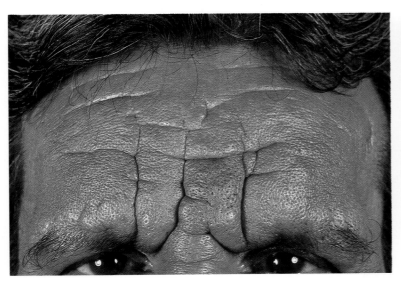

Fig. 13.12 Lepromatous leprosy. Involvement of the forehead has produced deep fissuring, so-called 'leonine facies'.

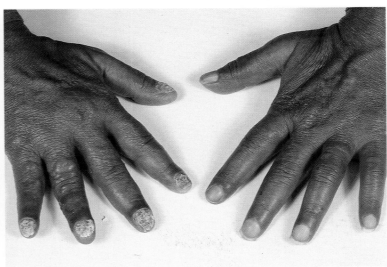

Fig. 13.13 Lepromatous leprosy, neuritis and tinea of the nails. Two lepromata are present on the fingers of the right hand. There is gross tinea of the nails secondary to immunosuppression. There is wasting of the small muscles of the hands.

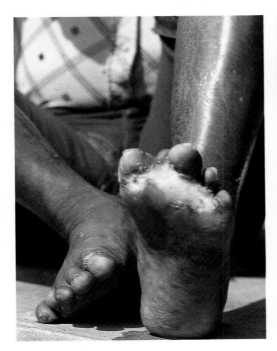

Fig. 13.14 Lepromatous leprosy. Destruction of the digits is an end result of glove and stocking anaesthesia.

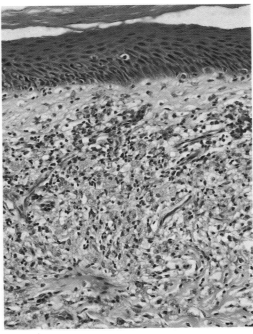

Fig. 13.15 Lepromatous leprosy. A diffuse infiltrate of foamy histiocytes (lepra cells) is separated from the epidermis by a grenz zone of sparing.

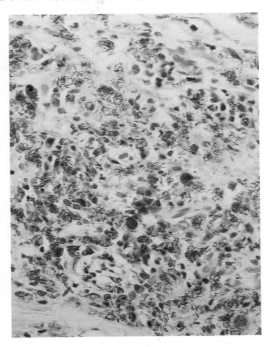

Fig. 13.16 Lepromatous leprosy. Innumerable red-staining bacilli may be demonstrated. The larger intracellular aggregates are sometimes known as globi. (Wade-Fite stain.)

CUTANEOUS LEISHMANIASIS (Oriental Sore, Baghdad Boil)

This condition results from bites by sandflies infected with the protozoan, *Leishmania tropica*. It is common in the Middle East, subtropics and tropics, but also may occur in Mediterranean countries, especially North Africa, so it is increasingly encountered in holiday makers. The exposed parts (Fig. 13.17) are the most common sites to be bitten, resulting in papules and nodules which break down, ulcerate and crust (Figs. 13.18 and 13.19). They subsequently heal within a year, but with considerable scarring. The organism may be demonstrated in skin smears. Leishman Donovan bodies are seen within large histiocytes on skin biopsy (Fig. 13.20). Treatment with pentavalent antimony compounds may be effective.

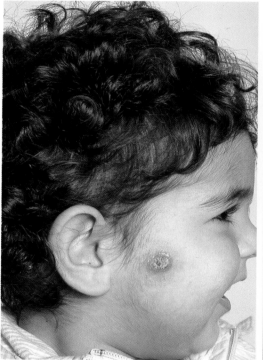
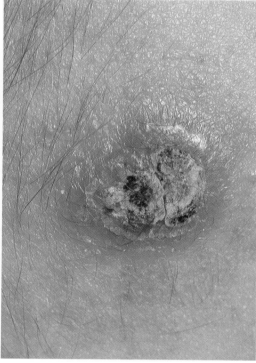

Fig. 13.17 Cutaneous leishmaniasis (Baghdad boil). This little boy was bitten on the face by an infected sandfly. The close-up shows a crusted ulcer.

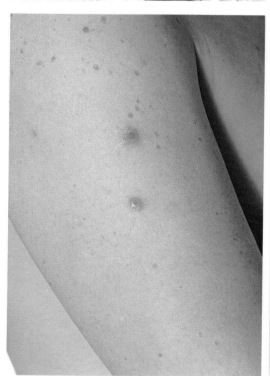
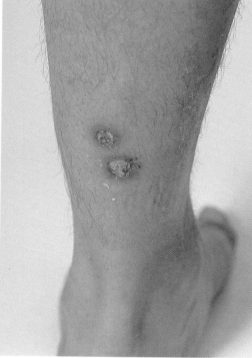

Fig. 13.18 Cutaneous leishmaniasis. This man received multiple infected sandfly bites whilst working in the Middle East. The initial lesions on the arm are red, slightly crusted papules. The red lesions on the legs have ulcerated and become indurated.

LARVA MIGRANS

This is caused by hookworm larvae from the faeces of infected dogs. The condition occurs in the Caribbean and New World, and anyone walking barefoot or sitting on a contaminated beach is at risk. *Ancylostoma braziliensis* is the most common hookworm responsible. The site of entry (usually the buttocks or foot) is itchy at first and subsequently the patient notices a linear moving eruption (Figs. 13.21 and 13.22) which is intensely itchy and may become secondarily infected. The condition responds to topical application of thiabendazole.

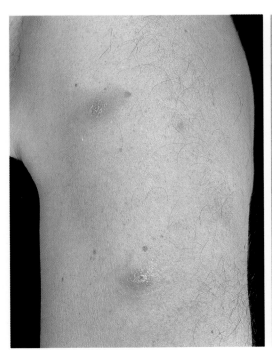
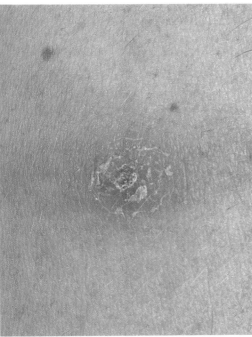
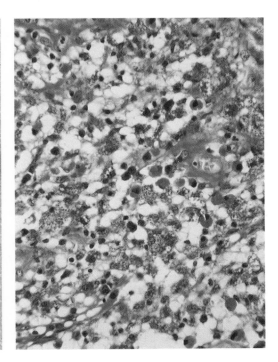

Fig. 13.19 Cutaneous leishmaniasis. Red nodules with a central crusted area are present.

Fig. 13.20 Cutaneous leishmaniasis. The dermis is extensively infiltrated by large numbers of macrophages containing numerous *Leishmania* organisms. In addition, scattered, intensely eosinophilic Russell bodies are evident. The latter represent plasma cells distended by immunoglobulin.

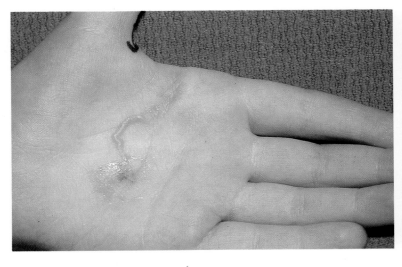
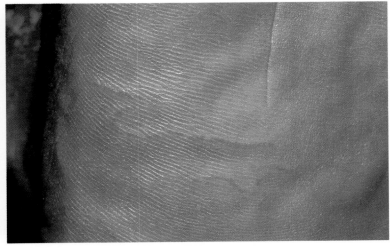

Fig. 13.21 Larva migrans. Linear mobile tracks occur. The disorder is due to canine hookworm larvae penetrating the skin.

Fig. 13.22 Larva migrans. This man contracted this infection in his foot on a Caribbean beach where infected dogs roam free.

ONCHOCERCIASIS

This is an infestation with larvae of the roundworm *Onchocerca* (*Onchocerca volvulus* in Africa or *Onchocerca caecutiens* in Central America). Gnats (*Simuliidae*) transmit the disease by biting human skin and injecting the larvae, which then mature into worms and produce subcutaneous nodules. The condition is extremely pruritic and widespread papules and lichenification occur (Fig. 13.23) particularly around the shoulders and upper arms and buttocks and thighs. Microfilariae invade the dermis and destroy the elastic tissue so that the skin may hang in folds, especially in the groin. Scarring and pigmentary changes are frequent.

The most important consequence of the disease is invasion of the eye as it may result in blindness. The condition is known as 'river blindness' because the gnats breed close to rivers. The disorder is thus more likely to be contracted in rural rather than urban areas.

The microfilariae (Fig. 13.24) may be found by examining strips of skin in saline. There is frequently an eosinophilia and the filarial complement fixation test is positive. The disorder may be treated with diethylcarbamazine (banozide) or suramin. Nodules may be excised.

BURULI ULCER

This is a tropical disease caused by *Mycobacterium ulcerans*. Buruli is a swampland district in Uganda. The organism is harboured by spiky grasses and can be inoculated into the bare legs of a passer-by. The condition is most often seen on the legs of young children. It presents as an ulcer with a deeply delineated edge (Fig. 13.25). The diagnosis is made by a skin biopsy and by culture of the organism from the skin. The condition does not respond to standard anti-tuberculous therapy and the ulcer needs to be widely excised and grafted as early as possible.

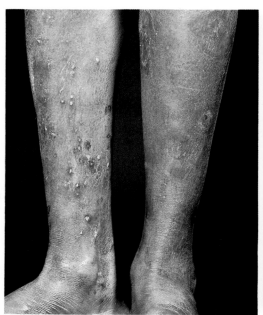 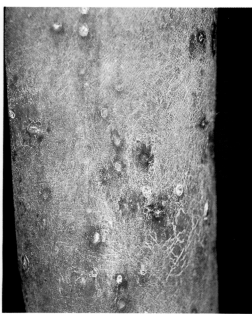 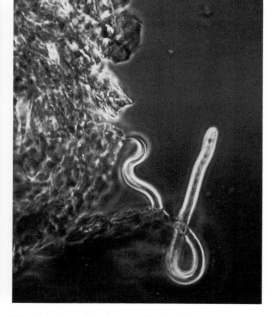

Fig. 13.23 Onchocerciasis. This is caused by bites from gnats infected with the larvae of the *Onchocerca* roundworm. The condition is extremely pruritic and widespread excoriated papules, lichenification and post-inflammatory hyperpigmentation occur. The skin is very dry. The lower limbs are commonly affected. By courtesy of Dr. Roger Clayton, St. Mary's Hospital.

Fig. 13.24 Onchocerciasis. The microfilariae may be demonstrated in strips of skin in saline. By courtesy of Dr. Roger Clayton, St. Mary's Hospital.

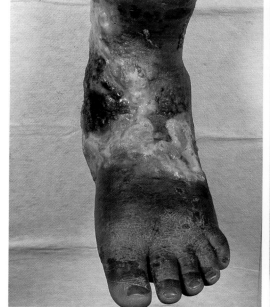 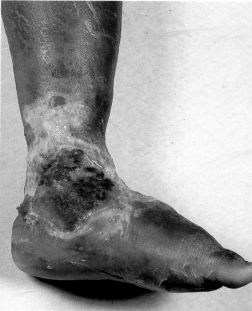

Fig. 13.25 Buruli ulcer. Children most commonly acquire this infection on the legs from contact with contaminated grasses. Extensive ulceration has occurred here and a large eschar is present. The condition is caused by *Mycobacterium ulcerans*. The infection must be widely excised and grafted.

14 Drug and Toxic Eruptions of the Skin

Toxic reactions affecting the skin are common and are the most frequent reason for a dermatology consultation involving a hospitalized patient. Sometimes the clinical appearance is a specific one, such as a fixed drug eruption, where there will be no cause other than a drug. However, more often, the clinical appearance could be produced by a drug or by some other toxic 'agent'. In the commonest cutaneous reaction of all, the exanthem or toxic erythema, it may be difficult to separate out a possible drug reaction from the infection for which the drug had been given. For this reason, such reactions of the skin are considered together with drug eruptions in this chapter.

The diagnosis of a drug eruption and the detection of the culprit may be difficult. Drug eruptions may mimic skin disorders, for example penicillamine may cause an eruption which is indistinguishable from pemphigus vulgaris. Sometimes the mimicry is not quite perfect and the true diagnosis will therefore be suspected, e.g. the psoriasiform eruption caused by practolol and the lichenoid eruption caused by gold.

Frequently patients are taking more than one drug, so the identification of the one causing the eruption is based on experience. Thus, antibiotics are probably the most common offenders, whereas digoxin rarely produces a cutaneous react-ion. Perhaps the most problematic aspect of drug eruptions is proving the case. At present there are no tests other than giving the suspected drug to the patient again in an attempt to reproduce the rash. This, however, is extremely hazardous as the patient may develop a lethal anaphylaxis or an uncontrollable exfoliative dermatitis and therefore it is not to be recommended. Thus, in the final analysis, unless the patient is taking only one drug, the most likely agent must be incriminated and the patient and family doctor warned about it.

Drugs may cause a skin eruption as a secondary effect, for example candidosis as a consequence of taking systemic steroids or antibiotics. Drugs may aggravate a condition but not actually cause it, for example lithium and psoriasis.

There are other problems. The word 'drug' may be misinterpreted by many patients and an enquiry should be made about everything that the patient is taking, whether it is prescribed by the general practitioner or bought at the pharmacy. For example, laxatives are not considered by the general public to be drugs and yet they are the most common cause of the fixed drug eruption. Patients also believe that medications which they have taken for many years can be exonerated, but this is a fallacy. Finally, doctors fail to appreciate that a skin eruption may

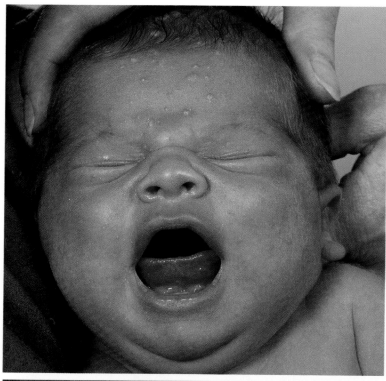

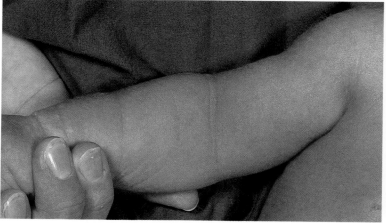

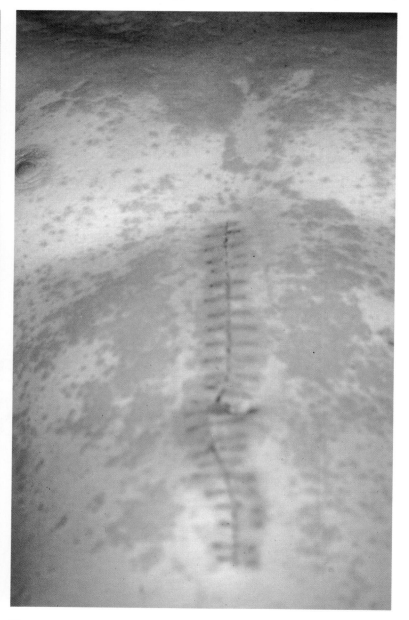

Fig. 14.1 Erythema toxicum neonatorum. This is a common evanescent 'toxic' erythema of unknown cause occurring in the first days of life. Pustules may be superimposed.

Fig. 14.2 Toxic erythema. This young woman had been given ampicillin post-operatively. By courtesy of St. Bartholomew's Hospital.

develop after treatment has ended. For example, eruptions due to ampicillin can take up to fourteen days to develop, even though the patient may only have taken the drug for five days.

Although the mechanisms for many reactions in the skin are not defined, so that they are still best described according to the clinical picture produced, some may be explained within the framework of classical immunology.

IMMUNOLOGICAL CONSIDERATIONS
Type I Immediate Hypersensitivity
This reaction results in the production of urticarial wheals in the skin. The antigen, for example penicillin, results in the production of IgE antibodies. These have an affinity for the membranes of mast cells and basophils, which results in the release of histamine and kinins. If the degranulation of these cells is massive, anaphylaxis occurs. This consists of bronchiolar constriction, oedema of the larynx and glottis, vasodilatation and shock, in addition to urticaria. Unless immediate resuscitative measures are taken with subcutaneous adrenaline (0.5 ml given slowly over several seconds) death may ensue. It is for this reason that if penicillin sensitivity is diagnosed, the patient should be informed of the hazardous nature of the allergy.

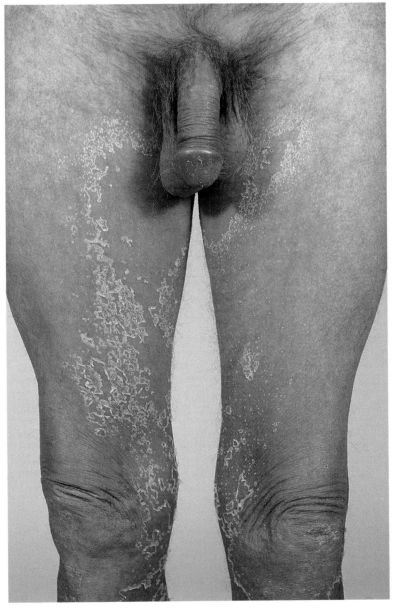

Fig. 14.3 Toxic erythema. The erythematous skin desquamates as it heals. By courtesy of St. Mary's Hospital.

Type II Cytotoxic Hypersensitivity
In this situation, the antigen attaches to the cell membrane and the resulting antibodies (either IgG or IgM) together with complement cause destruction of the target cell. This is the mechanism responsible for the production of purpura by the hypnotic sedormid. The target cell is the platelet.

Type III Immune Complex Sensitivity
The antigen and antibody (IgG or IgM) form complexes with complement and precipitate either within or without blood vessels. The vasculitis can occur locally in the skin and is known as Arthus' phenomenon, as exemplified by erythema nodosum. The circulating immune complexes may produce a constitutional upset, which is known as serum sickness. There is fever, arthralgia, lymphadenopathy and, most significantly, nephritis occurring about ten days after exposure to the antigen, usually penicillin or a sulphonamide. The eruption is either urticarial, maculopapular or vasculitic. The degree of nephritis resulting from deposition of the immune complexes in the glomeruli determines the outcome of the disorder.

Type IV Cell-mediated Reactions
Unlike the preceding reactions, humoral antibodies are not involved in this type. The reactions are exemplified in the epidermis by the production of a contact dermatitis, for example to a topically applied agent such as chloramphenicol, or in the dermis by a granulomatous reaction, for example to an intradermally-injected antigen such as Kveim or BCG. Sensitization takes about 10–14 days and then the reaction develops from 24–72 hours after subsequent exposure to the allergen. The antigen combines with proteins and is processed by Langerhans' cells and macrophages, and transported via the lymphatics to the paracortical zone of the lymph nodes. In this area, thymus-derived (T) lymphocytes proliferate, leave the node via the lymphatics, reach the bloodstream and then react with the antigen.

TOXIC ERYTHEMA (Exanthem)
This is the commonest cutaneous reaction and practically all of the body surface is affected. Red macules, which may become papular, are the hallmark of the eruption but the lesions merge into one another so that a general impression of redness is given (see Figs. 4.18–4.20). It may be caused by a drug or an infection or there may be no demonstrable cause, in which case it is referred to as a 'toxic erythema'. A common example is *erythema toxicum neonatorum*, which is a short-lived general erythema during the first few days of life (Fig. 14.1).

Drug eruptions occur a few days after commencing treatment with the agent, classically on the tenth day. The most common is an antibiotic such as ampicillin (Fig. 14.2). Indeed, 10 per cent of the population will react to this drug and 100 per cent will react if ampicillin is given to a patient with infectious mononucleosis or lymphatic leukaemia. Although it is never wise to give a drug a second time, patients who have recovered from glandular fever and inadvertently are given ampicillin again, do not usually react the next time. Barbiturates, especially phenobarbitone, sulphonamides, including septrin, chlorpropamide, phenylbutazone and amitriptyline also produce exanthems. The eruption is often very pruritic and will last a week to ten days, desquamating as it heals (Fig. 14.3). It is mandatory to discontinue the drug for fear that an erythroderma may develop. Symptomatic treatment with oral antihistamines and topical calamine is usually all that is required, but sometimes systemic steroids are necessary.

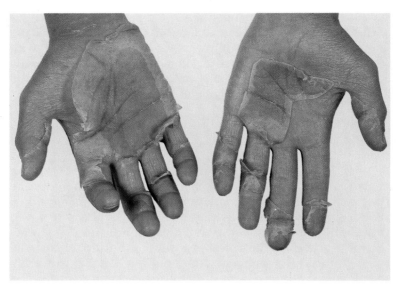

Fig. 14.4   Desquamation of the palms and soles. Marked shedding of the palmar and plantar skin may occur following a drug eruption. This patient had taken an overdose of barbiturates.

A toxic erythema may follow a streptococcal infection. The erythema may be quite faint and not noticed by the patient until desquamation occurs, particularly on the palms (Fig. 14.4) and soles and around the mouth (Fig. 14.5).

Viruses frequently produce a toxic erythema. The diagnosis is usually presumptive in the absence of confirmatory laboratory tests, but sometimes the pattern of the eruption may suggest the virus responsible. In *Fifth disease* the eruption is on the cheeks which look as if they have been slapped (Fig. 14.6 left), buttocks (Fig. 14.6 right), knees, elbows and extremities. The clinical picture is rather characteristic. A parvovirus is responsible.

EXFOLIATIVE DERMATITIS

This term is synonymous with erythroderma. It implies universal involvement of the skin with erythema and scaling (Fig. 14.7). There may be loss of nails and hair and sometimes lymphadeno-pathy. Psoriasis and eczema are the most common causes of exfoliative dermatitis but a drug may be suspected if the patient has never had either of these diseases, and if there is a drug that can be incriminated. Any drug can potentially produce the condition but the most common offenders are barbiturates,

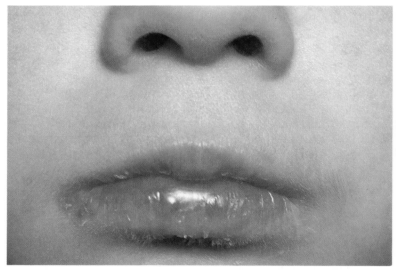

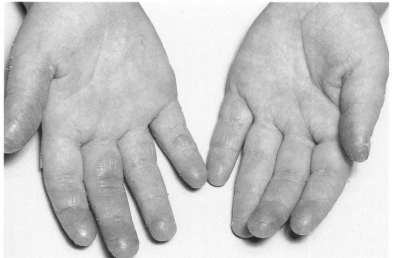

Fig. 14.5   Toxic erythema. Desquamation of the lips and peeling of the palmar skin is quite characteristic following a streptococcal infection. They were the first cutaneous abnormalities noticed by this child's mother, and she did not associate them with the preceding tonsillitis.

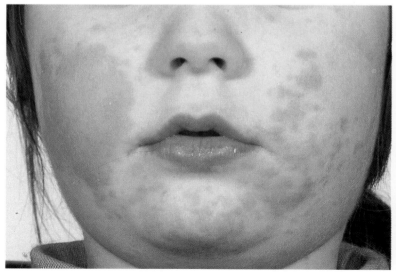

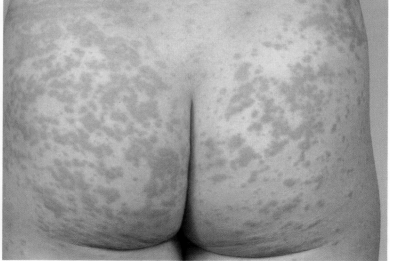

Fig. 14.6   'Slapped cheek' (Fifth) disease. Many viruses produce a toxic erythema of the skin. Some patterns are recognizable. This parvovirus produces an erythema of the cheeks (left), buttocks (right) and extremities.

sulphonamides, phenylbutazone, streptomycin and gold. Eosinophilia and fever may be present. The patient becomes severely debilitated by the loss of heat, fluid, protein and minerals from the skin leading to electrolyte imbalance. Cutaneous and systemic sepsis may occur. Cardiac decompensation is a hazard in those with pre-existing heart disease. The exfoliation may not cease immediately on stopping the drug and the condition may be fatal. Systemic steroids are usually required.

ANNULAR ERYTHEMA

This is a term used to describe the appearance of one or several erythematous rings on the body. The margin of the ring is red and very slightly raised (Fig. 14.8). The central area heals and may look quite normal. There is usually no surface change but sometimes a fine, thin line of scale occurs towards the edge of the erythema (Fig. 14.9) and the condition is then known as *erythema annulare centrifugum*. It is obviously important to exclude a ringworm infection, but scrapings are negative. In most cases no cause can be found for the annular erythema and the disease may run a protracted course but ultimately resolves spontaneously. However, occasionally blood dyscrasias and carcinoma can give rise to annular erythema. Equally rarely, a moderately severe ringworm infection of the foot can set up a widespread annular erythema on the body. Finally, annular erythema may be found on the trunk and hands of children with rheumatic fever. The lesions develop swiftly and are evanescent. This condition is better known as *erythema marginatum*.

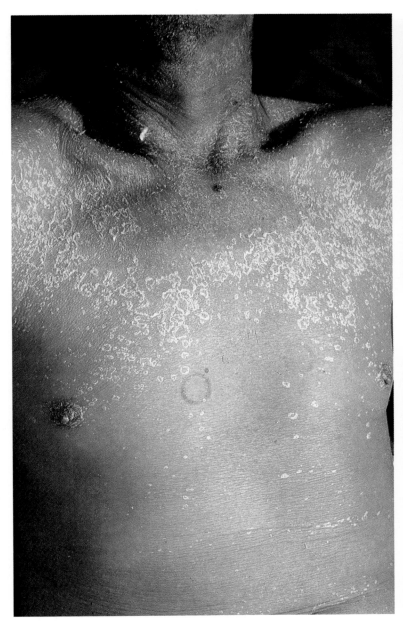

Fig. 14.8 Annular erythema. Red, ring-shaped lesions may occur on the body without known cause.

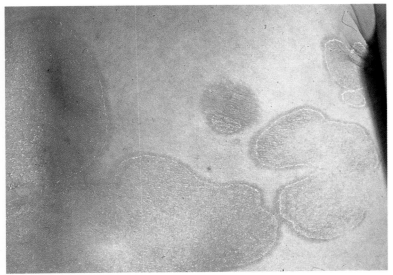

Fig. 14.7 Exfoliative dermatitis. Universal erythema and desquamation may result if the responsible agent (in this case an antiarrhythmic drug) is not discontinued. By courtesy of St. Bartholomew's Hospital.

Fig. 14.9 Erythema annulare centrifugum. In addition to the annular erythema there is a fine, thin, scaly line towards the edge of the lesion. The cause is unknown. By courtesy of St. Mary's Hospital.

URTICARIA AND ANGIO-OEDEMA

This is one of the most common of all skin reactions. Penicillin or aspirin may be the cause, but it is peculiarly frustrating that in the majority of patients who suffer from it chronically, no cause is found. The condition comprises intense irritation associated with swellings on the skin. These vary in size and shape (Fig. 14.10) and have a smooth surface. They take the form of wheals which are red (Fig. 14.11), particularly at the periphery, with a tendency for central pallor (Fig. 14.12). They are short-lived, lasting only for a few hours. Indeed, if urticarial lesions last longer, a vasculitis may be more likely. Frequently, when the patient is seen by the doctor, there are no abnormal physical signs and the diagnosis has to be made from the history. The patient often describes the lesions as blotches or blisters, although they do not contain fluid. The lesions resemble the changes that occur after a nettle sting, so that this disorder is known colloquially as 'nettle rash' or 'hives'. The wheals occur anywhere on the body and may be associated with swelling of the face (Fig. 14.13) or a hand, so-called 'angio-oedema'. If this angio-oedema affects the throat, the disorder becomes life-threatening due to the possibility of asphyxia. Anaphylaxis may also occur. The swellings of the skin and mucous membranes are caused by an acute vasodilatation of capillaries associated with increased permeability of the vessel wall, so that fluid flows into the skin.

Urticaria, rather like eczema, is a physical sign. There are a number of possible causes and urticaria may be classified as follows:

Acute Urticaria

This would appear to be a manifestation of a Type I immediate hypersensitivity reaction secondary to an ingested, injected or occasionally inhaled antigen. The diagnosis is usually obvious

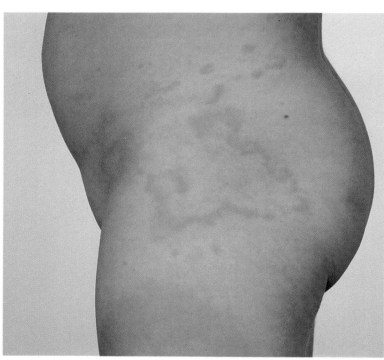

Fig. 14.10 Urticaria. The lesions are of various sizes and shapes.

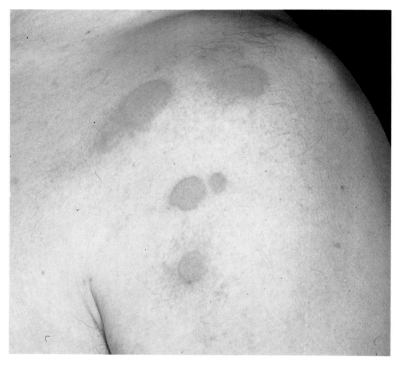

Fig. 14.11 Urticaria. The lesions are red and raised and have no surface scale. They persist for a few hours and disappear without trace. By courtesy of St. Mary's Hospital.

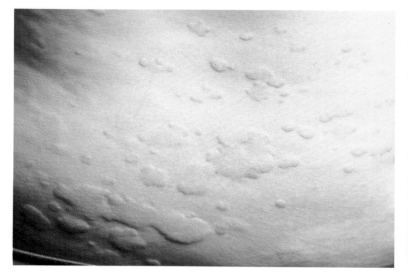

Fig. 14.12 Urticaria. The lesions are swellings which may be blanched centrally. By courtesy of St. Mary's Hospital.

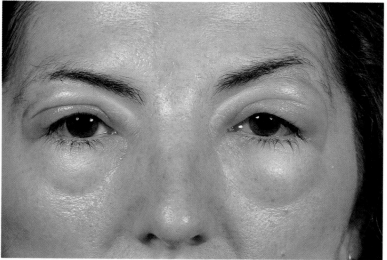

Fig. 14.13 Angio-oedema. There is considerable swelling around the eyes. By courtesy of Dr. Michèle Clement.

because the patient will give a history of having received a drug such as penicillin or aspirin, or an anti-serum such as anti-tetanus. Alternatively, the antigen may be food, for example crabmeat or strawberries, and the eruption may be associated with a gastrointestinal disturbance. The condition is short-lived, resolving within a few days. Insect bites and particularly bee stings present a similar problem, and in any of these cases the danger of anaphylaxis is present, therefore the antigen must never be given or taken again.

Physical Urticarias
Dermographism
This is a particularly common condition of young adults. It is an exaggerated response to trauma to the skin (Fig. 14.14), resulting in the release of histamine. These patients find that they can produce writing on their skin. It is temporary, but may last a few months or years. Systemic antihistamines may be of help.

Pressure Urticaria
After prolonged pressure, some patients develop painful sub-cutaneous swellings which may last for a number of hours. Typical sites are the buttocks and hands.

Solar Urticaria
This is a rare disorder that consists of urticarial wheals, usually occurring on areas of skin not normally exposed to ultra-violet light, so that it will appear on the skin a few minutes after being exposed to the sun. The eruption usually fades within an hour or so. Erythropoietic protoporphyria can sometimes present in this manner. In a polymorphic light eruption, urticarial wheals do occur, but they arise some hours after exposure to irradiation and last for several days.

Cold Urticaria
The development of wheals on exposure to cold is not particularly common, but when it does occur the patient must be warned to take special care against bathing in cold water, because ana-phylactic shock can occur.

Aquagenic Urticaria
Whealing can occur on exposure to water so that bathing becomes very uncomfortable and unpleasant. Small itchy wheals develop in contact with water, whatever the temperature, and last for ten to fifteen minutes.

Cholinergic Urticaria
This is a very distinctive kind of urticaria in that the wheals are very small indeed and there are a number of well-defined events which appear to precipitate it. Thus emotion, exercise and heat will set up a shower of intensely itchy wheals approximately two millimetres in size (Fig. 14.15), which last for about fifteen minutes. The condition appears to be particularly common in adolescence, and ultimately resolves. It is thought to be due to the release of acetyl choline from the sympathomimetic nerve endings, resulting in the release of histamine from mast cells.

Chronic Non-allergic Urticaria
This is probably the most common form of urticaria seen by the dermatologist. Chronic urticaria is defined as urticaria persisting longer than six weeks. Many patients have a personal or family history of atopy. Some find that aspirin and food additives aggravate the condition but in the main the cause is quite obscure. It ultimately disappears but may recur at a later stage. The condition is extremely distressing because of its itchy nature and there seems to be no way of predicting when or on which parts of the body the eruption may occur. Although exhaustive efforts may be made to determine whether there is a drug, food, physical, psychogenic or systemic reason for the eruption, in the vast majority of cases the cause is elusive. Prophylactic control with systemic antihistamines does give relief until the disease disappears.

HEREDITARY ANGIO-OEDEMA
This is a rare, autosomal dominant inherited disease. There is a deficiency of the esterase inhibitor of the first component of complement. It is neither a drug nor a toxic eruption, but since it does present in the skin as urticaria and angio-oedema it is included here. Deficiency of this enzyme allows the complement cascade to go unchecked and recurrent swellings of the skin, mucous membranes and gastrointestinal tract result. The cuta-neous swellings are frequently non-pruritic and the gastro-intestinal swellings may lead to obstruction. It is a serious disease because there is a significant mortality associated with laryngeal oedema. Fortunately, the disorder responds to danazol, an anabolic androgenic steroid which stimulates C1 esterase-inhibitor production. Tranexamic and epsi-aminocaproic acids also have some effect in this disease. The diagnosis is made by measuring the level of the C1 esterase-inhibitor.

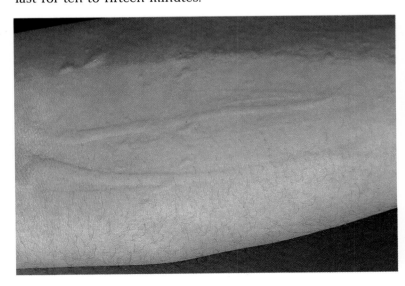

Fig. 14.14   Dermographism. This is an exaggerated response to trauma which results in whealing.

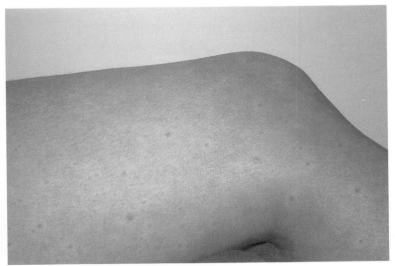

Fig. 14.15   Cholinergic urticaria. Very small, intensely pruritic wheals lasting for a few minutes occur with exercise, heat or emotion.

URTICARIA PIGMENTOSA

This is a rare disease distinguished by the accumulation of mast cells in the skin and occasionally in other organs (mastocytosis). It is not a reactive skin disorder but itching and urtication of the skin are its principle manifestations and it is convenient to include it here.

The most common form of urticaria pigmentosa presents in infancy, is usually confined to the skin and ultimately resolves. There are numerous reddish-brown macules (Figs. 14.16—14.18), papules or nodules which urticate spontaneously or on being rubbed. Isolated lesions occasionally occur.

A similar eruption may develop in adult life and may, very rarely, include involvement of the mast cells not only of the skin but also of the bones, liver, spleen, lymph nodes and gastrointestinal tract. Very rarely, a mast cell leukaemia may also be present.

A generalized eruption known as *telangiectasia macularis eruptiva perstans* occurs: widespread, confluent areas of telangiectatic macules (Fig. 14.19) develop in adults. This form appears to be limited to the skin only. An erythrodermic form of cutaneous mastocytosis with thickened infiltrated skin is extremely rare. Biopsy of the skin lesions will confirm the presence of excess

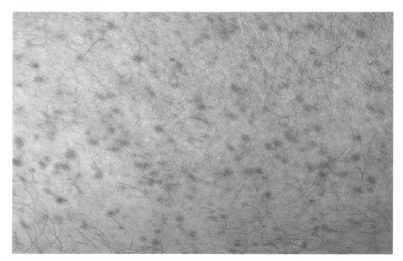

Fig. 14.16 Urticaria pigmentosa. There are numerous red-brown macules on the trunk and limbs. The commonest type occurs in infancy and resolves during childhood. By courtesy of Dr. R.H. Marten.

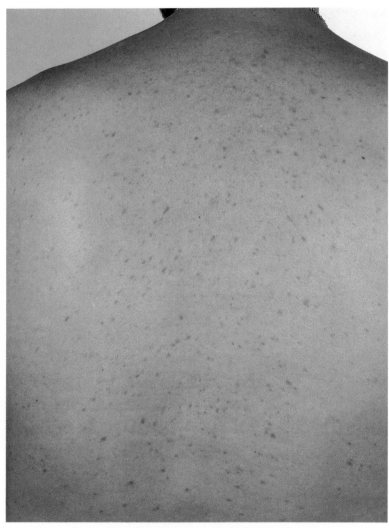

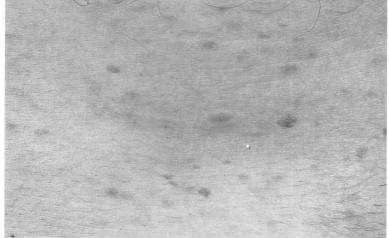

Fig. 14.17 Urticaria pigmentosa. In children the disorder remits spontaneously. In adults the condition is usually also benign. Very occasionally systemic involvement occurs.

Fig. 14.18 Urticaria pigmentosa. Numerous red-brown pigmented macules or papules occur (upper). In the close-up (lower) the central papule has been urticated by being rubbed.

mast cells (Fig. 14.20). Special stains aid this diagnosis.

There is no treatment for this disease, although the cutaneous form of urticaria pigmentosa is controllable with PUVA (photo-chemotherapy).

ERYTHEMA NODOSUM

This is an acute reaction which presents as red, painful nodules on the limbs. It is a set of physical signs which may be precipitated by a number of possible agents (Fig. 14.21).

The nodules are usually distributed symmetrically on the fronts of the shins (Figs. 14.22 and 14.23), but they occasionally occur on the extensor surfaces of the upper limbs and on the thighs. On the legs they may be associated with oedema of the ankles. The individual lesions last for a week or ten days and attain a diameter of three to four centimetres. They are bright red initially, but as they progress they change through shades of purple, blue, green to yellow, just like a bruise. The lesions are raised with no surface change and are tender to touch. They occur in crops and the attack is usually over within a month. The lesions do not ulcerate. The patient may feel unwell and have a fever and often arthralgia.

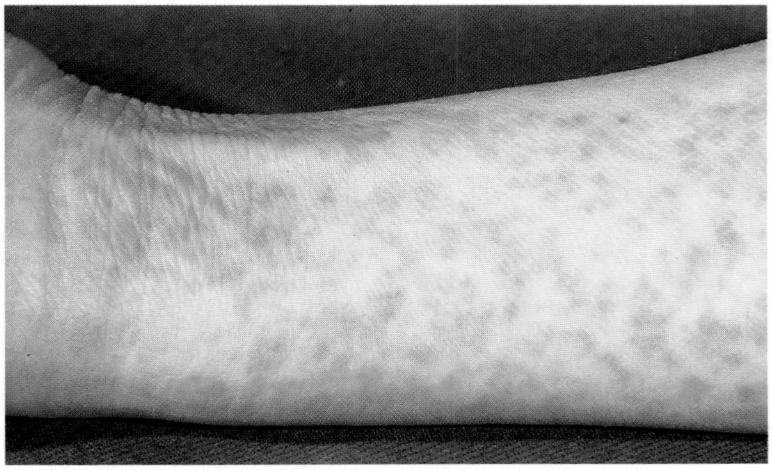

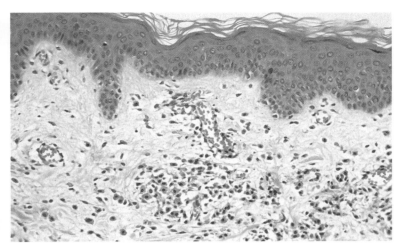

Fig. 14.19 Telangiectasia macularis eruptiva perstans. Confluent areas of telangiectatic macules occur.

Fig. 14.20 Urticaria pigmentosa. Numerous mast cells with intensely eosinophilic cytoplasm and small, uniform, hyperchromatic nuclei are present in the dermis.

Fig. 14.21 Causes of erythema nodosum.

Causes of Erythema Nodosum

Bacterial infections	Viral infections	Fungal infections	Drugs	Systemic disorders
Streptococcus	Vaccinia	Blastomycosis	Barbiturates	Sarcoidosis
Tuberculosis	Lymphogranuloma venereum	Coccidioidomycosis	Sulphonamides	Ulcerative colitis
Leprosy			Oral contraceptives	Crohn's disease
Syphilis	Cat scratch disease		Halogens	Hodgkin's disease
Yersinia infections	Glandular fever			

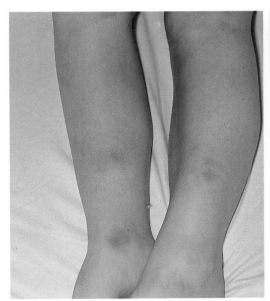

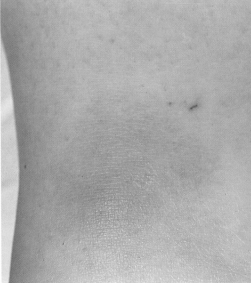

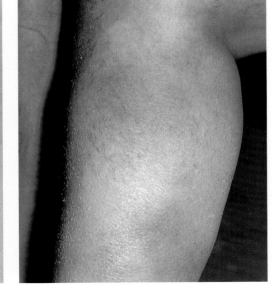

Fig. 14.22 Erythema nodosum. Painful red nodules occur mainly on the lower legs (left). The nodules are smooth, raised and tender (right). By courtesy of St. Mary's Hospital.

Fig. 14.23 Erythema nodosum. The nodules are bright red at first and then become purple and fade like a bruise.

This condition is the result of a panniculitis, that is, a vasculitis occurring in the fat (Fig. 14.24). It is probably mediated by immune complexes.

The diagnosis of erythema nodosum implies a search for the cause so that the appropriate treatment may be given. A variant of erythema nodosum is known as *erythema induratum* (Bazin's disease). In this condition the nodules appear predominantly on the backs of the lower legs, particularly in women. The lesions often break down and ulcerate, in contrast to erythema nodosum. This condition was seen more frequently in the past and was associated with active tuberculosis. Sometimes an identical picture is seen with an unusually high sensitivity to tuberculin testing but no overt tuberculosis is found. Some of these patients respond to anti-tuberculous therapy.

In a significant number of patients the erythema nodosum is chronic. The nodules are in every way identical to those of erythema nodosum but they persist indefinitely, waxing and waning in intensity. The condition is most common in women and is known as *nodular vasculitis*. Extensive investigations do not reveal a cause. The condition runs a benign course but it is difficult to treat. It may be necessary to control the disease with oral steroids.

ERYTHEMA MULTIFORME

Although this condition is not a disease in its own right, the pattern that it presents on the skin is readily recognizable. It is useful therefore to retain the name but to regard it as a reaction, the cause of which must be sought. It is a self-limiting disease of the skin and sometimes of mucous membranes, which usually lasts three weeks before complete recovery occurs. It may, however, vary from a mild inconvenient reaction to a potentially lethal disease. It may be precipitated by various agents which include infection (e.g. vaccinia, herpes simplex, orf, mycoplasma), malignant disease, radiotherapy or drugs such as sulphonamides, barbiturates and phenylbutazone. In a considerable proportion of patients no cause is found but the most common identifiable agent is herpes simplex. Recurrent attacks of erythema multiforme may follow each attack of herpes simplex resulting in a most debilitating condition.

By convention, three forms of erythema multiforme are described on the basis of the degree of damage done to the skin and mucous membranes. Not surprisingly, there is overlap between them.

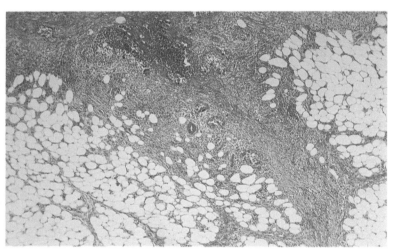
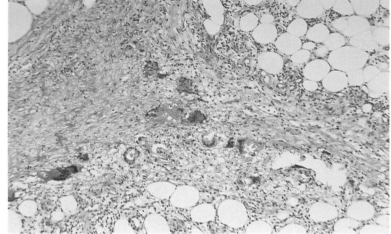

Fig. 14.24 Erythema nodosum. The essential features are those of a septal panniculitis: there is intense inflammation of the deep reticular dermis and fibrous septum with relative sparing of the fat lobules (left). Late stages of the disease are often characterized by a marked granulomatous component (right).

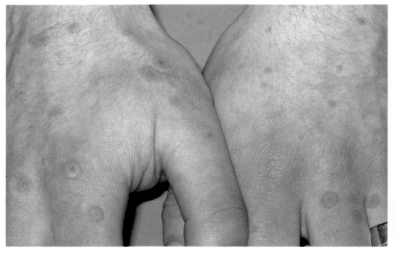
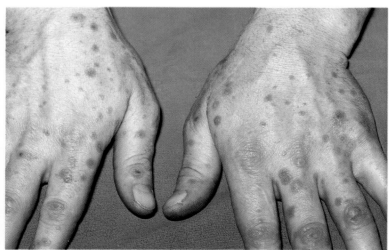

Fig. 14.25 Erythema multiforme. The lesions occur on the extremities, especially the hands and feet.

Fig. 14.26 Erythema multiforme. The lesions have a symmetrical distribution.

Iris Type

This is the commonest pattern of erythema multiforme. Symmetrical, round, red or purple lesions occur on the extremities and, in particular, on the backs of the hands (Figs. 14.25 and 14.26), forearms, palms, dorsa of the feet, soles and legs (Fig. 14.27). The characteristic feature of the annular lesions is that they resemble a target (Fig. 14.28) in that the central area is more involved than the periphery, probably because this has borne the brunt of the vascular damage.

Vesicular and Bullous Type

The degree of vascular damage is greater than in the simple type; there may be a vesicle (Fig. 14.29) or bulla (Figs. 14.30 and 14.31) in the central area of the target lesion, and the surrounding involved skin will show less damage. This type of eruption may be much more widespread with a large part of the body surface being involved. As the blisters break, raw, painful, denuded areas of skin result. The mucous membranes (Fig. 14.32) are frequently involved in this type.

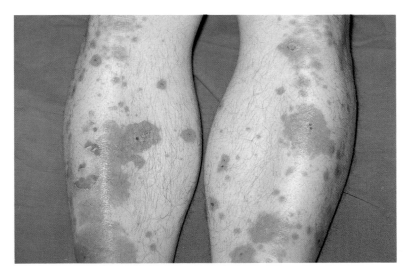

Fig. 14.27 Erythema multiforme. Multiform lesions may occur. This is the same patient as in Fig. 14.26.

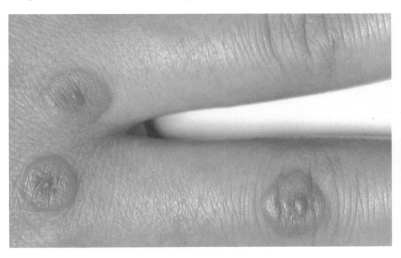

Fig. 14.28 Erythema multiforme. The central area of the lesion is more involved than the periphery so that it appears like a target. By courtesy of St. Mary's Hospital.

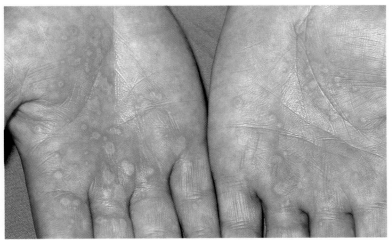

Fig. 14.29 Erythema multiforme. Vesicles may occur in the centre of the lesions.

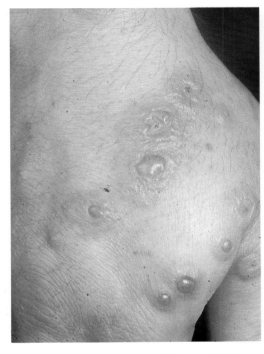

Fig. 14.30 Erythema multiforme. Bullae have occurred in the centre of oedematous lesions. The target-like appearance is still clear.

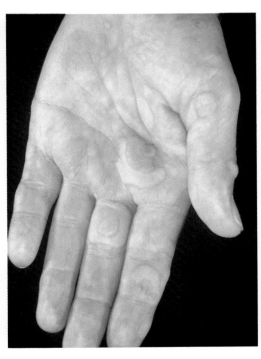

Fig. 14.31 Erythema multiforme. Large blisters are present with a target-like configuration.

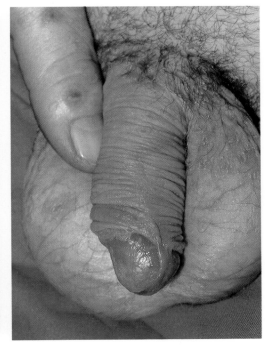

Fig. 14.32 Erythema multiforme. The genitalia are often involved. Target lesions may be seen on the patient's finger.

The Stevens-Johnson Syndrome

This is an eponymous term describing the most severe type of erythema multiforme, which has an appreciable mortality. There is serious involvement of the skin and mucous membranes, the joints, lungs, gastrointestinal tract and kidneys, causing profound systemic disturbance with a high fever. The blistering results in ulceration in the mouth (Fig. 14.33), making it almost impossible to eat, in the conjunctiva leading to corneal scarring and blindness, and on the genitalia and in the urethra causing urinary retention. Occasionally the skin is not involved at all.

The diagnosis of erythema multiforme is a clinical one. In the past, the blistering varieties (Fig. 14.34) were sometimes confused with bullous pemphigoid. However, although there may be a remarkably similar histology in that a subepidermal blister will be present, the immunofluorescence is positive in bullous pemphigoid and negative in erythema multiforme.

The management of the disorder depends on the severity of the illness. The offending agent must be identified if possible and treated or withdrawn. In more severe varieties of the disease systemic steroids may be helpful. Skilled nursing is essential. Sepsis is a major hazard both of the skin and of other organs, and should be identified and treated immediately. Parenteral nutrition and the correction of electrolyte imbalance are very important. The pulmonary, renal and ocular complications will require specialist management.

TOXIC EPIDERMAL NECROLYSIS (Lyell's Syndrome)

This is a rare but grave disorder; it usually afflicts adults, in contrast to the staphylococcal 'scalded skin' syndrome of childhood which responds rapidly to appropriate antibiotics. The condition is often a hypersensitivity to drugs such as phenylbutazone, sulphonamides, barbiturates or cytostatics. It is essentially a variant of erythema multiforme. Involvement of the eyes, mouth and genitalia usually occurs before the skin eruption. The skin becomes acutely tender with flaccid bullae

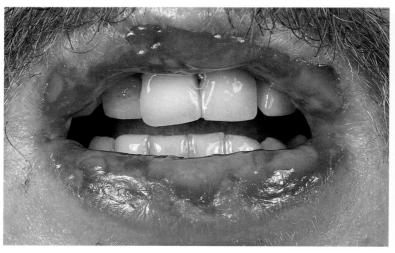

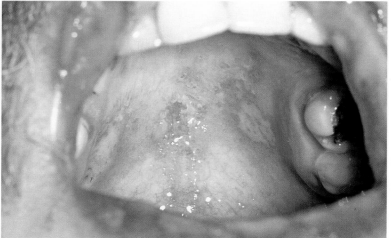

Fig. 14.33 Stevens-Johnson syndrome. Severe blistering and ulceration of the mucous membranes occur. Ulceration is present on the lips and in the mouth.

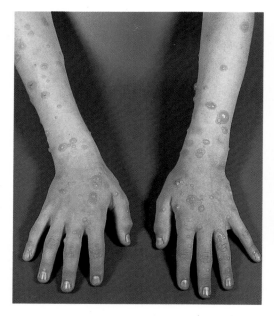

Fig. 14.34 Erythema multiforme. Large blisters similar to those of bullous pemphigoid are present. Immunofluorescence was negative however, and the eruption cleared within three weeks. Prior to immunofluorescence, these disorders were sometimes difficult to distinguish.

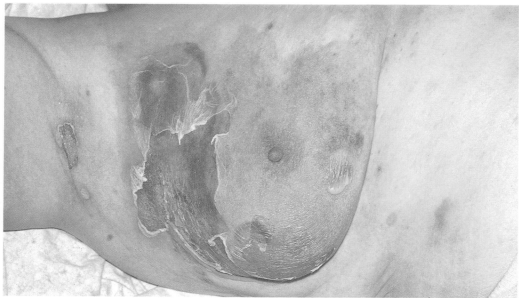

Fig. 14.35 Toxic epidermal necrolysis. There is 'sheeting' of the skin leaving a raw denuded area. This was secondary to a barbiturate. By courtesy of Dr. R. Staughton, St. Stephen's Hospital, London.

which begin to sheet all over the body leaving a red, raw, oozing, eroded surface (Fig. 14.35), very similar to the appearances of the skin following a burn. The lesions are particularly marked in the flexures and then become widespread. The patient is ill and feverish. The histopathology reveals sloughing of the whole of the epidermis due to the damage in the basal cell layer.

There is a significant mortality associated with the drug-induced toxic epidermal necrolysis, despite discontinuing the responsible noxious agent. The situation is identical to that of a severe burn and the management is similar to that of the Stevens-Johnson syndrome. Although systemic steroids are frequently given, their efficacy is not proven.

FIXED DRUG ERUPTION
The remarkable feature of this condition is that it appears in an identical site each time the drug is ingested. The eruption consists of a single (Fig. 14.36) or several (Fig. 14.37) well-demarcated, round, red or red-brown oedematous areas which

may become bullous. The lesion develops within hours and subsides fairly rapidly leaving very characteristic hyperpigment-ation of the skin (Fig. 14.38). It can occur anywhere on the body but especially in the mouth, on a limb, on the back of the hand or on the genitalia. Phenolphthalein in a laxative is the most common cause, but griseofulvin, phenacetin, barbiturates, tetracyclines and sulphonamides have all been incriminated. The mechanism of the reaction is obscure but the condition ceases if the allergen is identified and if the patient is prepared to avoid it.

PURPURA
Purpura is a term used to describe a physical sign in the skin, but it does not constitute a disease entity *per se*. The lesions are purple and do not blanche on pressure, unlike erythema. As the lesions age, their colour changes in a similar manner to those seen in a resolving bruise. If the lesions are small they are known as petechiae (Figs. 14.39 and 14.40) and, if large, as ecchymoses

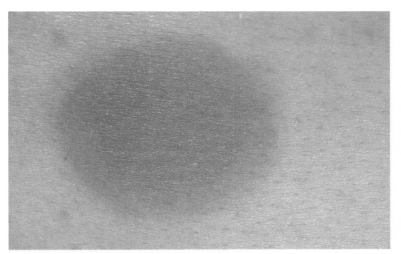

Fig. 14.36 Fixed drug eruption. The lesion is well-defined, reddish-brown and oedematous. It recurs in the same site each time the allergen is ingested.

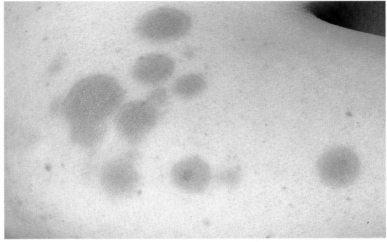

Fig. 14.37 Fixed drug eruption. Several lesions may occur with time if the allergen is not identified.

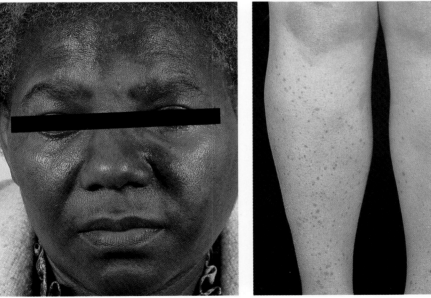

Fig. 14.38 Fixed drug eruption. Post-inflammatory pigmentation is characteristic of the condition.

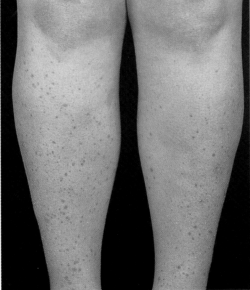

Fig. 14.39 Purpura. The lower limbs are the usual site. Small macules are known as petechiae. By courtesy of St. John's Hospital for Diseases of the Skin.

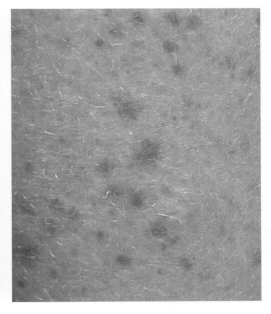

Fig. 14.40 Purpura. The lesions are purple and do not blanche on pressure (close up of Fig. 14.39). By courtesy of St. John's Hospital for Diseases of the Skin.

(bruises) (Fig. 14.41). The lesions occur symmetrically on dependent parts and in particular on the lower legs and buttocks where the back pressure on the capillaries is at its greatest. Purpura is due to either an abnormality of the blood vessels or a disorder of the blood. Causes of purpura are legion but the table shows a simplified classification (Fig. 14.42).

As a general rule, the coagulation defects produce ecchymoses rather than petechiae and the eruptions due to damage to the vessel walls produce a palpable purpura of the type described under vasculitis, rather than flat macules as in platelet abnormalities. The finding of purpura behoves a physician to investigate for a systemic cause. However, local factors may result in purpura. One of the most common causes is raised venous pressure and is found in association with varicose eczema around the ankle. Similarly, an acute inflammatory disorder such as a toxic erythema may result in purpura on the lower legs and ankles. This is known as *stasis purpura*.

Solar purpura is very common in the elderly and its recognition may save the patient from unnecessary investigation. Ecchymoses are seen on the backs of the hands and forearms. These changes are due to degeneration of the collagen which normally surrounds and protects the vessel walls. Although often referred to as 'senile purpura' it is quite clear that advanced age is not the prerequisite for this change, but rather excess exposure to ultraviolet light causing the degenerative changes in the collagen. It may thus be seen in relatively young people. Identical changes are seen in patients who have used excessive amounts of potent topical glucocorticosteroids on their skins.

DRUG ERUPTIONS SIMULATING SKIN DISORDERS
Drugs may occasionally simulate skin disorders such as eczema, psoriasis or lichen planus. The correct diagnosis may, however, be suggested because the rash is atypical and does not respond to the appropriate therapy for that disease.

Acneiform Eruptions
The most common drugs producing acne are the corticosteroids. The eruption occurs on the face and chest, but may well spread to the lower abdomen, lower back, upper arms and thighs. The individual lesions consist of papules or pustules, but the other features of acne vulgaris such as comedones, cysts and scars are not seen. Radio-opaque materials, ethambutol, anticonvulsants, isoniazid (Fig. 14.43) and ethionamide are regular offenders.

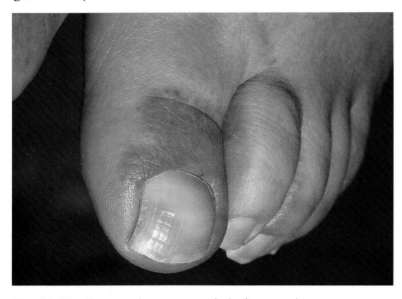

Fig. 14.41 Purpura. Large purpuric lesions are known as ecchymoses.

Classification of Purpura

Blood disorders

Platelet abnormalities
i) idiopathic thrombocytopenic purpura
ii) secondary thrombocytopenia
   bone marrow infiltration
   e.g. leukaemia or carcinomatosis
   bone marrow arrest
   e.g. drugs or irradiation

Coagulation abnormalities
e.g. haemophilia

Plasma protein abnormalities
e.g. macroglobulinaemia

Blood vessel defects

Congenital defects of vessel walls
e.g. Ehlers-Danlos syndrome

Increased vascular permeability
e.g. vitamin C deficiency (scurvy)

Fragility of the vessel wall
e.g. solar or corticosteroid purpura

Damage to the vessel wall
e.g. vasculitis or emboli

Fig. 14.42 Causes of purpura.

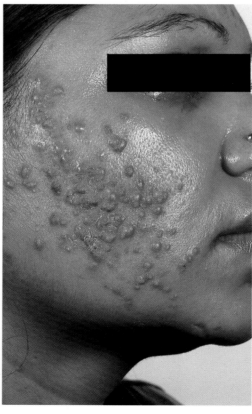

Fig. 14.43 Acneiform eruption. This severe eruption of papules and pustules on the face was caused by isoniazid.

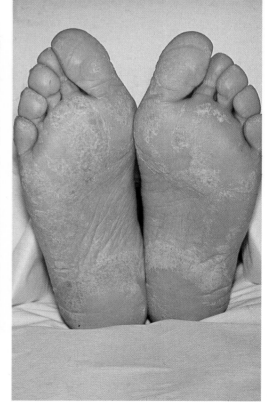

Fig. 14.44 Practolol eruption. Psoriasiform hyperkeratosis is present on the soles. By courtesy of Dr. A. Ive.

Iodides and bromides produce acne. Occasionally, particularly if the iodides are continued, bullous lesions occur which become haemorrhagic and ultimately develop into vegetating masses studded with pustules, which are extremely disfiguring.

Lichenoid Eruptions

These eruptions are similar to lichen planus and the most common offending agents are gold and arsenic, although they have also been described with chlorothiazide, phenothiazine, para-aminosalicylic acid and chloroquine. There was an epidemic of lichenoid eruptions during World War II when troops were given mepacrine as an antimalarial. Penicillamine causes a lichenoid eruption particularly affecting the mucous membranes, especially during the treatment of primary biliary cirrhosis.

Psoriasiform Eruptions

Practolol, a beta-blocking drug, was incriminated in producing an eruption which involved both the skin and the mucous membranes. The drug has largely been withdrawn as a result. The rash is partly psoriasiform but with features of lichen planus, eczema and lupus erythematosus. The eruption is widespread with a predilection for bony prominences. Hyperkeratosis of the palms and soles (Fig. 14.44) and around the fingers and toes is characteristic. Exfoliative dermatitis may result. The importance of the condition is not particularly the skin eruption, which is reversible on stopping the drug, but the involvement of mucous membranes, particularly those in association with the eye which lead in some cases to keratoconjunctivitis sicca and scarring. Very occasionally a sclerosing peritonitis occurs. Other beta-blocking agents may produce similar psoriasiform eruptions (Fig. 14.45).

Bullous Eruptions

Nalidixic acid may produce a bullous eruption, particularly on the lower legs. Individuals who have taken overdoses of barbiturates frequently develop blisters on areas of skin which have been under pressure from the patient lying immobile in an unconscious state.

Eczematous Eruptions

Contact dermatitis to topically applied agents is by far the most common form of eczematous drug eruption and the subject has been covered in Chapter 2. Eczematous eruptions following the ingestion of a drug are surprisingly rare. Methyldopa may produce the pattern of a discoid or a seborrhoeic eczema, often with palmar and plantar eczema. These patients often had constitutional eczema in the past. The rash responds to discontinuing the drug. Similarly, gold may produce a seborrhoeic or discoid type of eczema, or even simulate pityriasis rosea (Fig. 14.46). Fatal erythroderma may result. A stomatitis may precede or accompany the eruption and eosinophilia may be present.

Phototoxic Eruptions

Various disease processes are either exacerbated (for example lupus erythematosus), or induced (for example porphyria cutanea tarda or xeroderma pigmentosum) by ultra-violet light. The most common drugs causing phototoxic reactions are thiazides, phenothiazines, tetracyclines (especially demethylchlortetracycline) and benoxaprofen. The eruption consists of either a burn, i.e. erythema, oedema and blistering (Fig. 14.47) or eczema in light-exposed areas. Topical agents may also cause a photodermatitis.

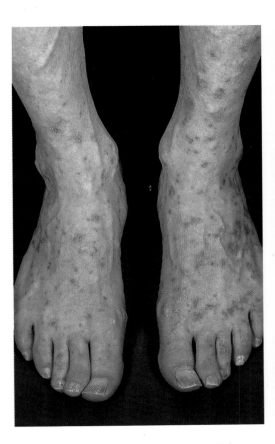

Fig. 14.45 Oxyprenolol eruption. This eruption was widespread. It had features of psoriasis, lichen planus and eczema but fitted none of these diseases completely.

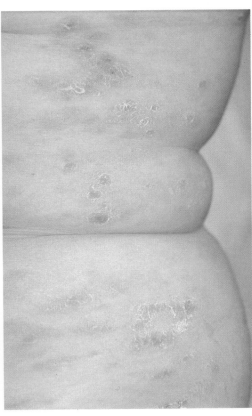

Fig. 14.46 Eczematous eruption. This eruption, which simulated pityriasis rosea, was secondary to gold injections.

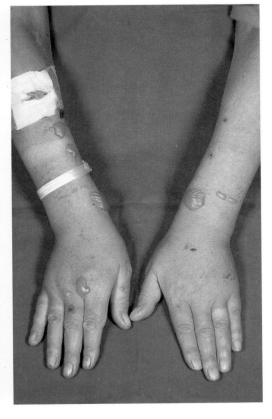

Fig. 14.47 Bullous eruptions. This was a phototoxic eruption. The patient had been sunbathing (her wrist-watch and ring areas are spared) and blisters developed. She was taking nalidixic acid.

The most common 'toxic' reaction to light is the *polymorphic light eruption*. Light-testing may reproduce the rash but it is unclear exactly which wavelength of light is responsible. It is not prevented by presently available sunscreens. It affects the areas of skin exposed to ultra-violet light but usually, for unknown reasons, spares the face. The condition begins in early or middle adult life and often occurs only in sunny climates on holiday. There is a tendency for the condition to lessen during the year as the patient acquires a protective tan. The lesions start 24–48 hours after exposure and are urticarial, oedematous papules (Figs. 14.48 and 14.49), plaques or vesicles.

The lesions clear within a week to ten days but can be very distressing and ruin a holiday. They recur each year and do not respond to topical steroids. The condition may be prevented by systemic steroids, chloroquine or photochemotherapy (PUVA).

A variant of light eruption is known as Hutchinson's summer prurigo: excoriated papules (Fig. 14.50) occur not only on exposed but also on covered areas, and sometimes persist through the winter months. It usually commences in childhood, unlike the polymorphic light eruption, and may or may not clear in adult life.

Pigmentation

Localized and generalized disturbances of pigmentation may occur. The contraceptive pill frequently produces melasma, a patchy hyperpigmentation seen on the forehead, cheeks, chin or across the bridge of the nose and upper lip. The condition is not necessarily reversible on stopping the drug. Localized hyperpigmentation can occur as the result of using hydroquinones in order to lighten the skin. Chronic use of cosmetics containing mercury can cause localized hyperpigmentation. Patients who have to take phenothiazines in high dosage on a long-term basis may develop generalized hyperpigmentation (Fig. 14.51) especially with chlorpromazine. The antimalarial mepacrine always

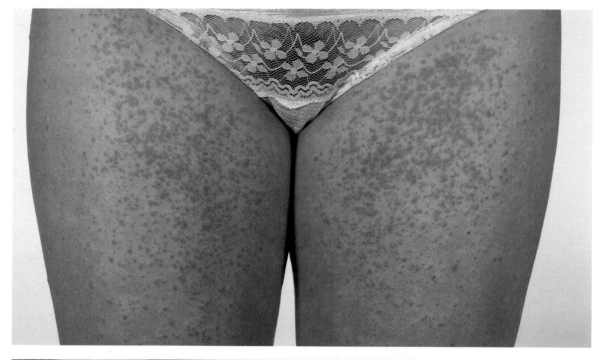

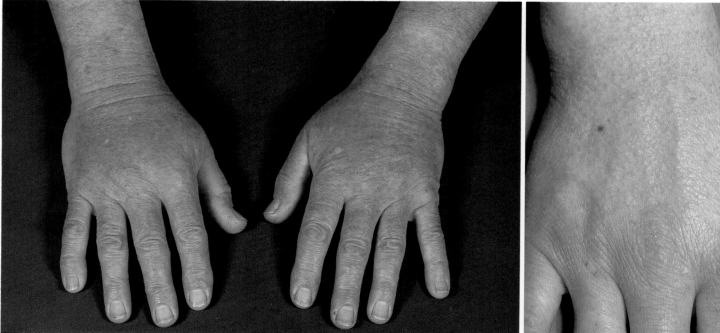

Fig. 14.48 Polymorphic light eruption. This young woman developed a widespread pruritic, papular eruption after using a sunbed.

Fig. 14.49 Polymorphic light eruption. Oedematous papules are present. The condition commences 24–48 hours after exposure to strong sunlight.

produces a yellow discoloration of the skin (Fig. 14.52). Arsenic causes a generalized hyperpigmentation with tiny macules of hypopigmentation and the appearance is sometimes termed 'rain drop' pigmentation.

Pemphigus

Penicillamine is the most common drug responsible for this eruption. This drug is used to treat Wilson's disease and, in lower doses, rheumatoid arthritis or primary biliary cirrhosis. Urticarial or morbilliform rashes are seen, but the most characteristic is a simulation of pemphigus vulgaris. The eruption may start as a stomatitis with flaccid blisters or erosions which bleed, are painful and show little tendency to heal. Similar erosions occur on the body. The vegetative form of pemphigus is also often seen. The histological and immunofluorescent changes are identical to those seen in pemphigus. The eruption does clear on stopping the drug but it may take many months. Captopril may produce a similar eruption.

Hair Changes

Loss of hair as part of the process of telogen effluvium is a common sequelae of a severe illness. Cytostatic agents, however, are common causes of hair loss, particularly cyclophosphamides, colchicine and methotrexate. The hair loss usually develops within a month or so of starting treatment. Anticoagulants also produce a diffuse alopecia, usually beginning after a couple of months and lasting for about six months. Similarly, drugs used in the treatment of hyperthyroidism may produce hair loss, either by inducing hypothyroidism or by unknown mechanisms of their own.

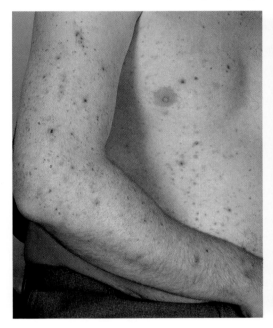

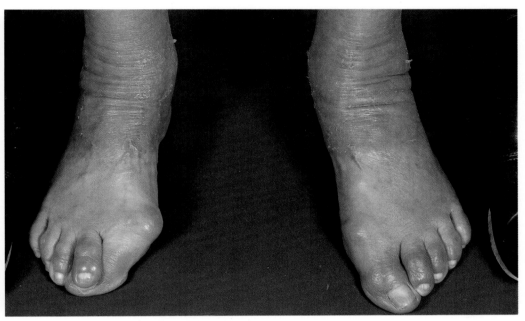

Fig. 14.50 Hutchinson's summer prurigo. Excoriated papules occur on both covered areas and parts exposed to light. It commences in childhood and may or may not go into remission in adult life.

Fig. 14.51 Hyperpigmentation. Hyperpigmentation may occur from persistent ingestion of a photosensitizing drug. Note the sparing of the skin protected by the patient's shoes.

Fig. 14.52 Mepacrine. This drug produces a yellow discoloration of the skin

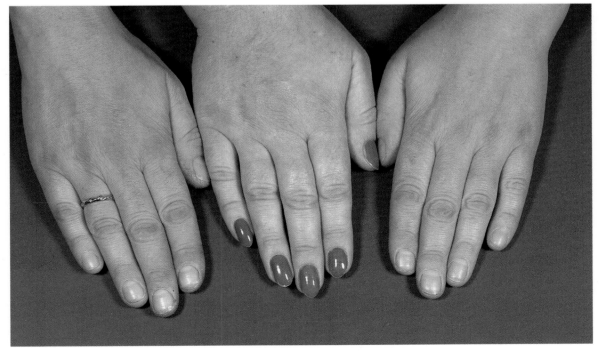

Pigmented Purpuric Eruption

Carbromal, a hypnotic which is now seldom used, produces a rather specific form of purpuric eruption, which is identical to a textile dermatitis produced by new khaki shirts during World War II. The chemical responsible for the latter was never identified. Petechiae, minute brown macules (due to haemo-siderin), and very small lichenoid papules start on the feet and lower legs (Fig. 14.53), but may spread all over the body. Some of the macules are arranged in round or oval patches. The disorder is due to capillary fragility.

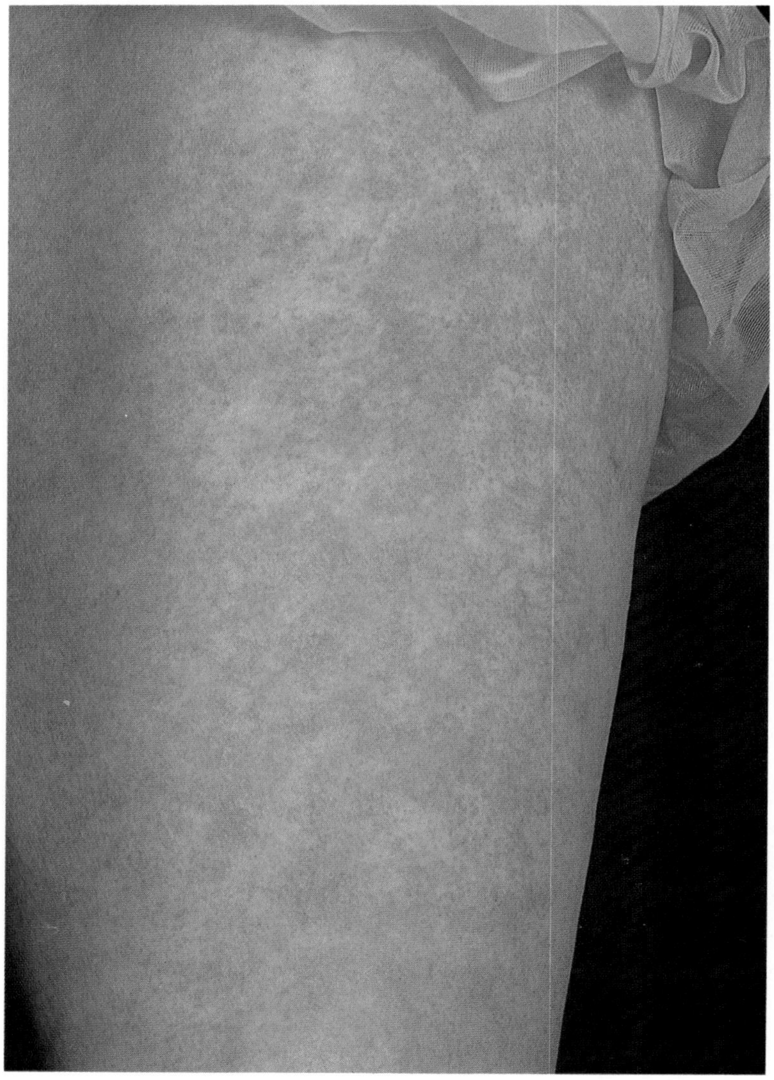

Nail Changes

The most common change in the nails seen following drug administration is onycholysis (Fig. 14.54). This separation of the distal part of the nailplate from the nailbed occurs particularly with the tetracyclines in association with exposure to strong sunlight. A similar change is common with the non-steroidal anti-inflammatory drug benoxaprofen.

Ichthyosis

Carbamazepine produces a dryness of the skin which may proceed to an exfoliative dermatitis. The eruption is widespread, very itchy, does not respond to emollients and is associated with an eosinophilia. It responds dramatically to withdrawing the drug.

TOPICAL GLUCOCORTICOSTEROIDS

Topical steroids have been the major breakthrough in the management of skin disorders and particularly eczema. However, if they are misprescribed or abused, side-effects are inevitable. The commonest problems associated with their use have been *perioral dermatitis* and exacerbation of rosacea. Acne and rosacea do not respond to steroids and indeed are made worse, and should never be prescribed. Steroids are powerful immunosuppressants and it is clearly inappropriate to prescribe them for infections of the skin (Fig. 14.55): they will inevitably exacerbate them. These conditions have been described and illustrated in Chapters 9–12.

Topical steroids are most commonly correctly prescribed for eczema and psoriasis. The choice of potency of steroid depends on the disease process and the site involved. Eczema on the whole responds to weaker steroids than psoriasis or lichen planus. Percutaneous absorption is much easier through the thin skin of the face or the warm occluded skin of the groin than through the thick skin of the palms or soles. These regional differences influence the choice of steroid. The prolonged use of too powerful a steroid for eczema in the groin or elbow flexures will inevitably lead to side-effects.

The potential side-effect of topical steroids is *atrophy* of epidermis, dermis (Figs. 14.56 and 14.57) and subcutaneous tissues (Fig. 14.58). The skin is thin and transparent such that the

Fig. 14.53 Carbromal eruption. Brown staining petechiae and macules occur on the legs and feet.

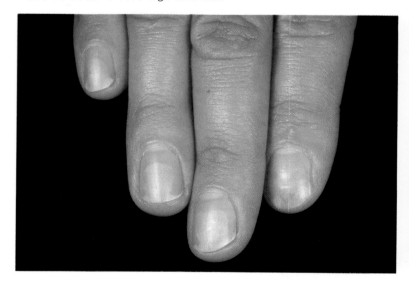

Fig. 14.54 Photo-onycholysis. Separation of the distal nailplate from the nailbed may occur as a result of a phototoxic eruption.

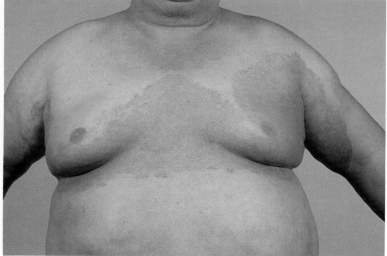

Fig. 14.55 Inappropriate use of topical steroids. Topical steroids are immunosuppressants and will cause infections such as tinea to flourish.

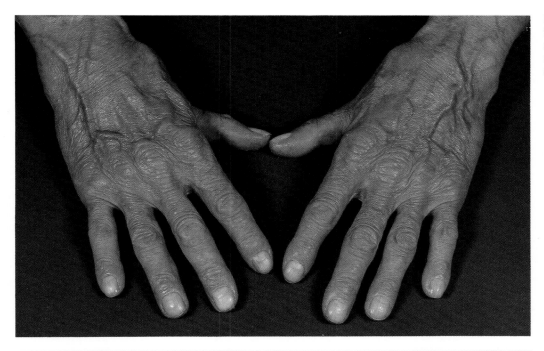

Fig. 14.56 Topical steroid atrophy. Gross thinning and a transparent erythema of the skin have occurred from the inappropriate use of clobetasol propionate on the backs of the hands.

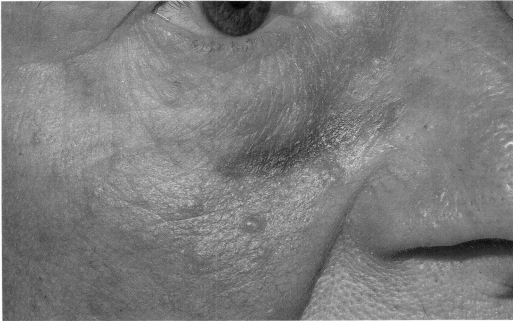

Fig. 14.57 Topical steroid atrophy. The skin becomes red and purpuric. The papules and pustules indicate that the patient has rosacea, which should not have been treated with topical steroids.

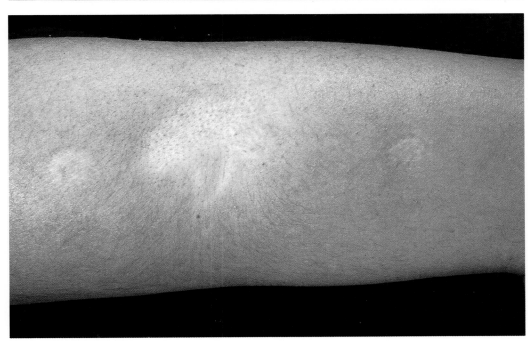

Fig. 14.58 Injected steroid atrophy. Subcutaneous atrophy and hypopigmentation have occurred as a result of a poorly given steroid injection. By courtesy of St. John's Hospital for Diseases of the Skin.

14.19

underlying blood vessels are visible (*telangiectasia*) and vulnerable to trauma, so that *purpura* occurs (Figs. 14.59 and 14.60). Dermal collagen is affected and *striae* result (Fig. 14.61).

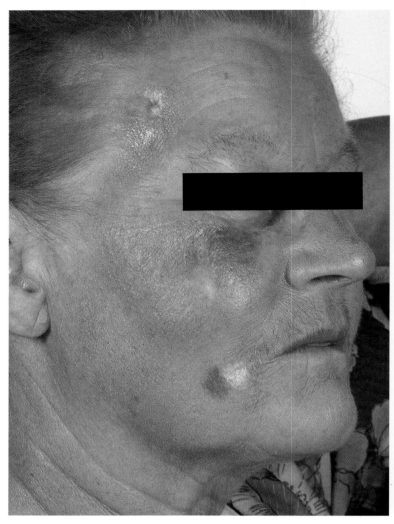

Fig. 14.59 Topical steroid purpura. Purpura is present from the persistent use of fluocinolone acetate on the face. The primary pathology was lupus erythematosus.

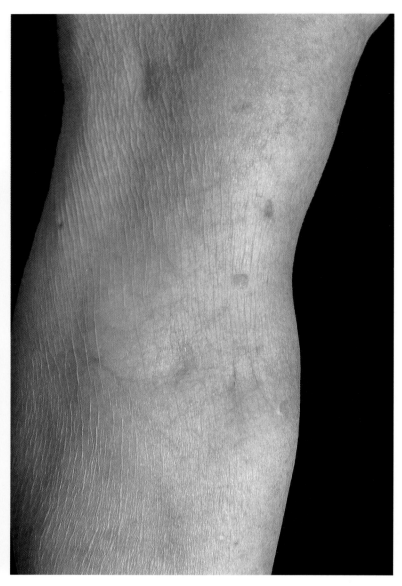

Fig. 14.60 Topical steroid atrophy. Thinning of the skin, telangiectasia and a small patch of purpura are visible. By courtesy of St. John's Hospital for Diseases of the Skin.

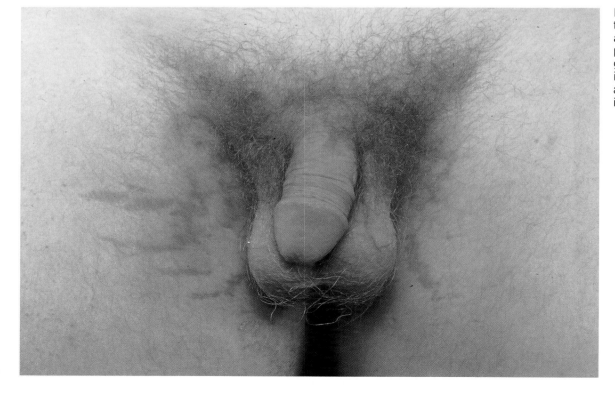

Fig. 14.61 Striae due to topical steroids. Gross striae are present due to the use of a powerful topical steroid in the groin to treat a fungus infection. Note the redness and scaling of tinea on the inner right thigh.

15 Blistering Disorders of the Skin

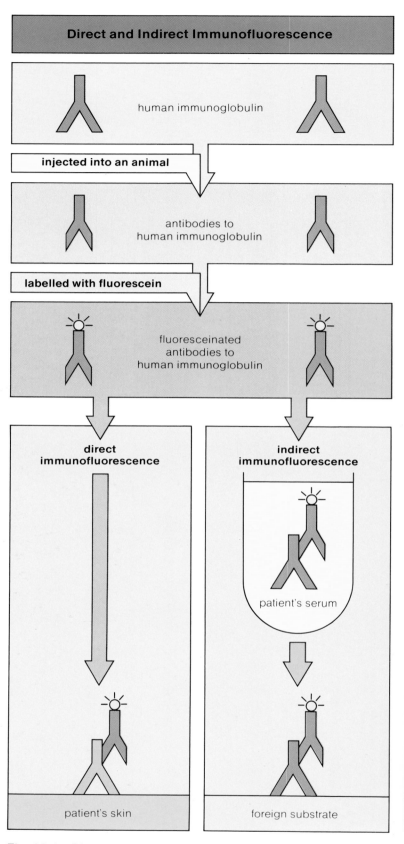

Direct and Indirect Immunofluorescence

human immunoglobulin

injected into an animal

antibodies to
human immunoglobulin

labelled with fluorescein

fluoresceinated
antibodies to
human immunoglobulin

**direct
immunofluorescence**

**indirect
immunofluorescence**

patient's serum

patient's skin

foreign substrate

Fig. 15.1 Direct and indirect immunofluorescence. The technique involves the raising of antibodies to human immunoglobulin by injecting it into an animal. These antibodies are labelled with a fluorescein marker which can then be incubated either with the patient's skin (direct immunofluorescence) or with the patient's serum and a foreign substrate, such as monkey oesophagus (indirect immunofluorescence). In the direct test, if antibody is present in the skin, it will be recognized by the fluorescein-labelled antibody which will be deposited as a pale green fluorescence. In the indirect test, if antibodies are present in the serum, the anti-human antibody will label them with fluorescein and be deposited at their target site on the foreign substrate, which will fluoresce.

Blisters are a common morphological disturbance of the skin and may result from disorders as diverse as insect bites, burns or impetigo. The diseases which are included in this chapter are uncommon, but are customarily grouped together because blisters constitute a principal manifestation of the eruption. Their nomenclature has been confusing, for example benign mucous membrane pemphigus was also known as ocular pemphigus. However, the definition of these diseases has been greatly clarified by the use of immunofluorescent techniques (Fig. 15.1). These probably represent one of the most important investigational aids to be developed in dermatology during the past two decades. Pemphigus and pemphigoid have been clearly shown to be autoimmune in nature and dermatitis herpetiformis, which occasionally can be difficult to diagnose, now has specific diagnostic immunofluorescent markers. These tests are probably more important than routine histopathology in blistering conditions and have markedly improved their management.

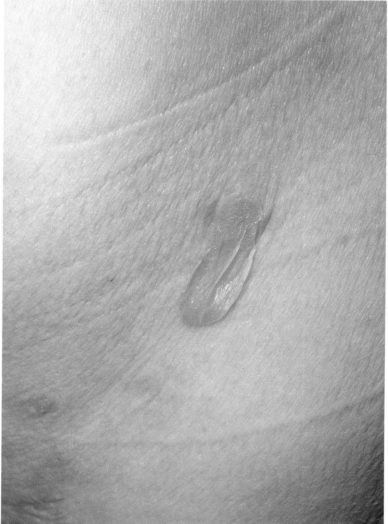

Fig. 15.2 Pemphigus vulgaris. The blisters are superficial, flaccid and break easily. By courtesy of Dr. L. Fry, St. Mary's Hospital.

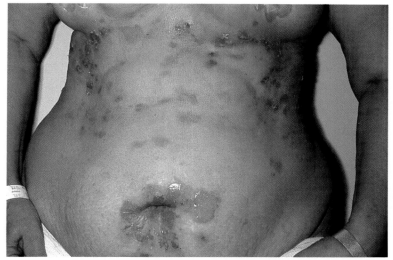

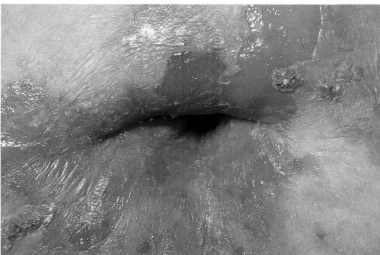

PEMPHIGUS

A set of rare autoimmune diseases are described under this heading. They have an appreciable morbidity and mortality. Certain drugs are capable of producing pemphigus-like syndromes.

Pemphigus Vulgaris

The disease tends to commence in middle age and is more common in Jews. It consists of superficial flaccid blisters (Fig. 15.2) which rapidly break and leave raw, denuded and eroded skin (Fig. 15.3) which may crust (Fig. 15.4) and has little tendency to heal spontaneously. The lesions do not itch, but are painful and tender to touch. A characteristic finding is the ability to slide the skin adjacent to a lesion over the underlying dermis (Nikolsky's sign). Scarring is not a feature of the condition when it is healing with treatment, but central clearing and post-inflammatory hyperpigmentation are characteristic (Fig. 15.5).

Fig. 15.3 Pemphigus vulgaris. The blisters leave raw, tender, denuded and eroded skin (upper), which has little tendency to heal spontaneously. The umbilicus is commonly affected (lower). By courtesy of Dr. L. Fry, St Mary's Hospital.

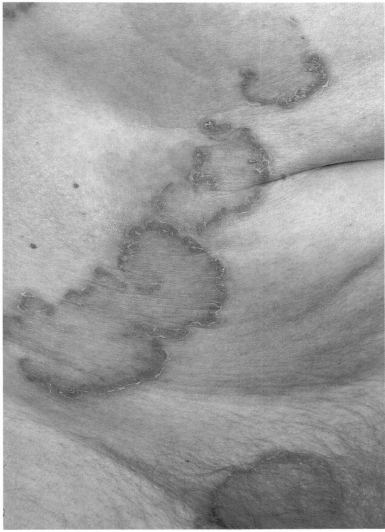

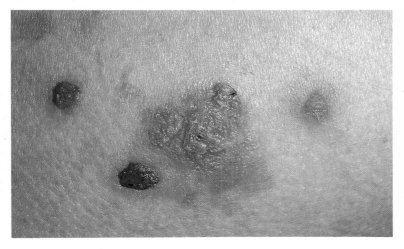

Fig. 15.4 Pemphigus vulgaris. The blisters may become crusted. By courtesy of Dr. L. Fry, St. Mary's Hospital.

Fig. 15.5 Pemphigus vulgaris. Spontaneous healing is slow. It tends to occur centrally with post-inflammatory pigmentation. The edge is slightly crusted and vesicular.

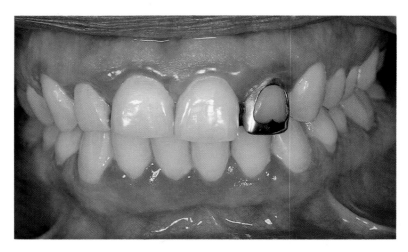

Fig. 15.6 Oral pemphigus vulgaris. The gums are denuded. Blisters are rapidly broken in the mouth and are not often visible.

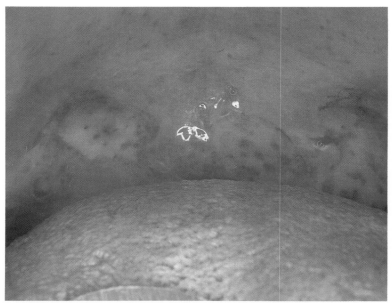

The disorder starts insidiously, usually in the mucous membranes, particularly of the oral cavity (Figs. 15.6 and 15.7) and pharynx, but also of the genitalia (Fig. 15.8), anus and eyes. Thus, the patient frequently presents to medical disciplines other than dermatology, but it is unusual for the diagnosis to be made until the skin becomes involved and a dermatological opinion is requested. Any area of the skin may be involved, but the trunk (Figs. 15.9 and 15.10), umbilicus, intertriginous areas and scalp are the most common sites. A considerable proportion of the body surface may be affected and the disorder is extremely distressing and debilitating. The situation is similar to that of severe burns in that there is considerable loss of fluid from the weeping, denuded skin, with the attendant dangers of disturbance in fluid balance and secondary sepsis. Prior to the introduction of systemic steroids the disorder was usually fatal. The prognosis is now much improved, but the use of systemic steroids in high doses and other immunosuppressants frequently bring hazards of their own.

The condition is autoimmune in origin and may be associated with other autoimmune diseases such as systemic lupus erythematosus, thyroid disease, myasthenia gravis and thymoma. Immunofluorescence of peribullous skin (direct immunofluorescence) has clearly demonstrated the presence of immunoglobulin (Ig) G and C3 in the intercellular region of the epidermis (Fig. 15.11). Immunoglobulin fixation and complement activation in some way damages the integrity of the intercellular junction with resultant keratinocyte disassociation. The squamous cells become separated and rounded often with intensely eosinophilic cytoplasm, a process known as acantholysis (Fig. 15.12). This may be demonstrated histologically (Figs. 15.13 and 15.14) and also by use of exfoliative cytology – the Tzanck test. The loss of cellular adhesion therefore results in the development of a blister. The roof of the blister is made up of only a thin layer of cells, and therefore the lesion appears flaccid and breaks easily, in direct contrast to bullous pemphigoid where the whole epidermis constitutes the roof of the blister such that it remains intact much longer.

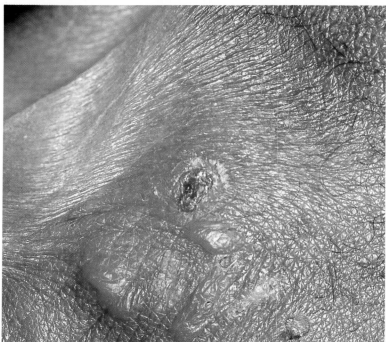

Fig. 15.7 Pemphigus vulgaris. Painful erosions were present on the tongue and palate (upper) some months before flaccid blisters developed behind the ear (lower).

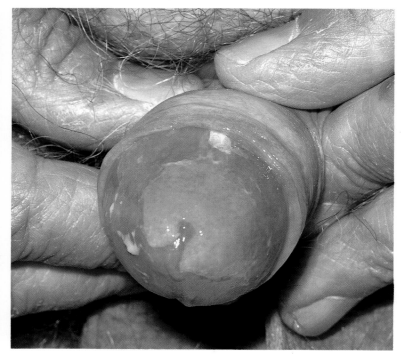

Fig. 15.8 Genital pemphigus. Denuded erosions on the genitalia may be the first sign of pemphigus. By courtesy of St. John's Hospital for Diseases of the Skin.

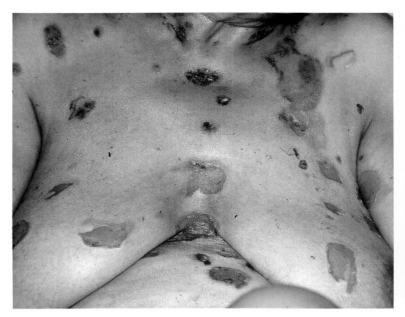

Fig. 15.9   Pemphigus vulgaris. The trunk and intertriginous areas are common sites. Many erosions are present. By courtesy of St. John's Hospital for Diseases of the Skin.

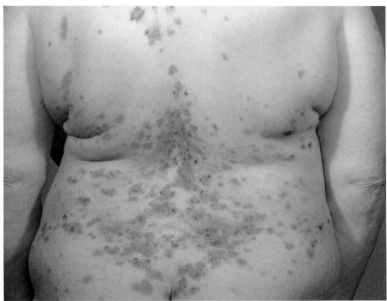

Fig. 15.10   Pemphigus vulgaris. Widespread erosions occur. Fluid loss, electrolyte imbalance and secondary sepsis are the major hazards as in burns.

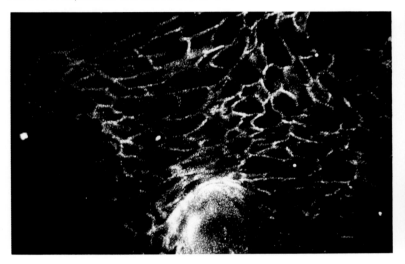

Fig. 15.11   Pemphigus vulgaris: direct immunofluorescence. Fluorescein labelled antibodies to human immunoglobulin are deposited between epidermal cells giving a fishnet appearance.

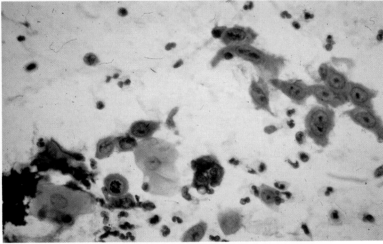

Fig. 15.12   Pemphigus vulgaris: Tzanck test. Acantholysis is demonstrated by exfoliative cytology.

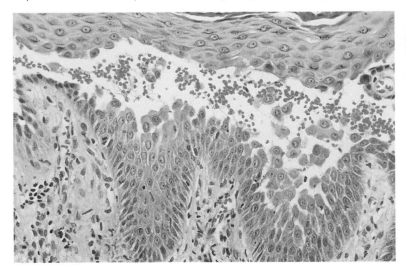

Fig. 15.13   Pemphigus vulgaris. The blister is intra-epidermal in location and is formed by loss of intercellular bridges between adjacent keratinocytes (acantholysis) seen best on the right of picture. A scattered chronic inflammatory cell infiltrate is present in the papillary dermis.

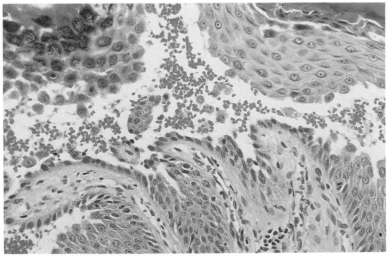

Fig. 15.14   Pemphigus vulgaris. Prominent dermal papillae project as villi into the blister cavity. They are covered largely by a single layer of basal cells: the 'tombstone' effect characteristic of suprabasal pemphigus.

Pemphigus Vegetans

This is a modified version of pemphigus vulgaris (Fig. 15.15) possibly related to an increased immunological resistance to the disease. The initial stages of the disease are similar to those of pemphigus vulgaris, in that flaccid weeping blisters dominate but subsequently the lesions heal by producing hypertrophic, warty and vegetative masses (Fig. 15.16) particularly in the flexural areas such as the axillae, groin and perineum. The mucous membrane lesions behave in the same way as pemphigus vulgaris.

Pemphigus Foliaceus

Although most cases are idiopathic, this is the variety of pemphigus which has been most frequently associated with penicillamine therapy (Figs. 15.17 and 15.18). It has also been described with rifampicin, captopril and phenylbutazone. Oral lesions are unusual and the antibodies attack cells higher in the epidermis so the condition is more superficial and less severe than pemphigus vulgaris. It may be difficult to identify blisters but instead shallow erosions, scaling and superficial crusting predominate (Fig. 15.19). The distribution of the eruption closely simulates that to be found in seborrhoeic dermatitis and may well be confused with this condition. Thus it is seen in the scalp, the face, the upper chest and back. The whole body surface may, however, eventually be involved. Itching is present in this condition and may well be severe and associated with burning. The Nikolsky sign is a helpful physical finding. The diagnosis is established by skin biopsy (Fig. 15.20) and immunofluorescence.

Pemphigus Erythematosus (Senear-Usher Syndrome)

This condition is similar to pemphigus foliaceus but more localized. The eruption on the face is reminiscent in distribution to lupus erythematosus. The immunofluorescent changes include both those to be found in pemphigus and those found in lupus erythematosus and the antinuclear factor is often positive. There is superficial blistering and crusting of the skin. The 'seborrhoeic' sites are predominantly affected (Fig. 15.21).

Management of Pemphigus

Pemphigus of whatever type is a serious disease, but pemphigus vulgaris is of particular importance. Very high doses of glucocorticosteroids are usually required to gain control of the blistering process in pemphigus vulgaris and 120mg of prednisolone daily would seem to be a minimum starting dose. Other immunosuppressants such as azathioprine, methotrexate and cyclophosphamide are worth incorporating into the treatment, but their action is delayed and they play little part in the acute management. Gold is also useful for the maintenance therapy of pemphigus vulgaris and for the control of the other types. Severe pemphigus must be managed in hospital. Skilled nursing care with attention to oral toilet, wet dressings to the skin, ripple beds and constant turning of the patient to prevent bed sores are essential. A constant watch must be kept for infection of the skin and elsewhere and for the side-effects of systemic steroids. The systemic steroids are reduced once the blistering process has ceased.

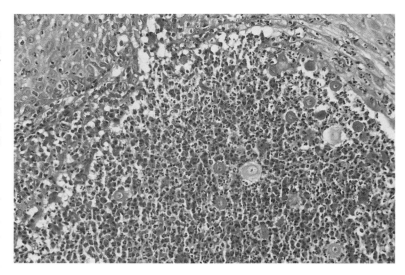

Fig. 15.15 Pemphigus vegetans. Although similar to pemphigus vulgaris in that suprabasal acantholysis is present, this is often masked, as here, by intra-epidermal abscess formation with conspicuous eosinophilia.

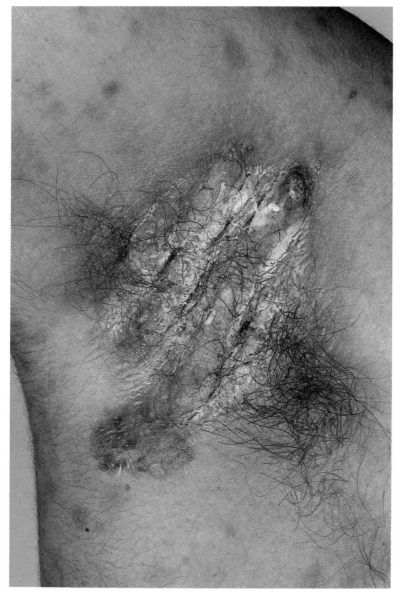

Fig. 15.16 Pemphigus vegetans. There is increased immunological resistance to the disease and the blisters heal with hypertrophic, warty and vegetative masses, especially in the flexures. By courtesy of Dr. R.H. Marten, King's College Hospital.

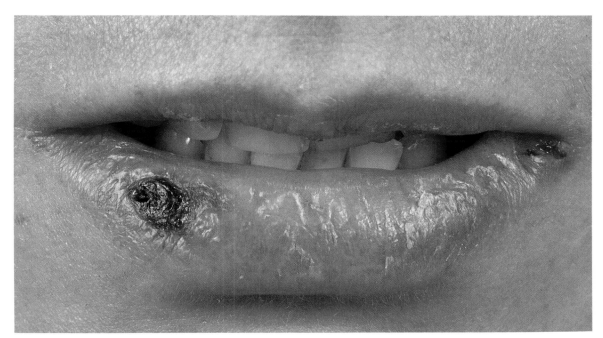

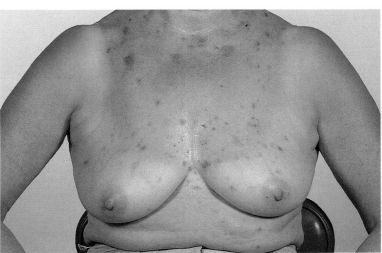

Fig. 15.18 Penicillamine-induced pemphigus. Shallow erosions and crusting occur over the trunk. Similarly this lady was receiving penicillamine for arthritis. By courtesy of Dr. R.H. Marten, King's College Hospital.

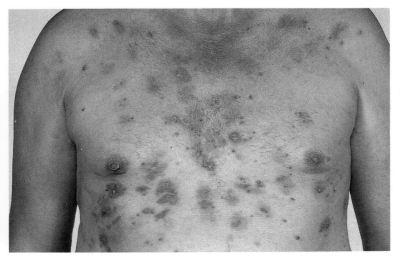

Fig. 15.19 Pemphigus foliaceus. It may be impossible to identify blisters but superficial crusting predominates. The chest is commonly involved. Biopsy for histology and immunofluorescence is necessary for diagnosis.

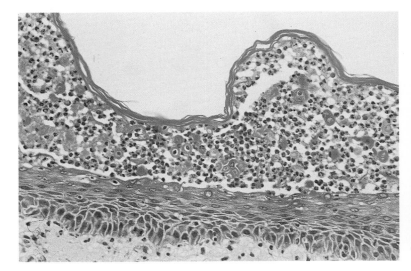

Fig. 15.20 Pemphigus foliaceus. The blister is situated immediately below the stratum corneum. In addition to neutrophils and scattered eosinophils, it contains numerous acantholytic keratinocytes.

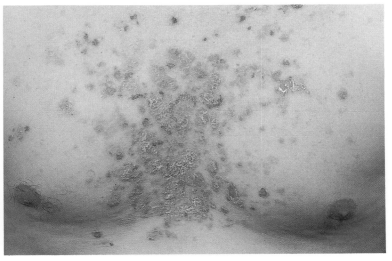

Fig. 15.21 Pemphigus erythematosus (Senear-Usher syndrome). Superficial blistering, erosions and crusting occur as in pemphigus foliaceus, to which it is identical clinically although more localized. However, immunofluorescent changes of both pemphigus and lupus erythematosus occur. The antinuclear factor is positive.

15.7

BULLOUS PEMPHIGOID

This is a disorder largely of the elderly. It is much more common than pemphigus, such that the average general practitioner should see several patients with this disease during a clinical career. There is no racial predisposition and the condition is not as serious as pemphigus. It presents as extremely itchy, tense blisters (Fig. 15.22), often on an erythematous base (Fig. 15.23), occurring on the limbs and particularly the inner aspects of the arms and thighs, but also on the trunk. The eruption is symmetrical (Fig. 15.24) and the blisters are tiny at first (Fig. 15.25), but rapidly achieve considerable size. They are tense and full of clear fluid, in complete contrast to the flaccid bullae of pemphigus. The blisters become haemorrhagic after a few days and break down, resulting in erosions (Fig. 15.26) which may become secondarily infected. The skin heals without scarring. Occasionally there is a prodromal itchy erythema with

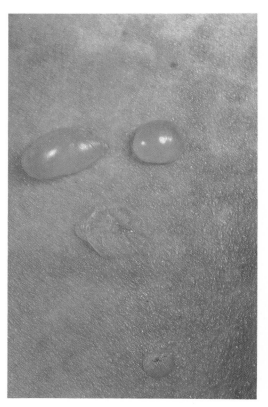

Fig. 15.22   Bullous pemphigoid. Large tense blisters are characteristic, in contrast to the flaccid blisters of pemphigus.

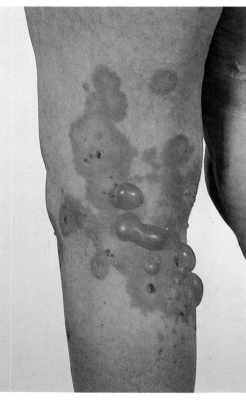

Fig. 15.23   Bullous pemphigoid. The tense blisters may be surrounded by erythema.

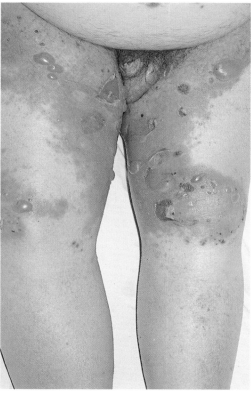

Fig. 15.24   Bullous pemphigoid. The eruption is symmetrical. The blisters take several days to burst, leaving eroded areas. By courtesy of St. Mary's Hospital.

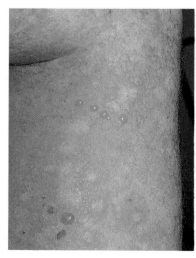
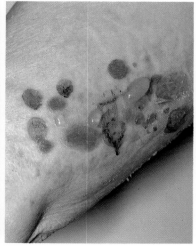

Fig. 15.25   Bullous pemphigoid. The blisters are initially tiny (left) but become larger and haemorrhagic after a few days (right).

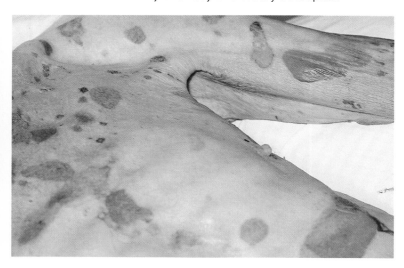

Fig. 15.26   Bullous pemphigoid. The blisters break and leave large areas of eroded skin.

features of urticaria, often of a figurate nature (Fig. 15.27), for several weeks before the blistering process commences.

Oral lesions (Fig. 15.28) do occur, but only in a minority of patients (unlike pemphigus) and other mucous membranes are not affected.

There is an uncommon variant of the disease whereby blisters recur in a localized area on the lower leg (Fig. 15.29). They are of an intermittent nature. Occasionally this type of pemphigoid does develop into generalized bullous pemphigoid.

Young patients are not infrequently referred to skin departments with the diagnosis of pemphigoid because they have a blistering eruption, but they turn out to have either insect bites or impetigo (formerly known as pemphigus neonatorum).

The blister of bullous pemphigoid is tense and remains intact for several days because the roof of the blister consists of the entire epidermis (Figs. 15.30–15.32).

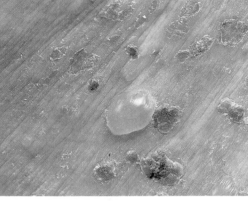

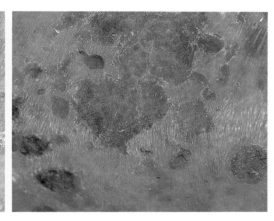

Fig. 15.27 Bullous pemphigoid. Occasionally an itchy figurate erythema or urticarial eruption (left) occurs for a few weeks before the blisters appear (middle). The blisters were secondarily infected in this man (right). By courtesy of St. John's Hospital for Diseases of the Skin.

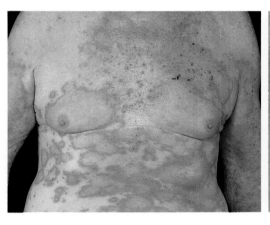

Fig. 15.28 Oral bullous pemphigoid. Blisters in the mouth are uncommon in bullous pemphigoid. They are probably more commonly associated with internal malignant disease.

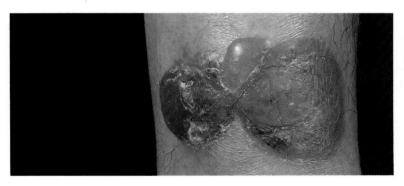

Fig. 15.29 Localized bullous pemphigoid. Intermittent bullous eruptions may occur in a localized manner, often limited to the lower leg and associated with positive immunofluorescence. Occasionally the disorder develops into generalized bullous pemphigoid.

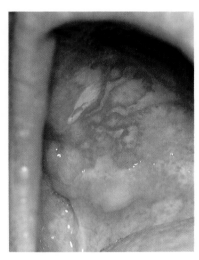

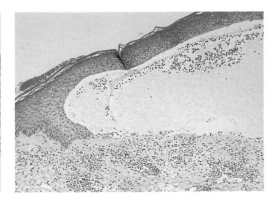

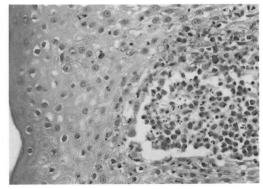

Fig. 15.30 Bullous pemphigoid. This low power view shows a typical intact blister. Note that the lesion is subepidermal in location and that the cavity is unilocular.

Fig. 15.31 Bullous pemphigoid (medium power view). The full-thickness of the epidermis forms the blister roof. Note the conspicuous eosinophils within the superficial aspect of the blister and also surrounding the dermal blood vessels. The connective tissue of the papillary dermis appears normal.

Fig. 15.32 Bullous pemphigoid. Eosinophil-rich dermal papillary micro-abscesses are characteristic of bullous pemphigoid.

Direct immunofluorescence usually demonstrates the presence of complement and IgG within the basement membrane region (Fig. 15.33). In bullous pemphigoid a split develops within the lamina lucida, thus producing a blister. Anti-basement membrane antibody is demonstrable in the serum by the use of indirect immunofluorescence, but unlike pemphigus the titre of the antibody does not relate to the activity of the disease.

The condition responds to systemic glucocorticosteroids and other immunosuppressant agents and much less heavy doses are required, for example 40mg of prednisolone may well be a reasonable starting dose. The condition quite frequently goes into spontaneous remission after either a number of months of treatment or couple of years. It is not as serious as pemphigus, but all the same there is appreciable mortality associated with it largely because the patients are elderly and the condition is debilitating. There is danger of fluid loss, secondary sepsis and septicaemia and of those complications arising from prolonged bed rest. The treatment with systemic steroids and other immunosuppressants is also hazardous; the patients frequently have other general medical illnesses which are further compromised by the treatment and occasionally malignant disease is associated with the condition. The latter is probably fortuitous, since bullous pemphigoid usually occurs towards the later stages of life when neoplasia is relatively common.

HERPES GESTATIONIS

This very rare, extremely pruritic disorder of pregnancy or occasionally the puerperium, has no relationship with herpes viruses. It usually begins in the second or third trimester and is identical both clinically and histologically to bullous pemphigoid (Figs. 15.34 and 15.35). Immunofluorescence shows deposition of C3 and sometimes IgG at the basement membrane zone and indirect immunofluorescence demonstrates a circulating factor which fixes C3 at the basement membrane. This factor can cross the placenta and temporarily affect the woman's offspring. The condition resolves after delivery but may recur with each subsequent pregnancy, often at earlier stages. Recurrences have also been reported with the oral contraceptive pill and during menstruation. The condition responds well to fairly small doses of systemic glucocorticosteroids.

BULLOUS PEMPHIGOID OF CHILDHOOD

This is a rare condition. The clinical picture of tense blisters resembles that of bullous pemphigoid and some of the immunofluorescent findings are identical. The blisters, however, have a different distribution (Fig. 15.36). They occur in the mouth, on the face, the lower abdomen, buttocks and genitalia. There appear to be two forms of the disease. In the first, IgG is found at the basement membrane and this condition is known as juvenile bullous pemphigoid. However, an identical clinical picture is associated with depositions of IgA at the basement membrane and this condition is known at present as *chronic bullous dermatosis of childhood*. Both diseases usually present in the pre-school age and remit spontaneously either after a few weeks or years and the condition is not serious but is steroid responsive.

CICATRICIAL PEMPHIGOID
(Benign Mucous Membrane Pemphigoid, Ocular Pemphigus)

This is a rare disease and the nomenclature is undoubtedly confusing. The condition is neither benign nor is it allied to pemphigus. However, it does appear to be related to bullous pemphigoid, but scarring (hence cicatricial) is a regular feature and the eyes and mucous membranes are usually involved, in contrast to bullous pemphigoid. The confusion in terminology has arisen because only a clinical description was possible initially. The advent of immunofluorescence has greatly clarified the situation.

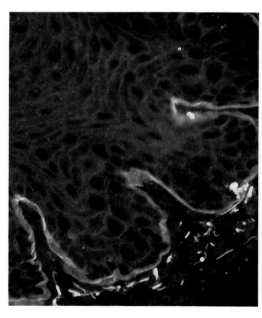

Fig. 15.33 Bullous pemphigoid: direct immunofluorescence. Fluorescein-labelled antibodies are deposited in the basement membrane separating the epidermis from the dermis.

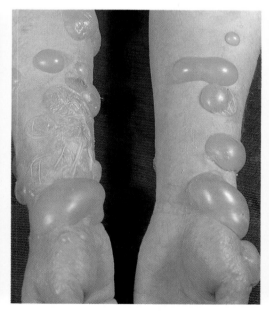

Fig. 15.34 Herpes gestationis. Blisters clinically identical to those of bullous pemphigoid may occur very rarely in pregnancy. Immunofluorescent changes are similar.

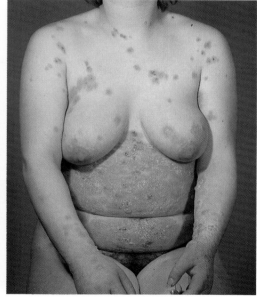

Fig. 15.35 Herpes gestationis. The condition recurs with each subsequent pregnancy and may be exacerbated by oral contraceptives.

Cicatricial pemphigoid is a chronic blistering disorder of middle years. It involves primarily the mucous membranes of the oral cavity (Fig. 15.37), nose, larynx, pharynx, oesophagus, ano-genital area and, of great importance, the eyes. The skin may or may not be involved and if it is, not to any great extent. The lesions are, however, identical to those of bullous pemphigoid in that they are tense blisters which are scattered, appearing either on a normal or erythematous surround. They may heal with scarring in contrast to bullous pemphigoid. They occasionally erupt briefly in a generalized manner similar to bullous pemphigoid, or recur in the same sites, usually the face and scalp (where a scarring alopecia may occur), (Fig. 15.38), neck, flexures and extremities. Periorificial skin involvement is a feature.

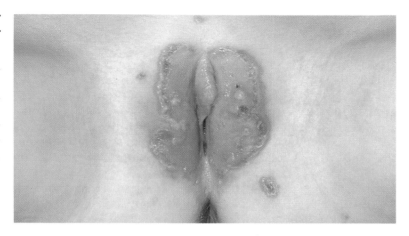

Fig. 15.36 Chronic bullous dermatosis of childhood. Tense blisters occur as in bullous pemphigoid, but the distribution is different. There are various forms and immunofluorescence is necessary to distinguish between them. By courtesy of Dr. A. Marsden.

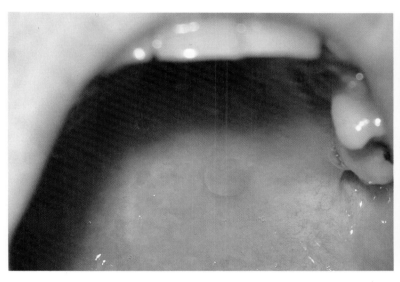
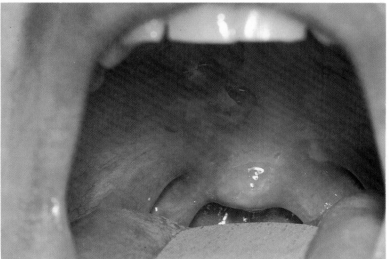

Fig. 15.37 Benign mucous membrane pemphigoid. Tense blisters in the mouth are common (left). The blisters break and result in erosion (right). By courtesy of Dr. R.H. Marten, King's College Hospital.

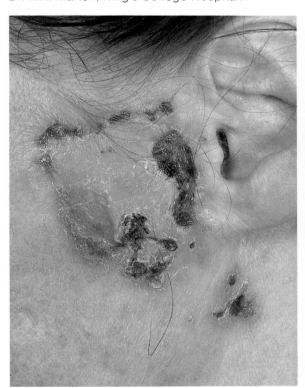
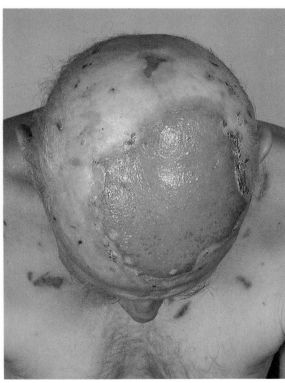

Fig. 15.38 Benign mucous membrane pemphigoid. Erosions secondary to blisters occur which heal with scarring. The face and scalp are common sites.

The scarring that may result, particularly around the mucous membranes, is often destructive, leading to strictures and, in the case of the eyes, to adhesions between the bulbar and palpebral surfaces – symblephara (Fig. 15.39). Blindness may occur, and therefore skilled ophthalmological supervision is required.

Although it is apparent that this condition differs clinically from bullous pemphigoid, the direct immunofluorescent findings in the skin and mucous membrane lesions are identical to those of bullous pemphigoid. However, circulating antibodies are found only occasionally. The relationships between the two conditions are thus inadequately understood at the present time. Treatment of this condition is far less satisfactory than for bullous pemphigoid. Systemic steroids are used in quite high doses, but the benefit varies and complications from long-term steroid therapy are frequent. Other immunosuppressives and dapsone may be tried.

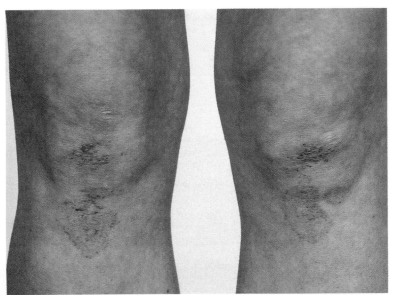

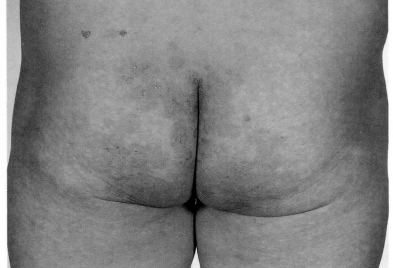

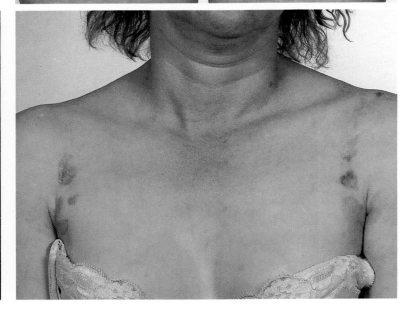

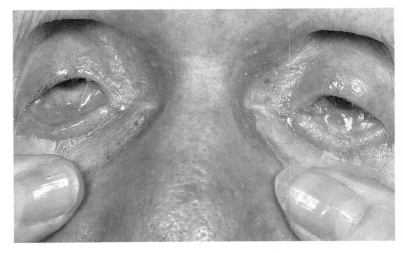

Fig. 15.39 Benign mucous membrane pemphigoid (ocular pemphigus). Adhesions result from the blistering process between the bulbar and palpebral surfaces. They are known as symblephara. The condition may lead to blindness. By courtesy of Dr. R.H. Marten, King's College Hospital.

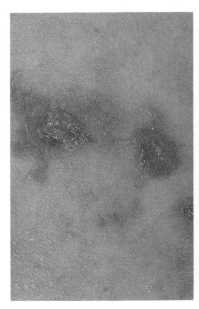

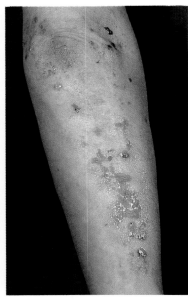

Fig. 15.40 Dermatitis herpetiformis. Grouped polymorphic lesions which include vesicles occur. They are intensely itchy.

Fig. 15.41 Dermatitis herpetiformis. The condition is intensely itchy. Vesicles may be difficult to discern, either because of the application of calamine or because of scratching. Excoriated urticarial papules are present.

Fig. 15.42 Dermatitis herpetiformis. The distribution is characteristic. The eruption is symmetrical. The fronts of the knees (upper), the buttocks (middle) and fronts of the shoulders (lower), are usually involved, as in this patient.

DERMATITIS HERPETIFORMIS

This is a rare chronic disorder of the skin which is associated with a gluten-sensitive enteropathy. It is characterized by the presence of intensely itchy, grouped (hence herpetiform), polymorphic lesions on the skin. These are characteristically in the form of vesicles (Fig. 15.40) rather than frank bullae. However, since the eruption is so intensely itchy the surface of the vesicles is frequently excoriated (Fig. 15.41). Urticarial lesions are common. Healing is often associated with post-inflammatory hyperpigmentation. The eruption is symmetrical (Fig. 15.42) and affects the scalp, scapulae, buttocks and the areas of skin just below the knees (Fig. 15.43) and elbows. Occasionally the mucous membranes are involved. The symmetry (Fig. 15.44) and distribution of the eruption coupled with intense pruritus usually suggests the diagnosis.

Although there is a characteristic histology in this disease of polymorphonuclear leucocyte infiltration of the dermal papillae causing a subepidermal blister (Figs. 15.45 and 15.46), immuno-fluorescence has superseded the importance of ordinary light microscopy. Deposits of IgA are found in the dermal papillae, either as granular deposits or in a linear manner (Fig. 15.47). These deposits should be looked for in skin which appears clinically normal. Remarkably, no circulating IgA antibodies have yet been demonstrated.

This is a disorder of younger age groups, often starting in the third or fourth decade and occasionally in childhood. It occasionally remits spontaneously but usually is a life-long predisposition. It appears to be genetic in origin in that certain HLA groupings are more commonly affected. Intense interest in this disorder has been generated by the finding of a gluten-sensitive enteropathy in association with the skin eruption. Overt malabsorption or indeed any symptom referable to the gastrointestinal tract is extremely rare, but jejunal biopsy in the vast majority of patients, and perhaps in all, shows changes similar to those described in coeliac disease. Indeed, some patients, who have had coeliac disease subsequently develop dermatitis herpetiformis and very rarely vice-versa.

The disorder responds rapidly to dapsone orally. A strict gluten-free diet will also induce remission of the disease after a number of months or occasionally years. However, relapse occurs on reintroduction of gluten. This finding of a relationship between diet, the gastointestinal tract and the skin has been of fundamental importance.

As a treatment, a gluten-free diet is unpleasant and many patients prefer to take dapsone. However, this drug is not without its hazards and haemolytic anaemia and methaemo-globinanaemia are common. An alternative drug is sulpha-pyridine but this also has side-effects. Lymphoma of the small bowel has occasionally been reported in association with dermatitis herpetiformis just as with coeliac disease.

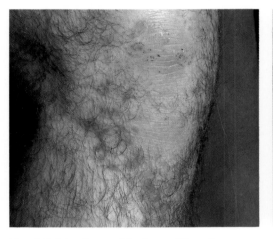

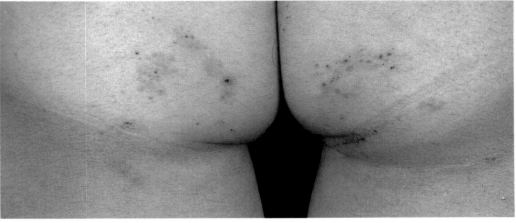

Fig. 15.43 Dermatitis herpetiformis. Excoriated vesicles occur over the fronts of the knees and lower legs. By courtesy of St. Mary's Hospital.

Fig. 15.44 Dermatitis herpetiformis. The lesions are grouped and symmetrical.

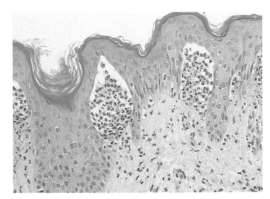

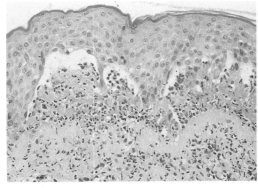

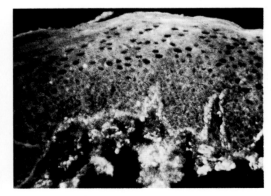

Fig. 15.45 Dermatitis herpetiformis. Neutrophilic dermal papillary microabscesses are typical of dermatitis herpetiformis.

Fig. 15.46 Dermatitis herpetiformis. The blister is multilocular and subepidermal in location. In addition to neutrophil polymorphs and eosinophils, abundant fibrinous material is present along the floor of the lesion. A mixed acute inflammatory cell infiltrate surrounds the superficial vascular plexus and leucocytoclasis is conspicuous.

Fig. 15.47 Dermatitis herpetiformis. Deposits of IgA in the dermal papillae and along the basement membrane are pathognomonic of this disease.

SUBCORNEAL PUSTULAR DERMATOSIS
(Sneddon-Wilkinson Disease)

This is a rare disorder occurring mostly in middle-aged women, which is characterized by a chronic relapsing benign eruption of flaccid pustules (Fig. 15.48) with a turbid nature. They may have a transient red erythematous margin. The pustules dry up after a few days and are followed by a superficial scale. The lesions tend to be grouped in an annular or serpiginous manner and post-inflammatory hyperpigmentation results (Fig. 15.49). The pustules appear to come in waves in the same places and particularly affect the flexures such as the axillae, under the breasts, groins and the flexor surfaces of the limbs. The mucous membranes are not affected and irritation is usually absent. The histology is quite distinctive, showing a collection of poly-morphonuclear leucocytes immediately below the stratum corneum. The eruption is symmetrical and tends to recur, although eventually it remits spontaneously. The immuno-fluorescence findings are not definitively defined. The disorder responds to dapsone.

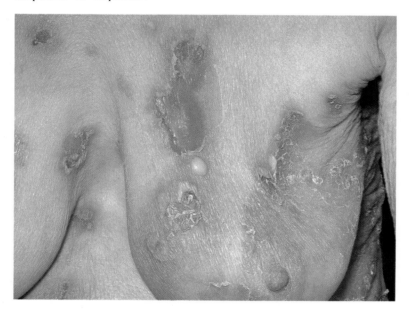

Fig. 15.48   Subcorneal pustular dermatosis. Pustules occur, followed by superficial scaling in an annular configuration.

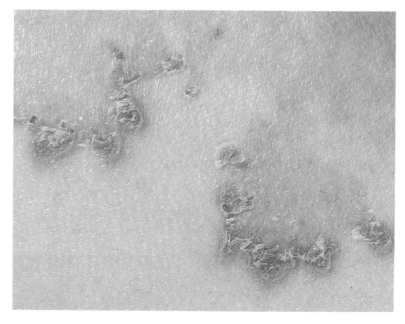

Fig. 15.49   Subcorneal pustular dermatosis. The lesions are annular. Very superficial flaccid blisters are visible at the edge, then scaling and crusting and post-inflammatory pigmentation.

16 Developmental Disorders of the Skin

ICHTHYOSIS

The term ichthyosis is derived from the Greek word for fish and refers to the scaly appearance of the skin. It covers a number of inherited disorders of keratinization which result in dryness and scaliness of the skin (Fig. 16.1).

Ichthyosis Vulgaris

This dominantly inherited condition is the most common variety of ichthyosis, occuring in about one in 250 individuals. It is often present at birth, but otherwise commences within the first few years of life. The skin is dry, rough and small fine white scales are found on examination (Fig. 16.2). Most areas of the body are affected, particularly the extensor surfaces of the limbs. There is, however, characteristic sparing of the flexures, especially those of the elbows and knees. The palmar and plantar creases and markings are often exaggerated (Fig. 16.3). The degree to which individuals are affected varies considerably. Milder cases are known as xeroderma, where there is a dryness but only slight scaling of the skin. The condition is frequently associated with atopic eczema and keratosis pilaris. It tends to be worse in winter than in summer and usually improves with age, although relapse is quite common in the elderly.

Histologically the epidermis is thin and can be distinguished from the other forms of ichthyosis because the granular cell layer is usually absent (Fig. 16.4). There is no specific treatment, but regular use of emollients including those containing urea is helpful.

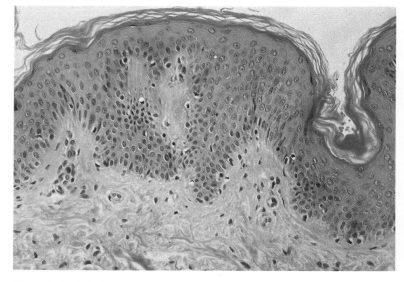

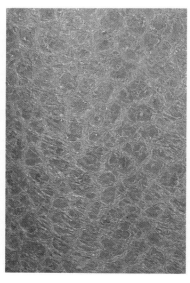

Fig. 16.1 Ichthyosis. The skin is fissured and individual white scales are seen. The scales resemble those of a fish. By courtesy of St. Mary's Hospital.

Fig. 16.2 Ichthyosis vulgaris. The skin is dry and rough. Small fine scales are present. By courtesy of St. John's Hospital for Diseases of the Skin.

Fig. 16.3 Ichthyosis vulgaris. The palmar creases are exaggerated. By courtesy of St. John's Hospital for Diseases of the Skin.

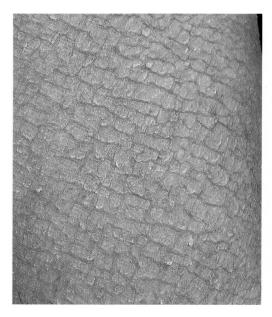

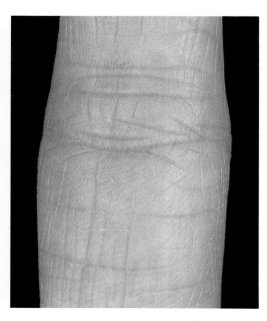

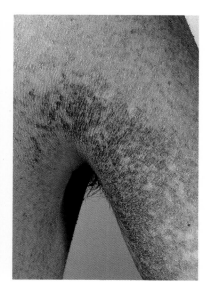

Fig. 16.4 Ichthyosis vulgaris. The changes of hyperkeratosis associated with an absent granular cell layer are subtle and easily overlooked.

Fig. 16.5 X-linked ichthyosis. The individual scales are brown.

Fig. 16.6 X-linked ichthyosis. The scales are coarser, larger and darker than those of ichthyosis vulgaris.

Sex-linked Recessive Ichthyosis

This is a rare condition which occurs in approximately one in 6000 male births. It is present at birth. The whole skin is involved and the hair may be coarse and dry. Sometimes the child is born encased in a collodion-like membrane. The scales are larger and darker than in ichthyosis vulgaris (Figs. 16.5 and 16.6), giving an appearance of dirtiness (Fig. 16.7), and the child is often falsely accused of not washing properly. It does not improve with age and there is no association with atopy.

The cause of sex-linked recessive ichthyosis is unknown. Histologically there is an increase in the horny and granular cell layers (Fig. 16.8). In some patients there appears to be a deficiency of steroid sulphatase. Because of a maternal failure to produce oestriol the cervix fails to ripen properly and labour is therefore delayed and prolonged, frequently necessitating caesarean section. Male infants are born post-mature.

The management of the disorder remains centred around the regular use of emollients. Topical cholesterol has been reported as being helpful. Oral retinoids such as Etretinate undoubtedly markedly improve the condition but their use may not be warranted in view of their potential side-effects on bone, liver and lipid metabolism.

Ichthyosiform Erythrodermas

These conditions are rare, severe and sometimes lethal. In addition to the scaling there is generalized erythema (erythroderma). The infant is frequently born encased in an armour of scales which may be so severe that it is incompatible with normal life (so-called ichthyosis fetalis or 'harlequin fetus'). In others (Fig. 16.9), the collodion membrane desquamates within a fortnight, leaving large scales with a background erythema

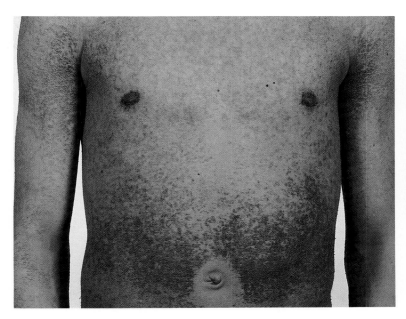

Fig. 16.7   X-linked ichthyosis. The dark scales give a false impression of dirt. The condition is confined to males and does not improve with advancing years.

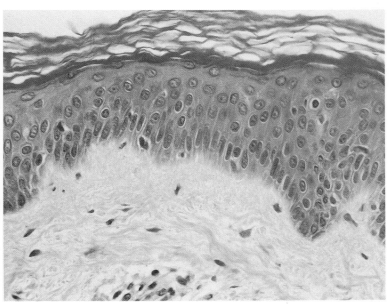

Fig. 16.8   X-linked ichthyosis. The lesion is characterized by hyperkeratosis associated with a normal granular cell layer. The epithelium is sometimes acanthotic.

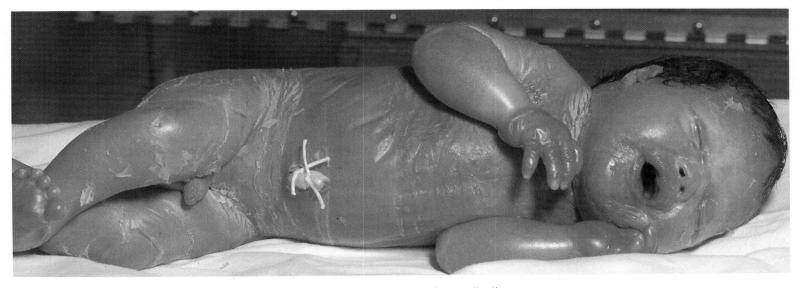

Fig. 16.9   Ichthyosiform erythroderma. The infant may be born encased in a collodion-like membrane which is shed after two or three weeks.

which continues throughout life (Fig. 16.10). Severe fissuring of the hands and feet occurs and the scales tend to be almost verrucous particularly around joints (Figs. 16.11 and 16.12).

The accumulation of scale occurs around hairs and may be accompanied by secondary sepsis which sometimes results in a scarring alopecia. The patients have abnormal nails, do not sweat effectively and therefore have difficulty with temperature regulation. Their nutritional requirements are important because of the loss of protein in the scale.

These conditions comprise a heterogenous group, probably inherited as autosomal recessives. Some can be divided into a non-bullous variant (lamellar ichthyosis), while others have a bullous (epidermolytic hyperkeratosis) form. The clinical features of ichthyosiform erythroderma vary. The skin is generally red all over, but particularly so in the flexures. The face and scalp are scaly and ectropion is usually prominent (Fig. 16.13). If the child survives, the erythroderma may fade in some cases, leaving prominent hyperkeratosis around the neck and limb flexures. The palms and soles may be markedly thickened.

In bullous ichthyosiform erythroderma the condition may be indistinguishable from the lamellar form at birth. Subsequently, however, blisters develop in addition to the erythroderma (Fig. 16.14). The latter may eventually subside, but the blisters frequently persist throughout life. Hyperkeratosis becomes prominent with time, especially around the flexures and on the hands and feet.

These diseases are extraordinarily rare and their management is complex. Undoubtedly the oral retinoids represent a major advance in therapy and can result in dramatic improvements in the conditions.

KERATOSIS PILARIS

This is an extremely common disorder and indeed many adolescents may have it temporarily, so that in these cases it is almost certainly physiological in nature. It is a disorder of follicular keratinization resulting in the formation of discrete horny papules around the exit of the hair follicles (Fig. 16.15). It particularly affects the extensor surfaces of the upper arms (Fig. 16.16), thighs and buttocks, but may be more widespread. The lesions are in many cases surrounded by erythema. The condition is often inherited in association with ichthyosis vulgaris; in these patients it is permanent, but gives rise to no significant symptoms other than its appearance. There is no specific treatment. A similar condition known as phrynoderma is seen in those who have gross nutritional disturbances. The lesions feel rough, like a nutmeg grater.

OTHER FORMS OF ICHTHYOSIS

Occasionally Hodgkin's disease and malabsorption disorders may present as an acquired ichthyosis. Another rare disorder which is interesting from an aetiological point of view is *Refsum's disease*. This is an autosomal recessive disease caused by an abnormality of phytanic acid alpha-hydroxylase metabolism, which allows the accumulation of dietary phytanic acid in tissues. It manifests as a syndrome consisting of retinitis pigmentosa, mental deficiency, peripheral neuropathy, hypogonadism and ichthyosis.

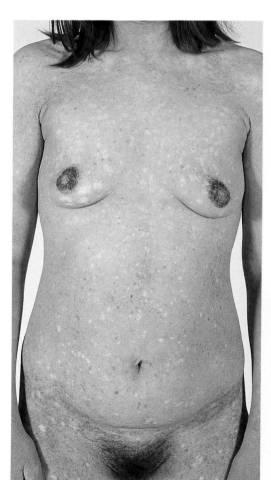

Fig. 16.10 Ichthyosiform erythroderma. There is background erythema with verrucous scaling which persists throughout life. By courtesy of St. Mary's Hospital.

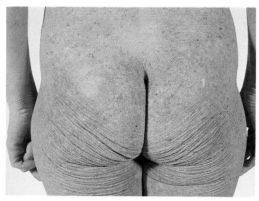

Fig. 16.11 Ichthyosiform erythroderma. The scaling is thick, almost verrucous and is most prominent around the flexures. By courtesy of St. Mary's Hospital.

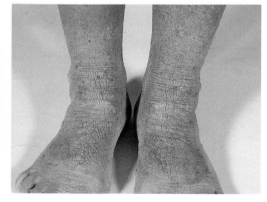

Fig. 16.12 Ichthyosiform erythroderma. The warty scaling and fissuring is particularly marked around the flexures. By courtesy of St. Mary's Hospital.

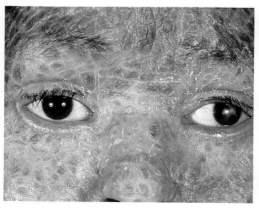

Fig. 16.13 Ichthyosiform erythroderma. Ectropion is usually prominent. By courtesy of St. Mary's Hospital.

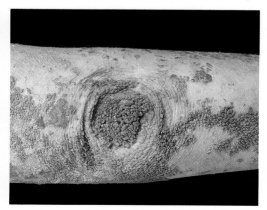

Fig. 16.14 Bullous ichthyosiform erythroderma. Erosions and hyperkeratosis are present. The erythroderma has disappeared. By courtesy of St. John's Hospital for Diseases of the Skin.

PALMAR PLANTAR KERATODERMA

This includes a number of conditions of the palms and soles, some of which may be associated with systemic manifestations. The most common form is inherited as an autosomal dominant characterized by a diffuse hyperkeratosis of the palmar and plantar skin, which ends abruptly at the sides of the hands and feet. It is symmetrical and the skin is very thick, often of a somewhat yellow colour (Fig. 16.17). It tends to crack (Fig. 16.18), particularly in the winter months, and the resulting fissures are painful and occasionally become infected. In addition to the diffuse varieties there are punctate and linear conditions seen particularly in negroes. These conditions are all persistent. A very rare acquired variety of diffuse keratoderma develops in familial association with carcinoma of the oesophagus (tylosis).

KNUCKLE PADS

These are seen more commonly in negroes and are often dominantly inherited. They consist of thickened skin overlying the dorsa of the interphalangeal joints and knuckles (Fig. 16.19). The pads appear during adolescence and are permanent. There is no treatment.

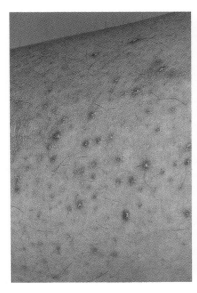
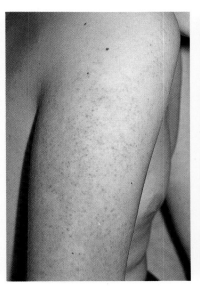
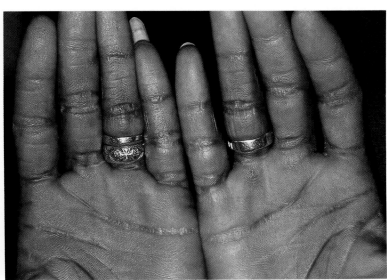

Fig. 16.15 Keratosis pilaris. Discrete follicular papules are present. The inherited varieties usually persist. By courtesy of Dr A.C. Pembroke.

Fig. 16.16 Keratosis pilaris. Discrete, rough, horny papules with erythema surround the hair follicles on the extensor surfaces of the limbs. This is common in adolescence and frequently disappears.

Fig. 16.17 Palmar keratoderma. Diffuse thickening of the palms and soles occurs.

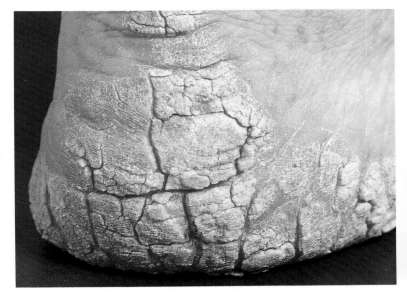
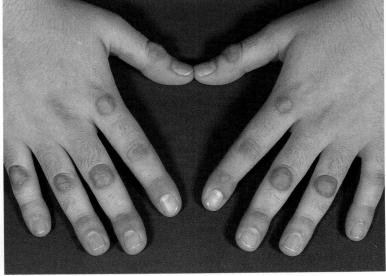

Fig. 16.18 Plantar keratoderma. The hyperkeratosis tends to fissure in dry, cold weather. There is an abrupt end to the eruption at the side of the foot.

Fig. 16.19 Knuckle pads. There is thickening of the skin overlying the interphalangeal joints. The condition is usually inherited. The cause is unknown. By courtesy of Dr R.H. Marten.

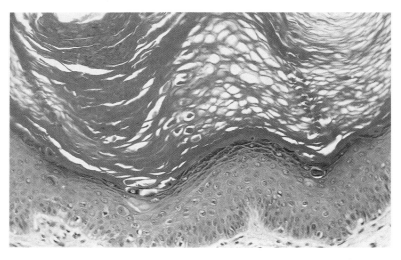

Fig. 16.20 Darier's disease. Darier's disease is characterized by an admixture of abnormal keratinization (dyskeratosis) and acantholysis. In this example of a very early lesion there is marked hyperkeratosis with a prominent parakeratotic tier (upper left quadrant). In the upper prickle cell and granular cell layers are several distinct abnormal keratinocytes showing marked cytoplasmic vacuolation and abnormal nuclei (corps ronds). Degenerate forms of the latter are also evident within the stratum corneum to the left and right of centre.

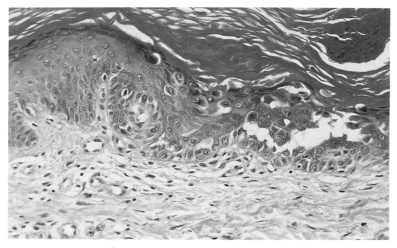

Fig. 16.21 Darier's disease. Supra-basal acantholysis has resulted in a cleft-like vesicle. Note the conspicuous parakeratotic tier on the far right.

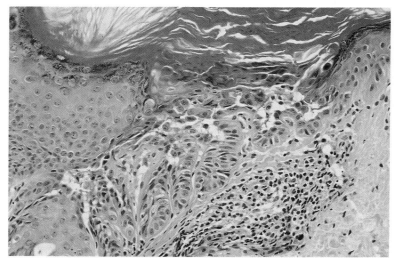

Fig. 16.22 Darier's disease. Dermal papillae project into the vesicle cavity. In addition to corps ronds, densely staining nuclear remnants (grains) can be seen in the keratin overlying the lesion. A chronic inflammatory cell infiltrate is present in the superficial dermis.

DARIER'S DISEASE

This rare, dominantly inherited disorder of keratinization begins in early youth and is caused by imperfect development of the tonofilament-desmosome complex. These inter- and intracellular structures are responsible for the attachment of one epidermal cell to another and to the basement membrane. Histologically, a split occurs above the basal layer and in the Malpighian layer (Figs. 16.20–16.22). Cells become separated from one another (acantholysis) and show signs of premature keratinization (dyskeratosis). Some are quite large with darkly-staining nuclei and a clear cytoplasm, and are known as 'corps ronds'. Later the cytoplasm shrinks and the cells become smaller, known as 'grains'. The surrounding epidermis is acanthotic, parakeratotic and hyperkeratotic.

The disease is characterized by a symmetrical and profuse eruption of small, firm and red-brown papules. They have a rather greasy, crusted and warty surface (Fig. 16.23). They are found on the face (particularly the forehead and ears), scalp, back, chest (Fig. 16.24) and in the body flexures, in a distribution rather similar to seborrhoeic dermatitis. In the flexures, the papules often coalesce into plaques which tend to vegetate and become secondarily infected and malodorous. The nails may be affected, developing longitudinal ridges which tend to break at their distal margin, producing a V-shaped notch (Fig. 16.25). Thickening occurs underneath the nails. Pits on the palms are a characteristic feature.

Secondary bacterial infection is common. Occasionally herpes simplex may become superimposed, resulting in Kaposi's varicelliform eruption. Vaccinia may produce a similar effect. The clinical features appear to be aggravated by exposure to ultra-violet light. Oral retinoids are helpful therapeutically.

HAILEY-HAILEY DISEASE (Familial Benign Pemphigus)

This is a relatively uncommon condition which is inherited as an autosomal dominant and commences in adolescence. It is similar to Darier's disease in that there is a fault in epidermal cell cohesion, resulting from an abnormal tonofilament-desmosome complex. However, the two produce different clinical appearances.

Histologically (Fig. 16.26), the condition is characterized by widespread incomplete acantholysis reminiscent of pemphigus vulgaris, hence its name, but has no relationship with it and is typified by negative immunofluorescent studies.

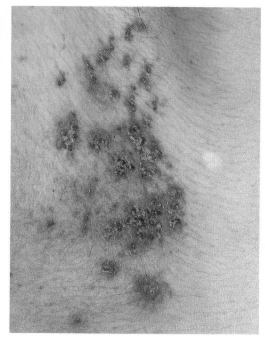

Fig. 16.23 Darier's disease. The lesions have a rather greasy and crusted surface.

Hailey-Hailey disease characteristically remits and relapses. The lesions consist of clear vesicles which tend to become turbid and then leave erosions and crusts. They tend to extend peripherally. Centrally the lesions may become macerated and rather typically fissured (Fig. 16.27). The flexural areas of the body are especially involved. Friction is an important precipitating factor and probably accounts for the involvement of the sides of the neck, axillae, groins and underside of the breasts.

However, any area subject to trauma, e.g. under a belt, may be affected. Ultra-violet light and infection are important exacerbating factors. The condition is likely to be pruritic.

There is no specific treatment for Hailey-Hailey disease. However, early treatment of infection, rest and weight reduction are of importance. Topical steroid-antibiotic preparations are useful. Occasionally excision and grafting of localized areas may be beneficial.

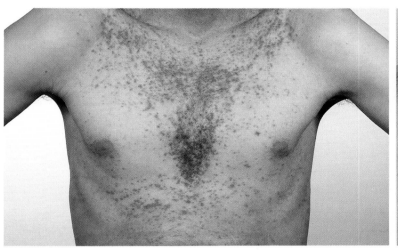

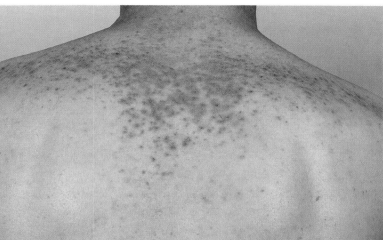

Fig. 16.24   Darier's disease. A symmetrical profuse eruption of small, firm, red-brown papules occurs on the chest and back. The distribution is similar to that of seborrhoeic dermatitis.

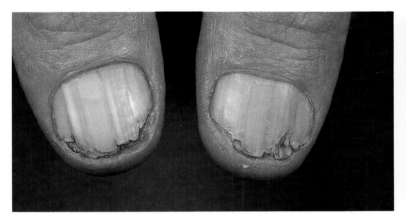

Fig. 16.25   Darier's disease of the nails. There are notches at the distal margins of the nails. This change is specific to this disorder.

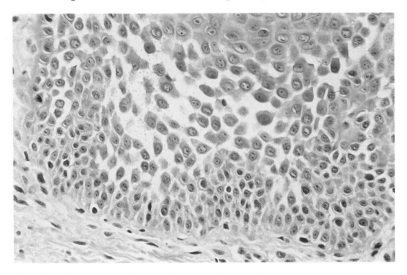

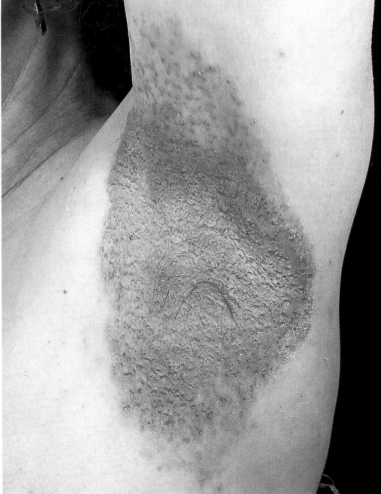

Fig. 16.26   Hailey-Hailey disease. The pathology has been likened to a 'dilapidated brick wall'. This degree of acantholysis with partial retention of cellular orientation is virtually pathognomonic of the disease.

Fig. 16.27   Hailey-Hailey disease. The skin is macerated and there is pronounced splitting or fissuring of the skin. The flexures are particularly affected, probably because of friction. By courtesy of St. John's Hospital for Diseases of the Skin.

EPIDERMOLYSIS BULLOSA

This general term is applied to a collection of inherited blistering disorders of the skin, characterized by increased skin fragility. Essentially there is a failure of proper cohesion between the epidermis and dermis (Figs. 16.28–16.30). Trauma, which may be relatively trivial, will induce separation of the two layers and thus cause the formation of blisters (Fig. 16.31). Electron microscopy of the skin has improved the classification of these disorders and is mandatory in the more serious varieties, for assessment of prognosis and facilitating genetic counselling. A clinical diagnosis may be made on the basis of whether the eruption is localized or generalized, heals with or without

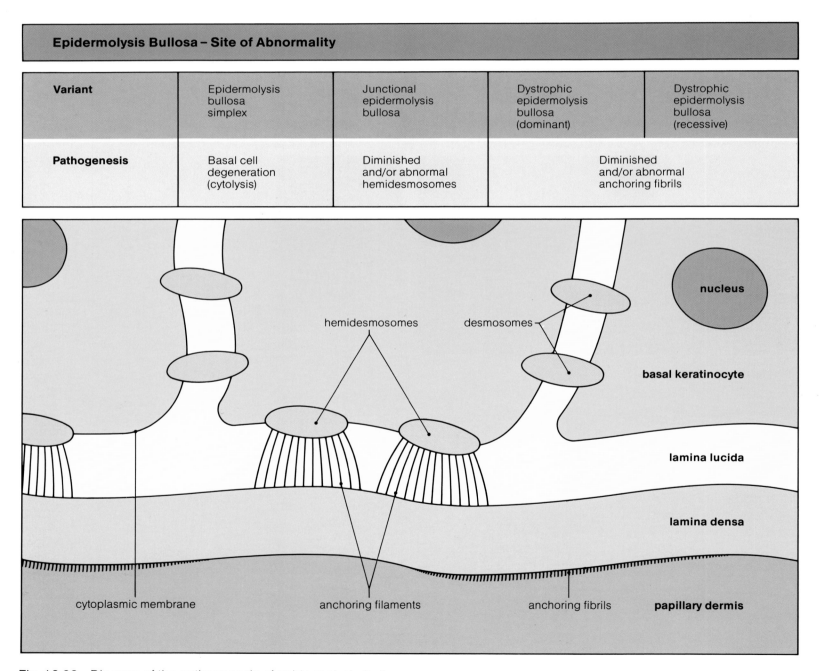

Epidermolysis Bullosa – Site of Abnormality

Variant	Epidermolysis bullosa simplex	Junctional epidermolysis bullosa	Dystrophic epidermolysis bullosa (dominant)	Dystrophic epidermolysis bullosa (recessive)
Pathogenesis	Basal cell degeneration (cytolysis)	Diminished and/or abnormal hemidesmosomes	Diminished and/or abnormal anchoring fibrils	

Fig. 16.28   Diagram of the pathogenesis of epidermolysis bullosa.

scarring, milia formation or hyperkeratosis and whether there is involvement of the mucous membranes, hair, teeth and nails.

Knowledge of the family history is helpful. The disorder is complex and patients with the generalized varieties should be referred to centres where electron microscopy is available. However, certain recognizable clinical pictures are as follows:

Epidermolysis Bullosa Simplex

This condition is inherited as an autosomal dominant and was described first by Weber and then by Cockayne.

It is localized to areas of trauma particularly the palms and soles. It occurs in childhood or later in life and is a result of excessive friction. Tense blisters (Fig. 16.32) occur on the palms

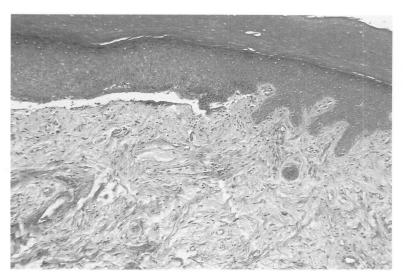

Fig. 16.29 Epidermolysis bullosa dystrophica. The lesions of epidermolysis bullosa (both congenital and acquired variants) are all characterized by blisters which appear at a light microscopic level to be situated subepidermally, usually containing only scattered red blood cells. At ultrastructural level, however, they can be seen to be located at various sites in relation to the basement membrane region, dependent upon their pathogenesis.

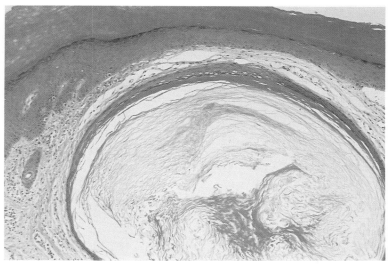

Fig. 16.30 Epidermolysis bullosa dystrophica – milia. The scarring forms of epidermlysis bullosa are characterized by the development of superficially located mini-epidermoid cysts (milia). Similar lesions are also a feature of bullous pemphigoid and porphyria cutanea tarda.

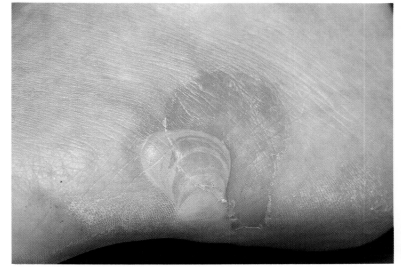

Fig. 16.31 Epidermolysis bullosa simplex. The feet are particularly affected. Exercise and the friction from footwear precipitate attacks of blistering. The condition is worse in hot weather. By courtesy of St. John's Hospital for Diseases of the Skin.

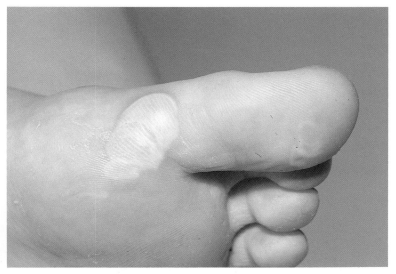

Fig. 16.32 Epidermolysis bullosa simplex. Tense blisters occur as a result of trauma. By courtesy of St. John's Hospital for Diseases of the Skin.

and soles and the lesions heal without scarring. They sometimes become secondarily infected. The condition tends to be recurrent, but is no more than an inconvenience. Light microscopy reveals a basally located 'intra-epidermal' bulla resulting from basal cell cytolysis. A more generalized variety exists but similarly there is no scarring and the lesions tend to occur at other sites of trauma.

Junctional Epidermolysis Bullosa (Epidermal Bullosa Lethalis)

This condition is inherited as an autosomal recessive and presents at birth. It is characterized by generalized blistering of the skin and mucous membranes. The tendency to heal is poor and scarring and milia formation result. Thus, extensive areas of eroded, oozing and denuded skin occur. The hands and feet are usually spared in this disease, unlike epidermolysis bullosa simplex, but periungual blistering and erosions are common. There may be severe oral and oesophageal involvement and the teeth are usually abnormal. This disease is commonly fatal.

The abnormality lies within the lamina lucida and is believed to be caused by an abnormality of the hemidesmosomes which connect the epidermis with the dermis.

Dystrophic Epidermolysis Bullosa
Autosomal Dominant Type

This condition begins at birth or in infancy. It is rarely fatal. Blistering occurs largely on the extremities (Figs. 16.33 and 16.34). Periungual blistering may lead to deformed nails (Fig. 16.35). Healing occurs with milia (Fig. 16.36) and scar formation. Oral lesions, if they occur, are mild and the teeth and hair develop normally.

The disease results from defective anchoring fibrils such that the lamina densa is separated from the underlying dermis. With light microscopy (stained by periodic acid-Schiff), the basement membrane can be seen to be attached to the roof of the blister. With electron microscopy the fibrils which anchor the basement membrane to the dermis are shown to be defective and/or diminished in number.

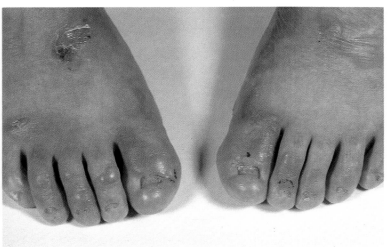

Fig. 16.34 Epidermolysis bullosa dystrophica. Blistering occurs mainly on the extremities and is induced by trauma. The blisters become erosions which heal with scarring.

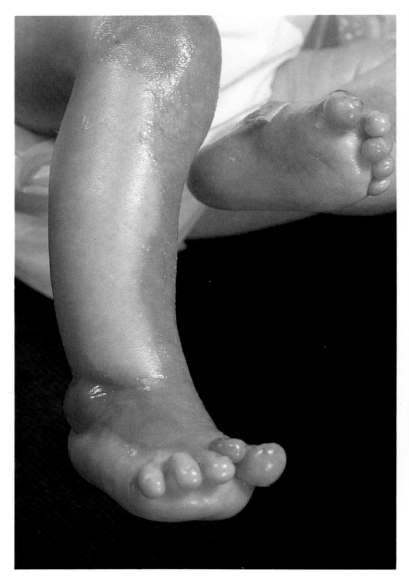

Fig. 16.33 Epidermolysis bullosa dystrophica. Tense blisters occur as a result of continual trauma. Severe cutaneous damage may occur. By courtesy of Dr. D. Atherton, Institute of Dermatology.

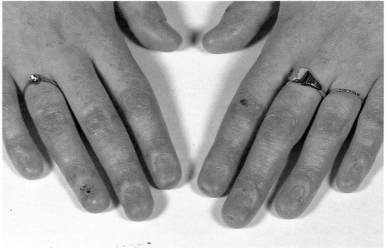

Fig. 16.35 Epidermolysis bullosa dystrophica. Periungal blistering leads to deformed nails.

Autosomal Recessive Type

There is considerable variation in the severity of affliction in subjects with this disorder. It is usually present at birth. Some neonates have a relatively localized blistering process limited largely to the extremities, in particular to the hands, feet, elbows and knees. Others have a much more widespread involvement.

The blisters which are slow to heal are frequently complicated by atrophic scarring and milia formation, especially around the hands and feet where fibrosis leads to fusion of the digits (Fig. 16.37). Flexural contractures occur at the knee, elbow, wrist and ankle joints. Mucous membrane involvement, not only of the oral cavity, but also of the epithelium of the whole gastro-intestinal tract is common and serious, producing difficulties with eating and defaecating and stricture formation subsequently develops. Morbidity and mortality are high in this depressing illness. Squamous cell carcinoma of the scar sites is reported in those who survive for a significant period.

The disease is associated with absent or diminished numbers of anchoring fibrils both in the blistered and non-blistered skin. In addition there appears to be an abnormality of collagen fibrils within the papillary dermis. Recessive dystrophic epidermolysis bullosa is associated with functionally abnormal collagenase, which can be partly responsible for the development of blisters.

Management

There is no specific treatment for these disorders. Those with the simplex form manage relatively well, especially when they are older and can take care to avoid trauma. The junctional and dystrophic types require specialized nursing and early treatment of infection. High doses of systemic steroids are often tried. An important advance in the management of the severe disorder is the use of the fetoscope to perform a skin biopsy *in utero* if there is a family history. Electron microscopy of the biopsy may determine whether or not the fetus is affected, so that abortion may be performed if necessary.

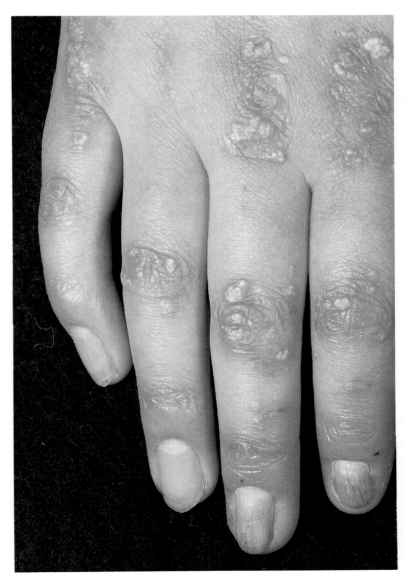

Fig. 16.36   Epidermolysis bullosa dystrophica. Milia (tiny white papules) occur after the blisters have healed. By courtesy of St. John's Hospital for Diseases of the Skin.

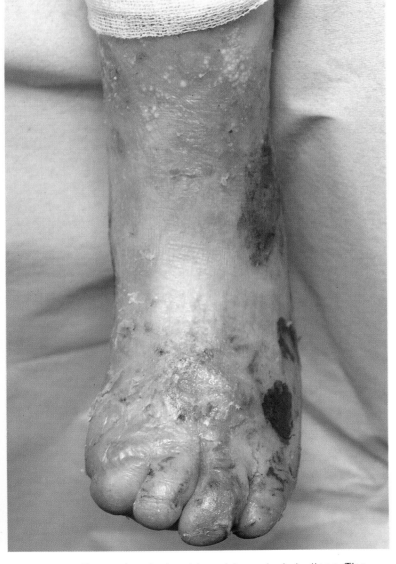

Fig. 16.37   Recessive dystrophic epidermolysis bullosa. The erosions are slow to heal. The scarring, which results, leads to fusion of digits. By courtesy of St. John's Hospital for Diseases of the Skin.

PEUTZ-JEGHERS SYNDROME

This condition is characterized by peri-oral and intra-oral pigmentation in association with polyps of the gastrointestinal tract. It is inherited as an autosomal dominant.

Round or oval macules between 1–5mm in diameter occur in profusion around the lips, especially the lower (Fig. 16.38). They may be brown, black or tan in colour. Macules may also be found elsewhere on the face and hands (Fig. 16.39), and on the feet. Within the mouth, the buccal mucosa (Fig. 16.40), gums and hard palate may be involved. The lesions are present at birth or in early childhood.

The importance of the condition is its association with polyps of the gastrointestinal tract and in particular of the small bowel, especially the duodenum. This may give rise to abdominal pain, bleeding and occasionally intussusception. Rarely, these polyps are premalignant.

Biopsy of the pigmented macules shows an increase in melanocytes in the basal layer and an increase in pigment-laden macrophages in the upper dermis.

GARDNER'S SYNDROME

This condition consists of multiple epidermoid cysts occurring on the face and neck, associated with mandibular bone cysts and polyposis coli. It is inherited as an autosomal dominant. The polyps are usually present by the second decade and there is a definite predisposition to malignancy such that prophylactic colectomy is recommended.

NEUROFIBROMATOSIS (von Recklinghausen's Disease)

This is a dominantly inherited disorder occurring in approximately 1/3000 births. It commonly occurs as a sporadic mutation. The condition is a result of an abnormal gene stimulating the excessive multiplication of cellular elements derived from the neural crest, i.e. Schwann cells.

Pigmented patches develop first during childhood (Fig. 16.41), but sometimes they are present at birth. The patches are usually several centimetres in size (Fig. 16.42), fawn-coloured and quite flat. Since they are a relatively common abnormality in otherwise normal people it is believed that the presence of six or more

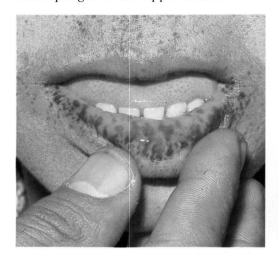

Fig. 16.38 Peutz-Jeghers syndrome. Round pigmented macules occur around the mouth and particularly on the lower lips. By courtesy of Dr. B. Leppard.

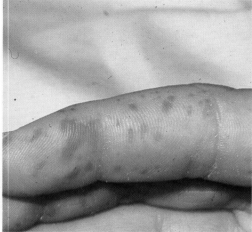

Fig. 16.39 Peutz-Jeghers syndrome. Pigmented macules may also be found on the extremities. The condition is associated with polyps of the gastrointestinal tract. By courtesy of Dr. B. Leppard.

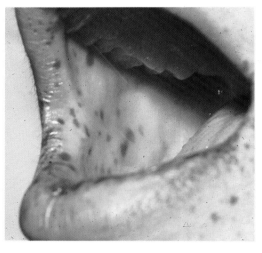

Fig. 16.40 Peutz-Jeghers syndrome. Pigmented macules occur within the mouth the disorder is inherited as an autosomal dominant. By courtesy of Dr. B. Leppard.

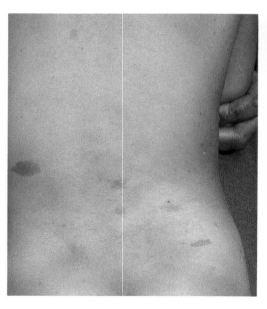

Fig. 16.41 Neurofibromatosis. Several 'café au lait' patches are present. They usually develop in childhood.

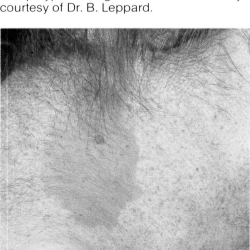

Fig. 16.42 Neurofibromatosis. A 'café au lait' patch is fawn-coloured and quite flat. They may occur in normal individuals, but several are usually present in von Recklinghausen's disease. By courtesy of St. Mary's Hospital.

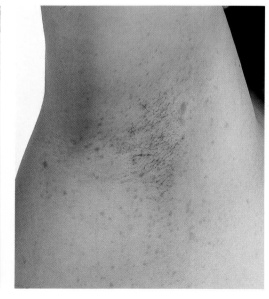

Fig. 16.43 Neurofibromatosis. Axillary freckling is virtually pathognomonic of the disease.

of these so-called 'café au lait' patches is necessary for the diagnosis of neurofibromatosis. Small pigmented macules, similar in appearance to freckles but unlike them in distribution, occur under the axillae (Fig. 16.43) and in the perineum. These are thought to be pathognomonic.

Neurofibromata, derived from peripheral nerves and their supporting structures, develop during childhood and adolescence. They are mostly painless and vary in size and quantity. They may be dermal and consist of soft, sessile, dome-shaped, sometimes pedunculated nodules (Fig. 16.44), usually less than 3cm in diameter, known as *mollusca fibrosa*. Subcutaneous neurofibromata consist of firm discrete nodules (Figs. 16.45 and 16.46) which are often attached to a nerve. A characteristic physical sign is that the lesions may be indented on pressure. Sometimes these nodules form large, grotesquely disfiguring pendulous masses. Neurofibromata may occur anywhere on the body surface, including the oral cavity.

The condition may vary from a minor to a gross disfiguring cosmetic problem with important systemic manifestations.

Intracranial neurofibromata may develop in the optic, trigeminal or acoustic nerves, or behave as a space-occupying lesion elsewhere in the brain. The spinal cord and peripheral nerves may be involved. Sarcomatous change may occur in any neurofibroma. Many other associated disorders are described in this disease and in particular endocrine and bony defects. There is no specific treatment. Symptomatic neurofibromata may be excised.

TUBEROUS SCLEROSIS (Epiloia)

This condition is inherited as an autosomal dominant and has sometimes been known by the acronym of epiloia: this stands for epilepsy (epi), low intelligence (loi), and adenoma sebaceum (a). Formes frustes are common and the cutaneous changes may be the only disorders present. An ovoid 'ash-leaf' patch of hypopigmentation (Fig. 16.47) is the first change to appear and may be easily seen by examination under Wood's light. There may be one or several of these either on the trunk or limbs. Although they may be white, they are different from vitiligo in that

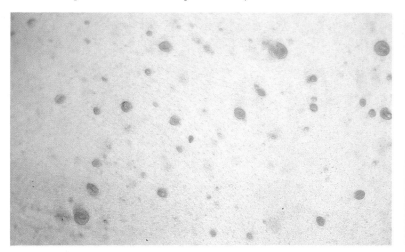

Fig. 16.44 Neurofibromatosis. Soft, sessile, pedunculated neurofibromata are known as mollusca fibrosa.

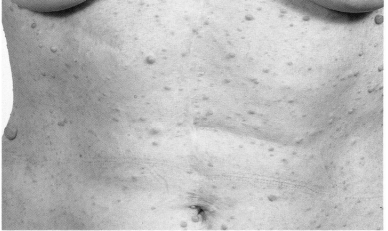

Fig. 16.45 Neurofibromatosis. Multiple neurofibromata are present. They vary in size and number.

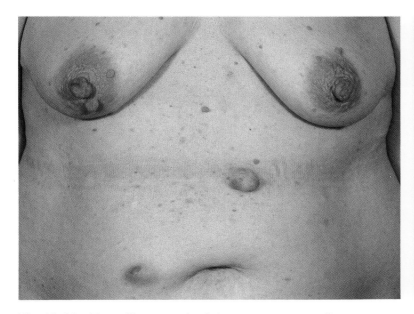

Fig. 16.46 Neurofibromatosis. Subcutaneous neurofibromata consist of firm discrete nodules.

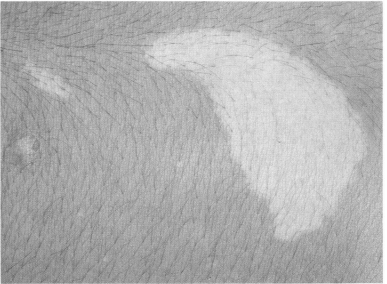

Fig. 16.47 Tuberous sclerosis. Ash leaf patch. An ovoid hypopigmented patch is characteristic. By courtesy of St. John's Hospital for Diseases of the Skin.

melanocytes are present in normal numbers but contain few melanosomes. In vitiligo, no melanocytes can be found. These patches of hypopigmentation occur in infancy. The so-called *adenoma sebaceum* are in reality angiofibromata appearing in childhood. They occur on the face, particularly around the sides of the nose (Fig. 16.48), but may also occur on the cheeks, chin and forehead. They consist of small red or yellow tumours (Fig. 16.49), about 2mm in diameter occurring symmetrically. *Periungual fibromata* are characteristic (Fig. 16.50). One or more connective tissue naevi may occur on the trunk, usually in the lumbo-sacral region. These lesions are skin-coloured but slightly raised, with a soft surface and an appearance similar to that of orange peel. They are caused by subepidermal connective tissue proliferation and are known as *shagreen patches* (Fig. 16.51). Fibrous nodules are also found on the gums, palate, tongue and in the larynx. Angiomyolipomata are found in the kidneys, and lung cysts are an important manifestation. Retinal phakoma is diagnostic and consists of a grey or yellow plaque near the optic disc. It may also be seen in neurofibromatosis.

EHLERS-DANLOS SYNDROME

These are a group of inherited disorders characterized by abnormalities in the synthesis of dermal collagen. Progress in understanding the biochemistry of these disorders is so rapid that fresh varieties of the syndrome are still being described. The conditions have the common symptom of hyperelastic skin (Fig. 16.52) which recoils immediately to its normal position, unlike the rare condition of cutis laxa. The skin is particularly fragile, bruising easily and healing poorly to leave unsightly scars (Fig. 16.53). The joints are hyperextensible (Figs. 16.54 and 16.55) and readily dislocate. Osteoarthritis eventually develops.

In some types the collagen of large vessels is disordered, so that dissecting aneurysms and spontaneous rupture of blood vessels may occur. There is no treatment for the condition, but genetic counselling may be valuable.

PSEUDOXANTHOMA ELASTICUM

This is a rare set of disorders characterized by an abnormality in the formation of elastic fibres. The condition affects blood vessels such that haemorrhage and its consequences are common.

The cutaneous physical signs consist of soft yellow papules with associated loose and thickened skin with a pebbled appearance on the sides of the neck (Fig. 16.56), under the axillae, in the groins, in the umbilicus and in the antecubital and popliteal fossae. Characteristic changes may be seen in the eyes due to the cracking of Bruch's membrane, producing angioid streaks. These are wider than blood vessels and extend across the fundus radially, away from the optic disc. The importance of this condition is that vascular involvement may result in gastrointestinal haemorrhage, bleeding from the urinary tract, hypertension due to involvement of the renal arteries, or occurrence of angina from coronary occlusion.

HEREDITARY HAEMORRHAGIC TELANGIECTASIA (Rendu-Osler-Weber Syndrome)

This is an autosomal dominantly inherited condition of recurrent haemorrhage, associated with multiple telangiectases of the skin and mucous membranes. It usually presents after puberty. Epistaxis and gastrointestinal haemorrhage are common but pulmonary and genitourinary haemorrhages may occur.

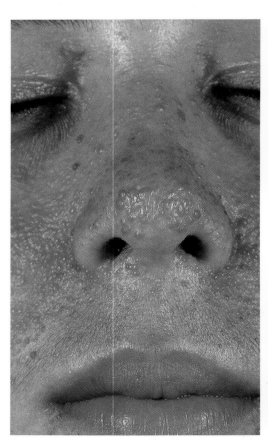

Fig. 16.48 Tuberous sclerosis. Angiofibromata occur particularly around the nose and spread to the cheeks.

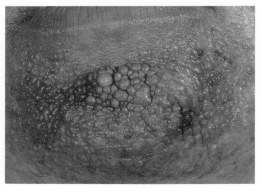

Fig. 16.49 Tuberous sclerosis. The angiofibromata are firm papules. By courtesy of Dr A.C. Pembroke.

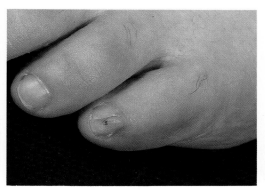

Fig. 16.50 Tuberous sclerosis. A fibroma is present on the fifth toe nail.

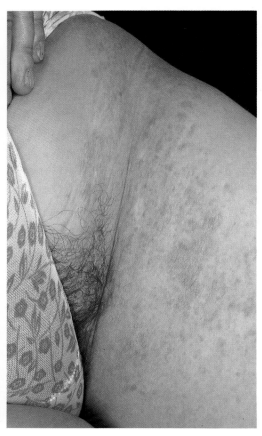

Fig. 16.51 Tuberous sclerosis. Slightly raised papules with a soft 'peau d'orange' surface are called shagreen patches. By courtesy of Dr A.C. Pembroke.

The cutaneous lesions consist of widespread, tiny telangiectases on the face, lips (Fig. 16.57), ears, hands, chest and feet. Oral lesions are almost always present, especially on the tip and dorsum of the tongue and on the palate. Lesions are found on the nasal septum and the nasopharynx.

There is no specific treatment for this syndrome except for supportive measures when bleeding occurs. The cutaneous, oral and nasal physical signs should point to the diagnosis in a patient bleeding from the gastrointestinal or nasal mucosa.

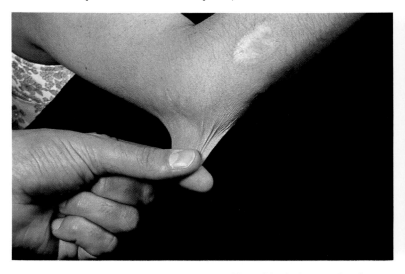

Fig. 16.52 Ehlers-Danlos syndrome. The skin is hyperelastic, but recoils to its normal position when released. By courtesy of St. Mary's Hospital.

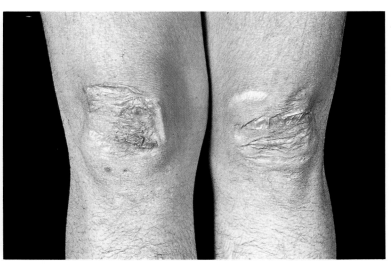

Fig. 16.53 Ehlers-Danlos syndrome. The skin is fragile and heals poorly with unsightly scars. By courtesy of St. Mary's Hospital.

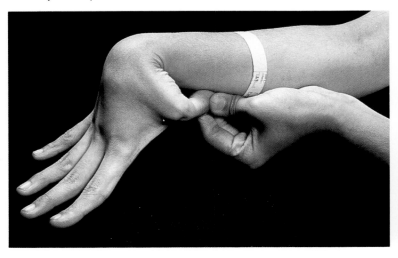

Fig. 16.54 Ehlers-Danlos syndrome. The joints are hyperextensible. By courtesy of St. Mary's Hospital.

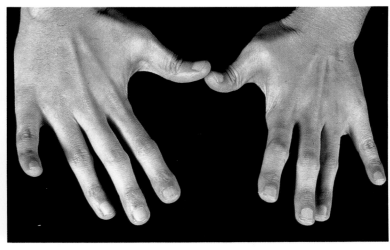

Fig. 16.55 Ehlers-Danlos syndrome. The joints are abnormal and dislocate readily. By courtesy of St. Mary's Hospital.

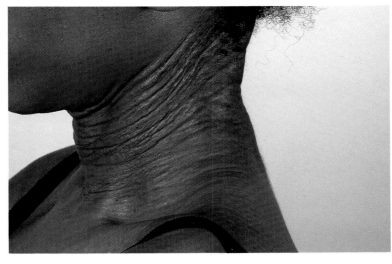

Fig. 16.56 Pseudoxanthoma elasticum. The skin is loose and thickened. The sides of the neck are characteristic sites. By courtesy of Dr R.H. Marten.

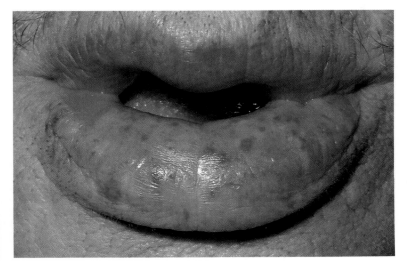

Fig. 16.57 Hereditary haemorrhagic telangiectasia. Tiny red telangiectatic lesions occur on the lips. Recurrent haemorrhage is common, especially from the nose and gastrointestinal tract.

ATAXIA TELANGIECTASIA

This is a very rare recessively inherited condition. There is distinctive cutaneous and conjunctival telangiectasia associated with cerebellar ataxia and recurrent pulmonary infections. There is a predisposition to malignancy, particularly of the reticulo-endothelial system, in adult life. The affected children are usually small in stature and present with difficulty in walking and other signs of cerebellar disease such as nystagmus and slurred speech. Mental retardation is frequent.

The cutaneous changes are usually present by the third or fourth year of life and consist of dilated blood vessels of a tortuous nature to be found over the eyeball (Fig. 16.58), eyelids, and in a butterfly distribution over the cheeks. Particularly characteristic is the telangiectasia over the backs of the ears and inside the helix. Telangiectasia is sometimes seen in the cubital and popliteal fossae. Occasionally it is also seen on the dorsa of the hands and feet.

The aetiology of the condition is unknown. Various disturbances of immunological function have been described. IgA is absent. There may be thymic atrophy, lymphocytopenia and consequent problems with humoral and cellular immunity. Abnormalities of DNA repair following radiotherapy are recognized.

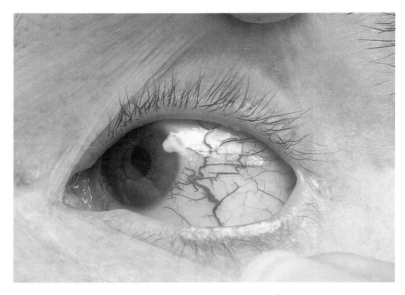

Fig. 16.58 Ataxia telangiectasia. Dilated, tortuous blood vessels occur over the eyeball. Similar lesions occur over the ears and cheeks. By courtesy of St. John's Hospital for Diseases of the Skin.

17 The Skin and Systemic Disease

There are a number of cutaneous disorders which may be associated with systemic disease. Not all such diseases are included in this chapter, for example Paget's disease of the nipple is described under skin tumours and dermatomyositis under collagen disorders, but several conditions not covered elsewhere may conveniently be collected here.

SARCOIDOSIS

This is a fairly uncommon but important multisystem disease with a predilection for the skin. Any organ may be involved, but especially the lungs, eyes, liver, spleen, lymph nodes and bones. The condition is of unknown aetiology, but a biopsy of involved tissue shows a non-caseating granulomatous infiltrate composed of epithelioid cells with occasional giant cells (Fig. 17.1). Special stains for tubercle bacilli and fungi are negative.

The disorder may present in the skin in a variety of ways. *Erythema nodosum* (Fig. 17.2) is the commonest presentation of sarcoidosis and affects young adults. It is associated with fever and arthralgia and has an acute onset. There are usually no pulmonary symptoms, but a chest X-ray will reveal bilateral hilar lymphadenopathy (Fig. 17.3) and this is sufficiently characteristic to confirm the diagnosis. Biopsy of the hilar glands reveals a non-caseating granulomatous infiltrate. Erythema nodosum is a vasculitis thought to be caused by circulating immune complexes. The prognosis is excellent, with clearing of the chest X-ray changes within a couple of years.

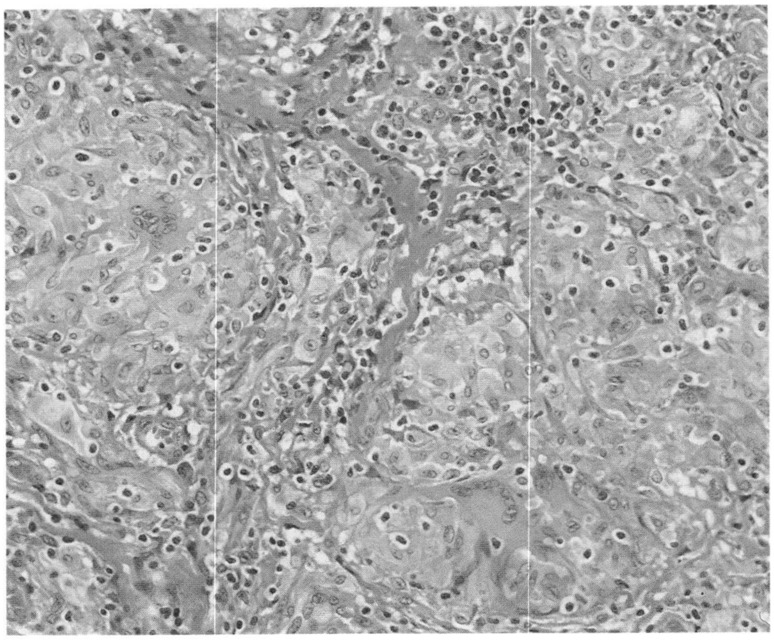

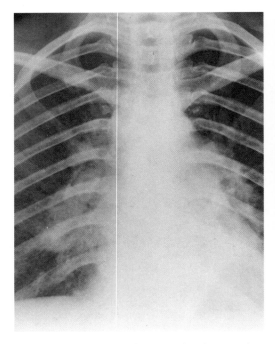

Fig. 17.1   Sarcoidosis. The section shows an extensive granulomatous infiltrate composed of well-defined clusters of epithelioid cells with occasional giant cells. Early scarring is seen in the centre of the field.

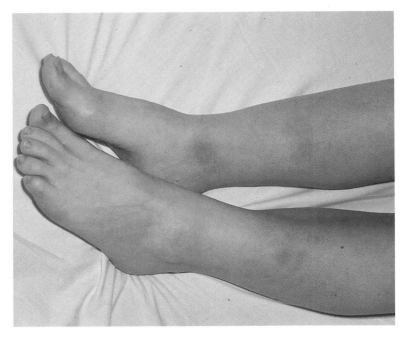

Fig. 17.2   Erythema nodosum. Painful red nodules on the shins may be associated with bilateral hilar lymphadenopathy. This is diagnostic of sarcoidosis.

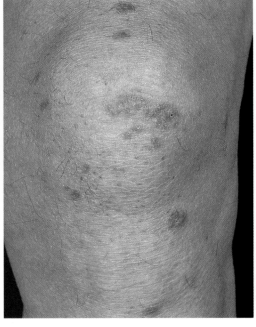

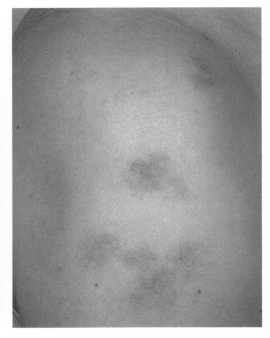

Fig. 17.3   Bilateral hilar lymphadenopathy. A chest X-ray is mandatory in a patient with erythema nodosum. The hilar adenopathy is asymptomatic. By courtesy of Dr. P. Gishen, King's College Hospital.

Fig. 17.4   Sarcoidosis. Persistent infiltrated papules occur. Biopsy is necessary to aid the diagnosis.

Fig. 17.5   Sarcoidosis. The nodules have a smooth surface.

The specific skin lesions of sarcoidosis are associated with multisystem involvement and tend to be chronic. They are an indication for general investigation and multidisciplinary consultation. Persistent infiltrated papules (Fig. 17.4), nodules (Fig. 17.5) and plaques (Fig. 17.6) are the most usual changes. They may be red-brown or purple in colour (Fig. 17.7) and are usually smooth-surfaced, since the pathology is wholly in the dermis without any epidermal involvement. The lesions can occur anywhere on the body, but the upper trunk (Fig. 17.8), arms and face (Fig. 17.9) are common sites.

Other variants of sarcoidosis are annular lesions, small facial papules and erythroderma. The invasion of old scars by sarcoid tissue is characteristic.

The granulomata may occur deep in the dermis involving subcutaneous tissues, such that a cyanotic hue develops on the surface. This is seen particularly in the variant of sarcoidosis known as *lupus pernio*. Thickened, purple plaques occur in an acral distribution on the cheeks, nose (Fig. 17.10), forehead, ears and fingers. These lesions are particularly persistent. Marked telangiectasia may occur on the surface of the lesions, in which case they are known as angiolupoid sarcoidosis. Lupus pernio is particularly associated with involvement of the upper respiratory tract and fibrosis of the lungs. Involvement of the nasal bones is common.

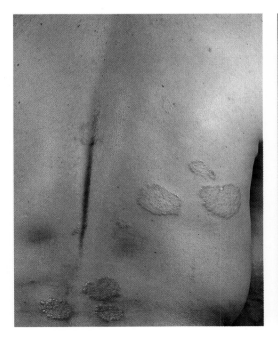

Fig. 17.6 Sarcoidosis. Annular plaques may occur. The trunk is a common site.

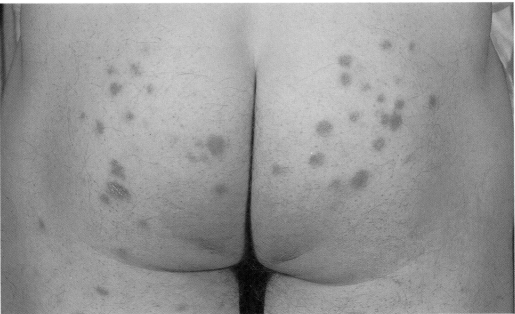

Fig. 17.7 Sarcoidosis. The lesion may be red-brown or purple and have a smooth surface.

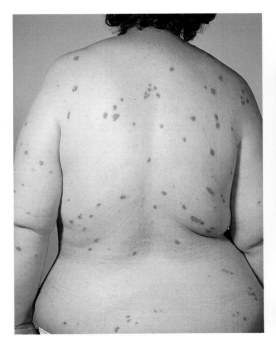

Fig. 17.8 Sarcoidosis. Widespread plaques may occur on the trunk.

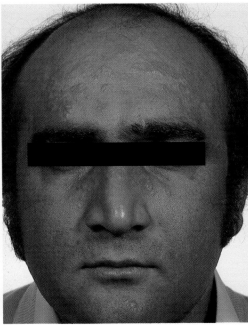

Fig. 17.9 Sarcoidosis. Small red or purple papules may occur on the face.

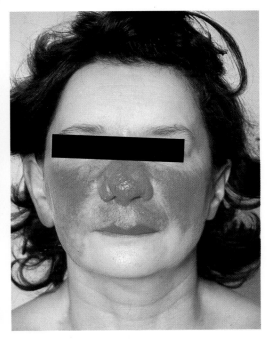

Fig. 17.10 Lupus pernio. Thickened purple plaques occur on the nose and are caused by granulomatous involvement of the dermis and subcutaneous tissues. By courtesy of St. Mary's Hospital.

In negroes the cutaneous lesions have a predilection for the face, particularly the eyelids and the area around the nose (Fig. 17.11). They are usually brown papules or nodules with a smooth surface (Fig. 17.12). They may be extremely disfiguring and very difficult to treat. Similar nodules may occur on the phalanges (Fig. 17.13), associated with cystic bone changes on X-ray (Fig. 17.14).

The diagnosis is made by biopsy of involved organs. Clearly, the skin is the most easily accessible for this procedure. The diagnosis may be confirmed by the Kveim test. A specially prepared antigen is injected intradermally at a marked site on the forearm. If the patient has sarcoidosis a granuloma will form and be apparent histologically when a biopsy of the site is performed six weeks later.

The prognosis of this disease depends on the extent and the site of systemic involvement. The cutaneous changes do not give rise to any symptoms other than disfigurement. However, the pulmonary infiltrates may lead to destructive fibrosis. Conjunctivitis and iridocyclitis may lead to serious impairment of vision so each patient must be treated accordingly. The disease is responsive to systemic corticosteroids. The cutaneous lesions also sometimes respond to intralesional steroids and to antimalarials or methotrexate.

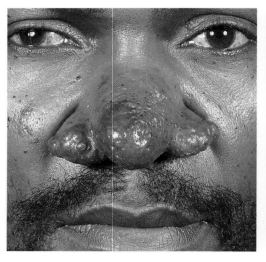

Fig. 17.11   Sarcoidosis. Infiltration of the nose may be extremely disfiguring and difficult to treat.

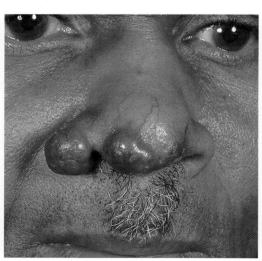

Fig. 17.12   Sarcoidosis. In West Indians the red-brown nodules occur particularly around the nose.

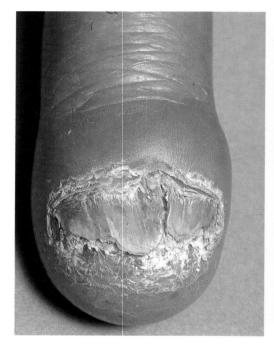

Fig. 17.13   Sarcoidosis. Nodules may occur on the fingers and cause discomfort. The phalanx is swollen and the nail is being destroyed.

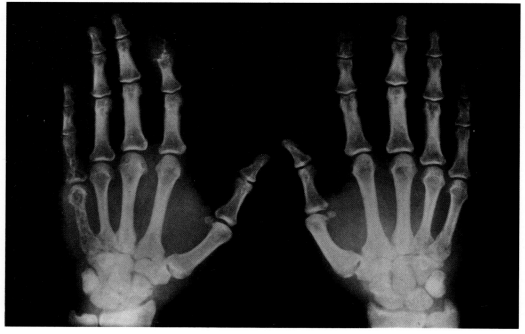

Fig. 17.14   Sarcoidosis. X-ray of the hands of the patient in Fig. 17.13 revealed erosions and bone cysts.

HISTIOCYTOSIS X

This is a rare collection of conditions characterized by a neoplastic proliferation of histiocytes in multiple systems. The syndromes are known as Letterer-Siwe disease, Hand-Schüller-Christian syndrome and eosinophilic granuloma of bone. There is considerable overlap between the conditions, so they are believed to be related. The retention of the original names is useful, however, because they do have different features. Quite characteristic cutaneous lesions occur in the first two conditions.

The aetiology is unknown (hence the letter X), but recent ultrastructural work has been revealing. The neoplastic cells are large (about four times the size of a small lymphocyte) and have a distinct cytoplasm (Fig. 17.15). Electron microscopy of these cells shows rod-shaped granules in the cytoplasm which are reminiscent of tennis racquets and appear to be identical to those found in the Langerhans' cell (Fig. 17.16). Thus, this condition is probably a proliferation, not of histiocytes, but of Langerhans' cells.

Letterer-Siwe disease is a disorder of infancy and has a tendency to an acute course. There is fever and anaemia associated with hepatosplenomegaly and lymphadenopathy. Pulmonary involvement is frequent. Infants are particularly prone to secondary infection, especially otitis media. The skin lesions are characteristic: they consist of discrete yellow-brown papules (Fig. 17.17)

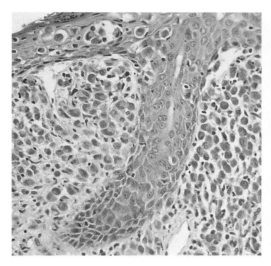
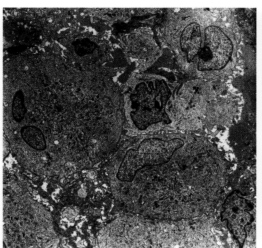
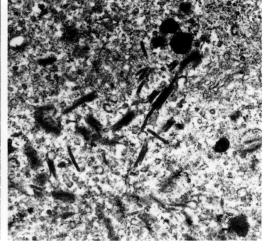

Fig. 17.15 Histiocytosis X. The dermis is infiltrated by large numbers of irregular histiocytes characterized by abundant eosinophilic cytoplasm and irregular vesicular and often reniform nuclei. Occasional eosinophils are also present. The infiltrate involves the epidermis.

Fig. 17.16 Histiocytosis X. In this example of Letterer-Siwe disease a small collection of Langerhans' cells is present in the mid epidermis (left). The high power view (right) shows abundant Langerhans' granules.

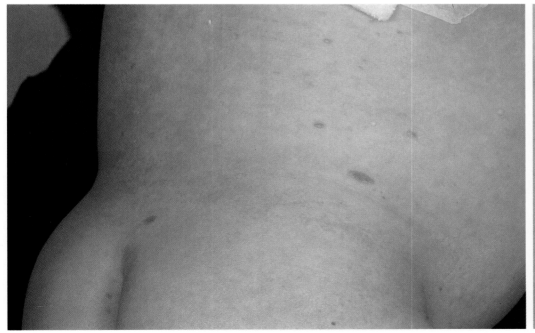
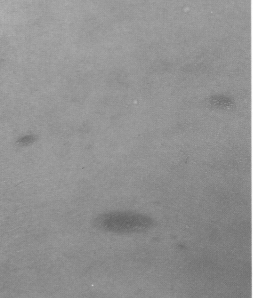

Fig. 17.17 Histiocytosis X. Discrete yellow papules and nodules are present on the trunk.

sometimes with a purpuric element, occurring in crops in the scalp (Figs. 17.18 and 17.19), on the face, neck (Fig. 17.20), trunk (Fig. 17.21) and buttocks. Lesions may occur in the napkin area (Fig. 17.22) and sometimes become necrotic.

Hand-Schüller-Christian disease occurs in children or young adults and classically involves bones, especially of the cranium, producing proptosis and diabetes insipidus. However, many systems may be affected and pulmonary and reticulo-endothelial involvement are common. The disorder tends to run a chronic course. The skin lesions are not quite as common but occur in a distribution similar to that of Letterer-Siwe disease and consist of macules and papules, often with a petechial element and sometimes with a surface scale. The distribution of the eruption is similar to that of seborrhoeic dermatitis. Secondary infection

of the cutaneous lesions is common and scarring may occur. Nodules may be present on the scalp in association with the bony defects.

Eosinophilic granuloma occurs in children and young adults and presents as an isolated bony lesion, usually in the cranium. Sometimes multiple lesions are found. Cutaneous signs are unusual but they are the same as those described for the other syndromes. The condition is usually benign.

The diagnosis is made with relative ease by performing a skin biopsy which would show the characteristic histology. Electron microscopy may also be helpful. Prognosis varies in these conditions and no specific treatment regimes exist, although various cytotoxic drugs are used.

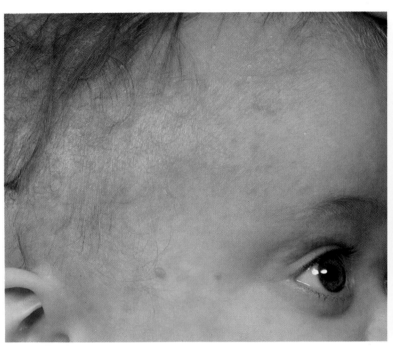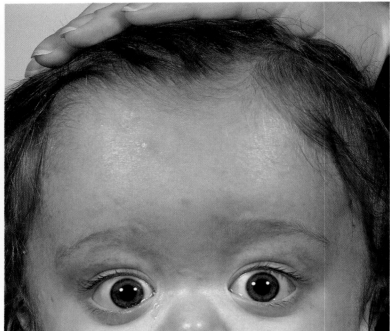

Fig. 17.18 Histiocytosis X. Discrete yellow papules are visible on the cheeks, forehead and in the scalp. Frontal bossing and proptosis are evident.

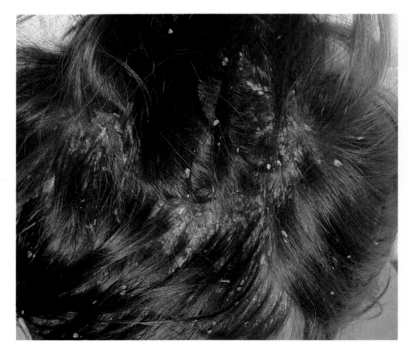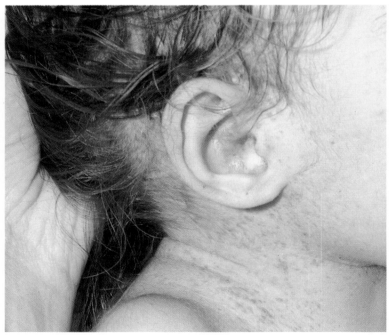

Fig. 17.19 Histiocytosis X. Yellow-brown papules in the scalp may give rise to crusting. The condition is easily misdiagnosed as cradle cap.

Fig. 17.20 Histiocytosis X. Closer inspection of the child in Fig. 17.19 reveals purpuric papules on the side of the neck. Skin biopsy revealed the true diagnosis.

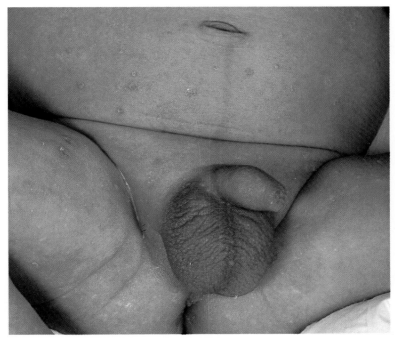

Fig. 17.21 Histiocytosis X. Discrete papules are visible over the body of the child in Fig. 17.19. She had Letterer-Siwe disease.

Fig. 17.22 Histiocytosis X. This child was misdiagnosed as having a napkin eruption. However, individual discrete papules can be seen encroaching on the lower abdomen. Skin biopsy confirmed the diagnosis.

METABOLIC DISORDERS
Porphyria

The porphyrias are a group of inherited, inborn errors of metabolism. Haem is formed from glycine and succinyl co-enzyme A in a complex series of reactions (Fig. 17.23). If an enzyme in the biosynthetic pathway is defective, an abnormality will occur. Certain porphyrin precursors are photosensitive, so that if they accumulate, a skin eruption occurs in a light-exposed distribution. The red cells or liver are also commonly affected.

Acute Intermittent Porphyria

The enzyme uroporphyrinogen I synthetase is missing so porphobilinogen accumulates. This is not a photosensitizer, so there is no skin eruption in this disorder. The condition gives rise to abdominal, psychiatric and central nervous system symptoms, usually precipitated by drugs or infections.

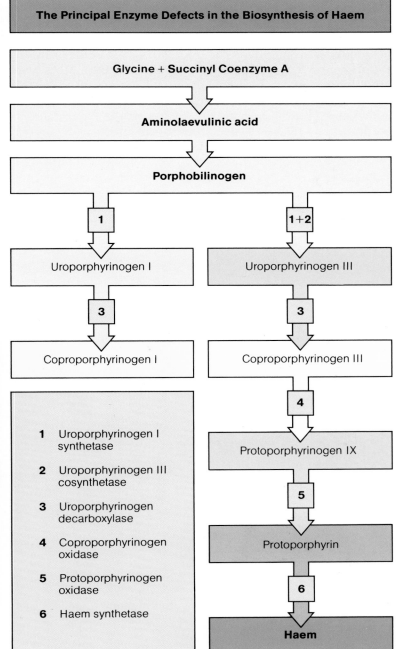

Fig. 17.23 Table illustrating the formation of haem.

17.7

Erythropoietic Porphyria (Gunther's Disease)

This is an extremely rare autosomal recessive disorder which presents in infancy. Uroporphyrinogen III cosynthetase is defective, therefore uroporphyrinogen I accumulates and is excreted as uroporphyrin I in the urine, discolouring the nappies pink or red (Fig. 17.24). Uroporphyrinogen I is a photosensitizer so blisters occur on exposure to sunlight (Figs. 17.25 and 17.26). The skin heals slowly and ulceration and scarring (Fig. 17.27) lead to mutilation (Fig. 17.28). Hypertrichosis is common and the teeth fluoresce red due to deposition in the dentine. This disease may have formed the basis of the werewolf legend. Uroporphyrin I accumulates in the red blood cells and haemolytic anaemia and splenomegaly result.

There is no effective treatment. Blood transfusion and splenectomy may be necessary. Photoprotection is critical and since porphyrins are maximally excited by long wave ultra-violet light, total sunblocks containing titanium dioxide are mandatory.

Porphyria Cutanea Tarda

This is the commonest form of porphyria. Uroporphyrinogen decarboxylase is defective so that both isomers of uroporphyrin accumulate. Uroporphyrins are found in excess in the urine and fluoresce red. Coproporphyrins are also increased. Most cases are inherited as an autosomal dominant but not all are clearly classified. The disorder is frequently precipitated by alcohol and sometimes by drugs, especially oestrogens. It commences in adult life and liver damage and cirrhosis result.

Blisters occur on sun-exposed areas (Fig. 17.29), especially the face and backs of the hands and the lesions heal with milia formation. The skin is very fragile and breaks with the slightest trauma (Fig. 17.30). Hypertrichosis and hyperpigmentation are common (Fig. 17.31). Sclerodermatous changes occur in some chronic cases.

It is imperative to stop further alcohol consumption or to discontinue the precipitating drug. Venesection is effective. It reduces the serum iron level which is increased in the disease. Chloroquine is also helpful.

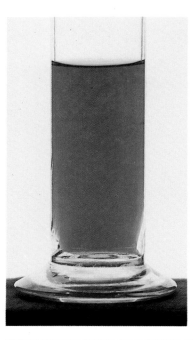

Fig. 17.24 Erythropoietic porphyria (Gunther's disease). The urine turns red or pink and discolours the infant's nappy. This may be the presenting complaint.

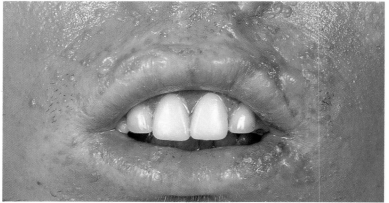

Fig. 17.25 Erythropoietic porphyria. Blisters occur on exposure to sunlight.

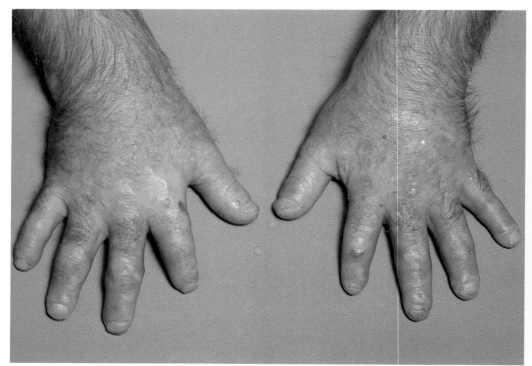

Fig. 17.26 Erythropoietic porphyria. Blisters occur on sun-exposed sites such as the backs of the hands and the resulting ulceration and scarring leads to destruction of the digits.

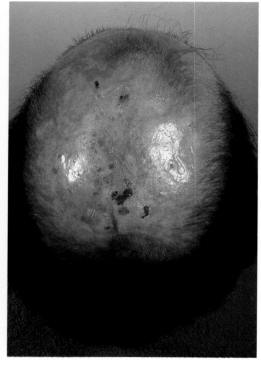

Fig. 17.27 Erythropoietic porphyria. The blisters heal slowly and often result in scarring. This man has a scarring alopecia as a result.

Erythropoietic Protoporphyria

This is a relatively common autosomal disorder. Haem synthetase (see Fig. 17.23) is defective and protoporphyrin accumulates in the skin, red cells, plasma and faeces. The red cells fluoresce pink. The condition begins in the first decade and the complaint is of itching, burning or stinging of the skin on exposure to sunlight. There may thus be no abnormal cutaneous signs. However, erythema and oedema, and occasionally an eczematous reaction may occur. Gallstones and cirrhosis may accompany the disorder. Photoprotection is essential and beta-carotene may reduce the photosensitivity.

Variegate Porphyria

This is an autosomal, dominantly-inherited disease which can be traced to a South African couple who married in the 17th century. Protoporphyrinogen oxidase is defective and protoporphyrin accumulates in the faeces; during acute attacks porphobilinogen accumulates in the urine. The condition has cutaneous features of porphyria cutanea tarda and neuropsychiatric and abdominal symptoms of acute intermittent porphyria. There are certain drugs which precipitate attacks, including barbiturates, sulphonamides, certain anaesthetics and alcohol, which must be vigorously avoided.

Hereditary Coproporphyria

This is a rare disorder inherited as an autosomal dominant. Coproporphyrinogen oxidase is defective and coproporphyrin III accumulates in the faeces. The clinical features are similar to acute intermittent and variegate porphyria, but photosensitivity occurs in some patients during acute attacks.

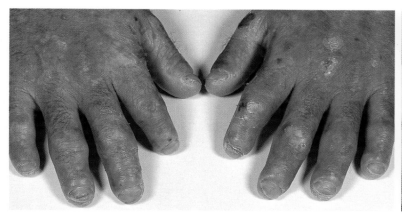

Fig. 17.28 Erythropoietic porphyria. The blistering process results in scarring and mutilation, in this case of the hands.

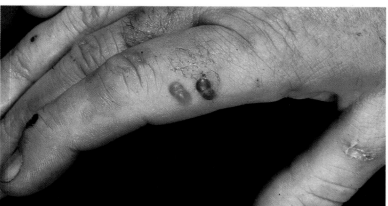

Fig. 17.29 Porphyria cutanea tarda. Vesicles or blisters are the hallmark of the eruption.

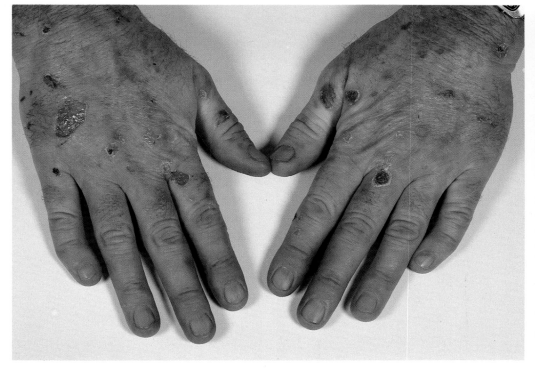

Fig. 17.30 Porphyria cutanea tarda. The sun-exposed areas are most severely affected. The skin is fragile and breaks with the slightest trauma, resulting in erosions and blisters.

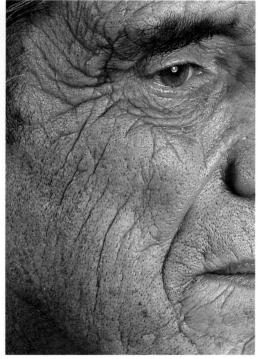

Fig. 17.31 Porphyria cutanea tarda. Hyperpigmentation and gross solar elastosis may accompany the disease.

17.9

XANTHOMATOSIS

The xanthomatoses are a group of disorders characterized by deposition of lipids in the skin. They result from hyperlipid-aemia, either due to a primary genetic defect or secondary to defective metabolism of lipids (Figs. 17.32 and 17.33). The lipids are deposited as flat, yellow plaques (known as *xanthelasmata*

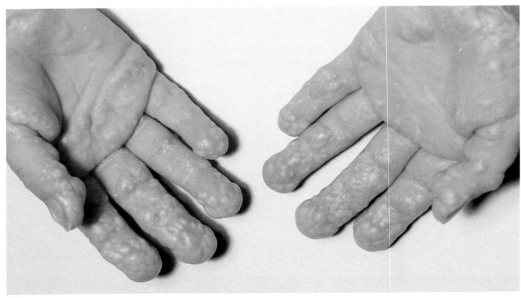

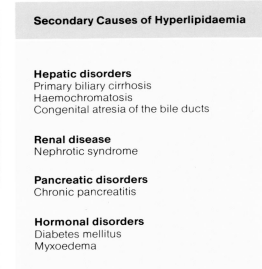

Secondary Causes of Hyperlipidaemia

Hepatic disorders
Primary biliary cirrhosis
Haemochromatosis
Congenital atresia of the bile ducts

Renal disease
Nephrotic syndrome

Pancreatic disorders
Chronic pancreatitis

Hormonal disorders
Diabetes mellitus
Myxoedema

Fig. 17.32 Hyperlipidaemia. This child had biliary atresia which resulted in gross xanthomata.

Fig. 17.33 Secondary causes of hyperlipidaemia.

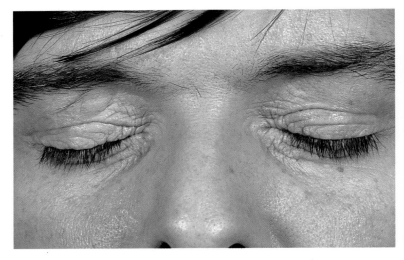

Fig. 17.34 Xanthelasmata. Flat yellow plaques are present around the eyes. This patient was jaundiced.

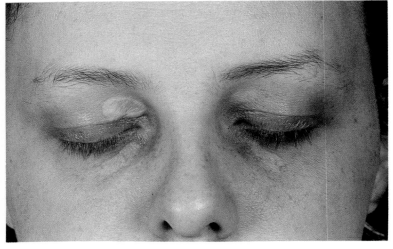

Fig. 17.35 Xanthelasmata. These may occur without hyperlipidaemia.

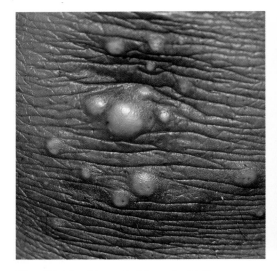

Fig. 17.36 Hyperlipidaemia. Yellow nodules (xanthomata) are present on the elbows of this West Indian lady. The elbows are a common site.

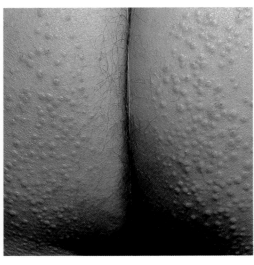

Fig. 17.37 Eruptive xanthomata. A myriad of yellow papules are present on the buttocks.

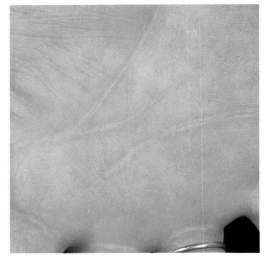

Fig. 17.38 Hyperlipidaemia. The palmar creases are filled with plane xanthomata. This is characteristic of type III hyperlipidaemia.

when occurring around the eyes, Figs. 17.34 and 17.35), yellow papules, or nodules (xanthomata, Fig. 17.36). Xanthomata may occur in an eruptive manner as a myriad of yellow papules which appear quite suddenly over the buttocks (xanthoma eruptiva, Fig. 17.37), thighs, arms, forearms, back, chest and face. Alternatively, they may present as lobulated nodules over the elbows and knees, or along the course of tendons, particularly over the backs of the hands and in the Achilles tendon (xanthoma tendinosum). Lipids may also be deposited in the creases of the palms (xanthoma planum, Fig. 17.38).

The primary hyperlipidaemias are not common. They are classified according to their pattern of lipoprotein electrophoresis and the subject is in a state of flux as new patterns emerge. The importance of the conditions is that they are potentially associated with arteriosclerosis and, in some, with diabetes mellitus.

Lipids are insoluble and are transported in the plasma as soluble lipoproteins. The four fractions of plasma lipoproteins can be separated out by electrophoresis or by ultracentrifugation into their respective densities. They are known as chylomicrons, pre-beta or very low density lipoproteins (VLDL), intermediate and beta or low density lipoproteins (LDL). Chylomicrons are the largest and scatter transmitted light, causing the plasma to appear milky when they are present in excess. They consist of 85% triglycerides and are induced by a fat-rich diet. Beta

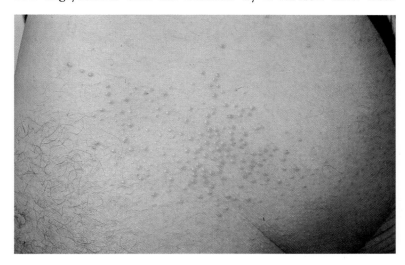

Fig. 17.39 Hyperlipidaemia. This man has eruptive xanthomata. Small, firm, yellow papules are present over the buttocks.

Fig. 17.40 Hyperlipidaemia. The eruptive xanthomata in Fig. 17.39 cleared with appropriate diet and a lipid-lowering agent.

lipoproteins are the smallest and consist of 50% cholesterol. Pre-beta lipoproteins are 50% triglycerides and 30% cholesterol, and intermediates are 50% triglycerides and 50% cholesterol. The hyperlipidaemias are divided into various types but they are not complete and their mechanisms are not fully understood.

Type I: Hyperlipoproteinaemia

This is an autosomal recessive disease which presents in childhood. There is a deficiency of the enzyme lipoprotein lipase, which is responsible for hydrolysing triglycerides to free fatty acids and glycerol. Chylomicrons accumulate and thus triglycerides. Eruptive xanthomata occur and the serum is lipaemic. Abdominal pain, hepatosplenomegaly and pancreatitis are usual. An increase in chylomicrons can be induced by diets which are rich in fat and the condition responds to restriction of dietary fat.

Type II: Hypercholesterolaemia

This is an autosomal dominant condition. There is a defect in the receptor mechanism for low density lipoproteins. Low density lipoproteins accumulate so that the cholesterol level is high (type IIa) and occasionally the triglyceride level is also raised (type IIb). Homozygotes tend to die in early adult life but heterozygotes develop cardiovascular disease and skin lesions later on. This disease is quite common, affecting approximately 1 in 500 individuals. Xanthelasmata, tuberous and tendon xanthomata and a premature corneal arcus are usually present.

The disorder is treated by weight reduction and restriction of dietary cholesterol. Substitution of unsaturated fatty acids for dietary saturated animal fats reduces the intestinal absorption of cholesterol. Lipid-lowering drugs are also used in an attempt to reduce the premature atherosclerosis and disperse the cutaneous deposits of lipid.

Type III Hyperlipidaemia

There is an accumulation of chylomicrons, pre-beta lipoproteins and intermediate lipoproteins. There is hypercholesterolaemia and hypertriglyceridaemia. The patients are obese, glucose-intolerant and develop premature atherosclerosis. Tuberous and tuberoeruptive xanthomata occur (Fig. 17.39) and palmar plane xanthomata are a striking feature. Reduction in weight, restriction of alcohol, carbohydrate and cholesterol and the use of lipid-lowering agents will return the skin (Fig. 17.40) and lipid levels (Fig. 17.41) to normal.

Lipoprotein Electrophoresis in Hyperlipidaemia			
Date (month/year)		Cholesterol (mmol/l)	Triglycerides (mmol/l)
9/82		21.3	8.0
11/82		5.3	1.2
2/83		10.2	2.6
9/83		5.2	1.1

Fig. 17.41 Hyperlipidaemia. The patient in Fig. 17.40 was shown to have a type III hyperlipidaemia on lipoprotein electrophoresis. This figure shows the return of the lipid profile, cholesterol and triglycerides to normal with treatment.

Type IV Hyperlipidaemia

The pre-beta lipoproteins are raised. There is often excessive carbohydrate ingestion and alcohol abuse which increases pre-beta lipoprotein synthesis in the liver of normal and type IV patients. The patients are frequently obese and have glucose intolerance and hyperinsulinaemia. The serum may be turbid. Eruptive and palmar xanthomata occur. Cardiovascular disease and pancreatitis are common. Restriction of calories and reduction of alcohol and carbohydrates are important. Lipid-lowering agents may be used.

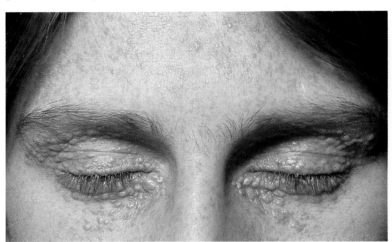

Fig. 17.42 Xanthoma disseminatum. Eruptive xanthomata may occur in the absence of hyperlipidaemia. By courtesy of St. Mary's Hospital.

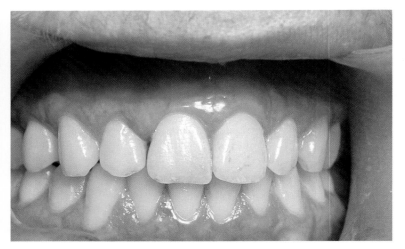

Fig. 17.43 Xanthoma disseminatum. Involvement of the gums, larynx and bronchi is characteristic of this rare histiocytic proliferative disorder. By courtesy of St. Mary's Hospital.

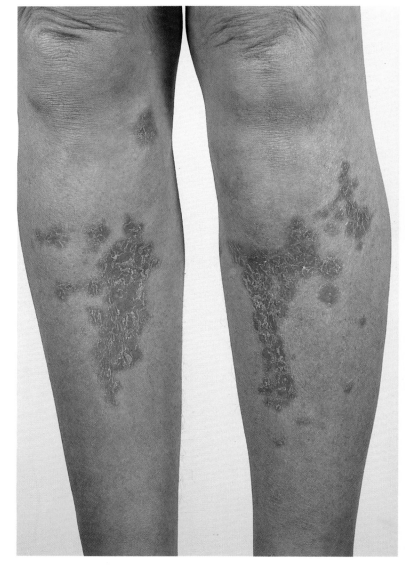

Fig. 17.44 Necrobiosis lipoidica. This condition occurs particularly on the lower limbs. It may or may not be associated with diabetes mellitus.

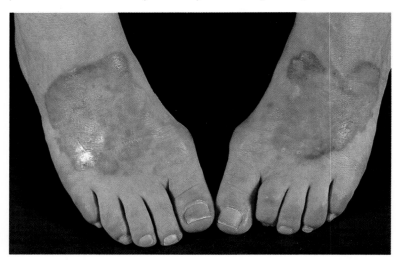

Fig. 17.45 Necrobiosis lipoidica. The lesions are usually relatively symmetrical. They are well-defined, slightly raised yellow plaques. They have a smooth waxy feel.

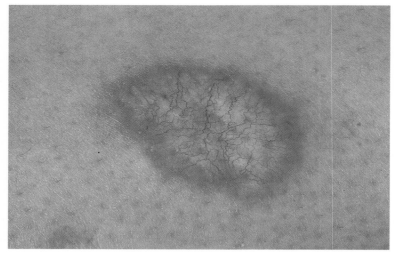

Fig. 17.46 Necrobiosis lipoidica. The plaque has a yellow colour with telangiectasia.

Type V Hyperlipidaemia

There are elevated levels of chylomicrons and pre-beta lipoproteins. Diabetes mellitus, hyperuricaemia and eruptive xanthomata result. Lipaemia, abdominal pain, hepatosplenomegaly and pancreatitis occur as in type I disease. Restriction of fat and carbohydrates and alcohol are important. Reduction in weight and lipid-lowering agents are employed.

Very rarely, diffuse involvement of the skin may occur with plane xanthomata in the absence of any demonstrable biochemical defect. This variety is often associated with an underlying multiple myeloma. Occasionally eruptive xanthomata may also occur with normal lipid profiles (Figs. 17.42 and 17.43). This condition is known as *xanthoma disseminatum*. It has some features in common with histiocytosis X.

DIABETES MELLITUS

Diabetics often have cutaneous complications. These are usually of an infective nature and are dealt with elsewhere. However, candidosis, particularly genital, is perhaps one of the more frequent presentations of diabetes in older women. There is said to be an increased incidence of tinea and also of staphylococcal infections of the skin. Atherosclerosis may lead to ischaemic changes in the skin and occasionally generalized pruritus may be a presenting feature of diabetes. Rashes may develop as a reaction to oral hypoglycaemiac agents and chlorpropamide in particular may produce a phototoxic eruption. Lipoatrophy of the skin may result from insulin injections.

Necrobiosis lipoidica and diabetic dermopathy are specific cutaneous associations with diabetes. Granuloma annulare is a rather dubious one but it is described here.

Necrobiosis Lipoidica Diabeticorum

This condition occurs more frequently in association with diabetes mellitus than by chance, but in many cases no association is found. The mechanism of the eruption is obscure. It consists of more or less symmetrical, well-defined plaques occurring on the shins (Fig. 17.44) and feet (Fig. 17.45). They have an irregular but well-defined margin, often of a brown-red or violaceous colour. The centre is yellow and atrophic, and has a characteristic waxy feel. Dilated blood vessels (telangiectasia) occur over the surface (Fig. 17.46). Occasionally the lesions ulcerate (Fig. 17.47). Intralesional steroids can sometimes be of benefit but the lesions rarely give rise to any symptoms except when they ulcerate. Under these circumstances excising and grafting the area may be helpful. If diabetes is present, treatment of this disease does not affect the necrobiosis.

Diabetic Dermopathy

Asymptomatic, atrophic, brown, small, well-circumscribed lesions occur on the lower extremities probably due to involvement of small vessels. The lesions are frequently not noticed by the patient.

Granuloma Annulare

The aetiology of this rather distinctive skin eruption is unknown and in the majority of cases there is no association with any underlying systemic disease. However, it has been reported to be more commonly associated with diabetes mellitus. The condition consists of a well-defined, red, annular lesion (Fig. 17.48), the margin of which may be made up of a number of individual, flat-topped papules (Fig. 17.49). The lesions occur most commonly over the backs of the hands, particularly the knuckles and

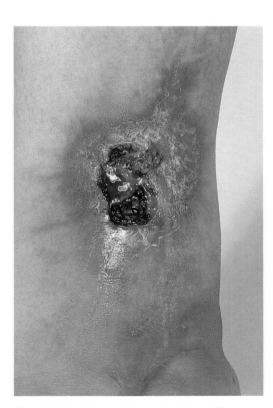

Fig. 17.47 Necrobiosis lipoidica. The lesion may ulcerate.

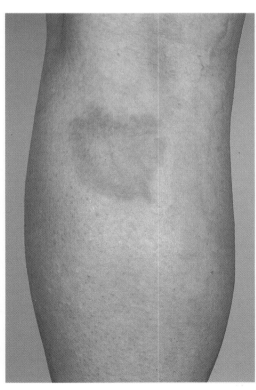

Fig. 17.48 Granuloma annulare. The lesions are annular and often mistaken for ringworm but there is no surface scale.

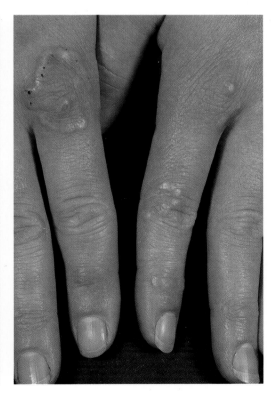

Fig. 17.49 Granuloma annulare. The margin of the eruption is made up of individual flat-topped papules. The knuckles are a common site.

fingers, as well as the feet, ankles (Fig. 17.50) and limbs (Fig. 17.51), but they may occur anywhere on the body. They may be tender if knocked. The aetiology is unknown but histologically a palisading granuloma is found in the dermis, so-called because there is focal destruction in the dermis surrounded by a histiocytic and granulomatous response. The lesions may disappear spontaneously. They respond to intralesional steroids but often recur.

DISORDERS OF JOINTS

Gout

Deposits of urates occur in gout, especially in the skin and cartilage of the pinna of the ear (Fig. 17.52) and around the joints. They are known as tophi, have a light pink colour and occasionally drain a white material which contains urate crystals.

Rheumatoid Arthritis

Although this disease rarely presents to the dermatologist, there are a number of cutaneous manifestations associated with rheumatoid arthritis, including vasculitis and pyoderma gangrenosum. Rheumatoid nodules are firm subcutaneous nodules,

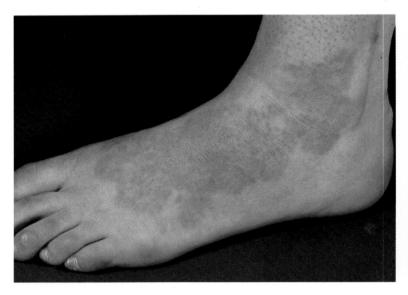

Fig. 17.50 Granuloma annulare. The dorsum of the foot or the ankle are common sites. The lesion is often quite flat in this area except for the margin which is slightly raised.

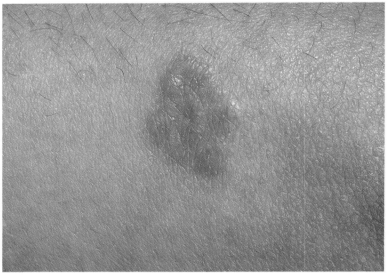

Fig. 17.51 Granuloma annulare. The margin of the eruption is most pronounced.

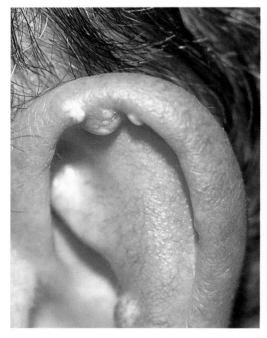

Fig. 17.52 Gouty tophi. Deposits of urates occur as hard papules around the pinnae.

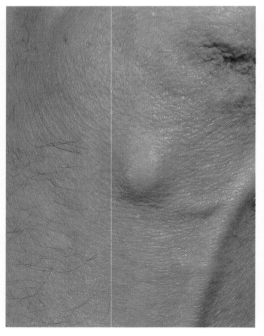

Fig. 17.53 Rheumatoid arthritis. Firm subcutaneous nodules occur particularly along the ulnar border of the forearms in rheumatoid arthritis. By courtesy of Dr. A.C. Pembroke.

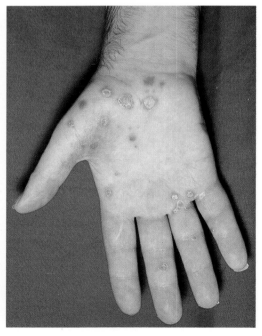

Fig. 17.54 Reiter's syndrome. Psoriasiform lesions occur on the palms and soles.

which occur along the ulnar border of the forearms (Fig. 17.53), backs of the hands and knees in particular. Psoriasis may develop, explaining the aetiology of a seronegative arthritis. Drug eruptions are the most common cause of a request for a consultation regarding a patient with rheumatoid arthritis. Aspirin, gold, non-steroidal anti-inflammatory drugs and penicillamine all cause cutaneous eruptions.

Reiter's Syndrome

This disorder presents with a tetrad of symptoms affecting the joints, eyes and skin, following shortly after either a venereal non-specific urethritis or an attack of dysentery. It is most common in young adult males. The arthritis is asymmetrical and affects the major weight-bearing joints. There is a high incidence of ankylosing spondylitis and sacro-iliitis in relatives, and the patients have the same HLA-B27 histocompatibility antigen as occurs in ankylosing spondylitis. The conjunctivitis is short-lived.

The skin lesions are psoriasiform and the palms (Fig. 17.54) and soles are especially involved. Initially the lesions are vesiculopustular but become hyperkeratotic and scaling. They are often conical (Fig. 17.55) and the appearance is known as *keratoderma blennorrhagica*. Psoriasiform lesions may occur on the skin and the scalp. Erosive and exudative psoriasiform lesions may occur on the penis and scrotum. The nails may also be involved.

Behçet's Syndrome

This is a triple symptom complex which may be associated with joint, pulmonary, vascular, intestinal and central nervous system involvement of a serious nature. It is a disorder of early adult life and is more common in males. The three symptoms which constitute the syndrome are recurrent ulcerations of the mouth (Figs. 17.56 and 17.57) and external genitalia (Fig. 17.58), and recurrent uveitis.

The oral lesions are similar to aphthous ulcers. They may be single or more frequently multiple, small or quite large. They persist for at least two weeks and frequently much longer. They have a yellow base with a red margin. Similar lesions occur on the genitalia, especially the scrotum, labia and around the root of the penis. Other cutaneous lesions are pustules (especially at sites of trauma, e.g. needle punctures) and erythema nodosum.

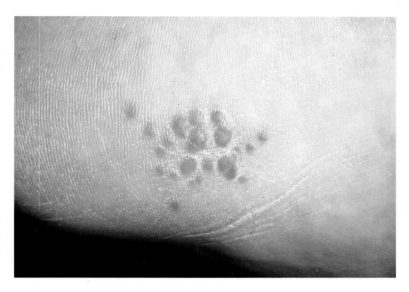

Fig. 17.55 Reiter's syndrome. Conical hyperkeratotic lesions are present on the sole. The appearance is known as *keratoderma blennorrhagica*. By courtesy of Dr. Barry Monk.

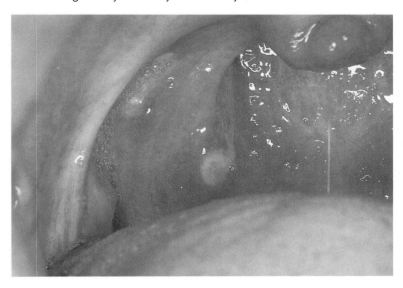

Fig. 17.56 Behçet's syndrome. There is an ulcer on the buccal mucous membrane and scarring of the uvula. By courtesy of Dr. J.J.H. Gilkes, Eastman Dental Hospital.

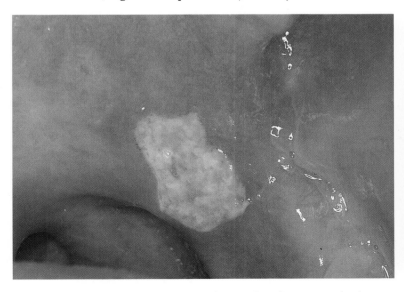

Fig. 17.57 Behçet's syndrome. A large ulcer is present in the mouth. By courtesy of Dr. J.J.H. Gilkes, Eastman Dental Hospital.

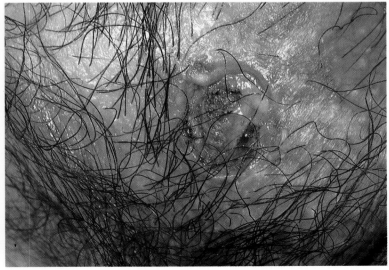

Fig. 17.58 Behçet's syndrome. There is a large ulcer on the scrotum.

17.15

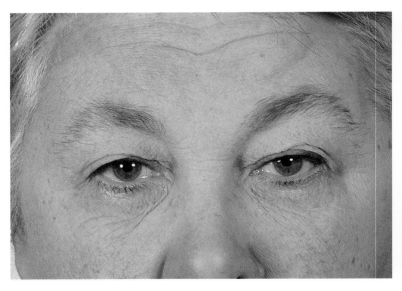

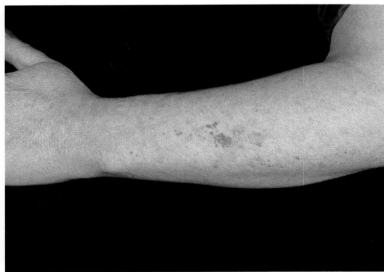

Fig. 17.59 Myxoedema. Thyroid disease is often diagnosed incidentally in a skin department. There is oedema around the eyes and the skin is yellowish. The patient's hair was thinning.

Fig. 17.60 Hypothyroidism. Purpura is occasionally the presenting complaint in hypothyroidism. By courtesy of St. Mary's Hospital.

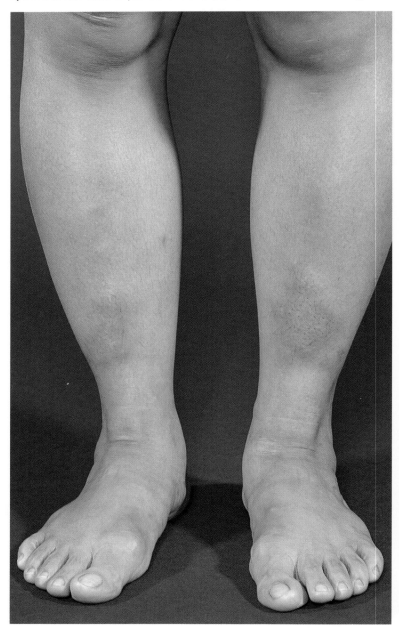

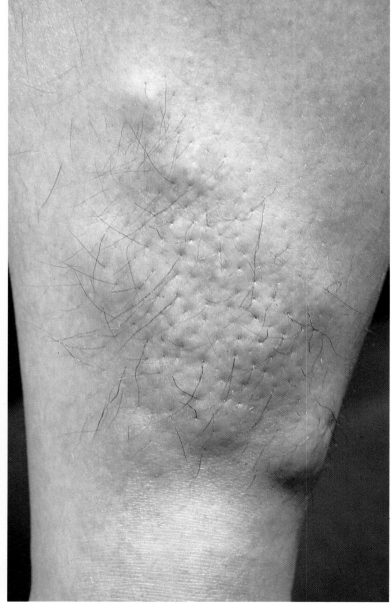

Fig. 17.61 Pretibial myxoedema. The plaques are relatively symmetrical and occur over the shins. By courtesy of St. Mary's Hospital.

Fig. 17.62 Pretibial myxoedema. The plaque is raised and nodular in part. The follicular orifices are patulous and there is hypertrichosis. By courtesy of St. Mary's Hospital.

HORMONAL DISORDERS

Thyroid Disease

Thyroid disease is often diagnosed in skin departments as a finding incidental to the patient's complaint (Fig. 17.59). However, generalized pruritus and diffuse hair loss are occasional presenting features of hypothyroidism. The skin is dry and yellow in colour, and the hair lacks lustre and is coarse. Purpura (Fig. 17.60)occasionally occurs. Leg ulcers which fail to heal and eczema craquelé are rare presenting features. The specific skin changes associated with thyroid disease are pretibial myxoedema and thyroid acropachy.

Pretibial Myxoedema

This condition is seen in thyrotoxic patients who have elevated levels of the long-acting thyroid stimulating hormone (LATS). There is infiltration of the dermis with mucin so that thickening and oedema of the skin occurs, particularly over the fronts of the shins (Fig. 17.61). This may also appear on the dorsa of the feet and calves. The lesions are quite well defined and are either yellow or skin-coloured with very prominent hair follicles and often associated hypertrichosis (Fig. 17.62). The treatment is

that of the thyroid disease, but the cutaneous changes do not necessarily respond to this. However, steroids may be helpful either under occlusion or by injection.

Thyroid Acropachy

Periosteal new bone formation may occur along the digits in association with exophthalmos, hyperthyroidism and pretibial myxoedema. This results in an appearance which simulates clubbing (Fig. 17.63).

Cushing's Syndrome

This is caused by either adrenal overactivity or excess stimulation by ACTH (adrenocorticotrophic hormone). Iatrogenic steroid therapy has made it commonplace. A full description of the disease is not appropriate here, but there is redistribution of subcutaneous fat, osteoporosis leading to kyphosis and a characteristic 'buffalo hump'. The face is plethoric and moon-shaped. Hirsutism and acne may occur. The skin is atrophic and bruises easily. Striking purple striae are seen over the trunk and limbs (Figs. 17.64 and 17.65).

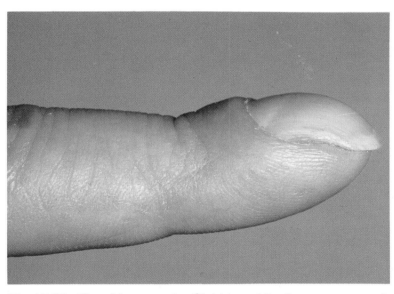

Fig. 17.63 Thyroid acropachy. Clubbing of the fingers may result from periosteal new bone formation in hyperthyroidism. By courtesy of Dr. T. Cundy, King's College Hospital.

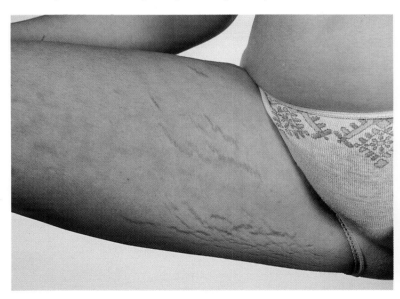

Fig. 17.64 Cushing's syndrome. This patient presented because of purple striae.

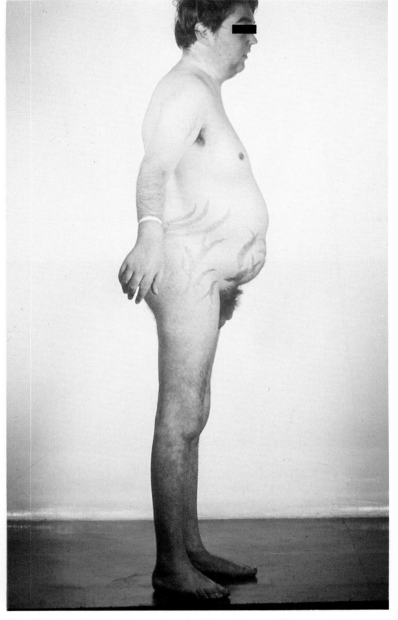

Fig. 17.65 Cushing's syndrome. There is a red face and obese torso. Striae are prominent. The upper back is humped due to kyphosis from osteoporosis. By courtesy of Dr. T. Cundy.

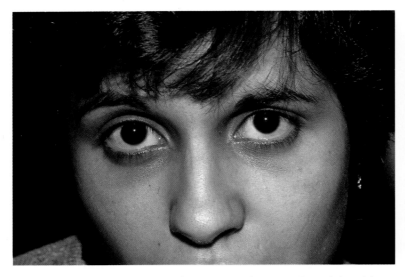

Fig. 17.66   Jaundice. There is a yellow discoloration of the skin and sclera.

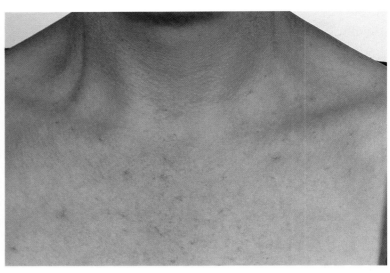

Fig. 17.67   Multiple spider naevi. Spider naevi are a common cutaneous manifestation of liver disease. However, the majority of spider naevi have no association with such disorders.

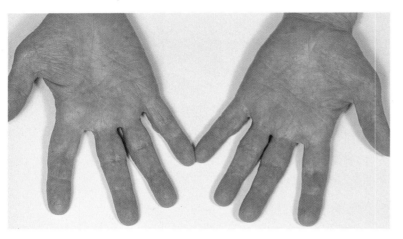

Fig. 17.68   Palmar erythema. An erythema of the palms may occur in association with liver disease.

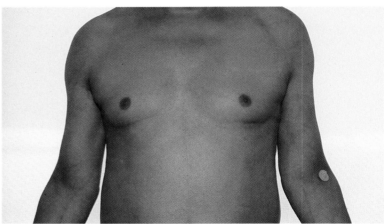

Fig. 17.69   Alcoholic liver disease. Loss of body hair and gynaecomastia occur as a result of liver failure to metabolize circulating hormones.

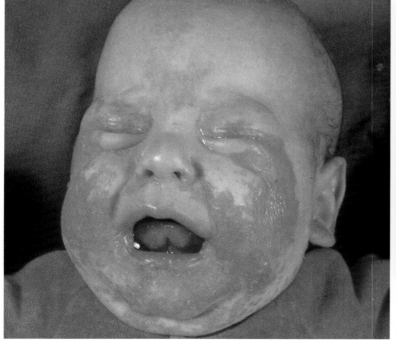

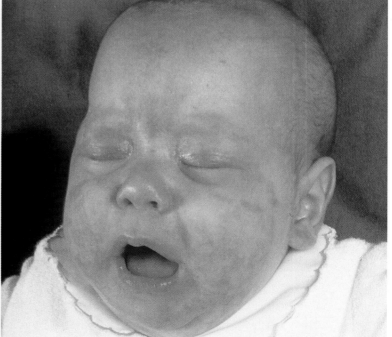

Fig. 17.70   Acrodermatitis enteropathica. There is a symmetrical oozing raw eruption around the eyes, mouth, cheeks and ears (left). The infant is shown two weeks after treatment with zinc sulphate (right). By courtesy of Dr. A.C. Pembroke.

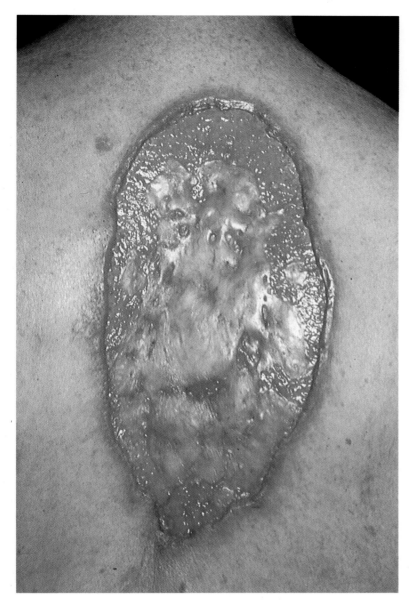

Fig. 17.71 Pyoderma gangrenosum. Large ulcers may evolve quite rapidly. A purple margin is characteristic. By courtesy of Dr. Roger Clayton, St. Mary's Hospital.

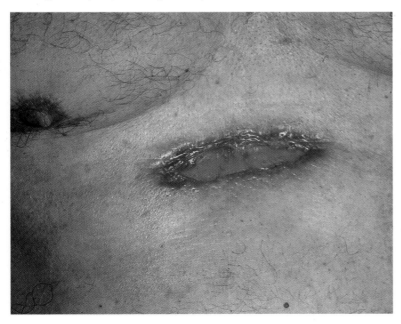

Fig. 17.72 Pyoderma gangrenosum. This patient also had a similar lesion on his chest. By courtesy of Dr. Roger Clayton, St. Mary's Hospital.

DISORDERS OF THE GASTROINTESTINAL TRACT

Many of the cutaneous associations of gastrointestinal disease are well known. In liver disease, for example, cutaneous stigmata such as jaundice (Fig. 17.66), spider naevi (Fig. 17.67), palmar erythema (Fig. 17.68), loss of hair (Fig. 17.69) and generalized pruritus are commonplace. Inflammatory bowel disease may occasionally present as erythema nodosum or as a widespread eczematous eruption. Crohn's disease may involve the mouth and perianal skin. Nutritional disorders frequently have cutaneous complications: scurvy causes purpura, particularly around the hair follicles, and twisted hairs are present; pellagra due to nicotinic acid deficiency presents as a photodermatitis.

Considerable interest in the connection between the gastrointestinal tract and skin disease has been generated by the finding of an association between dermatitis herpetiformis and a gluten-sensitive enteropathy. Many other skin disorders have been subsequently investigated for similar connections, but with less success. However, a major advance has occurred in the understanding and treatment of a potentially lethal condition known as acrodermatitis enteropathica.

Acrodermatitis Enteropathica

This is an extremely rare disease, but it is now known to be caused by an inherited disorder of zinc metabolism. Replacement of this essential trace element reverses the cutaneous, gastrointestinal and other effects of the condition. It presents in infancy or childhood following weaning as a failure to thrive and diarrhoea with malodorous pale and bulky stools. The child is miserable and unwell. The cutaneous changes are virtually pathognomic (Fig. 17.70). There is hair loss and vesico-bullous lesions which crust and erode around orifices such as the eyes, mouth, ears, nose, anus and genitalia. Similar lesions occur around the finger and toe nails producing a paronychia. Psoriasiform plaques may appear around the elbows, knees and buttocks. Secondary invasion of the skin by *Candida albicans* is common.

A similar clinical picture can arise if there is zinc deficiency due to inadequate parenteral feeding, malabsorption, or secondary to use of chelating agents such as penicillamine.

Pyoderma Gangrenosum

This is a rare condition which is sometimes associated with gastrointestinal disease, but there are also other causes. It consists of large ulcers (Fig. 17.71) which have a characteristic purple, overhanging edge (Fig. 17.72). They arise rapidly from a sterile pustule or tender nodule. There may be one or several lesions occurring particularly on the lower legs, abdomen or face. The exact aetiology is unknown. The prognosis and management depends on the underlying disorder (Fig. 17.73). The condition responds to systemic steroids.

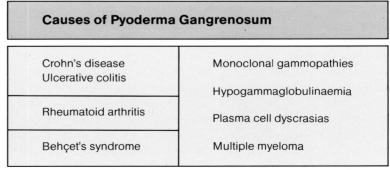

Causes of Pyoderma Gangrenosum	
Crohn's disease Ulcerative colitis	Monoclonal gammopathies
	Hypogammaglobulinaemia
Rheumatoid arthritis	Plasma cell dyscrasias
Behçet's syndrome	Multiple myeloma

Fig. 17.73 Causes of pyoderma gangrenosum.

DISORDERS ASSOCIATED WITH MALIGNANT DISEASE

Malignant disease may present in a variety of ways: generalized pruritus and secondaries (see Fig. 7.135) are quite common but acquired ichthyosis, thrombophlebitis migrans and the Leser-Trélat sign are rare. Acanthosis nigricans and necrolytic migratory erythema are specific conditions which are associated with malignant disease while Kaposi's sarcoma is a generalized malignant disease which usually presents in the skin. Skin lesions identical to those of classical Kaposi's sarcoma occur in the acquired immune deficiency syndrome (AIDS).

Thrombophlebitis Migrans

Recurrent migratory attacks of thrombophlebitis (Fig. 17.74) are a rare but well-documented association with carcinoma, especially of the lung and pancreas.

Sign of Leser-Trélat

An acute profuse eruption of seborrhoeic warts (Fig. 17.75) may be linked with internal malignant disease. It is an uncommon association, whereas seborrhoeic warts are very common.

Acanthosis Nigricans

This extremely rare condition is associated with underlying carcinoma, usually of the gastrointestinal tract, particularly the stomach. The eruption may precede the finding of a carcinoma by some time. It consists of pigmented, thickened skin (Fig. 17.76) with a velvety feel and occurs symmetrically in the flexures (Fig. 17.77) notably the axillae, umbilicus, groins and anogenital area. The backs of the hands can be involved and the palmar skin may be grossly thickened. Sometimes the eruption is almost universal. Skin tags and warty excrescences are common. The mouth may be involved. It is essential to identify the underlying malignant disorder and treat accordingly.

Pseudoacanthosis nigricans is much more common. It is clinically similar but is usually confined to the flexures. It occurs in perfectly fit individuals who are obese and is more common in coloured individuals.

Necrolytic Migratory Erythema (Glucagonoma Syndrome)

This is an extremely rare condition, but the eruption is characteristic (Fig. 17.78). Early diagnosis may lead to curative surgery of the associated glucagon-secreting tumour of the pancreatic islet cells. Patients often lose weight, are found to have diabetes mellitus and have a stomatitis which consists of circumoral crusting and glossitis. Annular or circinate lesions occur on the lower abdomen, in the groin and perineum and on the buttocks and thighs. These start as an erythema which blisters and erodes leaving post-inflammatory hyperpigmentation. The lesions are migratory. Each fresh lesion takes a couple of weeks to evolve and heal. The condition is associated with very high plasma glucagon levels.

Kaposi's Sarcoma

In 1872 Kaposi described a series of elderly men with blue-red nodules on their feet (Fig. 17.79) and oedema, some of whom subsequently died. The histopathology of the skin lesions revealed vascular proliferation, haemorrhage and haemosiderin deposition (Figs. 17.80–17.82). This is the classical form of the disease. It is largely confined to elderly men, especially of Jewish or Italian ancestry. The nodules are single or multiple and dark blue in colour. They usually occur on the lower limbs, especially the ankles, but may spread to the hands, ears and nose. They respond to radiotherapy. The disease frequently ends in Hodgkin's disease or some other lymphoproliferative process.

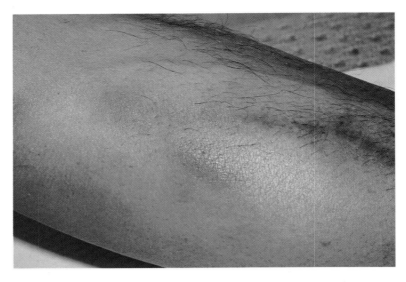

Fig. 17.74 Thrombophlebitis migrans. Recurrent painful red swellings along superficial veins may be associated with an underlying carcinoma.

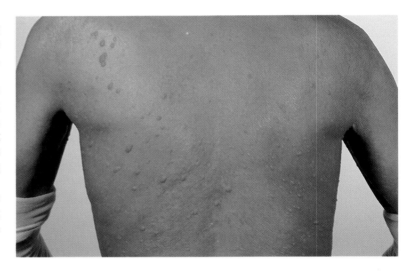

Fig. 17.75 Leser-Trélat sign. A sudden widespread eruption of seborrhoeic warts is occasionally associated with malignant disease. This man also had an erythroderma. He had a carcinoma of the colon.

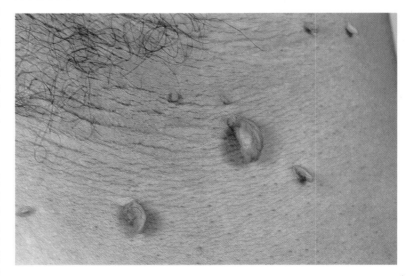

Fig. 17.76 Acanthosis nigricans. The thickened pigmented skin often has a smooth, velvety surface. Skin tags are often also present.

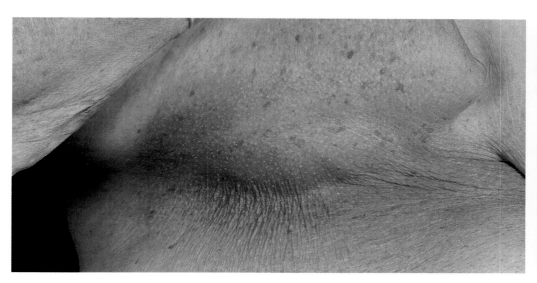

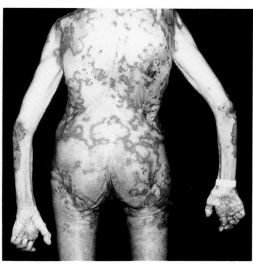

Fig. 17.77 Acanthosis nigricans. The skin is thickened and pigmented under the breasts. The axillae are another common site.

Fig. 17.78 Necrolytic migratory erythema. An annular migratory erythema occurs, which blisters and becomes eroded. By courtesy of Dr. C. Mallinson.

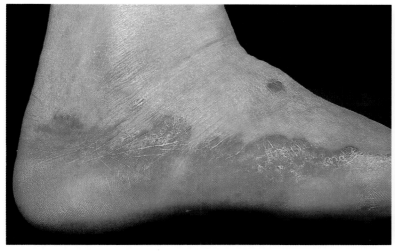

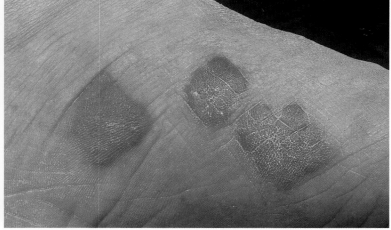

Fig. 17.79 Kaposi's sarcoma. Purple plaques and nodules occur particularly on the lower legs and feet. The close up (right) shows the detail of the lesion. By courtesy of Dr. Neil Smith, Institute of Dermatology.

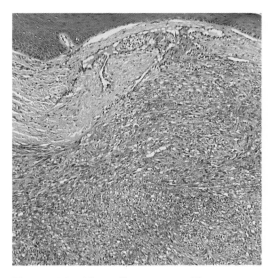

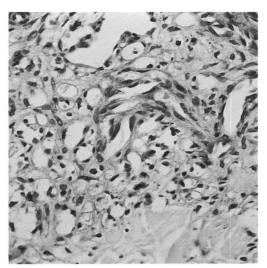

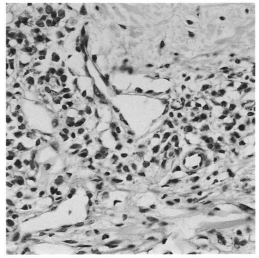

Fig. 17.80 Kaposi's sarcoma. The appearances of this established tuberous nodule are characteristic. Note the interlacing fascicles of spindle cells and the conspicuous red blood cell component.

Fig. 17.81 Patch stage Kaposi's sarcoma. The early stages of the evolution of Kaposi's sarcoma are characterized by the development of irregular cleft-like vascular channels lined by plump, slightly atypical and hyperchromatic endothelial cells.

Fig. 17.82 Patch stage Kaposi's sarcoma. A mononuclear (lymphocyte and plasma cell) infiltrate commonly surrounds these vessels.

17.21

A similar condition also occurs in equatorial Africa, particularly in the Congo and Uganda, but it spares the resident European community. It is common and affects younger individuals but also has a male preponderance. The nodular type occurs but there are also two locally aggressive processes. One type is a florid tumour which may invade the deep fascia. The other infiltrates particularly into bone. A generalized fulminant process without cutaneous involvement may involve lymph nodes, the mucosae, the gastrointestinal tract and lungs. This particularly affects young children.

Renal transplant patients and other individuals receiving immunosuppressive therapy have a much higher than expected incidence of Kaposi's sarcoma. Organs other than the skin are often involved and the prognosis is poor, although some have resolved on withdrawal of the immunosuppressive.

The situation has become further complicated because lesions identical to Kaposi's sarcoma may develop in individuals with the *acquired immune deficiency syndrome (AIDS)*.

Acquired Immune Deficiency Syndrome (AIDS)

The condition is a recently described entity. It is an acquired immune deficiency, probably of viral origin. It is most common in homosexual men, those who receive blood products, for example haemophiliacs, and those exposed to contaminated needles such as drug addicts. Haitian refugees have also been reported as being susceptible. Other risk factors are sexual promiscuity and amyl nitrite abuse. The disorder manifests as pneumonia, meningitis or encephalitis due to opportunistic infections which are not pathogenic under normal circumstances. Thus *Pneumocystis carinii*, cytomegalovirus, aspergillus,

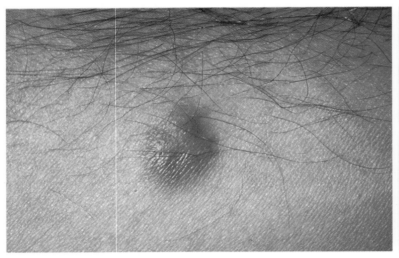
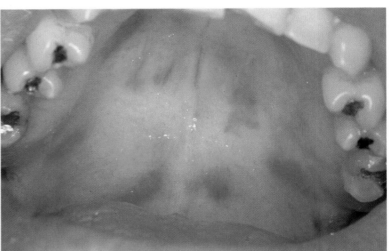

Fig. 17.83 Acquired immune deficiency syndrome. A purple nodule or plaque is characteristic (left). Several raised, purple patches are present in the mouth of this patient (right).

Causes of Generalized Pruritus	
Anaemia	especially iron deficiency
Obstructive liver disease	primary biliary cirrhosis, drug induced cholestasis, cholestatis of pregnancy
Chronic renal failure	
Carcinoma	
Lymphoma	Hodgkin's disease
Myeloproliferative disorders	polycythaemia rubra vera
Endocrine disease	myxoedema and thyrotoxicosis
Senile pruritus	
Psychological disturbance	
Delusional parasitophobia	

Fig. 17.84 Causes of pruritus.

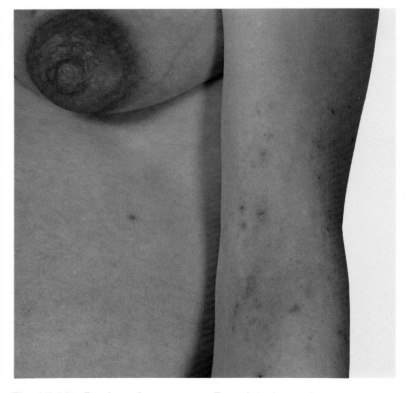

Fig. 17.85 Prurigo of pregnancy. Excoriated papules are present on the limbs. The condition is relieved by parturition. There are no maternal or fetal complications.

candida and cryptococcus are among the invading organisms. Lymphadenopathy, malaise, weight loss and fever occur. The skin lesions occur on the upper rather than lower half of the body but are otherwise identical clinically and histologically to Kaposi's sarcoma. The lesions are purple patches or indurated plaques (Fig. 17.83). The disease has a high mortality.

GENERALIZED PRURITUS

Itching is a common symptom of patients suffering from skin diseases. The term 'generalized pruritus' implies itching without evidence of any disorder of the skin. Thus, when the patient is examined, there are either no abnormal physical signs on the skin or there are solely excoriations as a result of scratching. It is thus important to exclude common itching disorders such as scabies, eczema, urticaria and lichen planus before extensive investigations are instigated. The more common causes of generalized pruritus are given in Fig. 17.84. A careful history and examination with appropriate investigations must be undertaken. In the final analysis there will be a number of patients for whom no systemic disorder will be found. This is particularly so in the elderly (*senile pruritus*). However, this may be suspected if there are abnormal physical signs, that is the skin is often dry, scaly and has lost its elasticity. It is postulated that the sensation of itching is a result of generalized arteriosclerosis affecting the blood vessels which supply the nervous tissue. Although the degree of irritation may be intense, it is remarkable how often there are no signs of excoriation on the skin.

PREGNANCY

The cutaneous consequences of pregnancy are considered here for convenience, although pregnancy can hardly be thought of as a systemic disease.

Most of the cutaneous changes in pregnancy are well known. Vascular changes such as spider naevi and palmar erythema are common and usually disappear after delivery. A generalized pigmentation occurs, particularly of already pigmented areas such as the areola, the genital area and the linea alba. Pigmented naevi may increase in number and in size and skin tags frequently develop. Striae are very common. Hair growth is more luxuriant in pregnancy and it appears that more hairs are in anagen than normal. There is frequently a compensatory precipitation of hairs into telogen after delivery, such that many women notice hair loss (telogen effluvium) three months or so after parturition. Itching is very common, particularly over the lower abdomen and some believe that it is caused by a mild cholestasis.

Prurigo of Pregnancy (Besnier's Prurigo Gestationis)

This is quite a common eruption. Small closely grouped pruritic papules occur mainly on the extensor surfaces of the limbs (Fig. 17.85) and sometimes the trunk. The lesions are excoriated. The condition is relieved by parturition but recurs in successive pregnancies. The mother is otherwise healthy and there are no fetal complications.

Polymorphic Eruption of Pregnancy (Toxic Erythema of Pregnancy or Pruritic Urticarial Papules and Plaques of Pregnancy)

This is a common, intensely itchy eruption. It tends to afflict younger women and is associated with excess weight gain during pregnancy and fetal distress and post-maturity. The itching begins in the abdominal striae (Fig. 17.86) and the lesions are symmetrical, discrete, red, urticarial papules (Fig. 17.87) which occur particularly on the limbs and extremities. It is relieved by delivery but recurs with successive pregnancies.

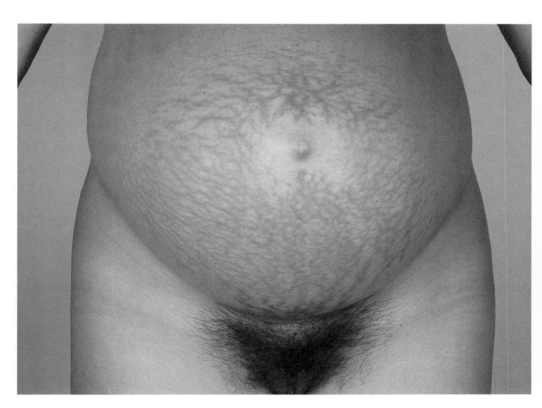

Fig. 17.86 Polymorphic eruption of pregnancy. Urticarial papules frequently appear in the abdominal striae.

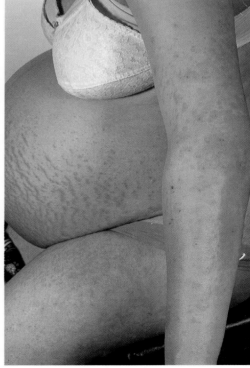

Fig. 17.87 Polymorphic eruption of pregnancy. The limbs and abdomen are affected. There are discrete red urticarial papules. The lesions are very itchy. It is associated with excess weight gain, fetal distress and prematurity.

Herpes Gestationis

This is an extremely rare condition but it is remarkable for its similarity to bullous pemphigoid clinically, histologically and immunologically. It can occur at any time during pregnancy and usually disappears some time after delivery. It tends to recur with each successive pregnancy and oral contraceptives can precipitate exacerbations (see Fig. 15.35). Fetal mortality and morbidity is increased.

Clinically, an itchy eruption occurs which consists of tense vesicles or bullae, often symmetrically distributed over the abdomen, back, buttocks and arms, although any site may be involved. Secondary sepsis may occur and urticarial lesions are common. Treatment with systemic steroids is normally necessary.

Impetigo Herpetiformis

This is also an extremely rare condition which is identical in its clinical manifestations to generalized pustular psoriasis and may occur in any pregnancy. It is a very serious condition associated both with fetal and maternal mortality.

18 Collagen Vascular Disorders and Vasculitis

LUPUS ERYTHEMATOSUS

This is a spectrum of disorders which varies from chronic discoid lupus erythematosus (which is completely confined to the skin) to a potentially fatal multisystem disease. The skin eruptions in systemic lupus erythematosus may sometimes be identical to those of the discoid variety. In between the two poles there is a subacute or widespread cutaneous group which is associated with immunological abnormalities and occasionally may develop into the systemic form of disease. Originally known as collagen vascular disorders, various autoimmune factors have been demonstrated, particularly antibodies to nuclear material and to DNA. Hypocomplementaemia, hypergamma-globulinaemia, positive rheumatoid factor, positive Wasserman reactions and LE cells are other abnormal immunological findings. Immunofluorescence reveals deposits of immuno-globulin in the basement membrane of involved and uninvolved sun-damaged skin. Most of these tests, except the immuno-fluorescence, are negative in the chronic discoid variety of lupus erythematosus.

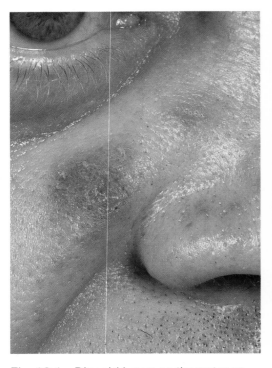

Fig. 18.1 Discoid lupus erythematosus. The cheeks are the most commonly affected site.

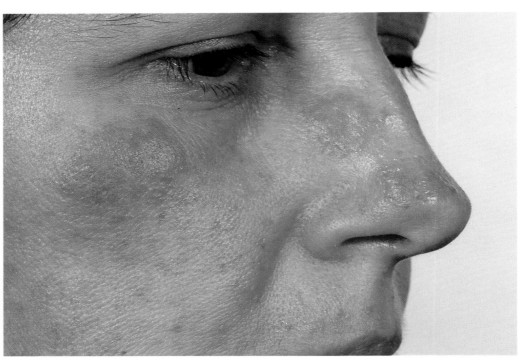

Fig. 18.2 Discoid lupus erythematosus. Well-defined, red, raised, disc-like plaques occur over the cheeks and nose.

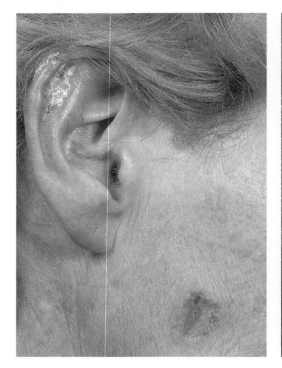

Fig. 18.3 Discoid lupus erythematosus. The ears and cheeks are common sites of involvement. Scaling is prominent.

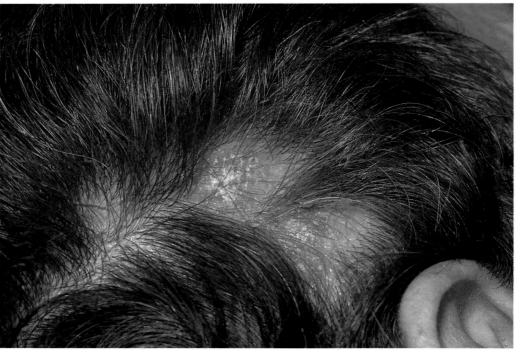

Fig. 18.4 Discoid lupus erythematosus. In the scalp there is complete loss of hair with erythema and scaling.

Chronic Discoid Lupus Erythematosus

This disorder is more common in women and frequently starts in early adult life. The eruption is largely confined to the face and scalp and ultra-violet light irradiation is an important factor in precipitating attacks. The condition is chronic and cosmetically disfiguring. It consists of well-defined disc-like plaques occurring over the cheeks (Fig. 18.1), the bridge of the nose (Fig. 18.2), forehead, preauricular area, ears (Fig. 18.3) and scalp (Fig. 18.4). Sometimes the lips and occasionally the inside of the mouth are involved (Figs. 18.5 and 18.6). The plaques are initially red and raised and sometimes oedematous (Fig. 18.7). Healing follows centrally with scaling, hyperkeratosis (Fig. 18.8) and sometimes scarring (Fig. 18.9). In the scalp this leads to

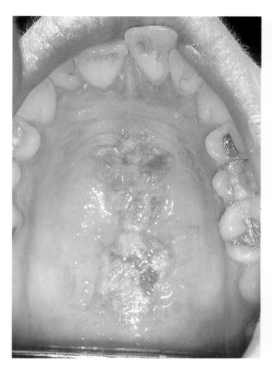

Fig. 18.5 Discoid lupus erythematosus. Well-defined discoid plaques may occur in the mouth.

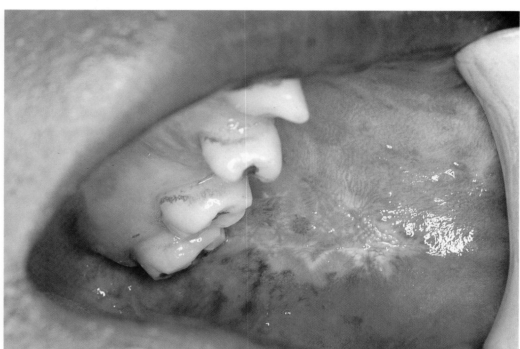

Fig. 18.6 Discoid lupus erythematosus. The diagnosis can be established by biopsy.

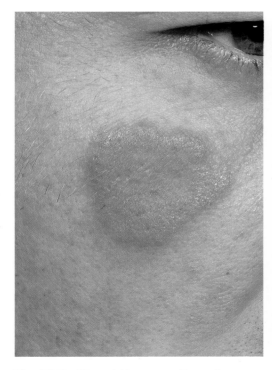

Fig. 18.7 Discoid lupus erythematosus. Initially the lesions may be red and oedematous.

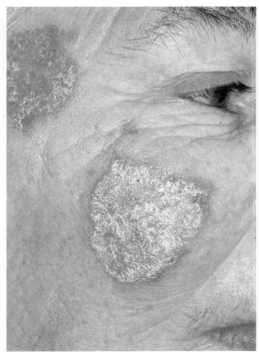

Fig. 18.8 Discoid lupus erythematosus. The lesions may have a thick and adherent scale.

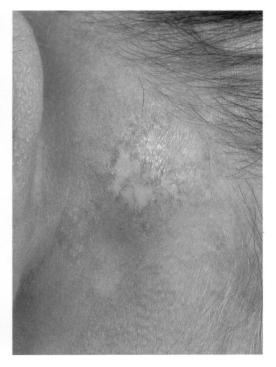

Fig. 18.9 Discoid lupus erythematosus. This lesion has resulted in scarring behind the ear.

18.3

permanent loss of hair (Fig. 18.10). The margin of the eruption is often hyperpigmented and there is depigmentation centrally (Fig. 18.11). Very occasionally the deep dermis and subcutis are affected such that nodules occur under the otherwise apparently normal skin. Destructive subcutaneous atrophy occurs with healing. This is known as *lupus erythematosus profundus* (Fig. 18.12).

The patient with chronic discoid lupus erythematosus is otherwise perfectly well. The disorder is limited to the skin and there are no antinuclear antibodies present. The histology (Figs. 18.13–18.17) reveals an admixture of lymphocytes and histiocytes, particularly around the skin appendages with oedema and hyalinization of the connective tissue. In the

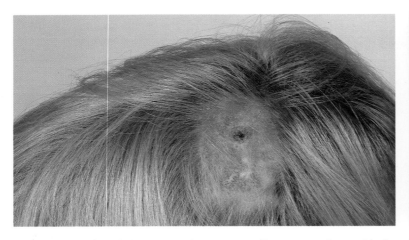

Fig. 18.10 Discoid lupus erythematosus. Permanent loss of hair results from scarring discoid lupus in the scalp.

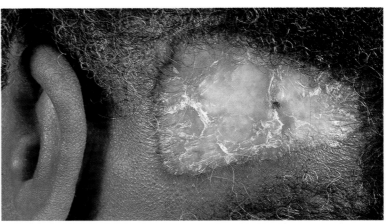

Fig. 18.11 Discoid lupus erythematosus. The margin of the eruption is often hyperpigmented. There is scarring centrally. By courtesy of St. Mary's Hospital.

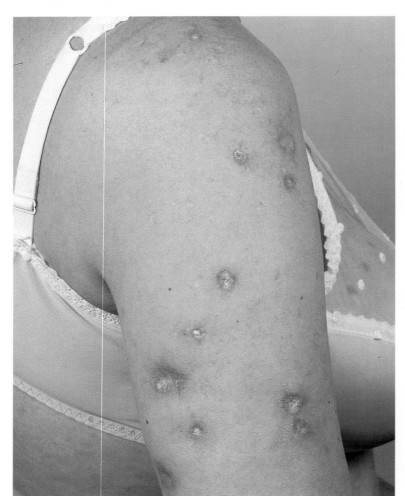

Fig. 18.12 Lupus erythematosus profundus. Subcutaneous atrophy results from lupus in the deep dermis and subcutis. By courtesy of Dr. R.H. Marten.

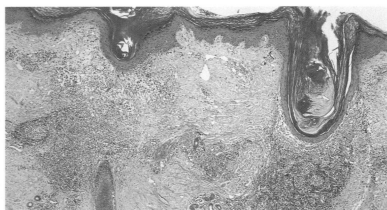

Fig. 18.13 Discoid lupus erythematosus. Low power view showing hyperkeratosis and conspicuous follicular plugging. A heavy chronic inflammatory cell infiltrate surrounds the adnexae.

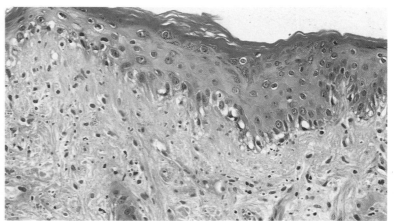

Fig. 18.14 Discoid lupus erythematosus. Marked basal cell hydropic degeneration is evident. Epidermal atrophy is present on the left side of this picture. Extravasated red blood cells are conspicuous in the papillary dermis.

epidermis there is damage to the basal cell layer with 'liquefaction degeneration' of individual cells, atrophy and hyperkeratosis with follicular plugging.

Widespread Chronic Discoid Lupus Erythematosus
In this group the skin is more widely involved and immunological abnormalities are demonstrable. Discoid lesions occur not only on the face (Fig. 18.18), but also on the upper limbs, particularly the forearms and hands (Fig. 18.19), and on the shoulders and back. These more widespread lesions (Fig. 18.20) are usually precipitated by exposure to ultra-violet light. Many patients are very susceptible to cold and Raynaud's phenomenon may occur.

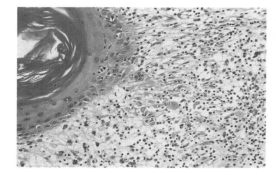

Fig. 18.15 Discoid lupus erythematosus. In addition to a heavy lymphocytic infiltrate and conspicuous melanophages, the superficial dermis contains scattered intensely eosinophilic degenerate keratinocytes (cytoid bodies) – markers of prior epidermal damage.

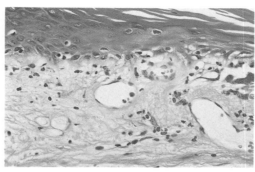

Fig. 18.16 Discoid lupus erythematosus. This field shows basal cell hydropic degeneration, scattered melanophages (indicating previous damage to melanocytes) and prominent ectatic blood vessels.

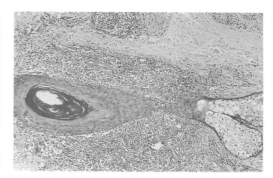

Fig. 18.17 Discoid lupus erythematosus. A heavy lymphocytic infiltrate surrounds this pilosebaceous unit.

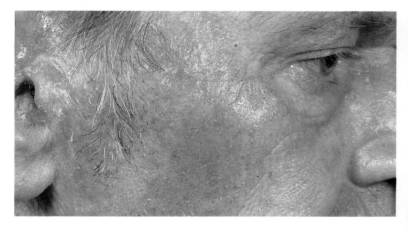

Fig. 18.18 Widespread discoid lupus erythematosus. Although the antinuclear factor may be weakly positive in the widespread forms of discoid lupus, the disease rarely becomes systemic.

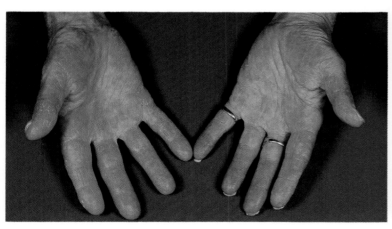

Fig. 18.19 Widespread chronic discoid lupus erythematosus. The lesions may be extensive and involve the palms.

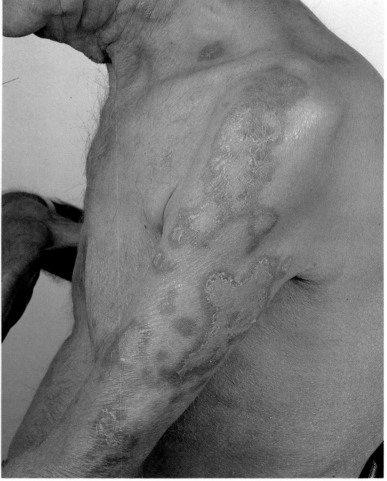

Fig. 18.20 Widespread chronic discoid lupus erythematosus. This is the same patient as in Fig. 18.19.

18.5

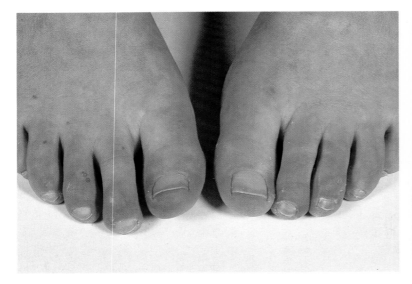

Fig. 18.21 Lupus pernio. Chilblain-like, painful purple lesions occur on the extremities.

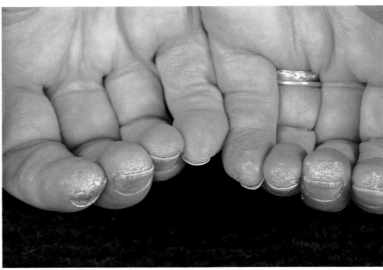

Fig. 18.22 Lupus pernio. Hyperkeratotic lesions occur under the finger tips. By courtesy of St. Mary's Hospital.

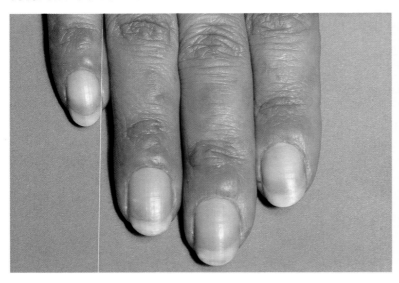

Fig. 18.23 Lupus pernio. Painful red plaques may occur on the fingers in association with exposure to cold weather.

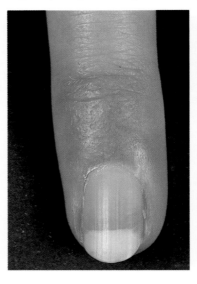

Fig. 18.24 Lupus pernio. Nailfold erythema is characteristic of collagen vascular disorders.

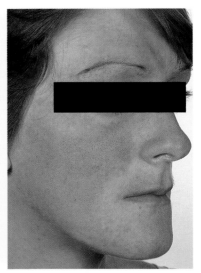

Fig. 18.25 Systemic lupus erythematosus. A diffuse erythema occurs over the forehead, cheeks and nose.

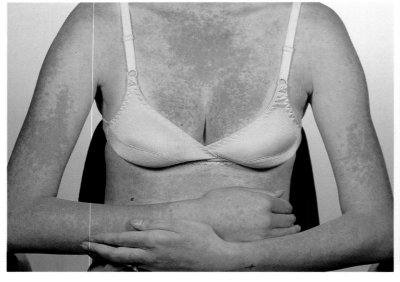

Fig. 18.26 Systemic lupus erythematosus. Both cutaneous and systemic lupus erythematosus may be exacerbated by strong sunlight. A diffuse blotchy erythema has occurred in the sun-exposed skin.

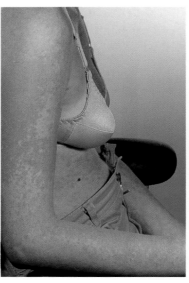

Fig. 18.27 Systemic lupus erythematosus. A diffuse alopecia is common in systemic disease and is often an indicator of disease activity.

Painful, red, vasculitic lesions known as *lupus pernio* or chilblain-type lupus occur on the hands and feet, particularly on the tips (Figs. 18.21 and 18.22) and the backs of the digits (Fig. 18.23). Nailfold erythema may be present (Fig. 18.24). It very occasionally may develop into systemic lupus erythematosus.

Systemic Lupus Erythematosus

This is a multisystem disease which often, but not always, affects the skin. The cutaneous involvement is characteristic and usually suggests the diagnosis which can be confirmed by the finding of antinuclear antibodies. The condition affects all races and is much more common in young women. It runs a remitting and relapsing course. The disorder is particularly precipitated by strong sunlight, but infection, physical or mental stress, menstruation, trauma to the skin and drugs may all be relevant. The disease affects the lungs, the central nervous system, the joints and the kidneys. The degree of the latter frequently determines the outcome. Fatigue is characteristic. Fever, lymphadenopathy, haemolytic anaemia, leucopenia and thrombocytopenia are common. The American Rheumatism Association has produced criteria based on these abnormalities which act as guidelines to establishing the diagnosis.

The skin manifestations may be identical to those occurring in chronic discoid lupus erythematosus. Often, however, there is an erythema over the cheeks and bridge of the nose (so-called 'butterfly rash') which heals without scarring (Fig. 18.25). A more widespread maculopapular eruption occurs on light-exposed areas, particularly the face, the 'V' of the neck and the arms (Fig. 18.26). Lupus pernio and a vasculitis affecting the extensor surfaces of the forearms, dorsa of the hands, small joints of the fingers, palms and periungual skin may occur. A diffuse alopecia is common (Fig. 18.27). The hair regrows as the disorder remits and is a good indication of disease activity. The diagnosis is confirmed by the finding of auto-antibodies (particularly to double-stranded DNA).

Management of Lupus Erythematosus

Clearly the management depends upon the severity of the disease. Systemic corticosteroids may be life-saving in systemic cases but are not indicated in the average case of discoid lupus erythematosus. Precipitating factors such as ultra-violet light should be strictly avoided, and photoprotective sun screens advised. Cold weather should be prepared for with warm clothing and central heating. Unnecessary medications such as sulphonamides or pyrazolones which are known to worsen the disease should not be given. Pregnancy and oral contraceptives may exacerbate the systemic disease.

Powerful topical corticosteroids are effective for chronic discoid lesions. Antimalarials may benefit more widespread lesions, particularly chloroquine and mepacrine. However, it must be remembered that chloroquine can cause retinal damage and mepacrine causes pigmentation, so these should be used with care. Immunosuppressives such as azathioprine may have a steroid sparing effect in systemic cases, but systemic steroids remain the mainstay of therapy for these cases.

DERMATOMYOSITIS

This is a rare disease and is about four times less common than systemic lupus erythematosus. It has a distinctive cutaneous eruption which is associated with a myositis affecting primarily the proximal limb muscles. The skin rash may precede the myositis by some months and very occasionally by years and the myositis may occur without cutaneous findings, in which case the disease is known as polymyositis. The cause is unknown but in the adult variety of the disease a significant proportion of patients have an underlying carcinoma. There are sometimes overlapping features of both lupus erythematosus and scleroderma, in which case the disease complex is known as mixed connective tissue disease.

The skin rash is usually diagnostic if there is periorbital oedema and a mauve erythema (Figs. 18.28 and 18.29). This

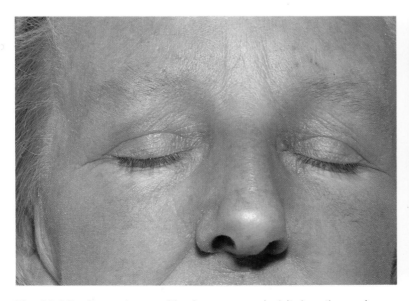

Fig. 18.28 Dermatomyositis. A mauve periorbital erythema is characteristic of dermatomyositis.

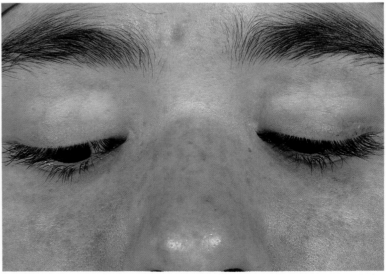

Fig. 18.29 Dermatomyositis. The changes may be subtle. Here the erythema is most marked over and under her left eye.

discoloration may extend to the cheeks (Fig. 18.30), forehead, around the neck (Fig. 18.31) and onto the extensor surfaces of the limbs (Fig. 18.32). A distinctive papular erythema occurs over the knuckles (Figs. 18.33 and 18.34), known as Gottron's sign. This erythema may also occur on the elbows, knees (Fig. 18.35) and ankles. Periungual erythema (Fig. 18.36) with cuticular splinter haemorrhages (Fig. 18.37) may also occur in lupus erythematosus, but are a helpful additional physical sign. The lesions may be followed by atrophic and pigmentary changes, so-called poikiloderma.

The affected muscles are sore and weak. The patient has difficulty combing the hair, climbing stairs, getting up from a chair and raising the neck when in bed, but distal muscle function is usually well preserved. Polyarthralgia may also be present.

The onset of the disease may be in childhood or in adult life. The juvenile variety may spontaneously remit especially if it is of acute onset. Alternatively, it may relapse and remit and the prognosis depends on the degree of muscle involvement and consequent atrophy. The cause of death is respiratory failure or aspiration of food or secretions due to respiratory muscle or pharyngeal involvement. Widespread calcinosis may occur in involved muscles (Fig. 18.38). In the adult, it is mandatory to search for an underlying malignancy: the most common are carcinoma of the lung, ovary, breast, stomach and cervix. Successful treatment of the malignancy can cure the dermato-

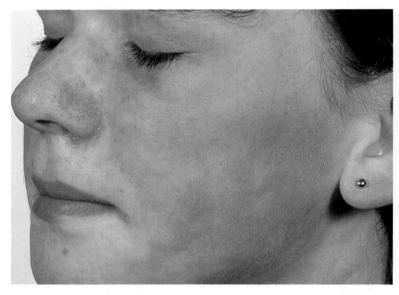

Fig. 18.30   Dermatomyositis. The eruption may spread onto the cheeks, in which case it is indistinguishable from systemic lupus erythematosus. Eyelid involvement is, however, characteristic.

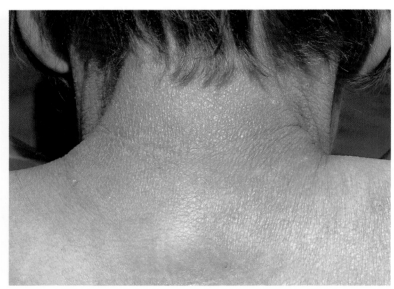

Fig. 18.31   Dermatomyositis. A mauve discoloration is characteristic.

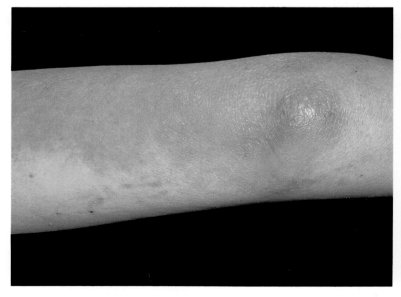

Fig. 18.32   Dermatomyositis. The arms and particularly the elbows are involved with a persistent erythema.

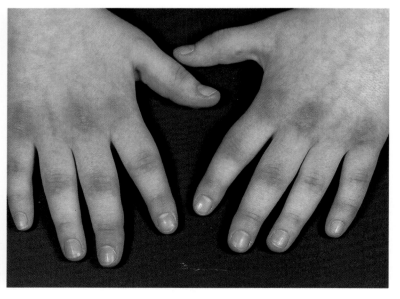

Fig. 18.33   Dermatomyositis. Erythematous papules over the small joints of the fingers are characteristic of this disease.

myositis. The incidence of malignant disease underlying dermatomyositis varies in different series, but it is certainly thought to be as high as 25%. Occasionally the malignancy may not be detectable until some years after the development of the disease. In patients where a malignancy is not found, management is the same as that for the juvenile type.

There is no specific diagnostic test for dermatomyositis comparable to the antinuclear antibodies in lupus erythematosus. The ESR may or may not be raised and the ANA may be positive in those with dermatomyositis as part of mixed connective tissue disease, but often is negative in dermatomyositis alone. The pattern of nuclear fluorescence is homogeneous or speckled rather than the rim fluorescence of lupus erythematosus.

Muscle enzymes, the aldolases, glutamic oxaloacetic transaminases, lactic dehydrogenases and creatine phosphokinases are raised if myositis is present. An electromyogram and muscle biopsy are important confirmatory tests.

Management of Dermatomyositis

Systemic glucocorticosteroids have profoundly influenced the prognosis of this disease and complete remissions may be produced with judicious use of the drugs. The usual starting dose is 60mg prednisolone and this is slowly reduced as muscle function returns and the enzymes are decreased. Methotrexate is sometimes used in addition. Rest is essential and physiotherapy is important to prevent contractures and wasting.

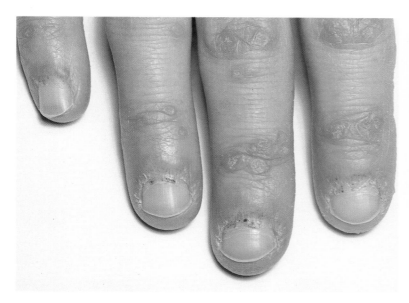

Fig. 18.34   Dermatomyositis. The mauve papules over the knuckles are known as Gottron's sign.

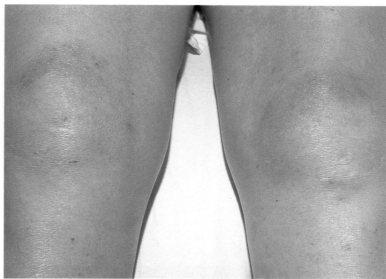

Fig. 18.35   Dermatomyositis. The knees may be affected.

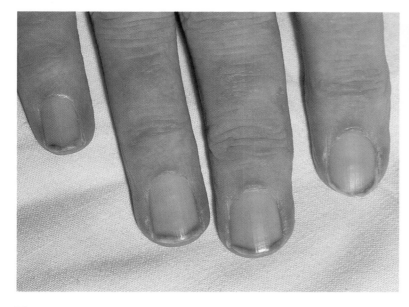

Fig. 18.36   Dermatomyositis. Periungual erythema is suggestive of dermatomyositis, but not diagnostic of this disease. Similar changes may be seen in systemic lupus erythematosus.

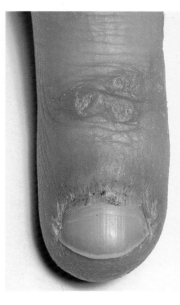

Fig. 18.37   Dermatomyositis. Periungual telangiectasia and cuticular splinter haemorrhages are present.

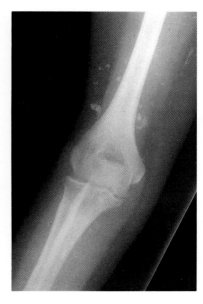

Fig. 18.38   Dermatomyositis. Widespread calcinosis may occur in affected muscles. By courtesy of St. Mary's Hospital.

SCLERODERMA

This is an uncommon disorder of unknown aetiology affecting women much more frequently than men. The condition involves not only the skin but also the gastrointestinal tract, heart, lungs and kidneys, although there is individual variation in the degree of damage to these organs and the prognosis is determined accordingly. Pathologically there is excess collagen deposition (Fig. 18.39) and arterial intimal thickening and often occlusion (Fig. 18.40). The most common presenting feature in the skin is Raynaud's phenomenon. On exposure to cold the fingers go white due to intense arteriolar vasoconstriction, then blue from cyanosis and lastly red, warm and painful following reactive vasodilation. There may be a chronic non-pitting oedema of the fingers. Some patients have pain and stiffness in the joints. Subsequent structural changes may take place in the hands so that a situation of acrosclerosis occurs (Fig. 18.41). The skin overlying the subcutaneous tissue becomes tethered so that it has a hardened (sclerotic) feel. There is loss of the normal skin creases (Fig. 18.42) and tapering of the fingers and thumbs due to atrophy of the pulp of the tips. Digital ischaemia leads to cutaneous infarction and ulceration and possibly gangrene of

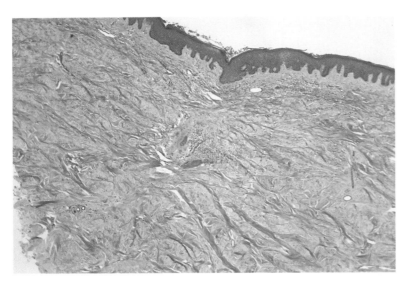

Fig. 18.39 Scleroderma. The typical alterations are seen in this low power view. The reticular dermis is grossly expanded by densely packed, broad bundles of relatively acellular collagen. Cutaneous appendages are markedly reduced in number and an atrophic hair follicle is seen in the middle of the picture. Eccrine sweat ducts are entrapped and compressed by the dense fibrous tissue. It is not possible to distinguish between morphoea and scleroderma using routine light microscopy.

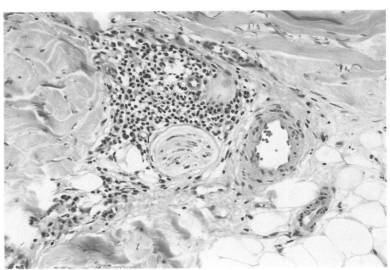

Fig. 18.40 Scleroderma. An inflammatory cell infiltrate often surrounds the vasculature, as seen in this field.

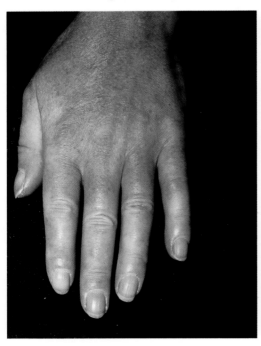

Fig. 18.41 Scleroderma. The condition frequently presents as Raynaud's phenomenon. The skin goes white in response to cold. Ultimately sclerodactyly results, with tapering of the fingers. By courtesy of St. Mary's Hospital.

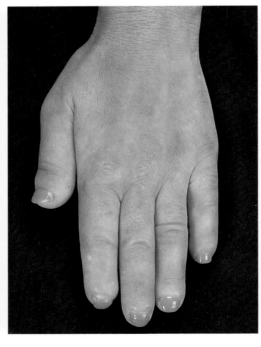

Fig. 18.42 Scleroderma. There is loss of the normal skin creases and loss of the pulp in the finger tips. By courtesy of St. John's Hospital for Diseases of the Skin.

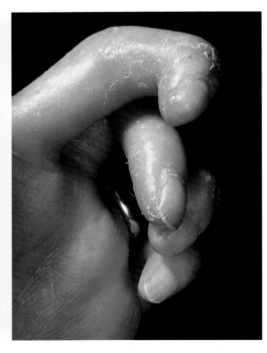

Fig. 18.43 Scleroderma. There is loss of the normal skin creases. The skin is tethered and hardened. Deformity has resulted. Finger tip vessel occlusion leads to ulceration, gangrene and loss of the digits. By courtesy of St. Mary's Hospital.

the finger tips. Deformity (Fig. 18.43) and dysfunction of the fingers results. The extent of this damage varies between patients. The skin of the face is also involved (Fig. 18.44). There is loss of the normal skin lines on the forehead, the skin feels hardened and it becomes impossible for the examiner to pinch the skin. There is loss of subcutaneous tissue so that the nose has a beak-like appearance. The oral aperture becomes smaller and there is difficulty in opening it to its full extent. Furrows radiating out from the mouth are typical.

Additional features are matt-like telangiectasia on the face and calcinosis, particularly in the fingers but also in the soft tissues elsewhere. Hirsutism and hyperpigmentation regularly accompany the disease. It has been said that patients with calcinosis, Raynaud's phenomenon, sclerodactyly and telangiectases (the CRST syndrome) have a more favourable prognosis.

Certainly there is great variation in the prognosis of this distressing disease. The outcome is determined by the degree of systemic organ involvement. Pulmonary disease may result in terminal fibrosis. Pericarditis, effusions, conduction defects and heart failure are fairly common cardiac complications. Renal failure and hypertension may occur. In the gastro-intestinal tract loss of peristalsis leads to difficulty swallowing and there may be malabsorption due to small bowel involvement. Diverticula may occur in the large gut.

The cause is quite unknown. There are no diagnostic tests so the diagnosis is a clinical one. However, it is related to rheumatoid arthritis, lupus erythematosus and dermatomyositis in that features of them all occur in mixed connective tissue disease. Other autoimmune disorders such as Hashimoto's thyroiditis and Sjögren's syndrome may occur in addition, and the rheumatoid factor and antinuclear antibodies are positive in a percentage of patients.

A scleroderma-like condition with systemic involvement including angiosarcoma of the liver occurs in workers exposed to vinyl chloride, particularly those who clean the reactors.

Scleroderma-like changes have also been described in patients with chronic graft versus host reaction following successful bone marrow transplants for a variety of disorders which include aplastic anaemia, acute leukemia and immuno-deficiency disease. These findings may lead to a better understanding of scleroderma in the future.

Treatment is most unsatisfactory, but systemic steroids, azathioprine, penicillamine and vasodilators are among a large number of drugs which have been tried in this disease. Intra-arterial injection of a variety of agents including prostaglandins have also been assayed.

MIXED CONNECTIVE TISSUE DISEASE

This is an overlap syndrome with features of rheumatoid arthritis, scleroderma, lupus erythematosus, dermatomyositis or polyarteritis nodosa. Many have a specific antibody to an extractable nuclear antigen (ENA) as well as a positive speckled antinuclear antibody. Raynaud's phenomenon and myositis are common, but skin lesions other than hair loss are less so. The condition is said to be less aggressive than most connective tissue disorders because the kidneys are infrequently involved and the condition responds well to systemic steroids.

MORPHOEA

This condition is described here in conjunction with scleroderma because occasionally patients with systemic sclerosis have patches of localized scleroderma (morphoea) in association with the typical cutaneous changes of scleroderma. However, in patients presenting with morphoea the likelihood of developing scleroderma is practically nil. A single oval or round plaque occurs with a smooth shiny surface (Fig. 18.45) and the skin is tethered as in scleroderma. There is loss of hair in the area and the margin is initially a lilac colour (Fig. 18.46), although it subsequently becomes brown. The plaque occurs anywhere on the body but particularly on the thighs, upper arms and trunk.

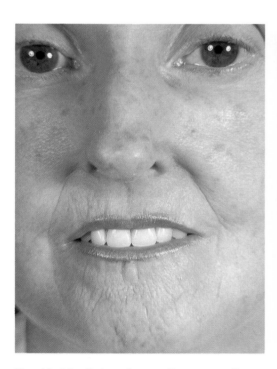

Fig. 18.44   Scleroderma. Furrows radiate out from the mouth which becomes shrunken. Matt-like telangiectasia may occur. The skin creases are lost. By courtesy of St. Mary's Hospital.

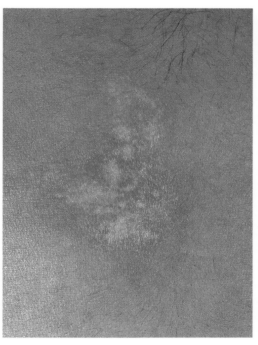

Fig. 18.45   Morphoea. A solitary sclerotic patch is present. The skin is tethered as in scleroderma.

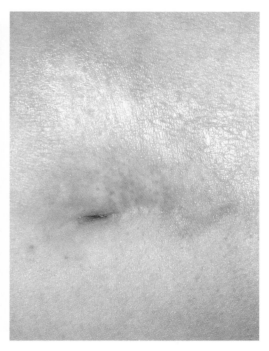

Fig. 18.46   Morphoea. The plaque has a shiny smooth surface. It is tethered. A lilac margin is characteristic.

After many years it may disappear. Linear forms do occur, particularly on the scalp and face with concomitant loss of subcutaneous tissue so that considerable cosmetic deformity results (Fig. 18.47). In this area the appearance has been likened to a 'coup de sabre'. Rarely, generalized involvement (Fig. 18.48) of the skin occurs with plaques of morphoea but without any systemic involvement or involvement of the extremities, such as the fingers, as in scleroderma. The cause is unknown and there is no effective treatment.

LICHEN SCLEROSUS ET ATROPHICUS

This is also an unusual but distinctive condition. There is no relationship with scleroderma, but the cutaneous lesions are scleroderma-like and hence the disorder is described here. It particularly occurs on the genitalia and around the anus and may or may not be associated with lesions elsewhere.

In the middle-aged female shiny, white and smooth-surfaced papules, which coalesce, occur in a symmetrical and well-defined manner around the vulva and the anus (Figs. 18.49 and 18.50). The papules may spread onto the skin of the inner aspect

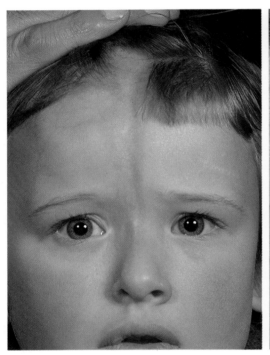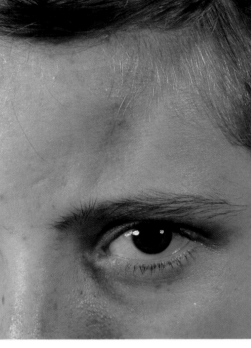

Fig. 18.47 Coup de sabre. Linear morphoea in the scalp and on the forehead leaves considerable deformity due to loss of subcutaneous tissue. It has been likened to a blow from a sabre.

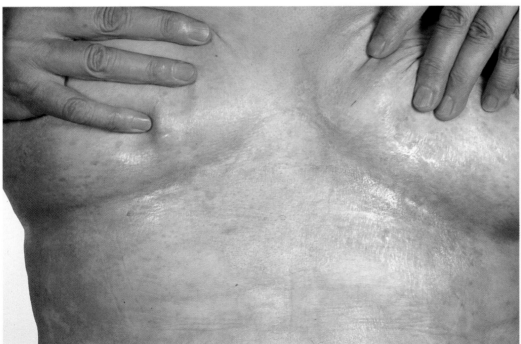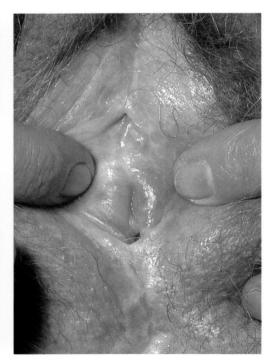

Fig. 18.48 Generalized morphoea. Widespread sclerodermatous plaques may occur, but without involvement of the fingers as in scleroderma.

Fig. 18.49 Lichen sclerosus et atrophicus. Ivory-white, shiny papules coalesce and surround the vulva. By courtesy of St. Mary's Hospital.

of the thighs. The lesions are atrophic and small telangiectasia may be seen. Because of the site and the attendant complications of friction, the area may become moist and macerated and break down. It is extremely pruritic. The accompanying atrophy of the skin leads to shrinkage of the vulval tissue so that there is obliteration of the normal features of the labia majora and minora and the introitus may become very small indeed. Very occasionally carcinomatous change may occur.

In the male the condition is sometimes known as *balanitis xerotica obliterans*. Identical ivory-white papules (Fig. 18.51) with telangiectasia occur on the foreskin and glans of the penis. The atrophy may lead to meatal stenosis (Fig. 18.52) and difficulty with micturition. It may become impossible to retract the foreskin and phimosis may occur. Once again, but extremely rarely, squamous cell carcinomatous changes may arise.

The extra-mucosal changes consist of white atrophic papules which coalesce into plaques (Fig. 18.53) occurring, usually symmetrically, on the fronts of the wrists (Fig. 18.54), neck, upper back, shoulders and around the umbilicus. They may occur in the absence of genital lesions.

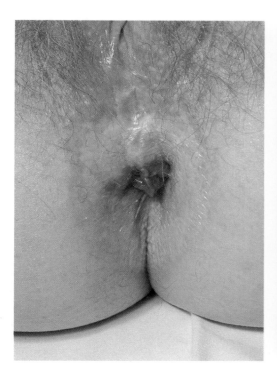

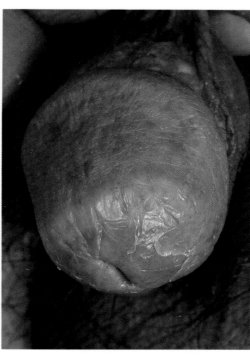

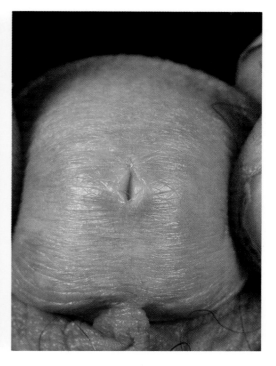

Fig. 18.50 Lichen sclerosus et atrophicus. Ivory-white, shiny papules coalesce and surround the anus. The condition is often very pruritic. By courtesy of St. Mary's Hospital.

Fig. 18.51 Balanitis xerotica obliterans. White atrophic patches occur on the glans.

Fig. 18.52 Balanitis xerotica obliterans. Meatal stenosis may result from lichen sclerosus et atrophicus.

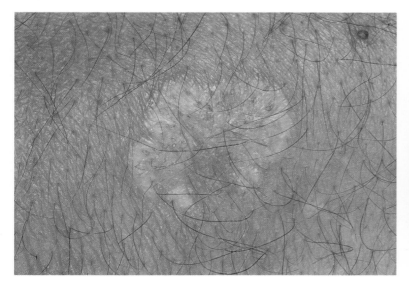

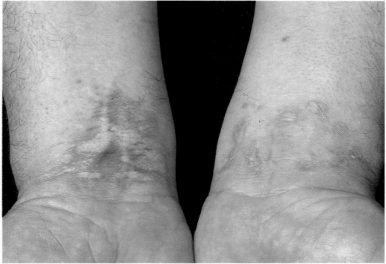

Fig. 18.53 Lichen sclerosus et atrophicus. White atrophic papules coalesce into plaques.

Fig. 18.54 Lichen sclerosus et atrophicus. Ivory-white papules surrounded by lilac occur symmetrically, especially on the wrists. By courtesy of St. Mary's Hospital.

The typical histological features comprise hyperkeratosis, variable epidermal atrophy and acanthosis, basal cell hydropic degeneration and hyalinization of the lamina propria or superficial dermis (Figs. 18.55–18.58).

The cause of this condition is compeletely unknown. Topical steroids sometimes help to alleviate genital soreness or discomfort. Surgery may be necessary for stenotic problems.

RELAPSING POLYCHONDRITIS

This is a rare inflammatory and subsequently destructive disease involving cartilaginous structures both in the joints and elsewhere. It is thought to be an autoimmune disorder and antibodies to mucopolysaccharides have been demonstrated.

The disorder can affect any cartilaginous structure, especially the nose, ears, joints, costochondral junction and larynx. The initial symptoms are of recurrent attacks of redness, tenderness and swelling of the affected area. The involvement of the ears (Fig. 18.59) and nose make a very characteristic picture and this is when the diagnosis is usually made. (The condition should be distinguished from *chondrodermatitis nodularis helicis* in which a single painful inflammatory nodule (Fig. 18.60) is localized to the helix or anti-helix.)

The patient is usually unwell and has a fever, anaemia and weight loss. Involvement and obstruction of the trachea and bronchial tree lead to respiratory difficulties and infection.

The cause of the condition is not known but it does respond to systemic steroids.

VASCULITIS

This is a term used to describe a reactive inflammatory condition of blood vessels which may affect the skin and various internal organs; classification depends on the size of the blood vessel and the predominant inflammatory cell involved. The cause of many of the diseases is unknown and a classification based on clinical pattern is used here.

ALLERGIC VASCULITIS (Anaphylactoid Purpura)

This form of vasculitis affects the superficial dermal capillaries, venules and small arterioles. Neutrophils are found in and around the blood vessels (leucocytolastic vasculitis). Many are degenerate and an appearance known as 'nuclear dust' is characteristic. There is fibrinoid necrosis of the vessels and surrounding tissues with extravasation of red blood cells (Figs. 18.61–18.63).

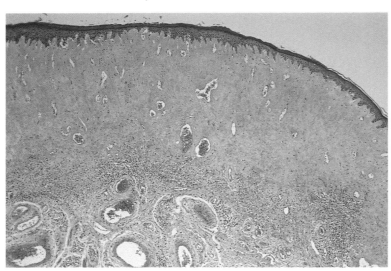

Fig. 18.55 Lichen sclerosus et atrophicus. Penile lesions showing marked hyperkeratosis, variable epidermal atrophy and irregular acanthosis. There is marked band-like hyalinization of the lamina propria and a chronic inflammatory cell infiltrate.

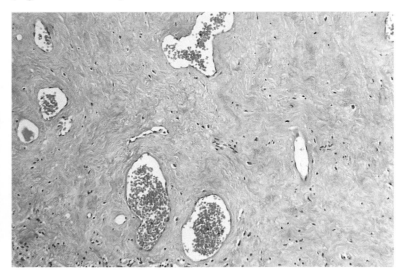

Fig. 18.56 Lichen sclerosus et atrophicus. In this field, conspicuous ectatic blood vessels are evident.

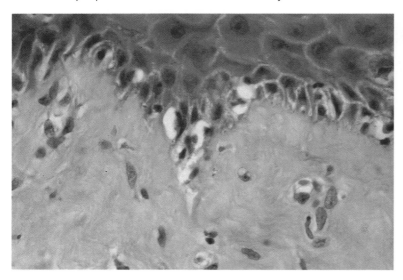

Fig. 18.57 Lichen sclerosus et atrophicus. Basal cell hydropic degeneration is seen on the right side of this high power view.

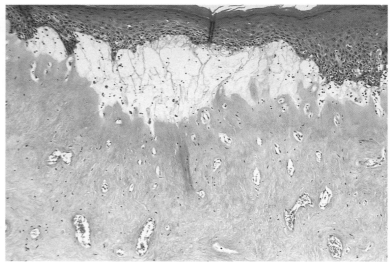

Fig. 18.58 Lichen sclerosus et atrophicus. Occasionally, intense oedema may result in subepidermal vesiculation.

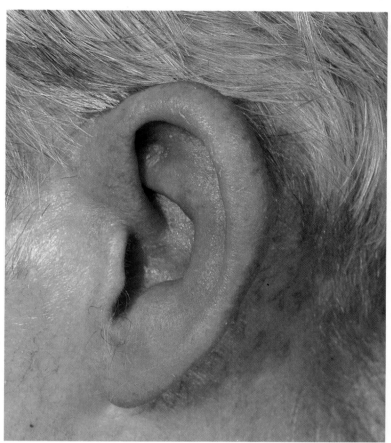

Fig. 18.59 Relapsing polychondritis. The upper helix is thickened. This patient had had recurrent attacks of redness, tenderness and swelling. By courtesy of Dr. A.C. Pembroke.

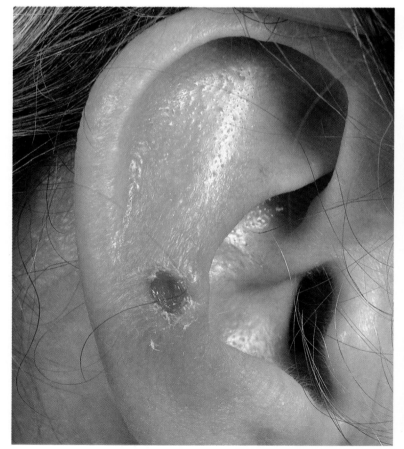

Fig. 18.60 Chondrodermatitis helicis nodularis. A single tender inflamed nodule is present on the outer helix. The condition probably results from repeated prolonged pressure on the helix or anti-helix whilst asleep.

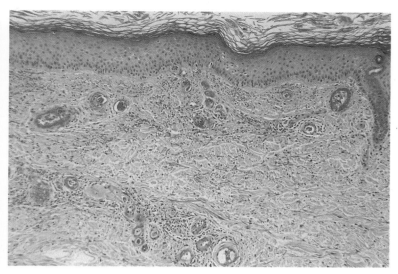

Fig. 18.61 Leucocytoclastic vasculitis. In this example of Henoch-Schönlein purpura, characteristic changes are present. The small blood vessels of both the papillary and reticular dermis are dilated and show florid fibrinoid necrosis. There is marked extravasation of red blood cells into the connective tissue.

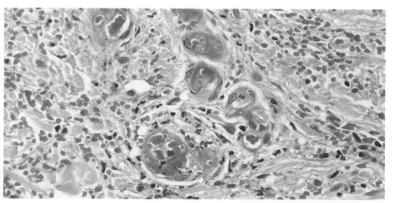

Fig. 18.62 Leucocytoclastic vasculitis. High power view to show partially occluded vessels and free red blood cells.

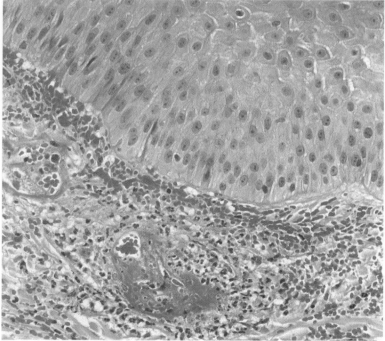

Fig. 18.63 Leucocytoclastic vasculitis. High power view to show infiltration of the venule wall and perivascular connective tissue by large numbers of neutrophil polymorphs. Note the presence of darkly staining nuclear dust (leucocytoclasis).

18.15

The condition may affect the skin alone or frequently also the joints, gastrointestinal tract and kidneys giving rise to haematuria (either macroscopic or microscopic), gastrointestinal haemorrhage and joint pains. The condition is then known as *Henoch-Schönlein purpura*. It is quite common in children. The skin rash is polymorphic and occurs largely on dependent areas such as the legs (Fig. 18.64), feet and ankles (Fig. 18.65), and the buttocks (Fig. 18.66). The hands, arms, face and trunk are sometimes affected. The lesions are essentially purpuric, but palpable lesions (Fig. 18.67) such as pustules, vesicles and

bullae occur with consequent necrosis and ulceration. In addition, urticarial wheals may be seen (Figs. 18.68 and 18.69). The degree of damage depends on the severity of the vasculitis. The lesions are painful and there is swelling of the peripheries, particularly the ankles, secondary to the inflammation.

It is important to establish the cause of the vasculitis (Fig. 18.70). The recent vogue has been to regard the disorder as part of an immune complex disease. Probably the most common identifiable antigen is the streptococcus.

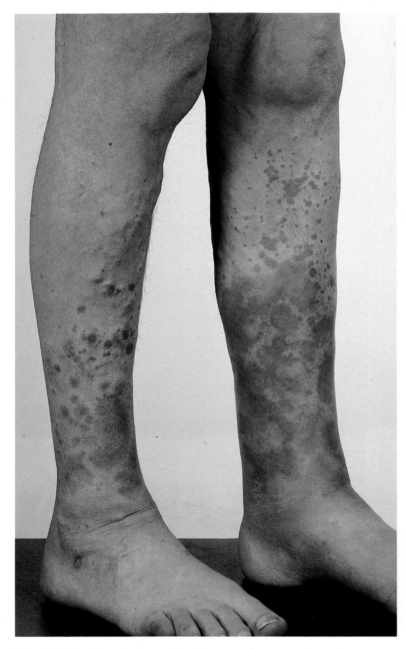

Fig. 18.64 Allergic vasculitis. The eruption occurs on the dependent parts especially the lower legs and feet.

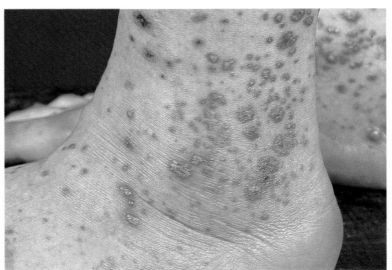

Fig. 18.65 Allergic vasculitis. Palpable purpuric lesions may be associated with renal, joint or gastrointestinal vasculitis when the symptoms complex is known as Henoch-Schönlein purpura. By courtesy of St. Mary's Hospital.

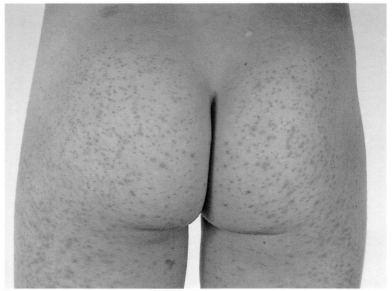

Fig. 18.66 Allergic vasculitis. Purpuric lesions on the buttocks are characteristic of Henoch-Schönlein purpura.

Those with Henoch-Schönlein purpura generally recover, but the prognosis in allergic vasculitis is related to the degree of renal damage. In a significant proportion of patients no cause is found and the disease will run a remittent, relapsing course. Bed rest and anti-inflammatory drugs are useful but systemic corticosteroids may be necessary to control exacerbations.

Fig. 18.67 Allergic vasculitis. Although urticarial, the lesions have a purpuric centre which suggests a vasculitic process.

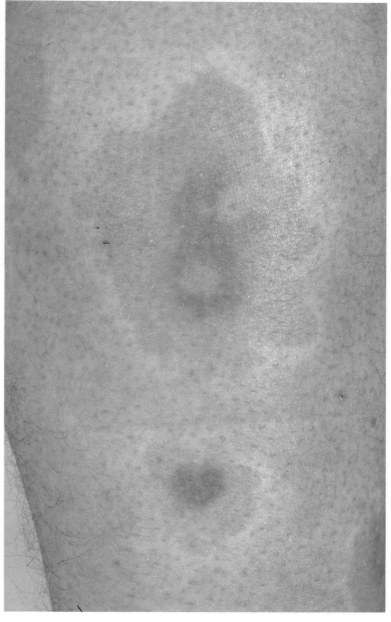

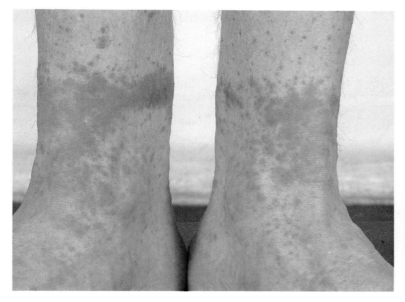

Fig. 18.68 Allergic vasculitis. Coalescent purpuric papules are present around the ankles.

Fig. 18.69 Allergic vasculitis. Urticarial lesions persist for several days unlike ordinary urticaria. Biopsy revealed a vasculitis.

Causes of Allergic Vasculitis

Infections	Drugs	Dysproteinaemias	Neoplasia	Collagen vascular disorders
Streptococcus	Sulphonamides	Cryoglobulinaemia	Hodgkin's disease	Sjögren's syndrome
Mycobacterium leprae	Penicillin	Macroglobulinaemia	Non-Hodgkin's lymphoma	Systemic lupus erythematosus
Hepatitis B virus	Others		Chronic lymphocytic leukaemia	Rheumatoid arthritis

Fig. 18.70 Causes of allergic vasculitis.

POLYARTERITIS NODOSA

This is a rare, very serious systemic disorder in which the skin is only sometimes involved. There is a necrotizing vasculitis of small and medium-sized vessels which consequently leads to thrombosis and infarction, embolism or rupture of the vessel wall (Fig. 18.71).

The condition usually begins in middle-age. The patient is unwell, has fever, loses weight and suffers from aching of the limbs and abdominal pain. Specific symptoms and signs are related to the organs involved. The gastrointestinal tract, pancreas, kidney, heart and muscles are most commonly affected. Thus, gangrene of the bowel, peritonitis, perforation and haemorrhage may occur. Pancreatitis is common, renal involvement is constant and infarcts are found. Hypertension results. Coronary thrombosis, pericarditis and pericardial haemorrhage are frequent developments. Mononeuritis multiplex and central nervous system disorders occur due to infarction.

The cutaneous lesions consist of nodules (Fig. 18.72) along the course of superficial arteries. They are usually between 0.5 and 1.5cm in size and often occur on the lower leg. Infarcts of the skin, particularly of the digits, may be found if embolization occurs.

The condition is of unknown aetiology but the hepatitis B antigen has been implicated in some cases. Systemic steroids may be of benefit.

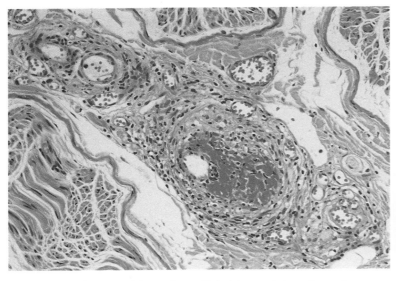

Fig. 18.71 Polyarteritis nodosa. This biopsy taken from deep subcutaneous fat shows a muscular arteriole adjacent to a small peripheral nerve (left). The arteriole shows intense fibrinoid necrosis accompanied by an acute inflammatory cell infiltrate.

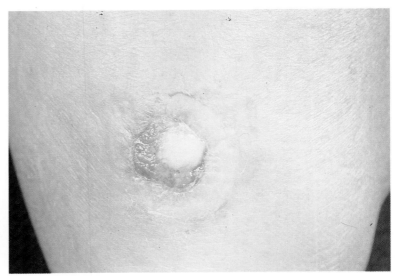

Fig. 18.72 Polyarteritis nodosa. Nodules may occur along the course of superficial arteries. By courtesy of St. John's Hospital for Diseases of the Skin.

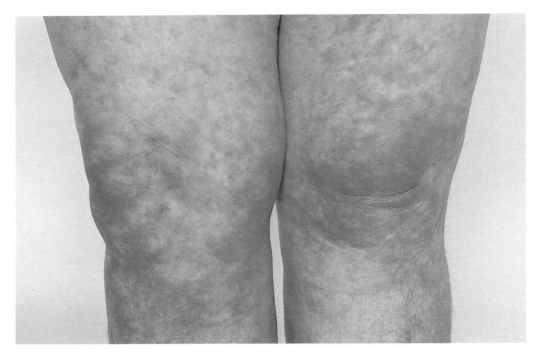

Fig. 18.73 Livedo reticularis. There is marked mottling of the skin of the thighs and lower legs. By courtesy of St. Mary's Hospital.

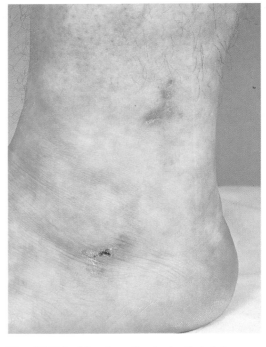

Fig. 18.74 Livedo reticularis. Painful purpuric lesions may develop into ulcers. The histopathology is similar to polyarteritis nodosa but the condition runs a benign course. By courtesy of St. Mary's Hospital.

LIVEDO RETICULARIS WITH NODULES OR ULCERATION

This is an uncommon disorder, usually affecting women. There is marked mottling of the skin of the thighs (Fig. 18.73) and lower legs, an appearance which is known as livedo reticularis. The patients develop painful nodules or ulcers, particularly around the ankles (Fig. 18.74) and lower legs, but occasionally elsewhere. The histology of the livedo is similar to that of the polyarteritis nodosa, but the condition runs a benign course and systemic involvement is most unusual. The aetiology of the condition is unknown.

PITYRIASIS LICHENOIDES ET VARIOLIFORMIS ACUTA

This uncommon condition has a distinctive clinical appearance. It is a vasculitis, possibly mediated by immune complexes, but the aetiology is obscure. The lesions can be limited or quite widespread over the limbs and trunk. They consist of vesicles and pustules which become haemorrhagic (Fig. 18.75) and necrotic (Fig. 18.76), leaving pitted scars. Some of the lesions are reminiscent of those seen in chickenpox and this accounts for its name. An attack may last a couple of months (Fig. 18.77) and the patient may have several episodes over a number of years. The condition is entirely confined to the skin. The disease overlaps with *pityriasis lichenoides chronica* in that similar lesions occur in both conditions.

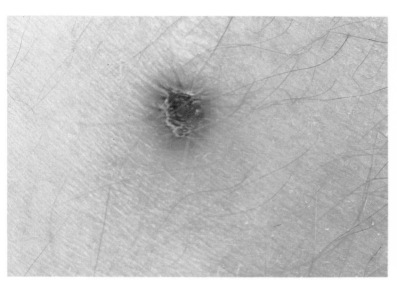

Fig. 18.75 Pityriasis lichenoides et varioliformis acuta. The individual lesion is quite haemorrhagic. By courtesy of St. John's Hospital for Diseases of the Skin.

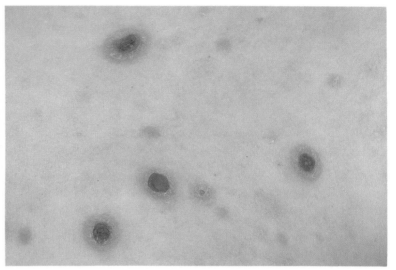

Fig. 18.76 Pityriasis lichenoides et varioliformis acuta. Haemorrhagic and necrotic papules occur. They may be quite limited and leave pitted scars and somewhat resemble chickenpox (hence varioliformis). By courtesy of St. John's Hospital for Diseases of the Skin.

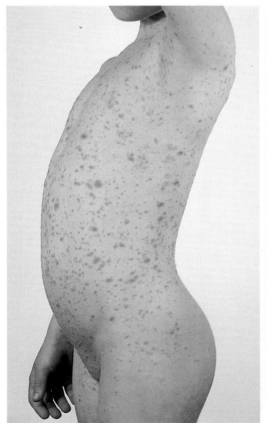

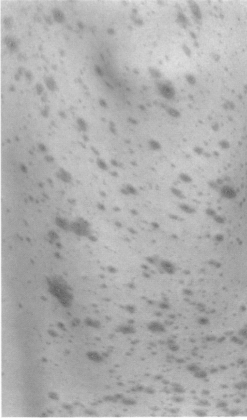

Fig. 18.77 Pityriasis lichenoides acuta. Acute eruptions of papules and plaques may occur on the trunk or limbs (left). The lesions are deep red and some have a crusted surface (right). The lesions cleared within a few weeks.

PITYRIASIS LICHENOIDES CHRONICA

This is an uncommon, completely benign, cutaneous condition of unknown aetiology. It is a chronic disorder of children and young adults. The lesions are symmetrical and favour the inner aspects of the limbs (Figs. 18.78–18.80) and sometimes the trunk. The lesions are small erythematous macules which become papules with a rather characteristic adherent scale which can be detached to reveal a brown surface (Fig. 18.81). Larger patches sometimes occur.

The histology is not very specific. Deposits of immunoglobulin and complement have been detected in the blood vessels in early lesions and the disorder is presumed to be mediated by immune complexes. Although a viral cause has been suspected there is no evidence in favour of this. There is no cure, but occasionally patients respond to antibiotics. Ultra-violet light is also helpful in suppressing the eruption.

GIANOTTI CROSTI SYNDROME (PAPULAR ACRODERMATITIS OF CHILDHOOD)

This is an unusual disorder of childhood. A profuse monomorphic eruption of deep red papules (Fig. 18.82) develops over a space of a few days. They first occur on the buttocks, thighs and legs (Fig. 18.83) and then spread to the arms and face.

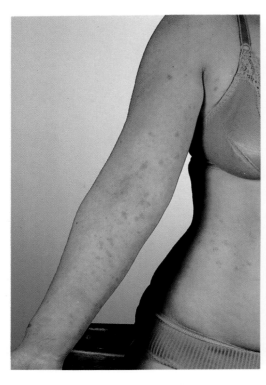

Fig. 18.78 Pityriasis lichenoides chronica. Small erythematous papules are present on the inner aspects of the limbs and the trunk.

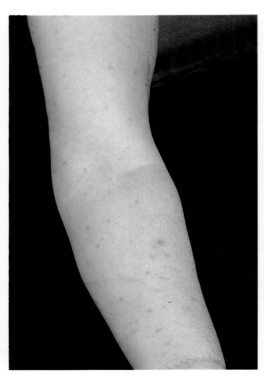

Fig. 18.79 Pityriasis lichenoides chronica. Many small scattered macules and papules occur more or less symmetrically on the limbs.

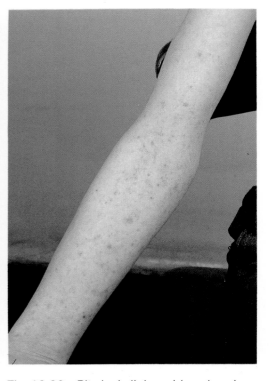

Fig. 18.80 Pityriasis lichenoides chronica. The condition is persistent although it may respond temporarily to ultra-violet light.

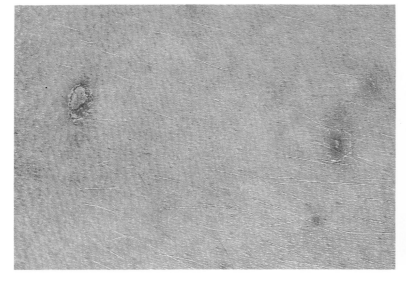

Fig. 18.81 Pityriasis lichenoides chronica. There are small erythematous papules with an adherent scale (left of picture) which when detached have a brown surface (right of picture).

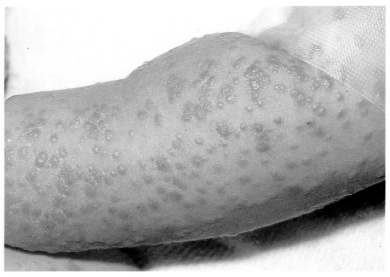

Fig. 18.82 Papular acrodermatitis of childhood. The papules are monomorphic and have a deep red colour.

The trunk is frequently spared (Fig. 18.84). There may be generalized lymphadenopathy. In the original descriptions of the condition hepatitis B was thought to be responsible but the child is often perfectly well. A perivascular infiltrate of lymphocytes and histiocytes is present. The condition resolves within a few weeks.

CAPILLARITIS (PIGMENTED PURPURIC ERUPTIONS)

These represent a number of chronic skin disorders which are uncommon but present as quite well-defined areas of petechiae in various patterns on the lower limbs (Fig. 18.85). They have a particularly confusing nomenclature (Schamberg, Gougerot-Blum and the Majocci's diseases), depending on the patterns produced on the skin. They are better regarded as variants of capillaritis – pigmented purpuric eruptions. The capillaries are dilated and predominantly surrounded by lymphocytes. Red cells escape and extravasate into the skin (Figs. 18.86 and 18.87).

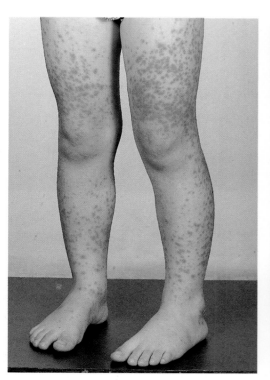

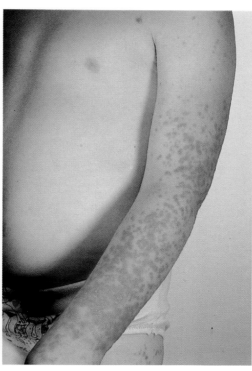

Fig. 18.83 Papular acrodermatitis of childhood. A profuse monomorphic eruption of deep red papules occurs over the legs.

Fig. 18.84 Papular acrodermatitis of childhood. The trunk is usually spared. This is the same child as in Fig. 18.83.

Fig. 18.85 Capillaritis. Multiple well-defined brown-stained petechial patches occur on the lower limbs. By courtesy of St. John's Hospital for Diseases of the Skin.

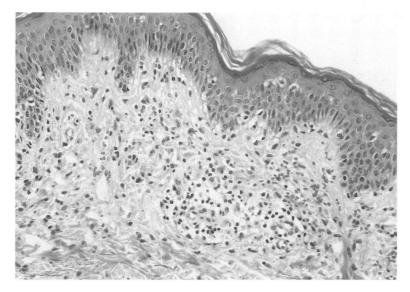

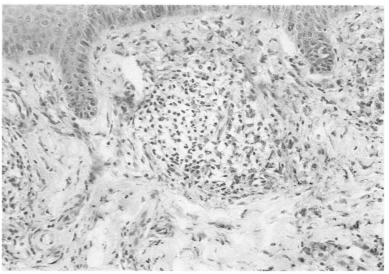

Fig. 18.86 Lymphocytic capillaritis. The typical changes are present in the papillary dermis. Slightly dilated capillaries are surrounded by a predominantly lymphocytic infiltrate. Free red cells (purpura) are conspicuous in the adjacent rather oedematous connective tissue.

Fig. 18.87 Lymphocytic capillaritis. Haemosiderin deposition (as shown by the blue granular material in this Perl's prussian blue reaction) is typical of the later stages of the disease.

The earliest petechiae are purple but later turn brown due to haemosiderin deposition (Fig. 18.88). Their cause is quite unknown and the patients are otherwise healthy. Reassurance is required for there is no treatment. Fortunately there are few symptoms. A similar clinical appearance occurs in stasis eczema, in khaki clothing dermatitis and as a reaction to carbromal.

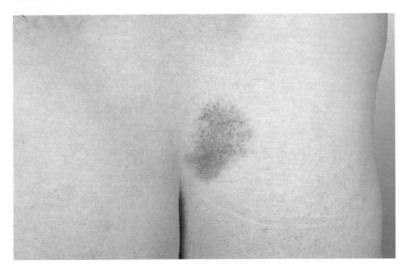

Fig. 18.88 Capillaritis. The earliest petechiae are purple but they become brown as a result of haemosiderin deposition. Various patterns occur.

19 Disorders of Circulation

VENOUS ULCERATION (Stasis, Gravitational or Varicose Ulcers)

Venous ulceration of the lower leg is a common problem particularly in women, who are often overweight. It is a disorder of lower socio-economic groups.

In the normal individual, blood is returned from the lower extremities to the heart via three sets of veins which are deep, superficial and inter-communicating. The powerful muscles of gastrocnemius and soleus are contained within a fixed fascial sheath and they pump the venous blood back to the heart as they contract with exercise. Valves in the veins prevent the blood from flowing back under the influence of gravity. If the system fails, venous hypertension results. This leads to capillary wall hypertrophy and consequent poor cutaneous nutrition due to impaired exchange of gases and metabolites. The most common cause of failure is damage to the valves or obstruction of the deep veins secondary to thrombosis. This is often clinically inapparent. It occurs particularly after a period of prolonged immobility, for example pregnancy, surgical operation or a fracture. As techniques for preventing venous thrombosis improve, the incidence of venous ulceration is reduced. In a minority of patients the valves are absent rather than damaged; this tendency is inherited and associated with varicose veins. Less often, the muscle pump itself is compromised, particularly in patients who have a neuromuscular disease such as polio, or a disorder such as arthritis, which lead to disuse and atrophy of the muscles.

Venous ulcers occur most frequently around the medial and lateral malleoli. The physical signs of venous hypertension are as follows:

Pigmentation

This is mainly due to haemosiderin secondary to extravasation of red cells but it is also a result of post-inflammatory melanin deposition (Figs. 19.1 and 19.2).

Eczema

This may occur in the presence or absence of leg ulceration (Fig. 19.3). Often a *dermatitis medicamentosa* (Fig. 19.4) may be superimposed: this is an allergic contact dermatitis to a topical application used to treat the eczema or ulcer. The most common offending agents are antibiotics, particularly neomycin (cicatrin) and soframycin. It is unwise to use these agents in the treatment of leg ulcers.

Atrophie Blanche

This is the end-result of necrosis of the skin and refers to small white plaques of sclerosis (Fig. 19.5) which have a characteristic surface stippling of dilated blood vessels. It often implies that thrombosis has occurred in the iliac veins or the inferior vena cava.

Oedema

This is a direct result of venous hypertension. Prolonged and neglected oedema ultimately leads to a woody induration and fibrosis of the leg, such that the skin feels and appears sclerodermatous. Infection (cellulitis, Fig. 19.6) is an early complication of the oedema from which fibrosis results. The eventual appearance of the leg is sometimes likened to that of an inverted champagne bottle, the upper and middle sections of the lower leg being swollen but the area around the lower third being tapered. The fibrosis tends to fix the ankle joint, which limits the action of the muscle pump and compounds the problem.

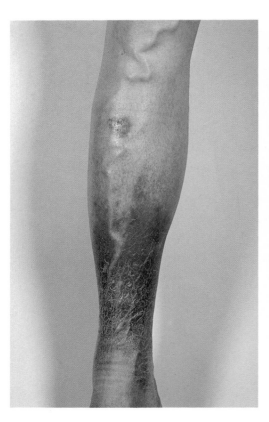

Fig. 19.1 Venous pigmentation. As a result of venous hypertension, red cells extravasate into the tissues and haemosiderin is deposited. Melanin is also present, secondary to inflammatory changes.

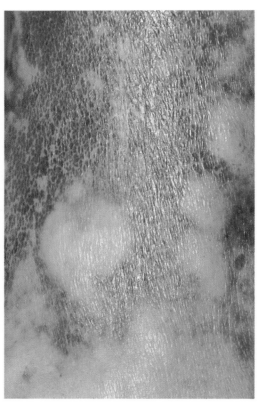

Fig. 19.2 Venous pigmentation. Pigmentation is present around the varicosities.

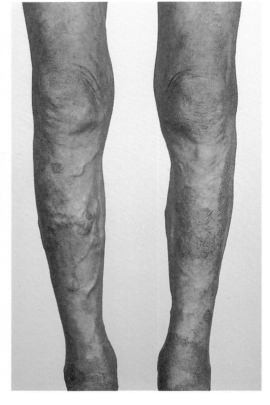

Fig. 19.3 Varicose eczema. Patches of eczema occur in association with varicose veins.

Ulceration

This is the final physical sign of cutaneous malnutrition and is usually precipitated by a minor injury. The ulcers vary in size and shape and may be very large indeed (Fig. 19.7). The margin of the ulcer is usually well-defined (Fig. 19.8) and the base of the

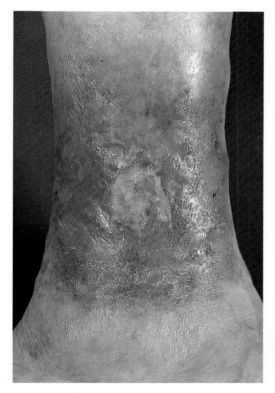

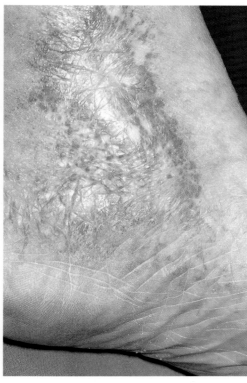

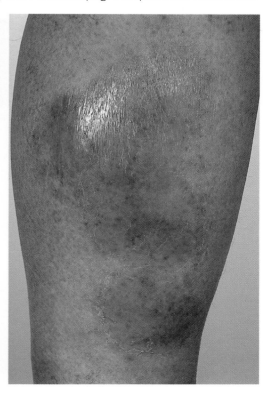

Fig. 19.4 Dermatitis medicamentosa. Contact dermatitis may result from medicaments used to treat varicose eczema or ulcers. This lady had become sensitized to cicatrin (neomycin).

Fig. 19.5 Atrophie blanche. White plaques of sclerosis occur as a result of necrosis of the skin. Hyperpigmentation and tortuous dilated veins are visible signs of venous hypertension.

Fig. 19.6 Cellulitis. Erythema and oedema are present around the varicosities.

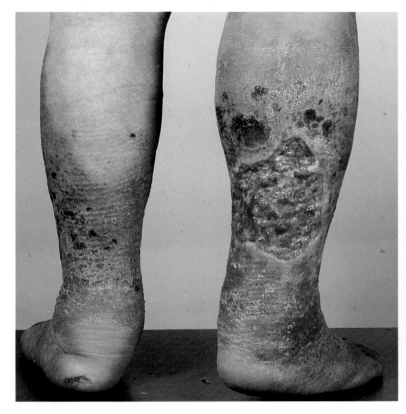

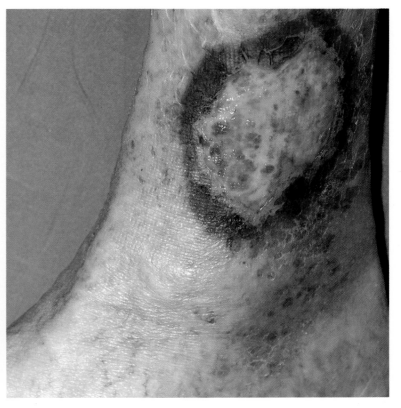

Fig. 19.7 Varicose ulceration. The ulcers may be quite large. This ulcer was completely healed after skin grafting, but broke down to its original state within a few weeks of discharge from hospital.

Fig. 19.8 Venous ulceration. The base of this ulcer has a yellow slough. The cutaneous nutrition is poor and healing will occur slowly.

ulcer varies from having a yellow slough oozing serum or pus to being red and haemorrhagic (Fig. 19.9). The latter state is the goal of all nursing techniques, for a clean red base indicates improved oxygenation of the blood and thus cutaneous nutrition. Ulcers are usually painless, but small ones are occasionally very painful indeed. Periostitis is sometimes found radiologically in association with ulceration.

Varicosities
These may or may not be present. However, tortuous dilated veins indicating venous hypertension are usually present on the feet (Fig. 19.10).

Management
It is important to overcome venous hypertension. Elasticated bandages or stockings are essential in providing an external force to combat gravity. Improvement of the muscle pump may be encouraged by active ambulation and heel-raising exercises. Elevation of the foot of the bed will improve venous flow at night. Eczema should be treated with topical steroids or medicated bandages, such as quinobands or calobands. Cellulitis requires systemic antibiotics, but infected ulcers often respond better to local preparations than to oral antibiotics. A variety of preparations are used for cleaning ulcers, particularly potassium permanganate soaks, aqueous gentian violet and half strength eusol (equal parts chlorinated lime and boric acid in solution). The general health of the patient should be considered, as patients often have accompanying medical conditions requiring treatment, such as anaemia and heart failure. Weight reduction is of great importance where obesity is present. Consultation with a surgeon may be necessary to consider removing incompetent perforating veins, tying them or injecting them. Ulcers often heal

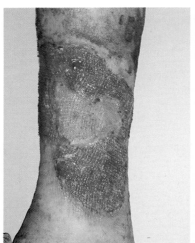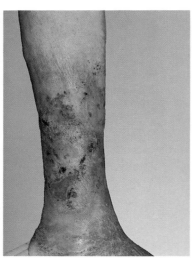

Fig. 19.9   Venous ulceration. The base of the ulcer is red and haemorrhagic (left). This indicates a reasonable blood supply and a favourable prognosis. The same leg is shown six weeks later (right).

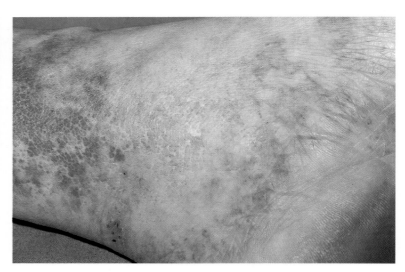

Fig. 19.10   Venous hypertension. Tortuous dilated veins on the medial sides of the feet indicate venous hypertension.

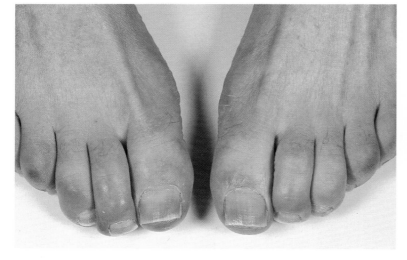

Fig. 19.11   Ischaemia. The toes are red and blue in colour, due to cyanosis from peripheral ischaemia.

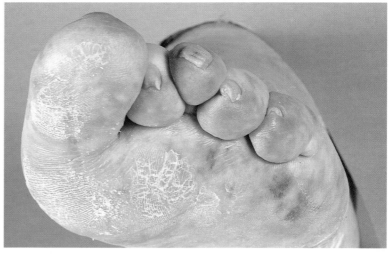

Fig. 19.12   Ischaemia. The toes are blue. This patient developed gangrene a few weeks later.

faster with rest in hospital, and hospitalization should be considered if treatment fails in an out-patient. Skin grafting, either with pinch grafts or split skin grafts, will accelerate healing in suitable patients.

ARTERIOSCLEROTIC LEG ULCERATION

Atheroclerosis is a generalized disorder of blood vessels which is common in Western civilized societies. It is associated with cigarette smoking, diabetes mellitus, hypertension, diets high in lipids, stress and genetic factors. It is a multi-system disease resulting in ischaemia and infarction due to tissue anoxia.

In the lower limb the patient may have symptoms of intermittent claudication. The peripheral pulses may be diminished or absent. The skin is thin, dry, scaly and shiny. Hair is sparse or absent. The colour of the skin is blue, purple (Figs. 19.11 and 19.12) or red due to cyanosis and the peripheries feel cold. Gangrene is the final stage of severe ischaemia (Figs. 19.13–19.15).

Healing is poor following injury and ulceration is common. The atherosclerotic ulcer is painful, particularly with the leg dependent and at night. The ulcers are found in sites which are unusual for a varicose ulcer, such as the dorsum of the foot, the shin and the back of the heels (Fig. 19.16) or legs. A characteristic finding is that the colour of the skin blanches with elevation of the leg.

The condition is properly managed in consultation with a vascular surgeon. Arteriography prior to vessel reconstruction may be necessary. Measures to control diabetes mellitus, hypertension, weight and smoking are imperative if relevant. Elastic stockings are contra-indicated in this disease.

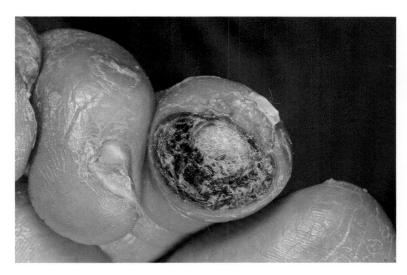

Fig. 19.13 Infarction. The skin is black and crusted. This man had severe peripheral vascular disease leading to gangrene of the toe.

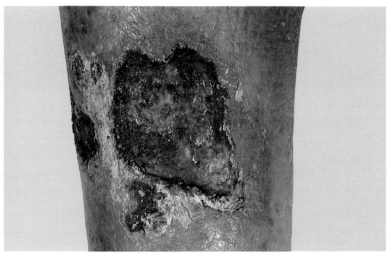

Fig. 19.14 Infarction. The skin nutrition on the lower leg is poor, hence the purple colour. There is a central ulcer with areas of gangrene in it.

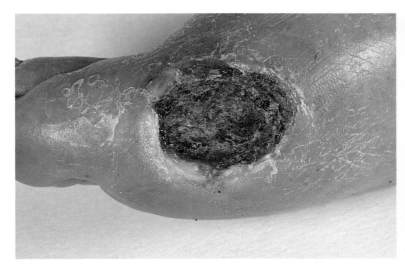

Fig. 19.15 Infarction. A black eschar is present in the ulcer and the surrounding skin is cyanosed. This is the same patient as in Fig. 19.14. The site is typical for peripheral vascular disease.

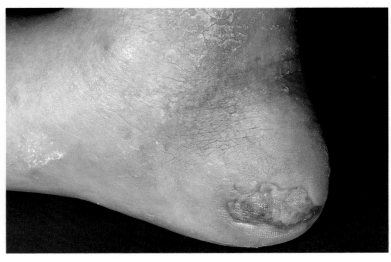

Fig. 19.16 Ischaemic ulcer. Ulceration has occurred on the heel. This is a characteristic site for arteriosclerotic disease, but not for venous disease.

'DECK-CHAIR LEGS'

This condition is caused by prolonged immobilization of the lower legs in a dependent position. Thus it occurs in those who tend to sleep in an armchair rather than going to bed at night. The term originated from those who found themselves homeless in World War II and spent long periods of time sitting in deck-chairs in London underground stations which were used as makeshift homes. The condition is a result of venous and

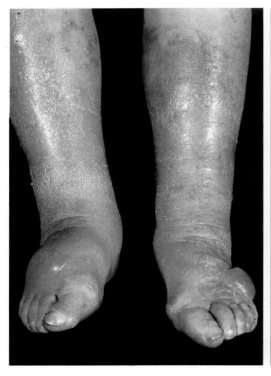
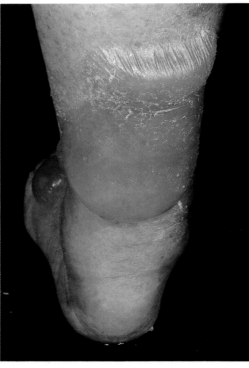
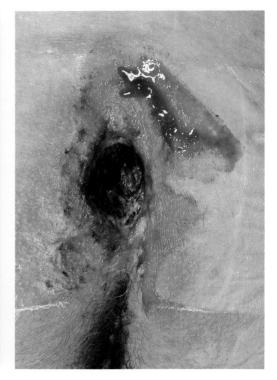

Fig. 19.17 'Deck-chair legs'. The legs are red and oedematous from prolonged immobilization (left). Blistering may result (right). Patients who lead an armchair existence are prone to this disorder.

Fig. 19.18 Neuropathic ulcer. This patient has disseminated sclerosis and no sacral sensation. The ulcer has developed partly because of this in addition to prolonged pressure and incontinence.

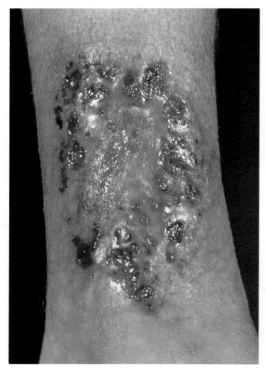
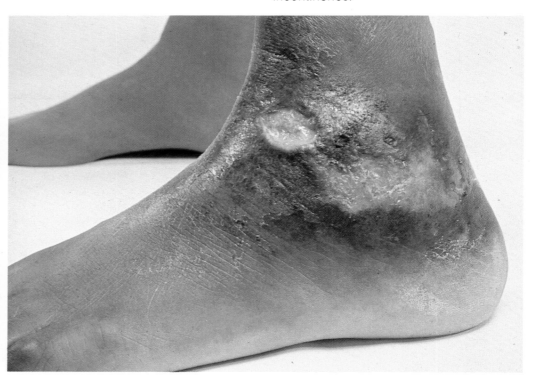

Fig. 19.19 Pyoderma gangrenosum. This ulcer has a blue, overhanging margin. The patient had ulcerative colitis.

Fig. 19.20 Sickle cell disease. This West Indian girl had no varicosities or venous hypertension to explain her ulcers, but had sickle cell disease. By courtesy of St. Mary's Hospital.

possibly lymphatic stasis, leading to persistent oedema coupled with an erythema (Fig. 19.17 left), probably due to a continual low grade cellulitis. Severe oedema may lead to blistering (Fig. 19.17 right). The condition is only rectified by restoring patients to an active life, although this is frequently impossible on account of their underlying chronic disease, such as heart failure or arthritis, which reduces them to an armchair existence.

DIFFERENTIAL DIAGNOSIS OF ULCERS ON THE LOWER LIMBS
The most common cause of ulceration in the lower legs is venous ulceration, but arterial ulceration is frequent and often there is a combination of both disorders. A neurological examination is essential to rule out a neuropathic ulcer (Fig. 19.18). Other causes of leg ulcers should be considered if these are not appropriate.

PYODERMA GANGRENOSUM. This is an ulcer with a characteristic blue overhanging margin (Fig. 19.19). It may occur anywhere on the skin, but the lower limb is a common site. There is usually an associated condition, such as rheumatoid arthritis, ulcerative colitis or myeloma.

HAEMATOLOGICAL DISORDERS. Haematological disorders, particularly sickle cell (Fig. 19.20) and spherocytic anaemia, give rise to ulcers on the fronts of the legs.

GUMMA. A gumma due to tertiary syphilis is a well-defined, characteristically punched-out lesion with a yellow base (Fig. 19.21) which is similar in appearance to chamois leather.

NON-HODGKIN'S LYMPHOMA. This may present in the skin as nodules which may break down and ulcerate (Fig. 19.22 upper). It is the finding of nodules that will aid the diagnosis (Fig. 19.22 lower), which can then be confirmed by biopsying the nodules. Biopsies of ulcers *per se* are frequently only characterized by non-specific features.

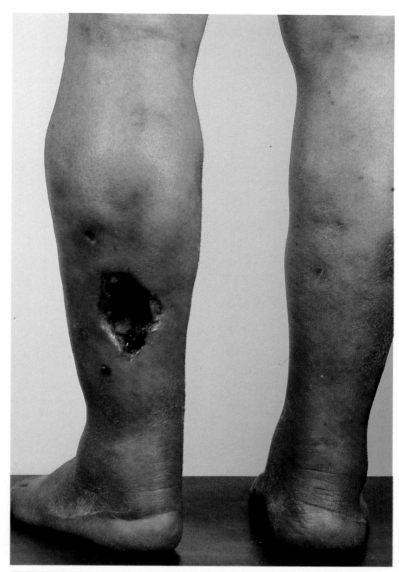

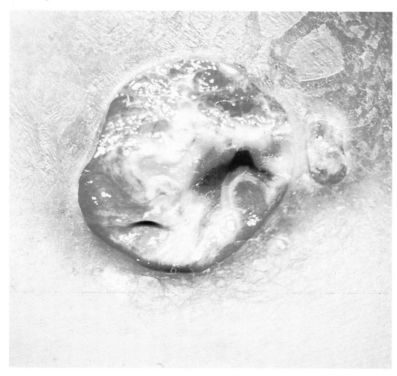

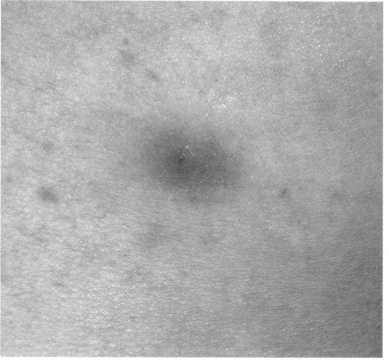

Fig. 19.21   Gumma. The ulcer is well-defined with vertical edges and appears 'punched out'. By courtesy of St. Mary's Hospital.

Fig. 19.22   Non-Hodgkin's disease. This patient (upper) presented these lesions to a surgeon who biopsied one ulcer. The histology was non-specific. Later biopsy of a nodule (lower) above the popliteal fossa showed non-Hodgkin's lymphoma.

NECROBIOSIS LIPOIDICA. Necrobiosis lipoidica, either in association with diabetes or *de novo*, consists of well-defined plaques on the front of the legs (Fig. 19.23), with a yellow appearance and a waxy feel on palpation, and dilated blood vessels on the surface. If this condition ulcerates, as it may, the cutaneous changes are sufficient to enable diagnosis.

VASCULITIS. This may ulcerate and in particular the nodular vasculitis or erythema induratum that occurs in association with tuberculosis, so-called Bazin's disease seen characteristically on the backs of the legs (Fig. 19.24).

TROPICAL DISORDERS. Tropical causes of ulceration such as yaws or Buruli ulcer (see Fig. 13.25) should be considered where appropriate.

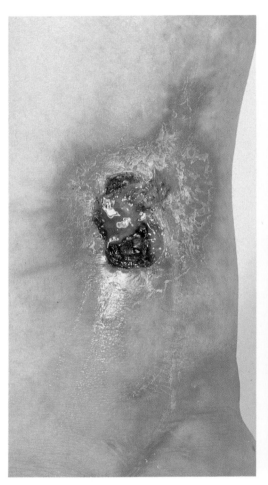

Fig. 19.23 Necrobiosis lipoidica. The lesion may ulcerate.

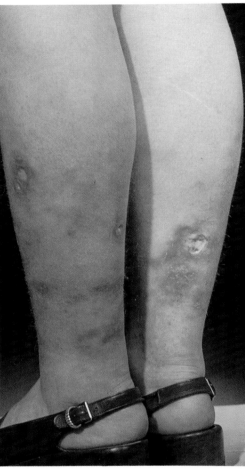

Fig. 19.24 Bazin's disease. Ulcerated nodules on the calves are particularly associated with tuberculosis.

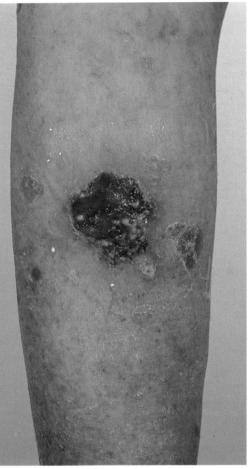

Fig. 19.25 Ulcerated basal cell carcinoma. This lesion occurred on the back of the leg. The margin of the ulcer is rolled and pigmented.

Fig. 19.26 Squamous cell carcinoma. This large ulcer with a purulent base and indurated margin had been misdiagnosed as a varicose ulcer.

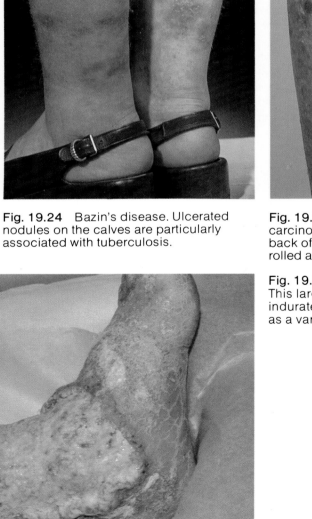

MALIGNANT DISORDERS. Occasionally a basal cell carcinoma may occur on the lower leg and ulcerate (Fig. 19.25). The diagnosis should not be difficult because the margin of the ulcer is rolled, pearly in colour with telangiectasia. Squamous cell carcinoma (Fig. 19.26) may also occur in this location. Rarely a long-standing varicose ulcer may turn into a squamous cell carcinoma.

KLINEFELTER'S DISEASE. Men with Klinefelter's syndrome are more prone to leg ulceration (Fig. 19.27).

CHILBLAINS (Perniosis)
These are localized swellings of the skin usually occurring on the fingers and toes as a reaction to cold. They occasionally occur on other acral areas such as the ears, buttocks and nose. Prolonged vasoconstriction is followed by hyperaemia. The lesions are itchy at first and become painful after rewarming occurs; they are small and dusky red or purple (Fig. 19.28). A similar condition occurs on the lower legs due to inadequate

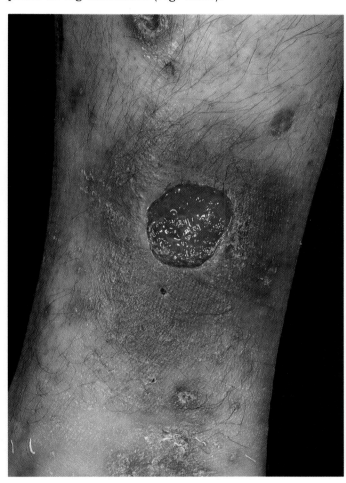
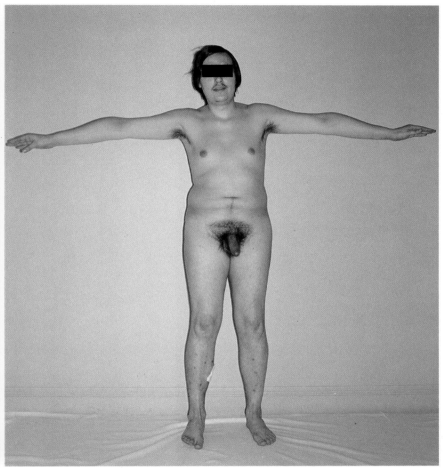

Fig. 19.27 Klinefelter's syndrome. Leg ulcers are unusual in young men. This man had XXY karyotype with associated undervirilization and excessive arm length (right). By courtesy of Dr. B. Monk.

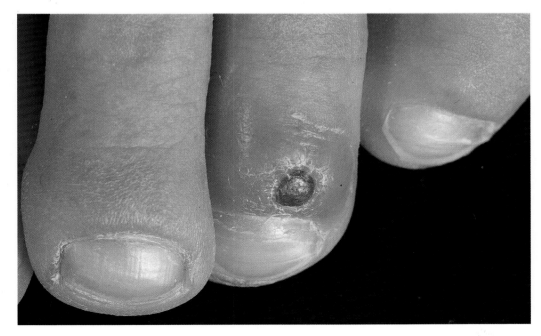

Fig. 19.28 Chilblains. Localized painful purple swellings occur on the extremities in response to cold. By courtesy of St. John's Hospital for Diseases of the Skin.

clothing. Young women and immigrants from warm climates (Fig.19.29) are mostly susceptible to the disease which is becoming less common as the standard of heating of houses has improved. Although chilblains develop on exposure to cold, damp living conditions predispose individuals to the condition. In severe cases the lesions may ulcerate. Perniosis is also a feature of systemic disorders such as lupus erythematosus. Treatment is directed towards better measures to keep the skin warm.

ACROCYANOSIS

This is a term for a common condition which consists of a persistent discoloration of the hands and feet (Fig. 19.30), but occasionally of the nose and ears, due to reduced peripheral circulation. The skin appears blue and feels cool or cold. It is a common condition and on the whole gives rise to few symptoms.

LIVEDO RETICULARIS

This appearance of the skin is extremely common in young adults: sluggish blood flow produces cyanosis which allows the

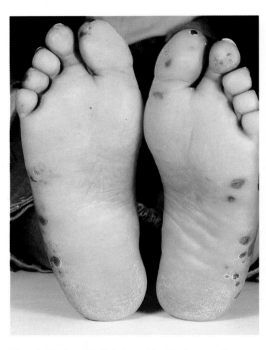

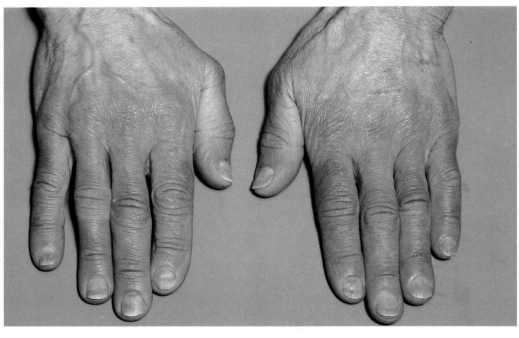

Fig. 19.29 Chilblains. Multiple small cutaneous infarcts occurred during this African woman's first winter in England. She was unprepared for the cold weather.

Fig. 19.30 Acrocyanosis. This term is used to describe persistent discoloration of the peripheral skin due to poor circulation. There is a marked contrast between the colour of the fingers and wrists.

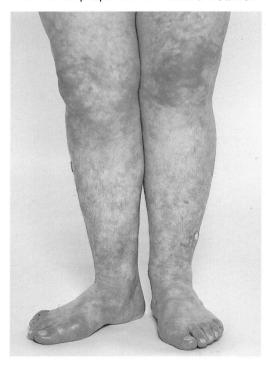

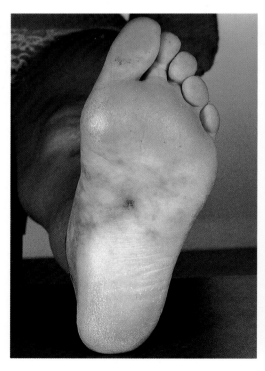

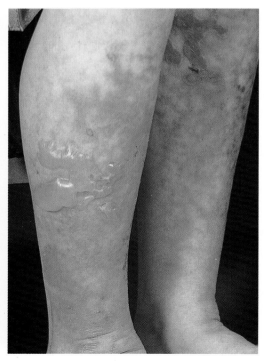

Fig. 19.31 Livedo reticularis. This is a mottled net-like pattern secondary to sluggish blood flow and producing cyanosis. By courtesy of St. Mary's Hospital.

Fig. 19.32 Livedo reticularis with ulceration. There is a central painful purpuric lesion. Livedo reticularis may occur as part of a vasculitis and is a cutaneous form of polyarteritis nodosa.

Fig. 19.33 Erythema ab igne. A permanent pigmented net-like pattern results from burns of the skin, in this case from sitting too close to a fire. Actual blisters from a recent burn are present.

net-like pattern of the blood vessels under the skin to become apparent. The condition is usually of no significance but is seen more commonly in patients who have a tendency towards acrocyanosis and perniosis. Occasionally, however, it is associated with lupus erythematosus or a cutaneous form of polyarteritis nodosa (Figs. 19.31 and 19.32). The drug amantadine used in the treatment of Parkinson's disease also causes livedo reticularis.

ERYTHEMA AB IGNE

This condition also highlights the distribution of the blood vessels in the superficial plexus under the skin, in that there is a permanent pigmented net-like pattern to be seen in the skin of the lower legs (Fig. 19.33). It usually occurs in elderly women who sit too close to a fire to keep themselves warm. It may occur on one leg more than the other and particularly on the outer side, corresponding to how the patient sits in front of the fire. The condition is of no significance, although occasionally this is seen in myxoedematous patients attempting to warm themselves. Rarely squamous cell carcinoma can develop in chronic erythema ab igne. A similar appearance can occur in response to any form of heat, particularly the application of a hot water bottle to relieve pain in the abdomen or back.

BEDSORES (Pressure Sores)

These lesions result from tissue anoxia. Prolonged immobilization, either as a result of unconsciousness or an illness, causes an impaired blood supply to the skin and subcutaneous tissue. Usually the patients are elderly and overweight. Necrosis and ulceration (Fig. 19.34) occur at the pressure points, which are most commonly the sacrum, backs of the heels (Fig. 19.35) and scapulae. If the patient is incontinent this compounds the problem on the sacrum (see Fig. 19.18).

Bedsores are extremely difficult to heal once they have occurred, therefore prevention of the condition is paramount. Any patient admitted to hospital who is unable or unwilling to shift his or her position constantly in bed is a candidate for bedsores. It is thus imperative that the patient is turned and moved at least every two hours by the nursing staff to prevent this. In many cases, however, the process of developing bedsores has already started before the patient is admitted.

EMBOLI

Fragments of atheromatous plaques or thrombi may leave a central location and occlude a peripheral blood vessel. If cutaneous vessels are occluded, small infarcts occur (Fig. 19.36).

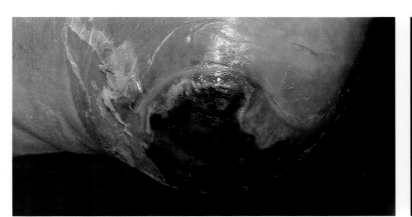

Fig. 19.34 Pressure sores. Necrosis of the skin has resulted from tissue anoxia caused by lying immobile for a prolonged period, resting on the heels.

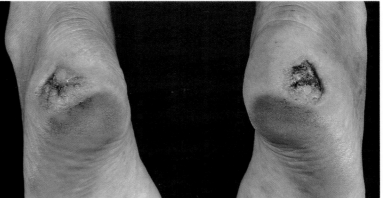

Fig. 19.35 Pressure sores. The backs of the heels are common sites. This lady was unconscious for 24 hours after a cerebral vascular accident. The resulting ulcers on the heels eventually required skin grafting.

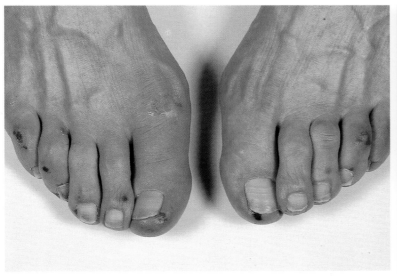

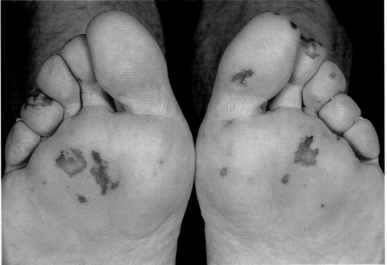

Fig. 19.36 Emboli. There are multiple small areas of cutaneous necrosis. This man was developing emboli from a mural thrombosis in an aneurysm of his left ventricle.

The most common sources of emboli are thrombi from the heart valves or wall, or from a plaque on a large vessel or aneurysm. Endocarditis, valvular disease, myocardial infarction, atrial fibrillation and congestive cardiac failure are the commonest causes.

RAYNAUD'S PHENOMENON

This condition is caused by intense spasm of the digital arteries in response to cold (Fig. 19.37). There is pallor of the tips of the fingers followed a few minutes later by cyanosis or reactive hyperaemia. Thus the fingers may go white, then blue and finally red. In severe cases there may be trophic changes with tethering of the skin and tapering of the fingers (sclerodactyly), and ulceration and gangrene as in scleroderma. The condition may occur without identifiable cause and is known as Raynaud's disease. Some of the causes are listed in the following table (Fig. 19.38):

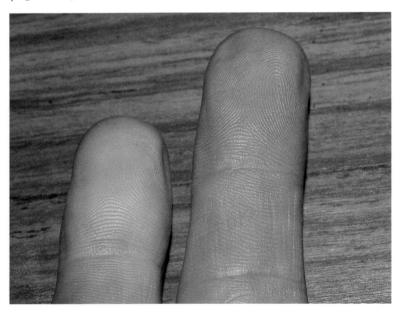

Fig. 19.37   Raynaud's phenomenon. There is pallor of the tip of the index finger, noticeable when compared with the middle finger.

Causes of Raynaud's phenomenon

Collagen vascular disease
Scleroderma
Systemic lupus erythematosus
Mixed connective tissue disease

Occupational
Pneumatic drills

Neurological disease
Cervical rib

Occlusive arterial disease
Buerger's disease

Immunoglobulin disorders
Cryoglobulinaemia
Cold agglutinins

Toxins
Ergotism
Heavy metals
Vinyl chloride

Fig. 19.38   Causes of Raynaud's phenomenon.

20 Disorders of the Sebaceous, Sweat and Apocrine Glands

DISORDERS OF SEBACEOUS GLANDS

Sebaceous glands are found throughout the skin except in the palms and soles. They are at a maximum in the scalp, the face and the anterior and posterior aspects of the trunk. They occur in association with hair follicles with which they share a common channel leading to the surface. The unit is known as the pilosebaceous apparatus. Sebaceous glands do occur on their own, e.g. the Meibomian gland in the eyelid, and in many people they are visible in the lips and buccal mucous membranes, where they are known as Fordyce spots (Figs. 20.1 and 20.2).

Sebaceous glands do not develop until puberty, apart from temporary activity during infancy as a result of maternal hormone stimulation. Animals require them for waterproofing their fur and perhaps the sebaceous gland was a necessity during the course of human evolution, but is now an unhelpful appendage. Sebum or grease is secreted by the gland as a holocrine process, in that the entire sebaceous cell is shed into the pilosebaceous channel. Sebum is a complex mixture of lipids. It is fungistatic, in that tinea capitis is rare after puberty, but the superficial yeast infection pityriasis versicolor thrives on sebum and does not occur until puberty. Over-production of sebum and its breakdown by bacteria results in acne, the most common disorder of the skin.

Acne

Acne is a disorder of the pilosebaceous apparatus. The physical signs of the disease are greasiness, comedones (Fig. 20.3), papules, pustules (Figs. 20.4 and 20.5), nodules (Fig. 20.6) and cysts on the face and the front and back of the chest. The condition may result in scarring (Fig. 20.7), which can vary from small pits to larger lesions. Occasionally, keloids may occur. Post-inflammatory hyperpigmentation is a problem in coloured skins (Fig. 20.8).

There are four factors involved in the aetiology of acne.

1) *Plugging of the Pilosebaceous Canal*

The pilosebaceous canal becomes blocked by a keratin plug, which is represented clinically by the blackhead. This is caused by a failure of the cells which line the channel to separate properly into the lumen, such that a keratin plug is formed. As a result of the blockage, the gland distends and various morphological changes take place. These range from whiteheads, which are closed comedones, to large cysts.

2) *Sebum*

There is an increased production of sebum, such that most patients with acne have a greasy skin. Pustules represent collections of sebum and are quite sterile, contrary to popular belief. The breakdown products of sebum are free fatty acids which are irritants. If they are injected into the skin they produce a sterile inflammatory response of polymorphs and lymphocytes. Thus, if sebum leaks into the surrounding tissues from the gland, inflammatory changes ensue. Red papules will result if the distension of the follicle is superficial, but if it is deeper, large, red, painful nodules occur. The deep inflammatory lesions may result in scarring.

3) *Bacteria*

Propionibacterium acnes (formerly known as *Corynebacterium acnes*) and *Staphylococcus epidermidis* and the yeast *Pityrosporum ovale* are found in the sebaceous follicles. *P. acnes* is probably the most important in the pathogenesis of acne. They all have lipase activity and break down sebum to fatty acids.

4) *Hormones*

Sebaceous glands are under hormonal control, particularly androgens. It is for this reason that eunuchs or pre-pubertal castrates do not develop acne unless they are given injections of testosterone. The sebaceous gland is very sensitive to circulating androgen. In females with acne, recent work suggests that the sex hormone binding globulin is reduced and, as a result, serum-unbound sex hormones are increased. Local factors at the level of sebaceous gland receptors for male hormones are important. 5-α-reductase is the enzyme responsible for the conversion of testosterone to dihydrotestosterone, which is a more active form. It may be that in acne there is greater local activity of this enzyme at the target organ, resulting in overactivity of the gland.

Relatively high does of oestrogens decrease the size of the sebaceous glands and the production of sebum. Progesterone has been implicated in the aetiology of acne, especially since many women report a premenstrual flare of their condition, but experimental work in this area has produced conflicting results.

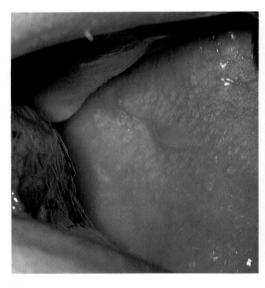

Fig. 20.1 Fordyce spots. Small yellow papules are present on the buccal mucous membrane. They represent sebaceous glands.

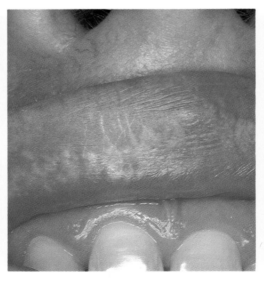

Fig. 20.2 Fordyce spots. Small yellow papules are present on the lips. They are extremely common, such that they may be considered to be a normal variant. Patients are sometimes anxious as to their nature.

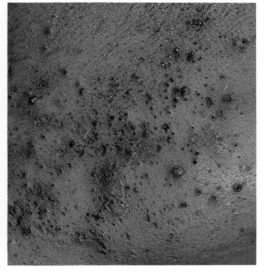

Fig. 20.3 Acne vulgaris. Comedones (blackheads) are plugs of keratin which block the pilosebaceous canal. They are a very common feature of acne. One pustule is present here.

Acne Vulgaris

This is the most common variety of acne and the appearance of spots is one of the first signs of puberty. It affects the face, chest (Fig. 20.9) and back and is a universal manifestation of adolescence, although individuals vary greatly in their degree of affliction. Acne usually peaks at about the age of sixteen or seventeen and most individuals are free of the condition by the early twenties, although there are many exceptions.

Post-adolescent Female Acne

This is a common problem. It is remarkably chronic and affects women in their twenties and thirties, who often report virtually no acne during adolescence. The acne particularly affects the chin (Fig. 20.10), jaw and cheeks. Painful, deep nodules are frequent and the condition is worse pre-menstrually. Some women relate it to either starting or stopping the contraceptive pill, but others have never taken an oral contraceptive. The aetiology of this kind of acne is uncertain but clearly there are hormonal irregularities, since the patients have low levels of the sex hormone transport globulin.

Infantile Acne (Milk Spots)

This is quite common and is due to the effects of maternal androgens in breast milk on the infantile sebaceous glands. The resultant acne (Fig. 20.11) usually clears by the age of three to six months. If it does not clear it may be a presenting sign of an adrenogenital syndrome.

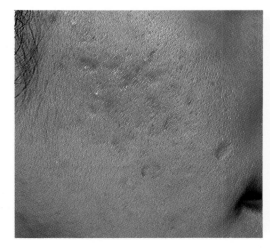

Fig. 20.4 Acne vulgaris. Greasiness is present with papules and pustules.

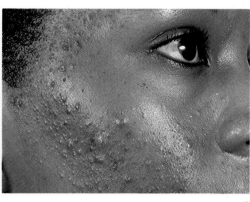

Fig. 20.5 Acne vulgaris. Papules, pustules and hyperpigmentation are present.

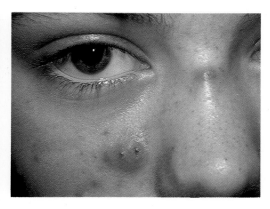

Fig. 20.6 Acne vulgaris. Painful nodules may occur.

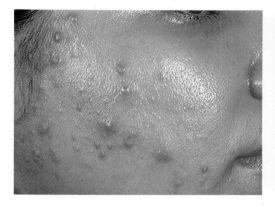

Fig. 20.7 Acne. Scarring occurs in some individuals and is permanent.

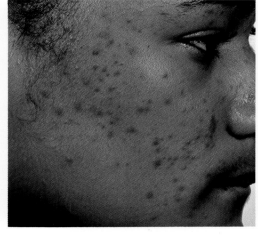

Fig. 20.8 Acne. Post-inflammatory hyperpigmentation may follow acne.

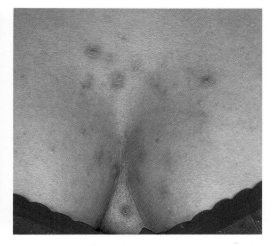

Fig. 20.9 Acne. Acne may occur on sites other than the face.

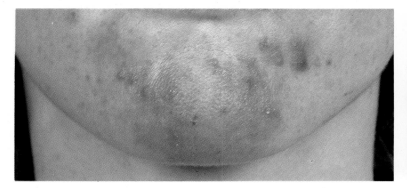

Fig. 20.10 Post-adolescent female acne. Papules and pustules occur, particularly on the chin. The cheeks and jaw may also be involved. The papules can be deep and painful and may be worse pre-menstrually. By courtesy of Dr. Michèle Clement.

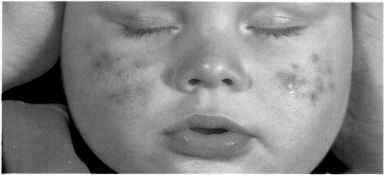

Fig. 20.11 Infantile acne (milk spots). Maternal androgens in breast milk stimulate the infantile sebaceous glands and produce acne. The condition disappears spontaneously within 3-6 months.

Tropical Acne

Many individuals suffer greatly from acne in humid and hot climates. They usually have a predisposition to acne but the environmental conditions exacerbate the disease. The condition may be extremely destructive and resistant to all therapy other than changing the environment.

Nodular Cystic Acne (Acne Conglobata)

This is an exceedingly unpleasant and chronic form of acne (Fig. 20.12) in which painful, red nodules (Fig. 20.13) and cysts occur in addition to the regular features of acne. The nodules may discharge serous-coloured material. They may dissect under the skin and form interconnections with other nodules. Unsightly scars may result (Fig. 20.14). The condition is more common in males and the face, chest and back may be involved either in isolation or together. Sometimes the lower back and buttocks may also be affected (Fig. 20.15). Occasional cases have been reported of males with this disease carrying an extra Y chromosome. The condition tends to persist for many years and, until the introduction of 13-cis-retinoic acid (Fig. 20.16), has resisted practically all forms of therapy.

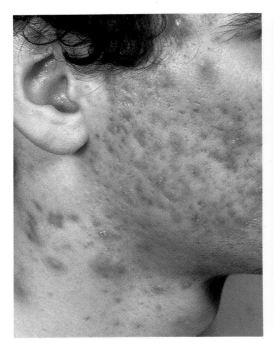

Fig. 20.12 Nodular cystic acne (acne conglobata). This is a destructive form of acne. Deep painful nodules leave disfiguring scars.

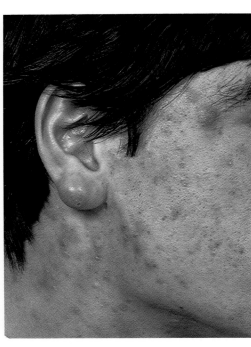

Fig. 20.13 Acne conglobata. Large inflamed cysts may occur. Surgical excision should be avoided.

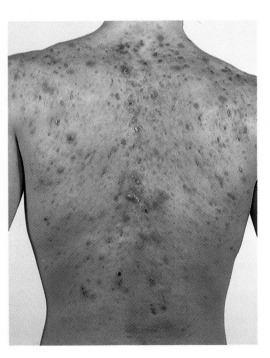

Fig. 20.14 Acne conglobata. Many deep nodules and scars are present. The back may be affected with little facial involvement and vice-versa.

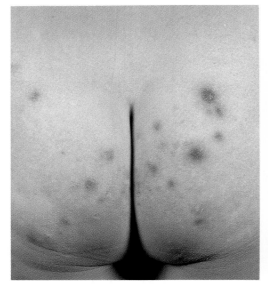

Fig. 20.15 Acne. The buttocks may occasionally be involved in acne, without evidence of the disease elsewhere.

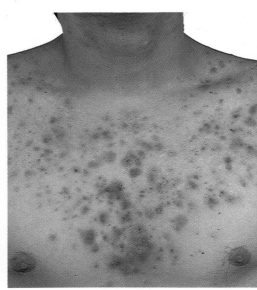

Fig. 20.16 Acne conglobata. 13-cis-retinoic acid has dramatically altered the management of this condition which does not respond well to conventional antibiotic therapy. This eruption (left) cleared within eight weeks (right).

Acné Excoriée des Jeunes Filles

This disorder is almost exclusively confined to women and presents as an obsessional desire to squeeze out or pick at lesions which they believe to be present on the face. There is some doubt as to whether these lesions do really exist but if they do, they represent a minor form of acne. However, the results of interfering with the skin do produce extremely unsightly excoriations (Fig. 20.17), post-inflammatory hyperpigmentation (Fig. 20.18) and scarring. The patients freely admit that they pick at their skin but it is virtually impossible to dissuade them from the habit. Psychotherapy seems to have little effect.

Acne Medicamentosa

Topical preparations may cause acne. Pomades used by negroes to grease the hair to make it more manageable or straighten it frequently spread onto the forehead and produce an acneiform eruption (Fig. 20.19) by occluding the orifices of the pilosebaceous follicles. Brilliantines and cosmetics can have the same effect and have been shown to produce comedones experimentally in animals.

Occupational Acne

Industrial workers develop acne when exposed to halogenated hydrocarbons (chloracne). If workers are exposed to these chemicals in a liquid form, the acne occurs on the forearms and thighs and if halogenated hydrocarbons are released as a vapour, acne appears on the neck, face and trunk. Exposure to oils and tars produces a similar clinical appearance on the limbs.

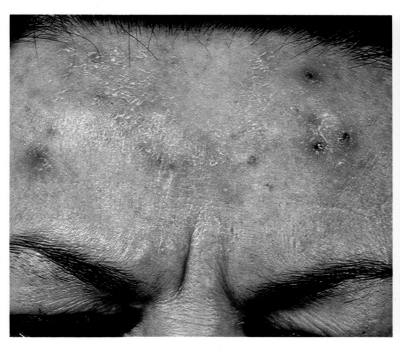

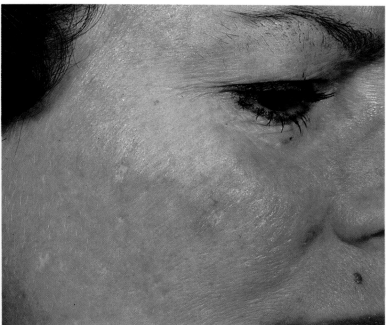

Fig. 20.17 Acne excoriée des jeunes filles. This is a chronic neurotic disorder of adult women, who pick and squeeze at their facial skin. The interference (which is freely admitted) leaves disfiguring scars (right).

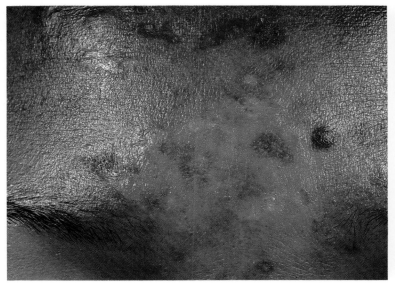

Fig. 20.18 Acne excoriée des jeunes filles. Fresh excoriations and hyperpigmentation are present. Evidence of acne is frequently absent.

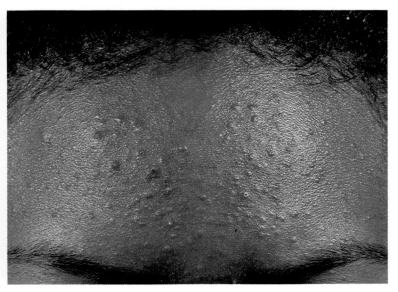

Fig. 20.19 Pomade acne. Greases used for the hair may spread onto the forehead and occlude the pilosebaceous orifices. This is common in negroes.

Drug-induced Acne

A number of substances are acnegenic. Halogens, in addition to being active topically, produce similar problems when taken orally. Iodides in cough mixtures, in radiological materials and in the treatment of thyroid disease may produce acne. Bromides cause similar eruptions (Fig. 20.20) and anti-epileptic drugs such as phenobarbitone and troxidone may also produce acne. Isoniazid may produce quite severe disease (Fig. 20.21).

Systemic steroids produce a rather characteristic acne situated largely on the trunk (Fig. 20.22), shoulders and upper arms. The lesions are monomorphic papules or pustules (Fig. 20.23). Histologically, this form of acne seems to differ from acne vulgaris in that there is an infiltrate of neutrophils around the hair follicles but no hyperkeratosis at the orifice of the hair follicle.

Topical steroids are frequently mistakenly applied to treat acne and will result in exacerbation of the disease (Fig. 20.24).

Sunshine Acne

A monomorphic eruption consisting of many red papules scattered all over the trunk, shoulders and limbs, sometimes occurs in fair-skinned individuals exposed to ultra-violet light. The cause is not known but histologically a folliculitis is found to be present, which is similar to that resulting from steroid therapy.

Acne as a Manifestation of Systemic Disease

Although not common as a presenting feature of internal disease, acne is present in endocrine disorders such as Cushing's syndrome, polycystic ovary syndrome and virilizing disorders. However, other features of virilization will be present.

Management of Acne

Topical agents are used for either their anti-bacterial or their desquamating effects or both. Sulphur, resorcinol and benzoyl peroxide are effective. Many patients do not like using them, however, because they produce redness and scaling, particularly on the face. Less frequent application sometimes surmounts this problem. Topical antibiotics, particularly erythromycin and clindamycin may be helpful. Retinoic acid is useful when many comedones are present. Ultra-violet light is of benefit in some patients, probably because of the desquamatory effect which follows the erythema. Cystic lesions may be helped by drainage and introduction of triamcinolone.

The mainstay, however, of treatment of moderate to severe acne is with long-term antibiotics (Fig. 20.25). Practitioners frequently err in giving only short courses. The minimum period of time that the antibiotic should be given for is six months, but since they are only a controlling therapy, they often need to be given for as long as the patient has the tendency to acne. Tetracyclines, erythromycin and septrin are all effective. Penicillin, however, has no effect. Smaller doses are used than would normally be prescribed for bacterial infections. Side-effects are uncommon. Candidosis occasionally occurs in females and clearly antibiotics, particularly tetracyclines (because of their effects on teeth), should be avoided in pregnancy. Patients are often particularly concerned lest long-term antibiotic therapy should lower their resistance to infection, but there does not appear to be any evidence for this. The mechanism of action of systemic antibiotics is not completely understood. They inhibit the growth of the follicular bacteria and thus reduce their lipolytic action and the breakdown of sebum into free fatty acids.

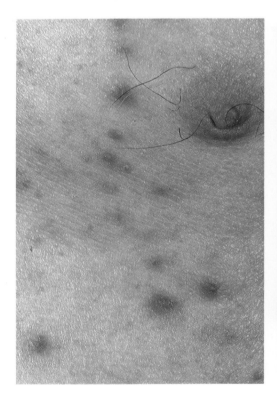

Fig. 20.20 This man had taken carbrital which contains bromide and may induce acne. By courtesy of Dr. R.H. Marten.

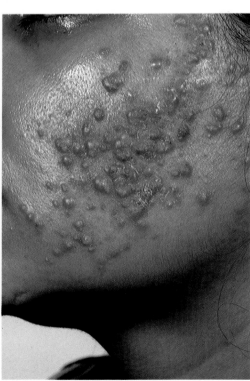

Fig. 20.21 Drug-induced acne. The lady has received isoniazid for tuberculosis and developed a very severe acne.

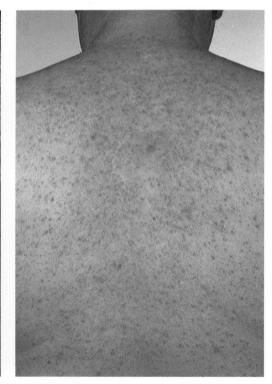

Fig. 20.22 Drug-induced acne. Topical and systemic glucocorticosteroids may induce acne.

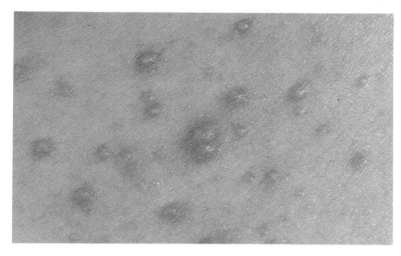

Fig. 20.23 Drug-induced acne. Steroid-induced acne is usually monomorphic. Pustules are predominantly represented here.

Cyproterone acetate is an anti-androgen which is active at the level of the target organ and improves acne. It should be given with ethinyloestradiol as a contraceptive, for it would otherwise cause feminization of the male fetus if a patient were to become pregnant. It obviously cannot be prescribed for males. Oestrogens themselves improve acne but require to be taken in high doses where the risk/benefit ratio may preclude their use. Effective topical anti-androgens may eventually become available.

13-cis-retinoic acid is proving to be a successful therapy, particularly for acne conglobata. The drug is given for a course of four months and may produce prolonged remissions. It is particularly effective on the face. Second courses are sometimes required. The drug causes dryness of the skin and lips and occasionally ataxia, headaches and temporary hair loss occur. The most serious side-effect is that the drug is a teratogen and must be used with the greatest of caution in women. The drug also increases serum lipids and is potentially hepatotoxic. The long-term side-effects are unknown.

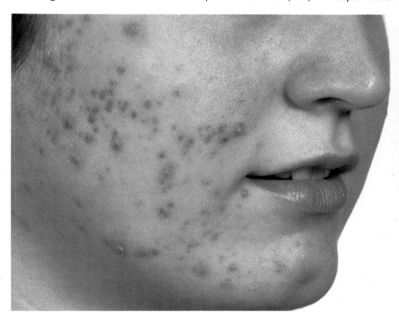
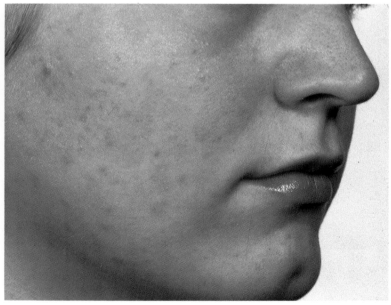

Fig. 20.24 Drug-induced acne. Acne is one of the first signs of incipient puberty and is occurring earlier than previously. This ten-year-old West Indian boy's acne was misdiagnosed and treated with topical steroids (left). It responded well to antibiotics (right).

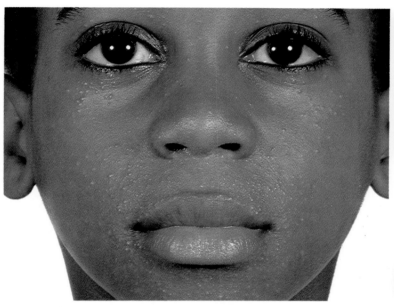
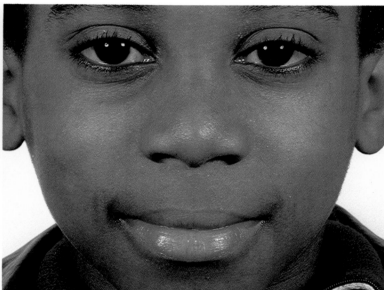

Fig. 20.25 Treatment of acne. Antibiotics are the mainstay of treatment of acne. They must be taken long-term otherwise relapse is frequent.

Rosacea

This is a common condition consisting of papules and pustules (Fig. 20.26) occurring with an erythema of the face. This condition usually starts in the fourth decade but may occur later in women at the menopause. It tends to persist indefinitely in most cases.

The lesions are distributed particularly in the central areas of the face. Papules and pustules are seen on the forehead, cheeks, over the bridge of the nose and on the chin (Fig. 20.27). The patients have a generally high colour and a tendency to flush easily (Fig. 20.28). Occasionally, the condition affects only the nose (Fig. 20.29) producing a marked erythema with very few papules and pustules elsewhere. Alternatively, there may be prominent sebaceous gland hypertrophy with overgrowth of the soft tissues of the nose, a condition known as rhinophyma (Fig. 20.30). This is more common in males and there may not be much concomitant rosacea.

The eyes may also be involved (Fig. 20.31). Patients complain of discomfort or a feeling of grittiness in the eyes. Conjunctivitis, blepharitis and keratitis with ulceration and vascularization of the cornea with potential visual impairment may be present. Lymphoedema may occur around the eyes (Fig. 20.32). The degree of rosacea may be quite minor in these ocular cases.

The cause of rosacea is unknown. Histology shows vascular dilatation and sebaceous hyperplasia. The patients have a vasomotor instability which is made worse by hot drinks, particularly tea and coffee. It is the temperature of the drinks not their caffeine content, which is the triggering factor. Hot or highly-spiced foods and alcohol also aggravate the condition. Indeed, rosacea may be a presenting feature of alcohol abuse. The ambient temperature and weather conditions may also aggravate the condition. Sunlight, cold winds and hot rooms all have an adverse effect.

Some authorities have implicated *Demodex folliculorum* in rosacea. It is a mite which is a normal inhabitant of the follicular apparatus and can sometimes be recovered in large numbers in rosacea. However, the appropriate treatment of rosacea does not appear to make any difference to the numbers of mites present.

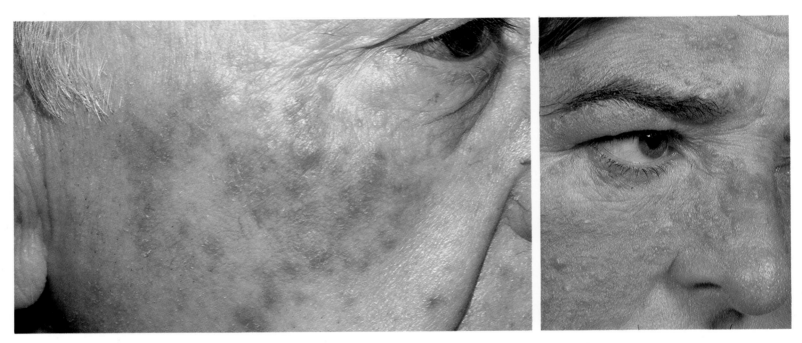

Fig. 20.26 Rosacea. Papules and pustules occur on the face. Comedones are not formed, unlike in acne.

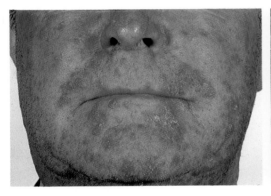

Fig. 20.27 Rosacea. The lesions occur on the forehead, cheeks, chin and nose.

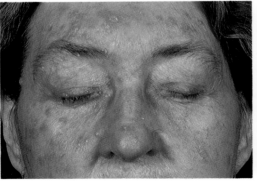

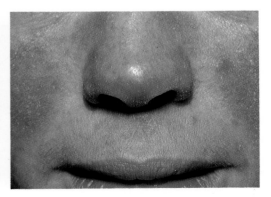

Fig. 20.28 Rosacea. Such patients tend to flush easily and there is often erythema of the face.

Rosacea, like acne, responds to oral antibiotics but does so much more quickly and effectively. However, the antibiotics usually have to be taken indefinitely, although most patients can adjust the dosage so that they only take one tablet a day or every other day. Tetracycline, erythromycin, septrin and metronidazole are all effective. Topical therapy with sulphur starting at doses of one percent but increasing up to ten percent may be a useful adjunct to therapy. Alcohol, hot drinks and spicy foods should be avoided or reduced. The eyes should be examined by an ophthalmologist if ocular symptoms are present. Oral antibiotics do benefit the eye complications but other medications may be required. Plastic surgery is the treatment of choice for rhinophyma.

Topical Steroids and Rosacea

In the late 1960s and early 1970s there was a widespread malpractice of prescribing powerful topical steroids to treat rosacea. The resulting condition (Fig. 20.33) is much less common now but patients do still use topical steroids which have been prescribed for other conditions, or have been given to them by well-meaning, often paramedical friends. Powerful topical glucocorticosteroids cause vasoconstriction of the skin and might therefore be thought to be helpful in a vasoactive disease such as rosacea. However, it is probable that a rebound vasodilatation occurs which makes the condition worse. Certainly, they appear to be effective at first but on stopping the steroids, the condition flares and the patient, presumably believing that the steroid has kept the condition under control, reapplies it and a vicious circle develops.

The face becomes very red and atrophic and papules and pustules (Fig. 20.34) develop over the areas where the steroid has been applied, which often includes the neck as well as the face.

It is important to inquire about the use of topical steroids in any patient with rosacea. Patients can be remarkably evasive in admitting to their use but the condition is easy to treat once the patient is made aware of the problem. Oral antibiotics are effective but it is important to warn the patient that there is likely to be a rebound worsening of the disease for a few days on stopping the steroid before the improvement takes place.

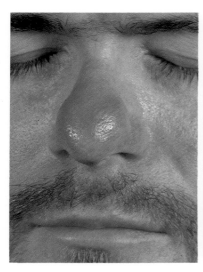

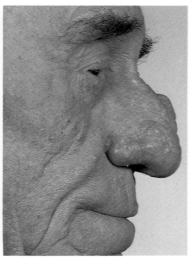

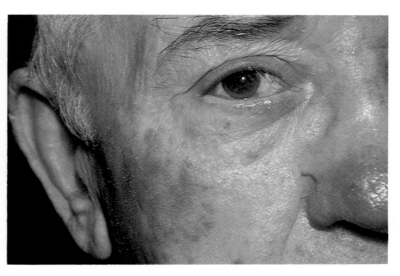

Fig. 20.29   Rosacea. Occasionally the nose may be red without involvement elsewhere. This variety does not respond well to antibiotic therapy unlike other types.

Fig. 20.30   Rhinophyma. This may occur in the absence of rosacea on the face. There is hypertrophy of the sebaceous glands and overgrowth of the soft tissues.

Fig. 20.31   Rosacea. This man has a red eye in addition to his rosacea. Eye symptoms and signs are common.

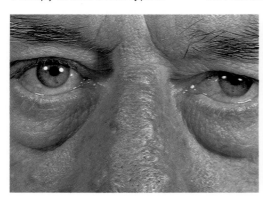

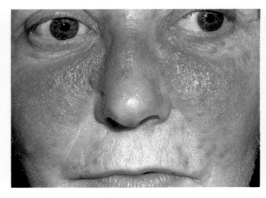

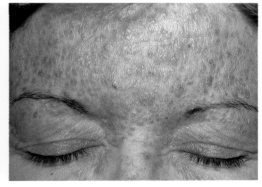

Fig. 20.32   Lymphoedema and rhinophyma. Lymphoedema of the eyelids may occur in addition to rhinophyma or rosacea.

Fig. 20.33   Topical steroid-treated rosacea. Topical steroids are contra-indicated in rosacea and exacerbate the condition.

Fig. 20.34   Topical steroid-treated rosacea. The condition responds initially to steroids but relapses on cessation of treatment. The patient therefore usually restarts applying them. The rosacea gradually worsens. Oral antibiotics are the correct treatment for rosacea.

Perioral Dermatitis

This has been a very common condition in the past. Papules and pustules occur around the mouth (Figs. 20.35 and 20.36) with erythema and sometimes scaling, and occasionally around the eye (periorbital dermatitis). It is caused by the misuse of the more powerful topical glucocorticosteroids on the face. There is some argument as to whether the condition was ever seen before the advent of these powerful therapeutic agents but certainly the condition has become widely recognized and a frequent occurrence since their advent. The condition has now become common knowledge among medical practitioners and the specialist does not see it so often. The original condition for which the topical steroids were prescribed is usually acne but sometimes seborrhoeic eczema.

The condition responds rapidly to stopping the topical steroids and commencing low-dosage antibiotic therapy. The underlying condition will require treatment; if this is acne it may be necessary to carry on the antibiotics for longer periods and if it is seborrhoeic eczema then topical hydrocortisone i.e. a weak steroid, is usually effective.

Acne Agminata (Lupus Miliaris Disseminatus Faciei)

This is an uncommon eruption of monomorphic, small, brown papules. It is of interest because the histology shows a granulomatous reaction, often with central caseation. In the past, it was thought to be a tuberculide but it does not respond to anti-tuberculous therapy and any relationship to this disease is now discounted.

The papules are distributed symmetrically on the forehead, temples, cheek, chin (Fig. 20.37) and, in particular, on the eyelids (Fig. 20.38) which is an unusual site for acne vulgaris. The papules are persistent but ultimately heal, often with unsightly scarring. The condition disappears after a couple of years and its aetiology is quite unknown. There is no particularly effective treatment although systemic antibiotics are worth trying and occasionally systemic steroids may help.

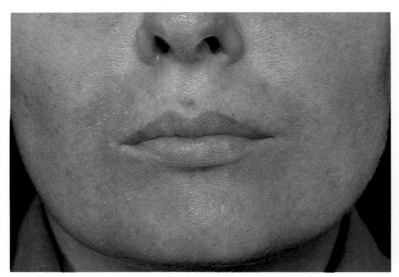

Fig. 20.35 Perioral dermatitis. Redness and scaling occurs around the mouth if powerful topical steroids are used to treat acne or seborrhoeic dermatitis. By courtesy of St. John's Hospital for Diseases of the Skin.

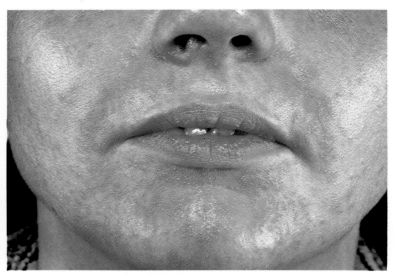

Fig. 20.36 Perioral dermatitis. Pronounced perioral erythema with papules and pustules results from the treatment of acne with powerful topical steroids. By courtesy of St. John's Hospital for Diseases of the Skin.

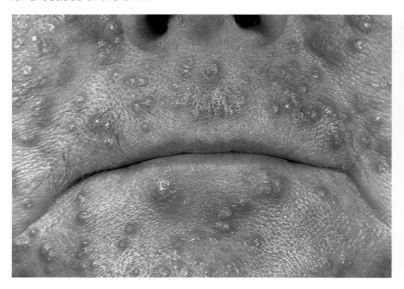

Fig. 20.37 Acne agminata. Monomorphic persistent small red-brown papules occur on the face. This is an uncommon condition. The histology shows a granuloma and the condition was previously thought to be related to tuberculosis, but this is now discounted.

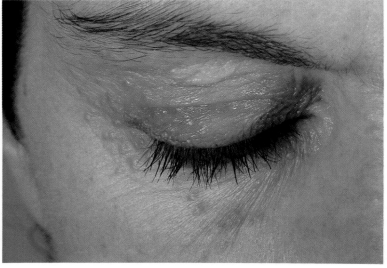

Fig. 20.38 Acne agminata. The eyelids are particularly affected in this condition. It ultimately resolves spontaneously.

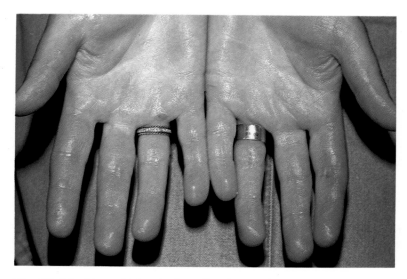

Fig. 20.39 Hyperhidrosis. Localized sweating may interfere with function, e.g. typing or writing with an ink pen, in addition to being embarrassing.

DISORDERS OF THE SWEAT GLANDS

Hyperhidrosis of the Skin

Localized excess sweating is a common disorder affecting either the axillae or the hands (Fig. 20.39) and feet. The cause is quite unknown and in severe cases may be extremely troublesome.

Management is not easy. There is a poor response to oral anticholinergic agents and the side-effects tend to outweigh the benefits. However, iontophoresis of these drugs via an electric current into the skin may be useful for cases limited to the hands and feet. Aluminium salts and formalin have a limited role as anti perspirants. Surgical excision of affected axillary skin is often very successful. Sympathectomy can sometimes be helpful in very severe cases affecting the hands and feet.

Pitted Keratolysis (Keratolysis Plantare Sulcatum)

This disorder occurs in patients who have considerable hyperhidrosis of the feet (Figs. 20.40–20.42). Occlusive footwear causes the skin to become damp and sodden. The macerated stratum corneum is invaded by organisms, either of the *Corynebacterium* or *Streptomyces* species. Circular, superficial erosions result on the soles and on the plantar surfaces of the toes. Treatment of the hyperhidrosis is necessary and formalin is often of benefit here. Topical fucidin may eradicate the organisms.

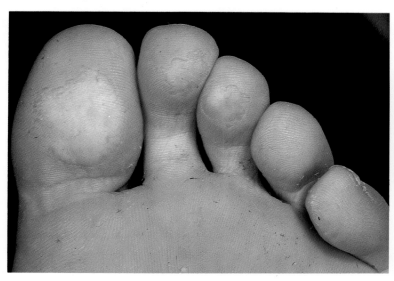

Fig. 20.40 Pitted keratolysis. The stratum corneum becomes macerated and sodden with plantar hyperhydrosis. Occlusive footwear accentuates the problem. By courtesy of Dr. A.C. Pembroke.

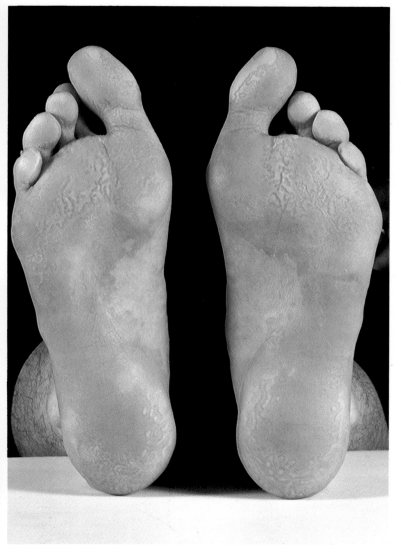

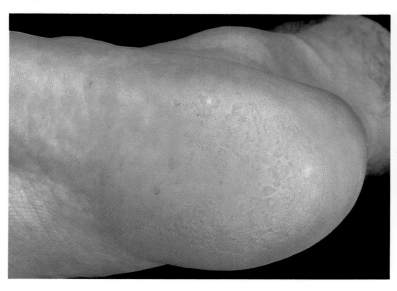

Fig. 20.41 Pitted keratolysis. Organisms invade the damp stratum corneum and superficial erosions result. By courtesy of Dr. A.C. Pembroke.

Fig. 20.42 Pitted keratolysis. The instep is usually spared.

Miliaria (Prickly Heat)

This is a common disorder in the tropics but is singularly uncommon elsewhere. The sweat duct becomes blocked by a keratin plug and the patient cannot sweat properly. In the form known as 'prickly heat' (*miliaria rubra*) the block occurs in the duct at the level of the epidermis. This results in a widespread, very itchy eruption consisting of red papulovesicles, particularly on the trunk. It responds quickly to cooling. In *miliaria crystallina* the duct becomes blocked at its orifice and then tiny, very superficial vesicles occur. This is seen in patients with an acute febrile illness and it subsides without symptoms in a matter of a few days.

DISORDERS OF APOCRINE GLANDS
Hidradenitis Suppurativa

This is a chronic disorder of the apocrine glands in the axillae and anogenital regions. The cause is unknown. Indolent, uncomfortable pustules and nodules occur (Figs. 20.43 and 20.44). They break down to form abscesses and sinuses (Fig. 20.45) which connect up with one another. Puckered scarring results. There is often concomitant acne and patients are sometimes overweight. There is no specific treatment but long-term antibiotics and intralesional steroids are sometimes helpful. Excision of local areas of affected skin and grafting (Fig. 20.46) can be successful if the disease is limited.

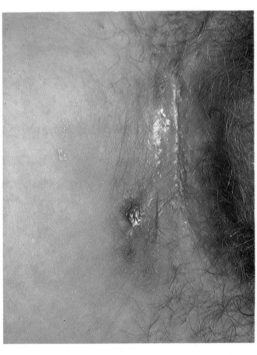

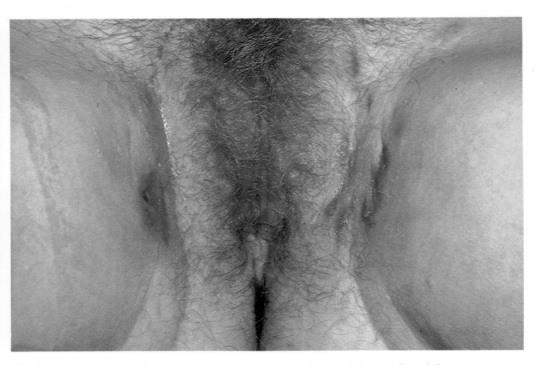

Fig. 20.43 Hidradenitis suppurativa. The groin is a common site.

Fig. 20.44 Hidradenitis suppurativa. Indolent painful pustules and nodules occur. Sinuses and scars result.

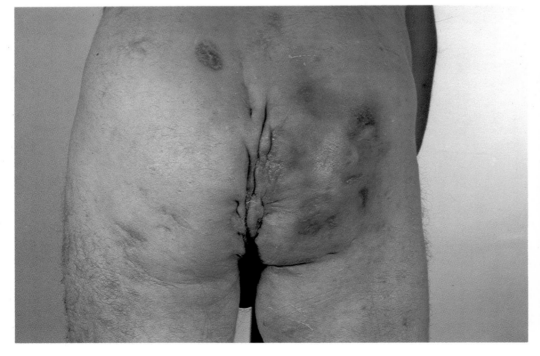

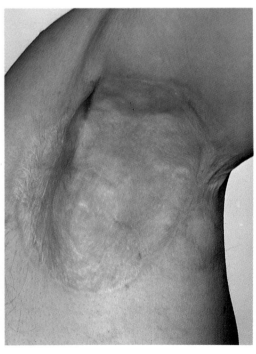

Fig. 20.45 Hidradenitis suppurativa. Severe scarring has resulted on this man's buttocks. Treatment is not very effective in this condition.

Fig. 20.46 Hidradenitis suppurativa. Excision of the apocrine glands and grafting may be extremely helpful in disease confined to the axillae or groins.

21 Disorders of the Nails

The nail protects the distal phalanx, facilitates the picking up of small objects and contributes to the appreciation of fine touch. The nailplate consists of hard keratin which is derived from an infolding of the epidermis on the dorsal surface of the finger. It lies on a bed, where it is firmly attached to the epidermis. It grows largely from a matrix, which extends from the junction of the roof and floor of the nailfold posteriorly to the foremost portion of the half moon (lunula). The latter is thought to be paler than the rest of the nailbed because keratinization is incomplete in this area and possibly the connective tissue is packed more loosely. The cuticle is an extension of the stratum corneum of the dorsum of the finger onto the nailplate and plays an important part in the protection of the potential space between the roof of the nailfold and its floor.

Under normal conditions the fingernails take about five months to grow out, but the toenails take considerably longer, between twelve and eighteen months. There is a variation in growth rates between individual fingernails and nails on the dominant hand grow fastest.

The diagnosis of nail disorders is difficult. Many abnormalities are untreatable, but it is always important to take clippings for mycological studies because fungal disorders are practically always treatable.

INFECTIONS AFFECTING THE NAILS
Acute Paronychia
This is usually a staphylococcal infection of the lateral or posterior nailfold (Fig. 21.1). Trauma is important in its aetiology and the patient is often a nail biter. The condition has an acute onset and presents as a painful red swelling of the nailfold. The pus may point (Fig. 21.2) and surgical drainage may be necessary, but broad spectrum antibiotics may be successful in the early stages. Sometimes an acute paronychia is superimposed on an existing chronic fungal infection (Fig. 21.3).

Chronic Paronychia
This is a very common condition which is more frequently mismanaged than misdiagnosed. *Candida albicans* is the most important organism involved. The condition is occupational and is almost exclusively a disorder of women. It is seen only in those males whose occupation involves having the hands frequently in and out of water. It is the continual immersion of the hands in water that sets up the scenario for the disease. The disease is thus most commonly seen in nurses, hairdressers, cooks, barmen and housewives. Water, especially alkaline, softens and eventually destroys the cuticle. This opens up a space between the posterior nailfold and the nailplate (Fig. 21.4). The consequent damp and occluded environment under the nailfold is ideal for colonization with *Candida albicans*. Candida is a skin commensal and acts as an opportunist, but occasionally the patient has vaginal thrush which may be the source.

The index and the middle fingers are most commonly involved and the patient usually presents with involvement of one finger only, but in neglected cases many or all of the fingers are affected. The physical signs consist of a red swelling of the lateral and posterior nailfolds (Fig. 21.5). The swelling is not particularly painful, although on occasion an acute paronychia may be superimposed and this is usually due to secondary infection either with staphylococcus, streptococcus, *Escherichia coli* or *Pseudomonas aeruginosa*. The cuticle is lost, the posterior nailfold is opened up and it may be possible to express a bead of pus. If this is not possible, the patient will frequently give a history that pus discharges from time to time. The nail itself is affected later on in the disease (Fig. 21.6) as a result of

interference with nail growth through involvement of the nail matrix under the posterior nailfold. This produces cross ridging of the nailplate (Fig. 21.7). The nailplate may also be invaded by the organism.

The successful management of this condition depends to a great extent on the co-operation of the patient in avoiding contact with water. The patient has to be fastidious about keeping the hands out of water and must dry them scrupulously should they become wet. The use of cotton gloves under rubber gloves is recommended for washing-up but even these should be kept on for a very short time, as the occlusive nature of the gloves will allow the fingers to become moist. Treatment of the condition with imidazole or nystatin ointments is important for the elimination of *Candida albicans*. Provided the patient grasps the significance of the detrimental effects of water, a cure is perfectly possible but it does take a number of months. The condition may be mismanaged because the significance of wet work is not appreciated and therapy involves treatment of the causative organism only, which in itself is not enough. Also, casualty medical officers have a penchant for incising the nailfold.

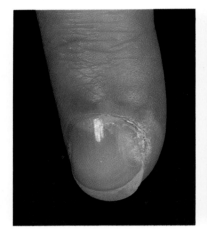
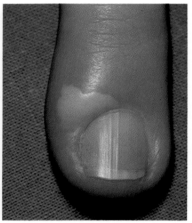

Fig. 21.1 Acute paronychia. The lateral and posterior nailfolds are red and swollen. *Staphylococcus aureus* is usually responsible. By courtesy of Dr. A.C. Pembroke.

Fig. 21.2 Acute paronychia. Pus and erythema are present. By courtesy of Dr. E.E. Glucksman, King's College Hospital.

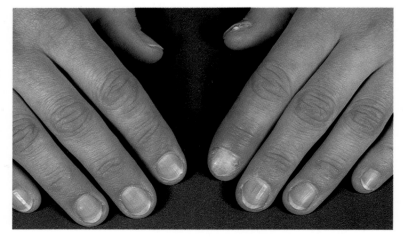

Fig. 21.3 Acute paronychia. This lady has a tinea infection of her left thumb and index fingernail. An acute paronychia is superimposed on the index finger.

Candidiasis of the Nailplate

Candidal invasion of the nailplate is not as common, but occurs as a result of chronic paronychia (Fig. 21.8) or may be super-imposed on the onycholytic changes secondary to psoriasis. Very much less commonly, invasion may occur in the absence of preceding paronychia or onycholysis. Several nails are usually involved and there appear to be two forms of dystrophy. In one form, the nail itself remains fairly normal to touch, but is over-curved in its long axis and appears rather brown. In the second form, the condition may be extremely difficult to distinguish clinically from tinea. This illustrates the importance of sending clippings of the nails to the laboratory before starting therapy for infections, since they do not respond to local measures. *Candida albicans* does not respond to griseofulvin and this will explain why some nails which appear clinically to be affected by tinea do not improve with this drug, when in reality they are infected by *Candida albicans*. The advent of ketoconazole has, however, remarkably transformed the situation since it is effective not only against tinea but also against *Candida albicans* (Fig. 21.9). Prior to this, it was virtually impossible to treat candidal infections of the nailplate in the absence of chronic paronychia as a cause. Hypoparathyroidism, acrodermatititis enteropathica and chronic mucocutaneous candidiasis pre-dispose the nail to invasion.

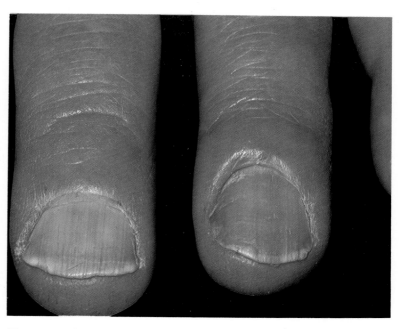

Fig. 21.4 Chronic paronychia. There is loss of the cuticle on the right, which has resulted in an opening into the posterior nailfold. Continual immersion of the hands in water results in breakdown of the protective cuticle.

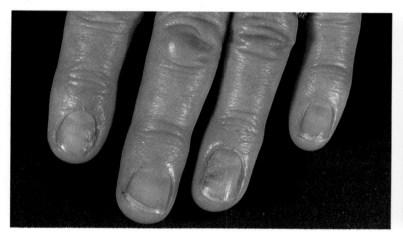

Fig. 21.5 Chronic paronychia. The lateral nailfolds are swollen and red. *Candida albicans* has invaded the nailfolds.

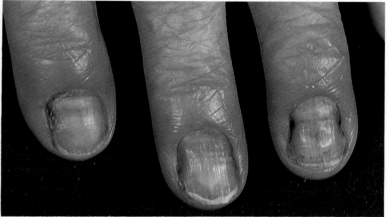

Fig. 21.6 Chronic paronychia. In neglected cases the nails become invaded by *Candida albicans*.

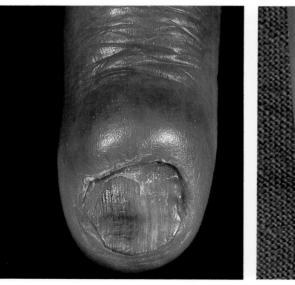

Fig. 21.7 Chronic paronychia. The posterior nailfold is swollen (bolstered) and the cuticle is lost. The nail is discoloured secondary to invasion by *Candida albicans*.

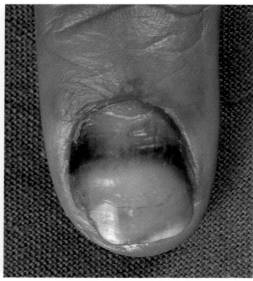

Fig. 21.8 Chronic paronychia. The lateral cuticle is lost. Considerable ridging and discoloration of the nailplate has occurred, secondary to invasion by *Candida albicans*.

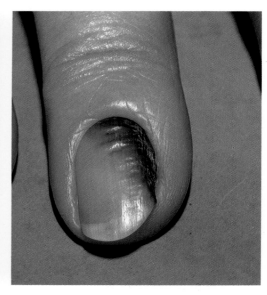

Fig. 21.9 Candida of the nails. Severe nailplate infections require treatment with oral ketoconazole and healing will occur within six months. Candida infections do not respond to griseofulvin.

21.3

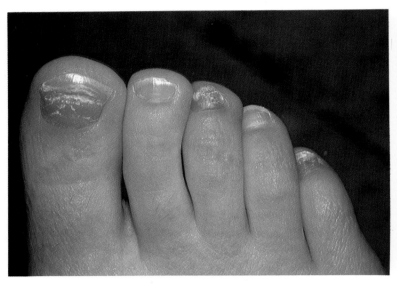

Fig. 21.10 Tinea of the nails. Three toenails are involved but two are completely spared.

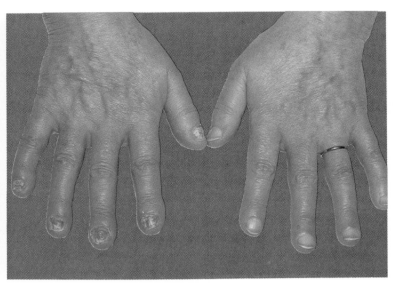

Fig. 21.11 Tinea of the nails. The involvement is asymmetrical. One hand is involved and the other is spared. The condition may remain unilateral for many years.

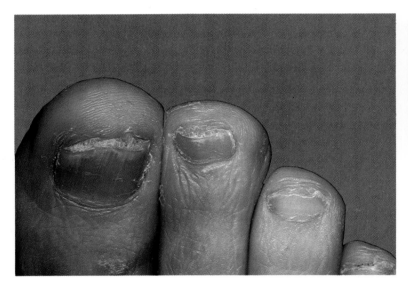

Fig. 21.12 Tinea of the nails. The infection begins at the sides of the nails. There is a brown discoloration and thickening of the nail.

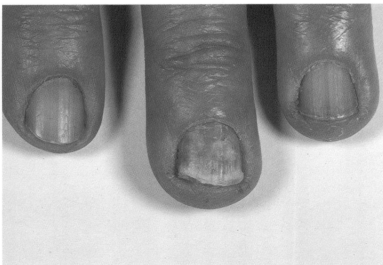

Fig. 21.13 Tinea of the fingernails. Onycholysis has occurred. The toenails were extensively involved. Clippings should be taken for microscopy and culture before treatment with griseofulvin is begun.

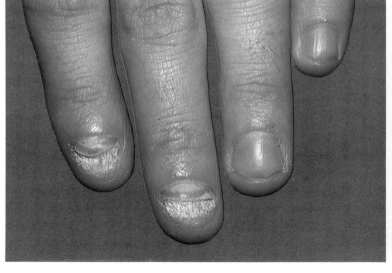

Fig. 21.14 Tinea of the nails. Partial loss of the nails may occur.

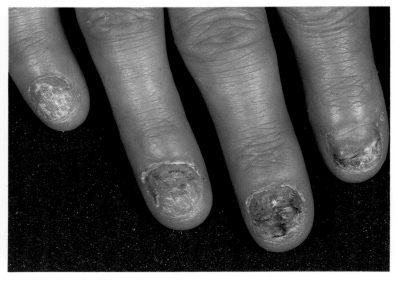

Fig. 21.15 Tinea of the nails. Gross destruction may occur in long-standing cases, resulting in loss of the nail.

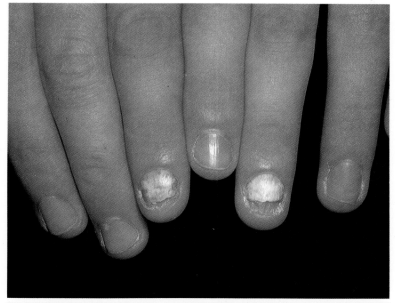

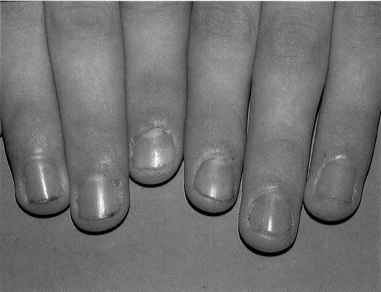

Fig. 21.16 Tinea of the nails. Ringworm infections of the nails do not respond to topical therapy. Griseofulvin is the treatment of choice for tinea (upper). The nails recover after 5–6 months of oral griseofulvin (lower).

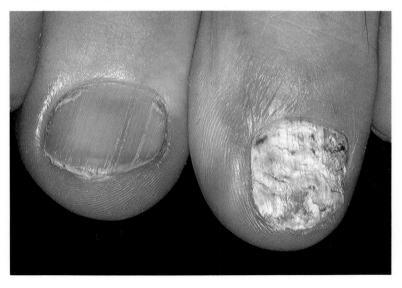

Fig. 21.17 *Aspergillus* invasion of the big toenail. The large toe is susceptible to continual trauma. *Aspergillus* species may invade the nail and produce a patchy white discoloration of the plate.

Tinea Unguium

Ringworm of the nails is a common malady which frequently affects the toenails and often goes unremarked by the patient. It is usually only when the fingernails become involved that medical advice is sought. Many such patients have a cold peripheral circulation.

The most common fungi to infect the nails are *Trichophyton rubrum* and *T. mentagrophytes* (var. *interdigitale*). Clinically there is no way of telling the species involved and culture of nail clippings is necessary. The involvement of the nails is asymmetrical and this is characteristic of tinea.

It is remarkable how several toenails may be extensively involved on one foot and yet one or two are totally unaffected (Fig. 21.10). Also the other foot may be much less involved. As regards the hands, it is an extraordinary and quite unexplained phenomenon that the fingernails of one hand may be infected with fungus for years before the other hand is affected, if at all (Fig. 21.11).

Usually the skin is involved in addition to the nails and these changes may raise the suspicion of the diagnosis (q.v.). However, sometimes there appears to be no involvement of the skin at all. The invasion starts as a brown discoloration at the edge of the nail (Fig. 21.12) and may then become widespread. Later the nail and its bed become thickened and as a result onycholysis occurs (Fig. 21.13).

The thickened nail crumbles easily and this is noticeable when taking clippings for mycology. In severely affected nails, part of the nail will break away completely (Figs. 21.14 and 21.15). Sometimes white patches are seen in the nailplate, probably secondary to pockets of air.

Tinea of the nails does not respond to any local therapy but requires many months of systemic therapy with either griseofulvin (Fig. 21.16) or ketoconazole. It is therefore imperative that the diagnosis is proven before starting on a treatment which might otherwise be fruitless and, certainly in the case of ketoconazole, not without risk in view of its hepatotoxicity. The diagnosis can be easily made by soaking clippings from the nails in 30% potassium hydroxide, after which it will be possible to find the fungal hyphae under the microscope. Cultures can also be made to determine the species, but the fungus does not always grow. Fingernail infections are always worth treating and require at least six months of therapy. It is more difficult to decide whether or not to treat toenail infections. It is usually necessary for the patient to take the drug for the best part of eighteen months to two years and even then there is no guarantee that the condition will not recur. It is probably worthwhile treating younger patients, but only if they are likely to be totally conscientious in taking the tablets every day. If the toenails have become severely damaged, particularly the large toenail, an ingrowing nail will sometimes occur during treatment. This is because the normally growing nail is wider than the nailbed, which has become smaller due to the shrunken nature of the diseased nail. Appropriate treatment is necessary.

Aspergillus Species

This is quite a common fungal infection affecting almost solely the great toenails. There is a patchy, white discoloration of the nail (Fig. 21.17). The organism is a secondary invader of a previously traumatized toenail and the big toenail is the most susceptible to such damage.

NAIL DISORDERS ASSOCIATED WITH CUTANEOUS DISEASE
Psoriasis

Psoriasis is a common skin disorder and the nails are probably involved in most psoriatic patients at some time in their lives. Occasionally nail changes identical to those seen in psoriasis occur in the absence of evidence of the disease on the skin, although cutaneous changes may subsequently occur. The diagnosis then has to be presumptive unless a nail biopsy is performed. The latter is a somewhat traumatic procedure and can leave a deforming scar, so it is often best avoided.

There are three forms of abnormality recognized with psoriasis.

1) Pitting

Tiny pits (Fig. 21.18) varying from just a few to a large number are seen on the surface of the nailplate, including over the lunula. They tend to be arranged in an irregular manner. Sometimes the arrangement may be uniform so that lines are produced, particularly along the length of the nails (Fig. 21.19). These pits are usually symmetrically distributed so that the corresponding fingernail of the other hand will show similar changes. The pits are believed to be due to parakeratosis (retention of nuclei in the nail keratin) similar to that which occurs in the stratum corneum in psoriatic skin. These areas of parakeratosis are presumed to be weaker than the surrounding nail and fall out leaving the pits behind.

2) Onycholysis

Onycholysis is the separation of the nail away from its bed (Fig. 21.20). It is a common feature in psoriasis. It usually involves the free edge of the nail and a considerable gap occurs between the nail and its bed (Fig. 21.21). Sometimes the separation occurs in the centre of the nail and a characteristic feature is a yellow margin discernible between the pink, normal-looking nail and the onycholysis. The involvement of the nails is usually symmetrical. The onycholysis is thought to be due to psoriasis underneath the nail (Figs. 21.22 and 21.23).

3) Gross Nail Dystrophy

The nail may be severely damaged by psoriasis and becomes most unsightly. It is thickened and discoloured (Figs. 21.24 and 21.25). This appears to start in the matrix underneath the cuticle. All the nails are usually involved to some degree and the state of the affliction may vary: one nail recovering and another deteriorating. Although recovery may occur, the prognosis is poor. It is common for patients who have psoriatic arthritis involving the distal interphalangeal joints to have gross nail changes (Fig. 21.26), but conversely, nail changes without joint abnormalities are much more common. In pustular psoriasis, either the generalized variety or the variety localized to the hands or feet, gross involvement of the nails commonly occurs and the nails may be lost altogether as a result of the process.

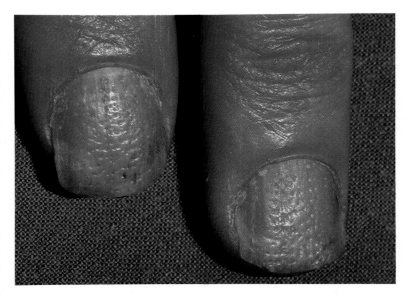

Fig. 21.18 Psoriasis. The fingernail is covered by multiple small pits and some onycholysis is present.

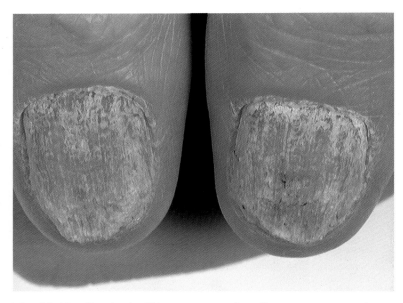

Fig. 21.19 Psoriasis. Pits may occur in a linear manner and produce longitudinal lines. Symmetry is a feature of psoriasis.

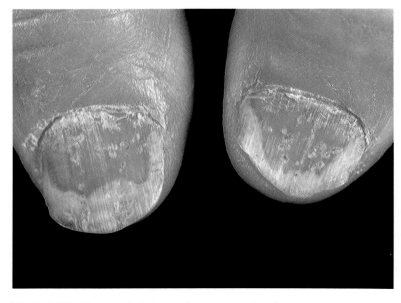

Fig. 21.20 Psoriasis. The nails are usually affected symmetrically. There is onycholysis and pitting

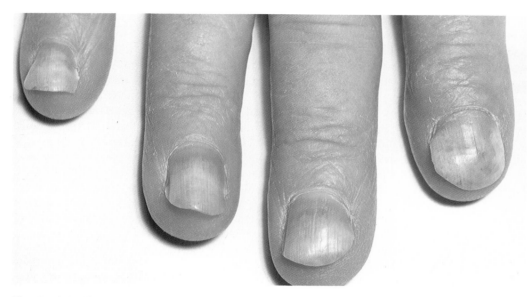

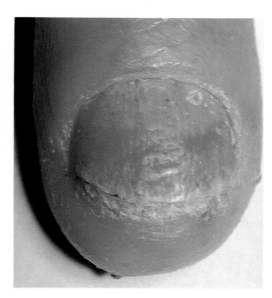

Fig. 21.21   Psoriasis. Extensive onycholysis is present. This may occur in the absence of psoriasis elsewhere and the diagnosis may be difficult. This patient developed cutaneous psoriasis one year later.

Fig. 21.22   Psoriasis. Psoriasis is present under the distal margin of the nail. Pitting is also visible.

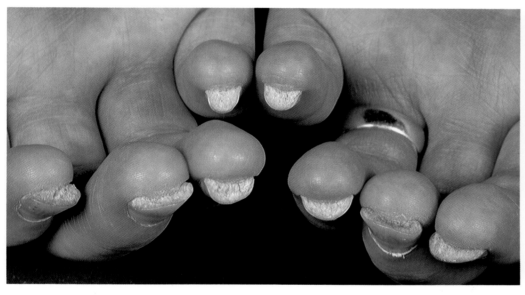

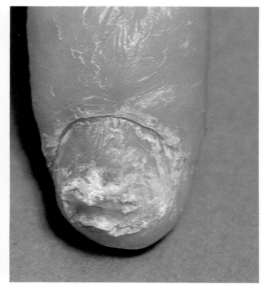

Fig. 21.23   Psoriasis. There is symmetrical hyperkeratotic psoriasis under the nails, which causes onycholysis.

Fig. 21.24   Psoriasis. Gross destructive changes are present.

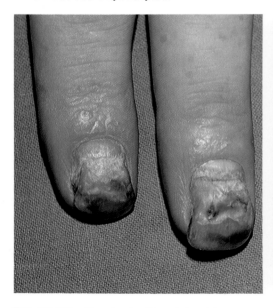

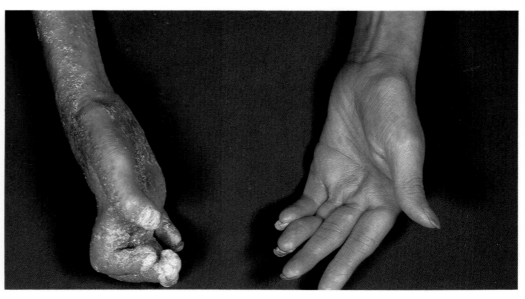

Fig. 21.25   Psoriasis. Considerable hyperkeratosis under the nail has led to severe onycholysis and discoloration.

Fig. 21.26   Psoriasis. It is common for patients with psoriatic arthritis to have gross nail changes, but the nails may be involved without any joint abnormalities.

The treatment of psoriatic nail changes is extremely disappointing. In the grosser varieties where the matrix appears to be involved it is worth injecting steroids, particularly via a Dermojet, or applying topical steroids under occlusion, because remissions may occasionally be induced. In those patients who have severe cutaneous psoriasis and receive systemic cytotoxic therapy, the nail involvement will recover completely (Fig. 21.27).

Onycholysis

The most common cause of onycholysis is psoriasis. However, a single or several nails may be involved (Fig. 21.28) without cutaneous evidence of the disease, or even a positive family history of psoriasis or arthritis. The cause is unknown, although trauma may be relevant. The condition often responds spontaneously. Certain drugs, particularly when associated with strong sunlight (Fig. 21.29), may cause onycholysis of all the nails. The tetracycline group and the non-steroidal anti-inflammatory drug benoxaprofen are examples. Thyrotoxicosis may be associated with a widespread onycholysis (Fig. 21.30).

Sometimes onycholysis may be complicated by secondary infection, particularly candidiasis and pseudomonas (Fig. 21.31).

Pseudomonas

Pseudomonas aeruginosa is a common secondary invader of diseased nails, especially those with onycholysis and chronic paronychia. It imparts a green discoloration to the nail (Fig. 21.32). 15% sulphacetamide is a useful remedy.

Nail Changes associated with Eczema of the Hands

Changes of the fingernails secondary to eczema are usually obvious because eczema is also seen on the fingers, particularly around the posterior nailfolds. However, occasionally patients will present with abnormalities in their nails some time after the eczema of the skin has healed. The physical signs are usually ridges across the nails (Fig. 21.33), quite similar to Beau's lines except that there is normally more than one ridge in eczema (Fig. 21.34). If the process has been severe, there may be temporary shedding of the nail, particularly as an end result of exfoliative dermatitis. Coarse pitting may occur in addition or occasionally on its own. Secondary infection with *Candida albicans* occasionally occurs, but in these cases the nails will be discoloured and nailfold abnormalities typical of candidiasis will be present (q.v.).

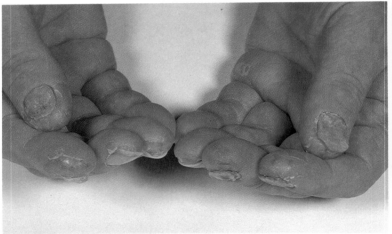

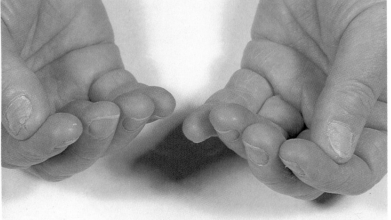

Fig. 21.27   Psoriasis of the fingertips and nails. Psoriasis of the fingertips is very painful and does not respond well to topical therapy (left). There is no local treatment for psoriasis of the nails. This man's skin and nails responded very well to an oral retinoid, etretinate (right).

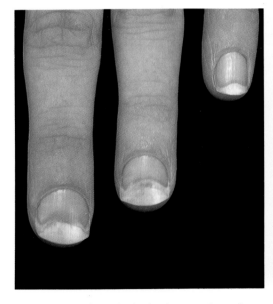

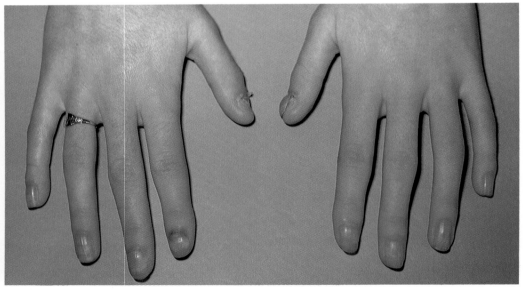

Fig. 21.28   Onycholysis. Loosening of the nail away from the nailbed may occur without obvious cause. By courtesy of St. John's Hospital for Diseases of the Skin.

Fig. 21.29   Photo-onycholysis. All the fingernails are involved and some are being shed. This patient was taking a tetracycline and had been holidaying in a sunny climate; a phototoxic reaction occurred.

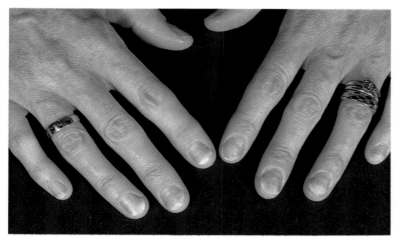

Lichen Planus

Nail changes occur only in a minority of patients with lichen planus, but when present they can be severe, resulting in permanent damage. The most commonly encountered abnormality is an increase in the longitudinal lines (Fig. 21.35) which develop into ridges. In other patients the nailplate becomes thin and atrophic and the cuticle grows forward onto the nailplate. This is known as *pterygium*. The atrophic nailplate is usually lost permanently (Fig. 21.36), but this is not always the case.

The damage in lichen planus appears to take place in the nail matrix; some authorities advocate the use of systemic steroids in early cases to prevent permanent scarring and loss of the nail. Occasionally nail changes typical of lichen planus may occur in the absence of a history, or the presence of lichen planus on the skin.

Fig. 21.30 Onycholysis. When all the nails are involved it is often possible to identify the cause. This lady had thyrotoxicosis.

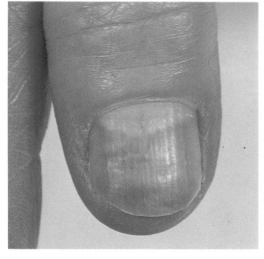

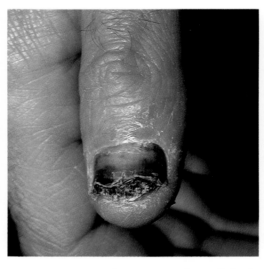

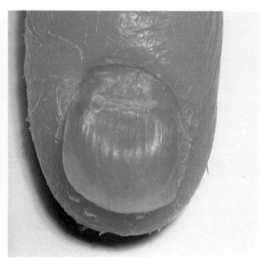

Fig. 21.31 Onycholysis. Solitary involvement is not uncommon in women. Minor trauma to long nails may be the cause. *Pseudomonas aeruginosa* frequently is a secondary invader and imparts a green colour.

Fig. 21.32 Pseudomonas and candidiasis of the nails. Pseudomonas produces a green discoloration of the nailplate. It is always important to take clippings from abnormal nails. Cultures grew *Candida* species. The nail completely recovered with ketoconazole.

Fig. 21.33 Nail changes and eczema. Eczema around the nailfolds produces horizontal ridging of the nails.

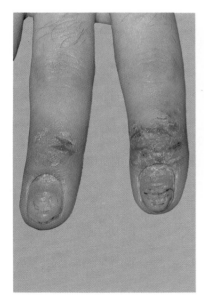

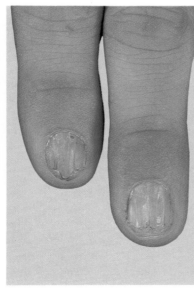

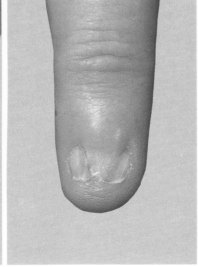

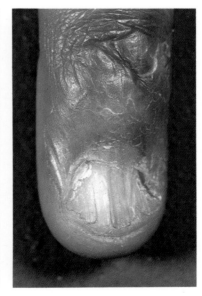

Fig. 21.34 Nail changes associated with eczema. Gross ridging may occur with severe eczema.

Fig. 21.35 Lichen planus. Longitudinal lines may sometimes occur on the nailplate (left). Adhesion may form between the epidermis of the posterior nailfold and the nailplate, resulting in pterygium formation. By courtesy of St. John's Hospital for Diseases of the Skin.

Fig. 21.36 Lichen planus. Permanent destruction of the nails may result.

21.9

Alopecia Areata

In addition to hair loss there may also be nail changes. Pitting similar to that in psoriasis is the most common abnormality, although rather than being irregularly distributed through the nailplate, the pitting often occurs in a regular manner either along the longitudinal (Fig. 21.37) or horizontal axis of the nail and sometimes both. Occasionally gross changes occur, particularly in association with alopecia universalis. No treatment is available for these disorders but the prognosis is quite good for the pitting variety.

Twenty Nail Dystrophy of Childhood

This is rather a characteristic condition in that all twenty nails are involved without any other disturbance (Fig. 21.38). The cause is quite unknown and the abnormality consists of excess ridging along the entire length of the nails. It is not present at birth and does not appear to occur in adult life. It usually improves during childhood, but may take a number of years.

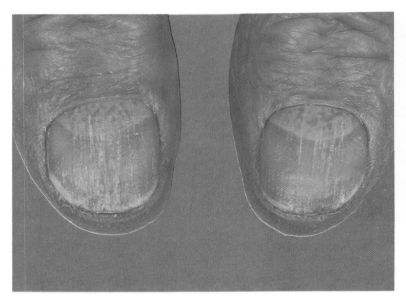

Fig. 21.37 Alopecia areata. Pitting is characteristic and is usually arranged symmetrically in longitudinal lines.

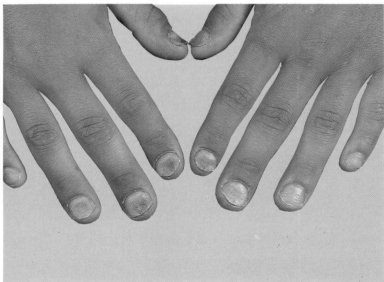

Fig. 21.38 The twenty nail syndrome. This is a disorder of unknown cause which is found in children. All twenty nails are involved. It usually resolves spontaneously.

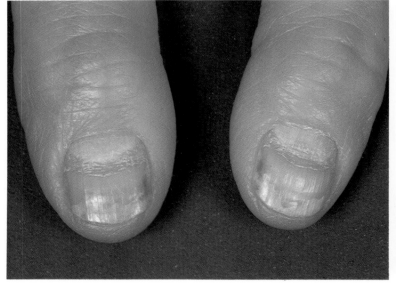

Fig. 21.39 Beau's lines. Severe illness temporarily interferes with the growth of the nails and a horizontal ridge occurs. It is not usually noticed until it is half way up the nailplate, some months after the illness.

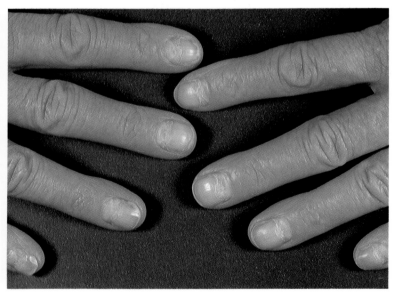

Fig. 21.40 Beau's lines. All the nails are involved.

NAIL CHANGES ASSOCIATED WITH SYSTEMIC CAUSES
Beau's Lines
These lines consist of a single depression across the horizontal axis of the nailplate (Fig. 21.39). They occur after any moderately severe physical or mental illness and are due to a temporary slowing in the rate of growth of the nails. All the nails are affected (Fig. 21.40), which will serve to distinguish the condition from local causes of horizontal ridging, such as eczema or trauma. In a very severe illness, the whole thickness of the nailplate may be involved and the nail temporarily shed (Figs. 21.41 and 21.42). Patients often present with the complaint some time after the illness, for the change is not immediately apparent, only appearing as the nail grows out.

Koilonychia
This abnormality is associated with iron deficiency anaemia and consists of a 'spooning' of the nailplate such that it is concave instead of its normal convex shape (Fig. 21.43). Similar changes may occur in association with Raynaud's phenomenon or may be congenital.

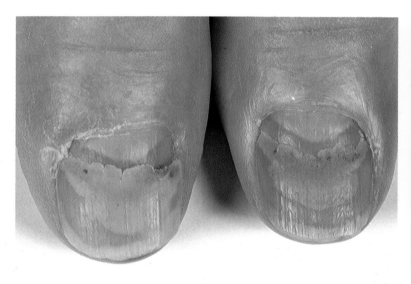

Fig. 21.41 Shedding of the nails. This may result after a severe illness.

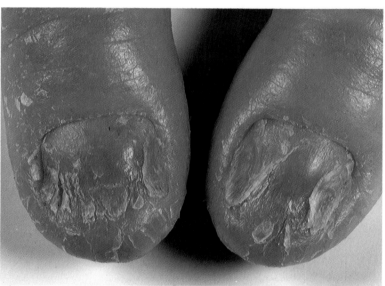

Fig. 21.42 Shedding of the nails. Total loss of the nails may occur after severe illness. This patient has exfoliative psoriasis.

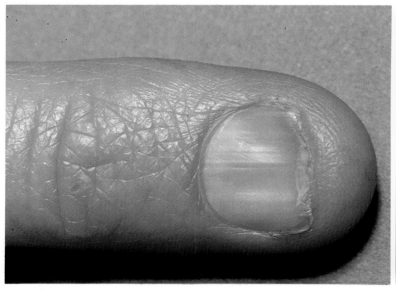

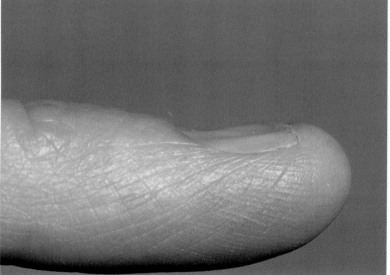

Fig. 21.43 Koilonychia. The nail is concave rather than convex and is thus 'spoon'-shaped. In this case the deformity was congenital. By courtesy of Dr. A.C. Pembroke.

Clubbing of the Nails

This is an extremely important physical sign and the cause should be vigorously sought (Fig. 21.44). It is not often noticed by the patient and it rarely presents to the dermatologist. It is usually readily recognized by the general physician during a medical examination. There is a loss of the normal angulation between the posterior nailfold and the nailplate such that it is 180° or more. The posterior nailfold overlying the nail matrix feels spongy. The distal phalanx enlarges as does the nail and its curvature becomes more pronounced (Fig. 21.45).

Splinter Haemorrhages

These are tiny subungual haemorrhages (Fig. 21.46). They occur particularly in acute bacterial endocarditis, systemic lupus erythematosus and trichinosis, but are more common secondary to trauma.

Broad White Lines

Broad white bands appear horizontally across the nails secondary to hypoalbuminaemia from whatever cause, particularly cirrhosis and renal disease.

The Yellow Nail Syndrome

This is a rare but distinctive disorder. The nails are discoloured yellow or yellow-green, thickened and excessively curved, particularly across the horizontal axis (Figs. 21.47 and 21.48). There is loss of the cuticle and a distinctive gap occurs between the skin and the nail, especially along the sides. The condition appears to be due to failure of the nail to grow or to grow sufficiently, and is associated with a deficiency of lymphatics draining the area. Occasionally lymphoedema may be seen in association with nail changes. The nail changes are associated with pulmonary abnormalities, especially chronic bronchitis, bronchiectasis or carcinoma of the lung. Sometimes an asymptomatic pleural effusion may be found.

Pigmentation of the Nails

Dark bands running along the longitudinal axis of the nailplates (Fig. 21.49) are very common in negroes but in the Caucasian they may be a sign of Addison's disease.

Causes of Clubbing		
Pulmonary	**Cardiovascular**	**Miscellaneous**
Carcinoma of the bronchus	Bacterial endocarditis	Cirrhosis
Bronchiectasis	Cyanotic congenital heart disease	Crohn's disease
Tuberculosis		Ulcerative colitis
Fibrosing alveolitis		Thyrotoxicosis
Asbestosis		

Fig. 21.44 Causes of clubbing.

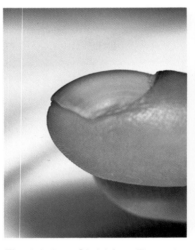

Fig. 21.45 Clubbing. There is loss of the normal angle between the posterior nailfold and the nailplate and the posterior nailfold feels spongy. The nail becomes more curved. This patient had pulmonary tuberculosis. By courtesy of St. Mary's Hospital.

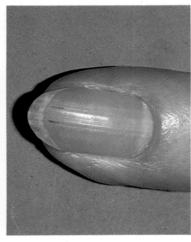

Fig. 21.46 Splinter haemorrhages. Tiny subungual haemorrhages result in pigmented linear splinter-like lesions. Trauma is the most common cause but they can also be a feature of certain systemic diseases.

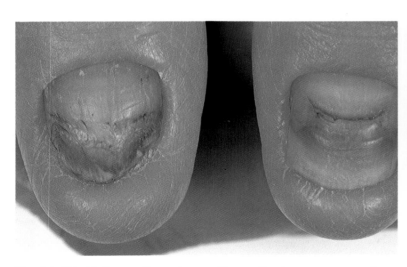

Fig. 21.47 Yellow nail syndrome. The nails do not grow at all. They are thickened and excessively curved across the horizontal axis and there is yellow discoloration. The changes are frequently associated with pulmonary disorders.

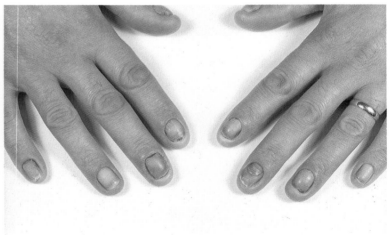

Fig. 21.48 Yellow nail syndrome. All the nails are involved. There is loss of the cuticles.

CIRCULATORY DISORDERS OF THE NAILS

Raynaud's phenomenon, peripheral vascular disease and perniosis may produce a thinned nailplate by virtue of the reduction in blood supply. All the nails are affected and are ridged longitudinally. Splits occur and the nail breaks easily (Fig. 21.50). The nail bed becomes more visible such that the nail appears redder than normal. Sometimes onycholysis occurs and the nail may become secondarily infected with bacteria or occasionally candida, resulting in pigmentary changes. Pterygium formation and occasionally permanent nail loss may occur.

The peripheries are cool or cold and appear blue. The condition of the nails often improves with the use of a vasodilator in addition to local measures to keep the hands warm.

NAIL TRAUMA

Acute trauma of a fingernail is usually obvious and the haemorrhage is visible underneath the nail, or if the haemorrhage is into the matrix area, within the nail. If it is considerable, the condition will be painful. Release of the blood by puncturing the nailplate with a hot needle will relieve the problem.

However, trivial injuries to nails, particularly the large toenail, are frequently forgotten and subsequently a consultation is made for the appearance of pigment within the nail (Fig. 21.51). In this case it is always important to distinguish the change from the pigment of subungual malignant melanoma. This is not usually difficult in that the discoloration is blue-black or purple, rather than the various shades of brown of the melanoma. Clipping back the nail or lifting it up may serve to identify the haemorrhage more clearly. Also the pigment of haemorrhage will grow forward with passing weeks.

Severe damage to the nail matrix may result in abnormalities of growth and in particular a split right down the length of the nail. The latter may be prevented if treated early enough by suturing the damaged matrix, although a permanent ridge will result.

Chronic traumatic effects on the nails are common. Hang nails (Fig. 21.52) are common in nail biters, although they may occur spontaneously and consist of skin which has split away from the sides of the nail.

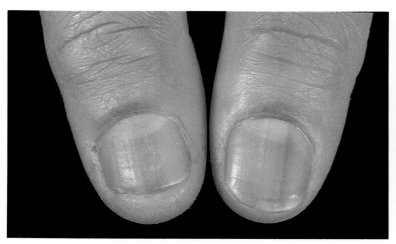

Fig. 21.49 Pigmentation of the nails. A longitudinal dark band is common in negroid nails. In Caucasians it may be a sign of Addison's disease. By courtesy of St. John's Hospital for Diseases of the Skin.

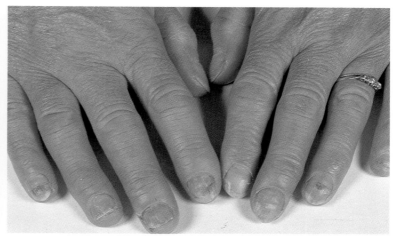

Fig. 21.50 Circulatory disorders. The nailplate becomes thinned if there is poor peripheral circulation. Onycholysis, ridging or splitting of the ends of the nails results.

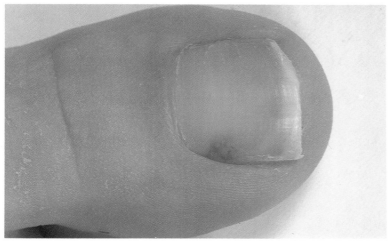

Fig. 21.51 Nail trauma. Minor trauma to the toes is usually forgotten, but the subsequent appearance of pigment under or in the nail gives rise to anxiety.

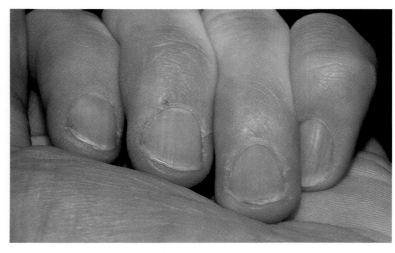

Fig. 21.52 Hang nails. Skin has split away from the sides of the nail.

Leukonychia

Leukonychia or white spots in the nails (Fig. 21.53) are very common and, contrary to the popular myth that they are due to calcium deficiency, the cause is not known. It is suspected that they are due to minor trauma.

Other less common nail disorders secondary to trauma are as follows:

Habit Tic

This occurs on one or both thumbnails and is due to the repeated scratching of the nailplate (or picking at the cuticle) with the fingernail of the index finger of the same hand. A longitudinal depression along the length of the nail is seen with cross ridges (Fig. 21.54). The habit is very difficult to break. Minor horizontal ridging (Fig. 21.55) may result from over-zealous pushing back of the cuticles. If the patient desists from this practice the condition is rectified.

Lamellar Dystrophy

This is an extremely common condition and results in splitting of the ends of the nailplate into layers (Figs. 21.56 and 21.57). It probaly occurs in both sexes, but it is mostly women who complain of this splitting. The most likely explanation appears to be that the nailplate is softened and then dried out by having the hands continually in and out of water, so that the cells of the nailplate do not adhere effectively and splits occur. The

condition thus occurs in housewives and can be rectified by advising them to cut down exposure to water and take protective measures

Nail Cosmetics

Stick-on nail dressings and artificial fingernails may cause nail dystrophies. These materials are not porous and prevent the normal free exchange of moisture between the nail and the atmosphere. When the dressings or nails are taken off, portions of the nailplate are pulled away with the adhesive. This produces an irregular surface and splits the nail into layers. Leuconychia and onycholysis may result.

Artificial fingernails may also be made by mixing a liquid monomer and powder acrylic polymer together on the nail. These are then shaped to improve the appearance of the nail. Acrylic is a potent contact sensitizer of the skin and if the patients do sensitize to it, onycholysis and sepsis may occur. Formalin is incorporated into nail hardeners and may cause onycholysis. Other chemicals including phenol are also added from time to time to nail cosmetics and occasionally epidemics of onycholysis and other nail disorders may occur.

Contact dermatitis may also occur to nail varnish. The nails themselves are unaffected, but dermatitis occurs on those areas of skin touched by the nails. These are usually on the face, especially the jaw, around the mouth and eyes and the neck.

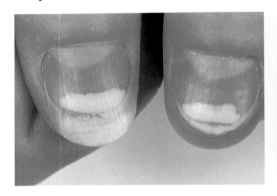

Fig. 21.53 Leukonychia. White spots in the nails are common. Gross examples may occur. The cause is unknown but trauma may be relevant.

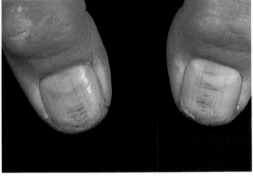

Fig. 21.54 Habit tic. Repeated scratching of the nailplate or picking at the cuticle produces a longitudinal depression in the nail.

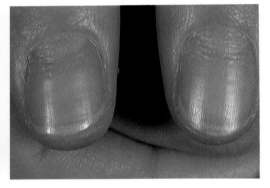

Fig. 21.55 Nail trauma. Minor horizontal ridges result.

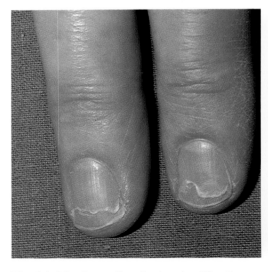

Fig. 21.56 Lamellar dystrophy. The tips of the nails are split into layers. This is probably caused by softening of the nailplate by continual immersion in water.

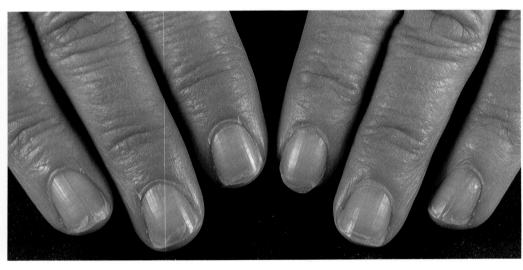

Fig. 21.57 Lamellar dystrophy. Usually all the fingernails are affected to some degree or another.

Ingrowing Toenails

This painful condition is related to chronic trauma. Ill-fitting shoes interfere with the normal growth of the big toenail, so that it grows abnormally into the surrounding skin. Nails should be cut horizontally rather than into the sides of the nail. Poor cutting of the nail may lead to small projections of the nail which cut into the lateral nailfold. This may produce discomfort and inflammatory changes, and subsequently granulation tissue occurs (Figs. 21.58 and 21.59). Sometimes the projecting area of the nail becomes detached and acts as a foreign body in the area. Ingrowing toenails may occur as a result of tinea infection or treatment of a long-standing fungal infection of the large toenail. The nailbed may shrink in chronic infections and cannot accommodate the normal regrowing nail after treatment.

Management consists of wearing shoes which do not exert any pressure on the toenail, cutting the nail horizontally, the use of potassium permanganate soaks as an anti-infective and the introduction of cotton wool under the edges of the nail to aid the nail to grow out straight. If there is an added foreign body it should be removed. Excess granulation tissue can be cauterized. Occasionally, operative procedures are needed.

Onychogryphosis

This condition usually affects the great toenail and once again, chronic trauma is probably an important feature. The nails are grossly thickened, hard and elongated (Fig. 21.60) and tend to be curved rather like a horn (Fig. 21.61); depending on the age of the patient the condition can either be kept in check by regular paring by a chiropodist or the nail can be removed. It will, however regrow abnormally again and removal will have to be repeated.

CONGENITAL DISORDERS OF THE NAILS

These are all extremely rare conditions and range from deficiency (Fig. 21.62) or complete absence of the nails from birth, to supernumerary digits and nails; often a family history of such abnormalities is present. Changes may be seen as a result of a generalized disorder of the skin such as epidermolysis bullosa, where the nails are destroyed secondary to the blistering process. Alternatively, the nails may be involved as part of a generalized ectodermal disorder where the nail changes are really of secondary importance, for example Darier's disease. These are dealt with elsewhere.

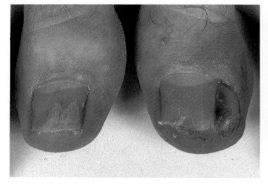

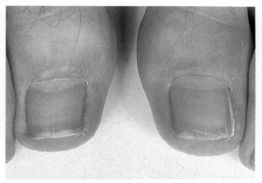

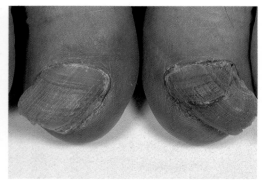

Fig. 21.58 Ingrowing toenails. Heaped-up granulation tissue occurs at the side of the big toe. Ill-fitting shoes resulting in chronic trauma are the commonest cause. This man also had a tinea infection resulting in abnormal nail growth.

Fig. 21.59 Ingrowing toenail. The condition shown in Fig. 21.58 responded to surgery and treatment of the tinea with griseofulvin.

Fig. 21.60 Onychogryphosis. Chronic trivial trauma ultimately interferes with the nail growth of the big toes. The nails grow outwards and are thickened and discoloured.

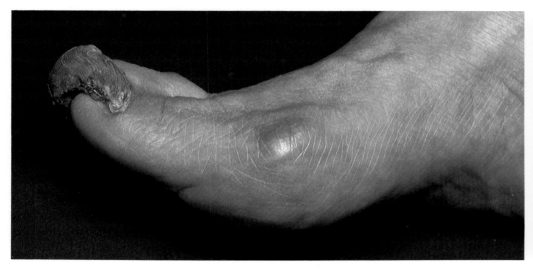

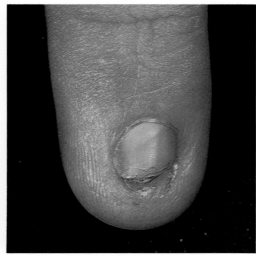

Fig. 21.61 Onychogryphosis. The nails may become grossly thickened and excessively curved.

Fig. 21.62 Micronychia. Nails may be partially or totally absent resulting from a congenital defect. By courtesy of Dr. A.C. Pembroke.

Nail Patella Syndrome

This is an autosomal dominant condition where the patellae (Fig. 21.63) are either rudimentary or absent, with similar changes in the nails. The thumbnails are always involved (Fig. 21.64) and often the rest of the nails but not to such a great degree. Either the nail is totally absent or grows only partially which makes picking up small objects virtually impossible. Abnormalities also occur in the elbow joints and iliac horns. The cause is quite unknown.

Nail en Raquette

This disorder is inherited as an autosomal dominant. It is due to a failure of development of the distal phalanx of the thumb such that it is shorter and wider than normal and consequently the nail is similarly affected (Fig. 21.65). There are no related abnormalities.

Median Nail Dystrophy

This is an uncommon condition which can affect any fingernail, but most often occurs in the thumbnail. A split starting at the cuticle develops in a longitudinal manner along the nail. Splits also occur off the main ones, giving an appearance resembling the branches of a fir tree (Fig. 21.66). The condition does recover and grows out with the nail, but relapses are frequent. The cause is quite unknown, but because the lunula is often much larger than normal, the matrix may be more vulnerable to trauma.

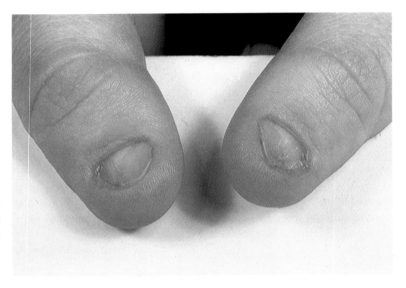

Fig. 21.64 Nail patella syndrome. The thumbnails are always involved. They may be absent or partially formed. Other nails may be involved to a lesser extent. This makes picking up small objects virtually impossible.

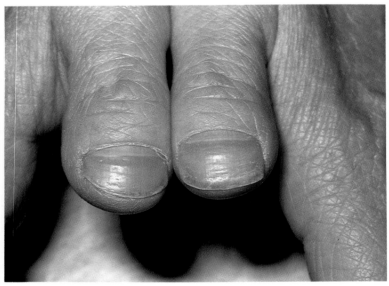

Fig. 21.65 Nail en raquette. The distal phalanx of the thumb fails to develop fully, so it is shorter and wider than normal, as is the nail.

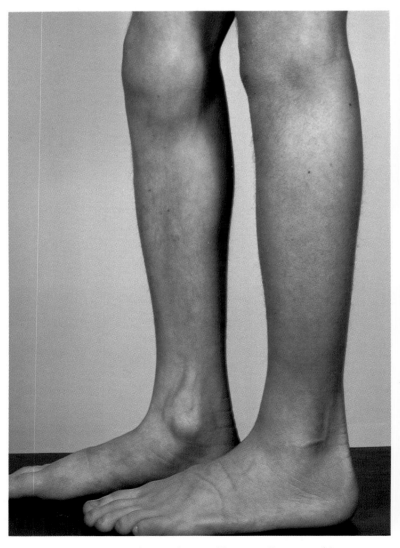

Fig. 21.63 Nail patella syndrome. The patellae are either rudimentary or absent.

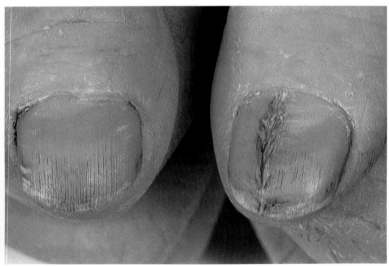

Fig. 21.66 Median nail dystrophy. A longitudinal split is present, and is likened to an inverted fir tree in appearance. The thumbnails are most often involved. By courtesy of Dr. Michèle Clement.

22 Disorders of the Hair

Hair is keratinous. It is a protein manufactured by the cells at the bulb of the hair follicle. The hair follicle is an invagination of the epidermis and the bulb is at its base and encloses an area of the dermis which is highly vascular. The cells of the hair bulb are the most mitotically active and are very susceptible to arresting influences such as cytotoxic drugs. The hair shaft itself consists of several layers. The bulk is made up of a cortex which may have a central medulla. Surrounding the cortex is a cuticle and an inner and outer root sheath. The keratinized cells of the hair shaft are tightly bound together. It is a dead structure and can be invaded by superficial fungi.

There are three types of hair. Lanugo hair is present *in utero* and is shed at approximately the age of seven months. It is therefore normally only seen in the premature baby. Vellus hair is a fine down which covers the entire surface of the body except for the palms and the soles. This hair is capable of being transformed under hormonal influences into terminal hair. Terminal hair is the thick pigmented medullated hair of the scalp, eyebrows and eyelashes. With secondary sexual development terminal hairs appear in the beard area, axillae, pubic region and on the body.

Human hair grows in an asynchronous manner unlike animal hair which falls out synchronously in the form of a moult. There are three phases of hair growth. *Anagen* is the longest phase, lasting up to four or five years and the majority of the hair is in this phase at any one time. Following anagen, cell division ceases and involution occurs (*catagen*). The follicle regresses and the hair shaft is shortened, becoming club-shaped. Catagen lasts a few weeks and is followed by *telogen*, during which hair is shed; this period lasts three or four months.

TELOGEN EFFLUVIUM

If the hair cycle is interrupted, loss of hair results. Telogen effluvium occurs when anagen hairs are prematurely precipitated into catagen and subsequently telogen. A severe illness, whether physical or psychological is usually responsible (Figs. 22.1 and 22.2). At the time of the illness the hair stops growing and enters the catagen phase. Since this is the resting phase of several weeks, it is not until after this time that the hair falls out. Patients tend, therefore, not to associate their illness with the hair fall. The hair loss (Fig. 22.3) is of a diffuse nature and is alarming, but recovery starts to occur some three or four months later. Patients may also note abnormalities in their nails (see Fig. 21.39), particularly horizontal ridging (Beau's lines). A similar occurrence is noticed, to a greater or lesser extent, by many women three months after parturition. During pregnancy those hairs which should enter catagen do not but continue to grow. As a result, most women will remark that their hair is more luxuriant during pregnancy. However, with parturition all those hairs which should have entered catagen during pregnancy do so at once and three months later fall precipitously as they enter telogen. Recovery is usual three or four months later.

ANAGEN EFFLUVIUM

Anagen effluvium is loss of hair secondary to mitotic arrest. Drugs used in cancer chemotherapy, such as cyclophosphamide, induce acute hair fall within a few days. Various procedures including icepacks applied to the hair are used to minimize the loss. Heparin, carbimazole and overdosage with vitamin A may also precipitate such hair loss.

MALE PATTERN ALOPECIA AND HIRSUTISM

Both *male pattern alopecia* and *hirsutism* are features of virilism, but usually they are genetically determined and there are no other features of virilism. Male pattern alopecia is inherited as an autosomal dominant and may begin in early adult life.

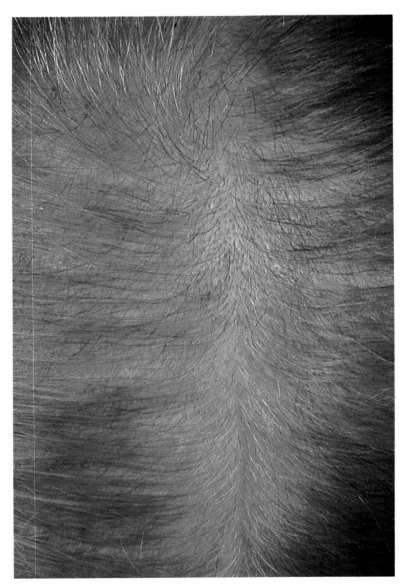

Fig. 22.1   Telogen effluvium. This lady's hair fell out precipitously three months after a serious illness. By courtesy of St. Mary's Hospital.

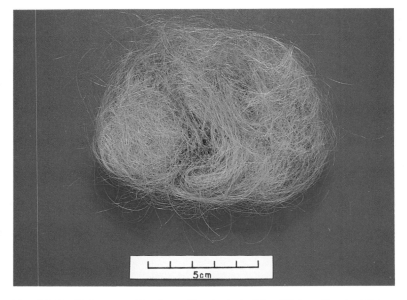

Fig. 22.2   Telogen effluvium. The lady in Fig. 22.1 collected this amount of hair during a few days. By courtesy of St. Mary's Hospital.

Temporal recession usually occurs first and subsequently there is loss of hair from the vertex and frontal regions. There is retention of hair, however, around the occiput and the sides of the head. Transplantation of occipital hair follicles to areas of hair loss will result in hair growth. Often there is associated seborrhoea.

In pre-menopausal females, hair loss does occur but it is not as noticeable as in the male (Fig. 22.4). There is normally a family history of hair loss which is manifest as diffuse thinning rather than complete loss of hair over the vertical, frontal and temporal areas. However, once the protective effect of oestrogens is lost after the menopause, hair loss may be very marked (Fig. 22.5) but, paradoxically, hair may grow on the face (Fig. 22.6).

It is thought that the hair loss results as an increased hair follicle sensitivity to dihydrotestosterone produced from testosterone by 5-alpha reductase. Constitutional hirsutism is explained in a similar manner.

The growth of secondary sex hair results from the change of vellus hairs to terminal hairs. It is under the control of growth hormone and androgens. Pubic and axillary hair are the earliest secondary sex hairs to be developed. They will not develop in hypopituitarism, will be minimal before puberty and will be diminished with advancing years and in adrenal failure. In the latter instance the sparsity of hair will be much more marked in the female than in the male where testicular androgens will still be operative. At puberty androgens are secreted by the Leydig cells of the testis as testosterone, and by the adrenals as the weak androgenic steroids androstanedione and dehydroepiandrosterone. (Pubic and axillary hair are very sensitive to androgens and are maximally developed in both sexes.) Adrenal androgens (males and females) and testosterone (males only) control the growth of the lower triangle of pubic hair and testosterone alone controls the upper triangle of growth towards the umbilicus (Fig. 22.7). This explains the different distribution of pubic hair in males and females.

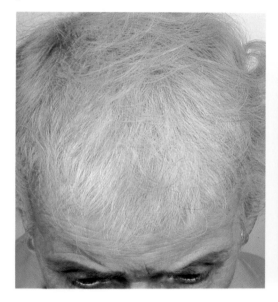 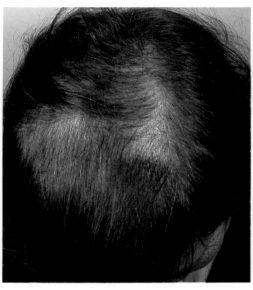 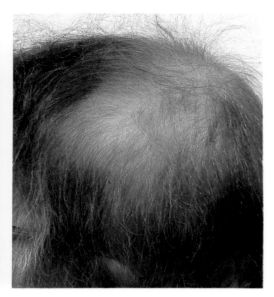

Fig. 22.3 Telogen effluvium. This lady lost a great deal of hair three months after an episode of generalized pustular psoriasis. It had completely regrown within the next three months.

Fig. 22.4 Male pattern alopecia in a female. Diffuse hair loss began in this lady in her late twenties. Her father was completely bald.

Fig. 22.5 Male pattern alopecia in a post-menopausal female. After the menopause, hair loss in a female may be very marked indeed.

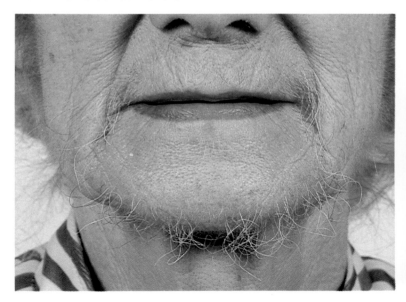 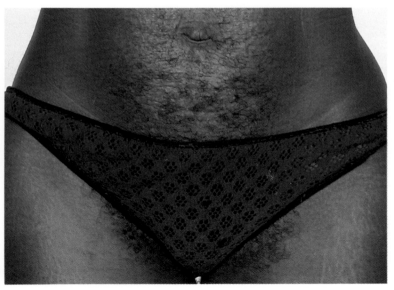

Fig. 22.6 Hirsutism in a post-menopausal female. Facial hair growth is common after the menopause.

Fig. 22.7 Male escutcheon in a female. The upper triangle of pubic hair growth towards the umbilicus is under the influence of testosterone only and in a female may indicate a hormonal irregularity.

Testosterone is a powerful androgen and males are maximally virilized by testosterone such that no further hair growth will occur even if adrenal androgens are produced in excess as, for example, by an adrenal tumour. Thus, virilization is a term only applicable to a child or a female.

Virilism results in clitoromegaly, acne, seborrhoea, hirsutism, male pattern alopecia and escutcheon, deepening of the voice, muscle hypertrophy and amenorrhoea. Hirsutism only constitutes a problem in females (Fig. 22.8) and is dependent on local cultural influences. Certain races are more susceptible to hirsutism than others. For example the Japanese and Chinese have minimal secondary sex hair and hirsutism is rare, whereas Mediterranean, Middle Eastern, Indian and negro races often have considerable facial and body hair. This may be of no moment in their own environment but once subjected to Western influences it becomes of great significance.

In deciding whether to investigate a patient presenting with hirsutism the cessation or irregularity of periods is a useful indicator (Fig. 22.9). Abnormalities of pituitary, adrenal and ovarian function should be ruled out and the most helpful basic investigations include a full blood count, plasma testosterone level, plasma cortisol studies and 24 hour collections of urine for estimation of hydroxycorticosteroids and ketocorticosteroids. X-ray of the pituitary fossa is also indicated. The more common causes of hirsutism are listed in Fig. 22.10 and the reader is referred to general medical texts for full accounts of these disorders.

The treatment of hirsutism is dependent upon its cause but the management of constitutional hirsutism is unsatisfactory. Shaving is aesthetically disturbing to most females. Bleaching, plucking, waxing and depilatories are all second-best treatments. Electrolysis (Fig. 22.11) is time-consuming and expensive but produces the best results in skilled hands as the effect is likely to be permanent. Small doses of glucocorticosteroids such as prednisolone, 5 mg every night, will suppress adrenal androgens but the treatment is not without risk from the long-term effects of excess steroids. Oestrogen therapy to suppress androgen production is justified in the teens and early adult life before maximum androgen production and hirsutism has occurred. Anti-androgens such as cyproterone acetate are increasingly being used for constitutional hirsutism. Since they will feminize a masculine foetus they are usually given combined with oestrogens to prevent pregnancy.

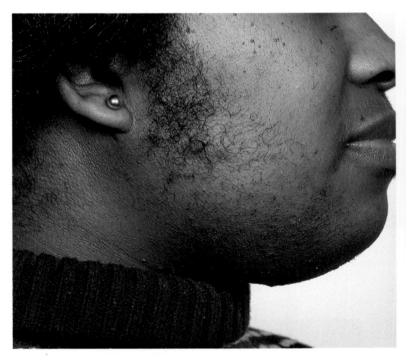

Fig. 22.8   Hirsutism. This young woman developed terminal hairs over the beard area. In her own country this might not have presented a problem but in Westernized societies it does.

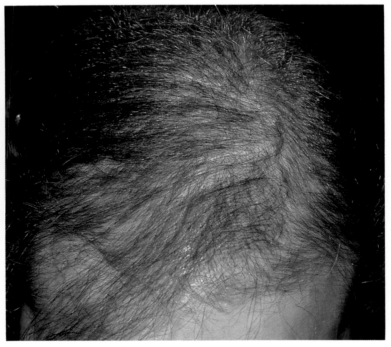

Fig. 22.9   Male pattern alopecia in a female. Pronounced male pattern hair loss and hirsutism (Fig. 22.11) had occurred in this young female. She had oligomenorrhoea and polycystic ovary syndrome.

Causes of Hirsutism

Constitutional	Excess production of cortisol	Adrenal virilization	Ovarian virilization	Ovarian failure	Androgenic drugs
	Hyperpituitarism	Adrenogenital syndrome	Polycystic ovary syndrome	Post-menopausal	Testosterone
	Adrenal tumour or hyperplasia		Ovarian tumour	Post-oophorectomy	Anabolic steroids
	Steroid therapy				Danazol

Fig. 22.10   Table showing causes of hirsutism.

HYPERTRICHOSIS

This term refers to a growth of terminal hair in a site which is not normally hairy. It can occur in a localized manner, such as in naevi (see Fig. 5.11), or generalized as in anorexia nervosa or porphyria. Certain drugs such as corticosteroids, diazoxide and penicillamine may be responsible.

ALOPECIA AREATA

This is a common disorder of unknown aetiology, although an autoimmune mechanism seems likely since it occurs more commonly in association with organ-specific autoimmune disorders such as Hashimoto's thyroiditis or pernicious anaemia and a lymphocytic infiltrate occurs around the hair follicles. The condition is also common in Down's syndrome (Fig. 22.12).

It can commence at any age although early adult life is most usual. It ranges from one or two circular patches of complete hair loss on the scalp (Fig. 22.13) or in the beard area (Fig. 22.14) to loss of the majority of the hair on the scalp and face (alopecia totalis) to complete loss of hair (alopecia universalis, Fig. 22.15).

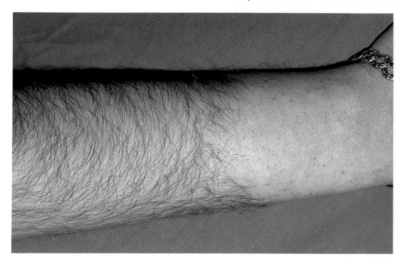

Fig. 22.11   Hirsutism treated by electrolysis. Electrolysis, although time-consuming, produces the most permanent results.

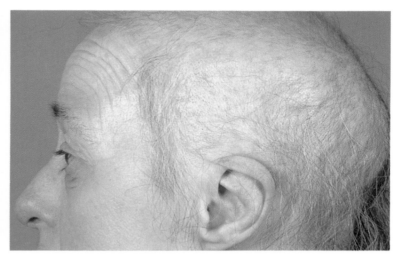

Fig. 22.12   Alopecia areata. Alopecia is common in Down's syndrome.

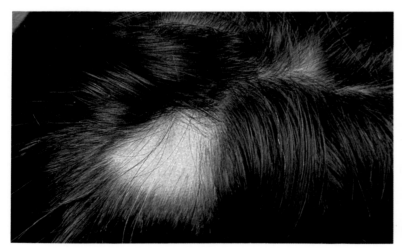

Fig. 22.13   Alopecia areata. One or two circular patches of complete hair loss occur. Recovery is usual within a year.

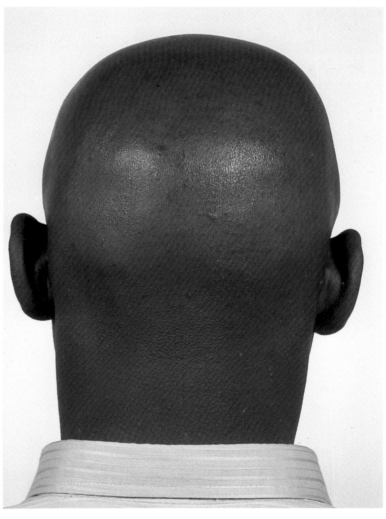

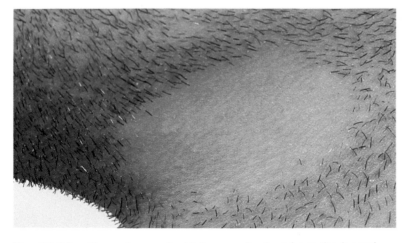

Fig. 22.14   Alopecia areata. Hairs may be lost from the beard area. The skin appears quite normal.

Fig. 22.15   Alopecia universalis. Hair may be lost from every part of the body. The chances of recovery are slim.

The eyebrows (Fig. 22.16) and eyelashes (Fig. 22.17) may be lost separately or in addition. Examination of the scalp or other affected areas shows the skin to be perfectly normal in appearance and texture. Within the patches of alopecia 'exclamation mark' hairs may be found. These are a few millimetres long. The stump of the hair appears normal but the proximal portion nearest the scalp is thin and has lost pigment. These hairs indicate activity of disease and that the condition may deteriorate. In the majority of cases, the patient recovers completely within a period of nine months or so (Fig. 22.18). However, the prognosis becomes guarded the earlier the onset of the condition (viz. in childhood), the more rapid the onset and the greater the extent of involvement. The number of affected areas, recurrences, associated atopic eczema, involvement of the occiput (Fig. 22.19) and alopecia totalis are bad prognostic signs. It is rare for patients with alopecia universalis to recover. In those patients where recovery is occurring, the hair commences to regrow without pigment, thus appearing white (Fig. 22.20). There is an uncommon form of alopecia areata whereby the patient seemingly becomes white-haired overnight (Fig. 22.21). This condition is seen in adults who have normally an admixture of white and black hairs. There appears to be a preferential loss of the black pigmented hairs, leaving behind the white hairs and thus producing a somewhat dramatic effect. Occasionally, ridging and pitting of the nails may occur in association with the alopecia (Fig. 22.22).

Since the condition resolves spontaneously the results of treatment are not always easy to interpret. Certainly, intralesional steroids may produce a rather convincing picture of hairs growing at the sites of the injections (Fig. 22.23). Systemic steroids cause regrowth, even in alopecia universalis but the hazards of these drugs, which have to be taken long-term, outweigh the benefits of treatment. Many other therapies have been used from inflammatory approaches, such as ultra-violet light irradiation, photochemotherapy (PUVA) to immunological techniques such as producing a contact dermatitis with dinitrochlorobenzene (Fig. 22.24).

The diagnosis is comparatively simple but other causes of localized areas of hair loss have to be considered. The main distinguishing feature is that the skin in the area affected shows no sign of inflammation or scarring, the surface remaining perfectly normal.

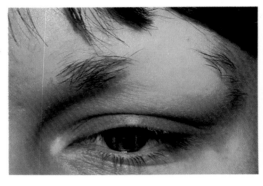

Fig. 22.16 Alopecia areata. Hair may be lost from the eyebrows.

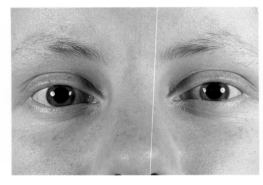

Fig. 22.17 Alopecia areata. The eyelashes may fall out. There is often total or universal hair loss but the eyelashes may be only partly affected.

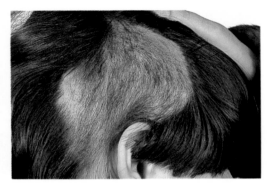

Fig. 22.18 Alopecia areata. Recovery usually occurs within a year.

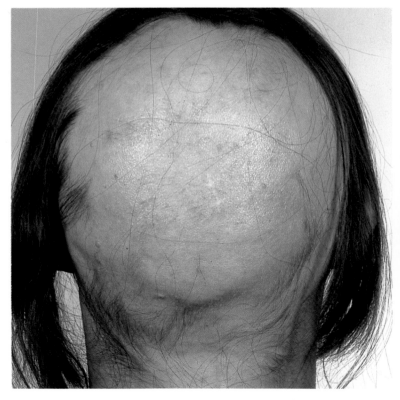

Fig. 22.19 Alopecia areata. Occipital loss of hair (ophiasis) is associated with a poor prognosis.

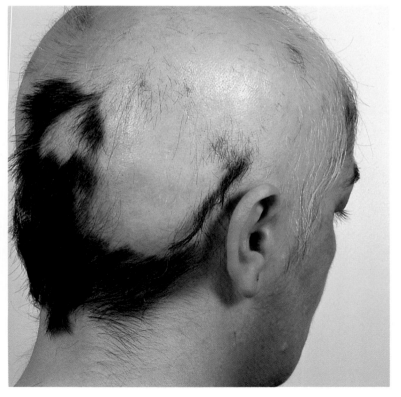

Fig. 22.20 Alopecia areata. The hair is just beginning to regrow white on the right side of this woman's head.

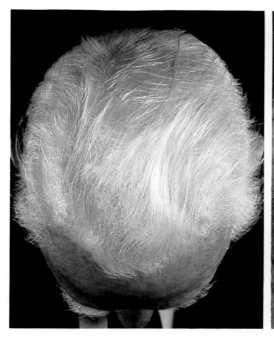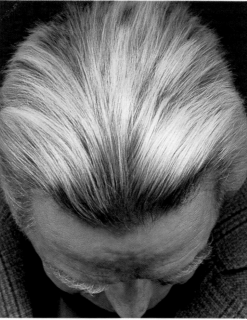

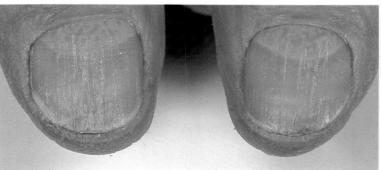

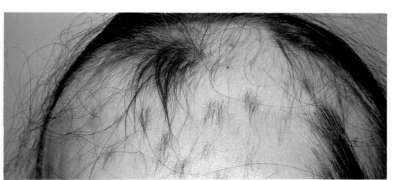

Fig. 22.21 Alopecia areata. A patient may go white 'overnight' (left). There is a preferential loss of the pigmented hairs which can be seen when he recovered (right). By courtesy of St. John's Hospital for Diseases of the Skin.

Fig. 22.22 Alopecia areata of the nails. Linear ridging of the nails although not common may occur in association with alopecia.

Fig. 22.23 Alopecia areata treated with intralesional steroids. Hair is regrowing at the sites of previous steroid injections. Fresh injection sites are also visible.

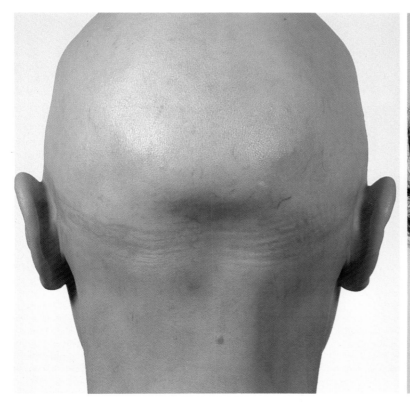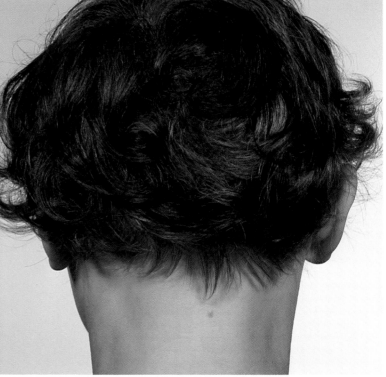

Fig. 22.24 Alopecia universalis. This woman's universal alopecia recovered completely with dinitrochlorobenzene. This is exceptional. The hair began to fall out in patches four years later.

DIFFERENTIAL DIAGNOSIS
OF COMMON SKIN DISORDERS AFFECTING THE SCALP
Most of these disorders have been dealt with elsewhere but are
included together here to aid differential diagnosis.

TINEA CAPITIS. Ringworm of the scalp is characterized by localized
patches of hair loss similar to alopecia areata but there are
varying degrees of erythema and scaling present (Fig. 22.25).

PSORIASIS. It is most unusual for hair loss to occur in psoriasis.
The patches are well-defined, deep red with a silver scale
(Fig. 22.26) and are symmetrical.

PITYRIASIS CAPITIS. Hair loss may occur as a part of associated
male pattern alopecia but otherwise is not a feature of pityriasis
capitis. The patches are pink, not so well-defined and there is a
fine scale (Fig. 22.27). There may be signs of seborrhoeic
dermatitis elsewhere. Dandruff is a fine scaling of the scalp
without erythema.

PITYRIASIS AMIANTACEA. This is a relatively common condition of
adolescents and young adults. There is considerable build-up of
scale in patches on the scalp. The scales are attached to the hair
shafts (Fig. 22.28). It may result from psoriasis or a severe pityriasis capitis. It does not respond to topical steroids but it does to
tar-containing preparations. Temporary hair loss usually follows.

TRICHOTILLOMANIA. This results from a habit tic of fiddling with
the hair and there is a unilateral loss of hair without overt
alopecia (Fig. 22.29). The hairs are broken off at various lengths
above the surface. There are no inflammatory changes on the
scalp.

LICHEN SIMPLEX. This results from rubbing and scratching the
scalp. The skin is thickened and lichenified and hair is lost
(Fig. 22.30).

SCARRING ALOPECIA
Permanent hair loss results from any process which leads to
scarring and destruction of the hair follicles. *Discoid lupus
erythematosus* is a common example (Fig. 22.31). *Favus* and very
occasionally *lichen planus* cause a scarring alopecia. *X-irradiation
of the scalp* for ringworm used to be a common cause.

    Pseudopelade is a name given to scarring alopecia of unknown
origin. The hair loss occurs in patches. The scalp is atrophic,
tethered and punctuated by islands of tufts of hair growing out
of these areas (Fig. 22.32). Sometimes pustules are present, in
which case the condition is known as *folliculitis decalvans*. These
are rare conditions.

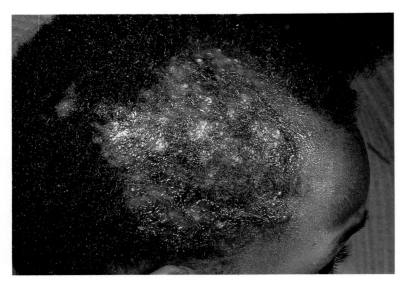

Fig. 22.25 Tinea capitis. There is weeping and crusting of the
skin in addition to hair loss.

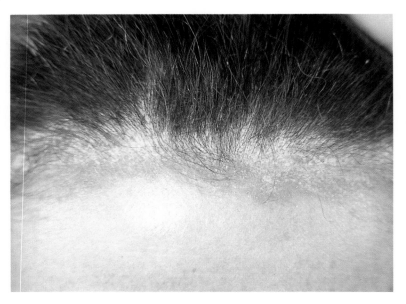

Fig. 22.26 Psoriasis. There is redness and a thick silvery scale.
It is not usual for there to be any loss of hair.

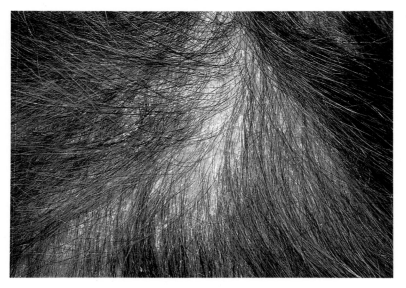

Fig. 22.27 Pityriasis capitis. The scales are finer and pinker
than in psoriasis.

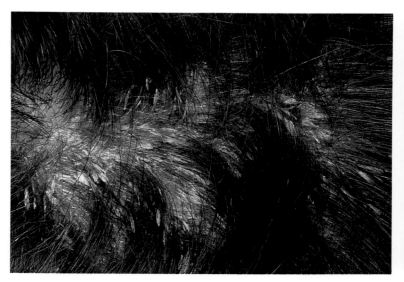

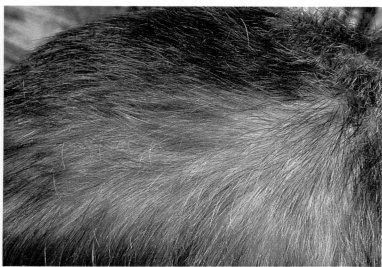

Fig. 22.28 Pityriasis amiantacea. Thick scales are attached to the hair shafts. The condition does not respond to topical steroids but it does to tar-containing medicaments. Temporary hair loss usually follows.

Fig. 22.29 Trichotillomania. There is a unilateral thinning of the hair. The hairs are broken off at various lengths above the surface.

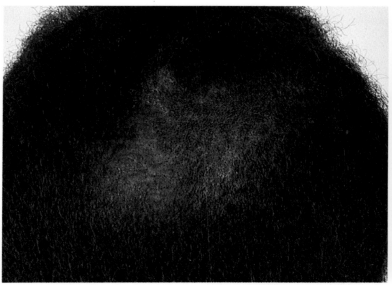

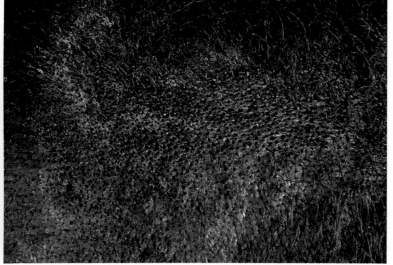

Fig. 22.30 Lichen simplex. There is hair loss (left) and a well-defined patch of lichenification (right) from continual rubbing and scratching of the scalp.

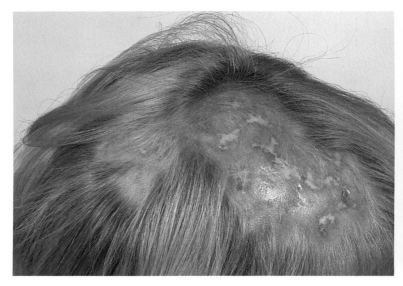

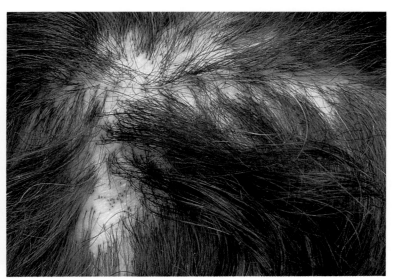

Fig. 22.31 Scarring alopecia. Discoid lupus erythematosus is a common cause of scarring permanent alopecia.

Fig. 22.32 Pseudopelade. The cause of this scarring alopecia is unknown. The scalp is punctuated by islands of tufts of hairs growing out of the scarred areas. By courtesy of St. John's Hospital for Diseases of the Skin.

TRAUMATIC HAIR LOSS

The most common form of traumatic hair loss is that which occurs on the occiput of an infant secondary to friction between the back of the head and the mattress (Fig. 22.33). Probably all babies develop this temporarily.

Hairstyles which exert a pull on the hair follicles may result in hair loss. Frontal recession of hair may result from having the hair tied tightly in a pony-tail or bun. The West Indian custom of plaiting hair in 'cornrows' may result in alopecia if done over-zealously (Fig. 22.34). Recovery does not always occur, particularly in adults (Fig. 22.35). The use of hot combs to straighten the hair and permanent waves to do the opposite may result in hair loss due to disturbance of the protein molecule of hair.

STRUCTURAL DEFECTS OF HAIR
Monilethrix

This is usually a dominantly inherited defect of the hair shaft. The thickness of the shaft varies due to intermittent absence of the medulla, such that a beaded appearance occurs (Fig. 22.36). Depending on the degree of abnormality, the hair will break at the thin, non-medullated parts of the shaft so that the affected individual may have quite short hair or indeed alopecia (Fig. 22.37). All the scalp hair may be affected but more usually the affliction is patchy. Occasionally other sites are affected. There is considerable variation in the severity of the disease between individuals. Some make a complete recovery, others remain abnormal permanently.

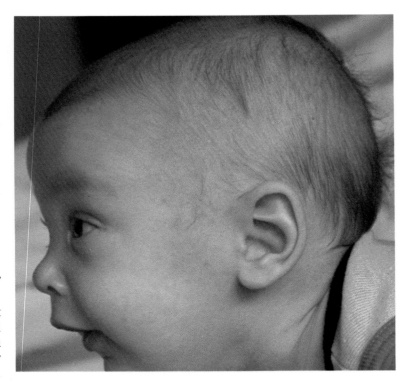

Fig. 22.33 Traumatic hair loss. Infants lose hair from around the sides and back of the scalp through rubbing.

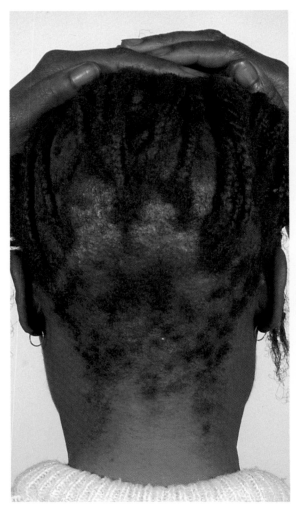

Fig. 22.34 Traction alopecia. Plaiting may exert undue traction of the hair follicle and hair loss results.

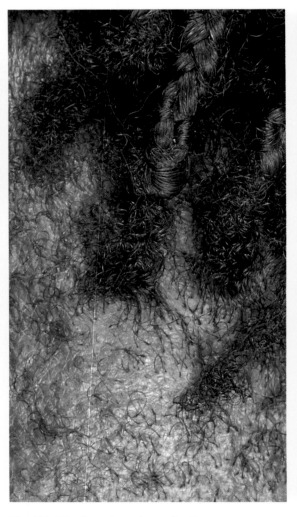

Fig. 22.35 Traction alopecia. Recovery may not occur after this variety of traction alopecia. This is a close up of 22.34.

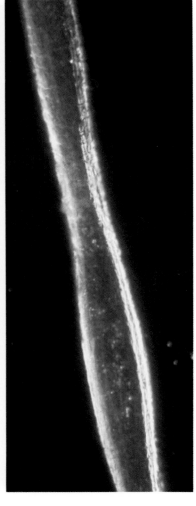

Fig. 22.36 Monilethrix. The thickness of the shaft varies due to intermittent absence of the medulla. By courtesy of Dr. R.P.R. Dawber, Oxford.

Pili Torti

This is a twisting of the hair shaft along its long axis (Fig. 22.38). The resultant hair is fragile (Fig. 22.39) and breaks easily. It is usually inherited as an autosomal dominant disorder. It may occur as an isolated finding or sometimes in association with other abnormalities including mental retardation. A rare condition is *Menke's kinky hair syndrome* where various structural defects of the hair may occur including monilethrix and trichorrhexis nodosa but most commonly pili torti. The disorder is inherited as a sex-linked recessive and there is a failure to absorb copper from the intestinal tract. The condition presents in infancy as failure to thrive with central nervous system abnormalities. The hair is initially normal but is shed after a month or so and the structural abnormalities develop.

Trichorrhexis Nodosa

Small grey-white nodules occur along the hair shaft in this condition (Fig. 22.40). Under the light microscope the nodules consist of partial fractures of the hair shaft. Probably the most common cause is excessive brushing or perming of the hair, i.e. as a result of trauma and will recover on cessation of these procedures. In other patients, however, there seems to be a structural abnormality.

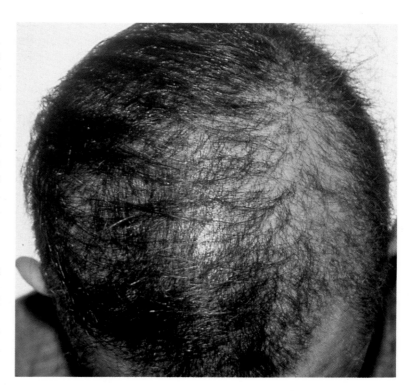

Fig. 22.37   Monilethrix. The hair may break at the non-medullated parts producing patchy shortened hair. By courtesy of Dr. R.P.R. Dawber, Oxford.

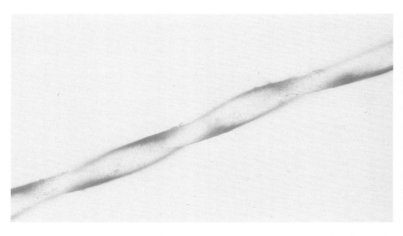

Fig. 22.38   Pili torti. Twisting of the hair occurs along the long axis. By courtesy of Dr. R.P.R. Dawber, Oxford.

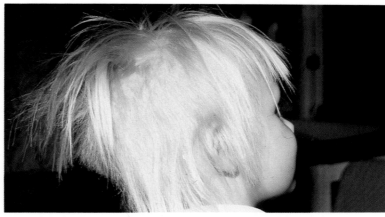

Fig. 22.39   Pili torti .The resultant hair is fragile and breaks easily. By courtesy of Dr. R.P.R. Dawber, Oxford.

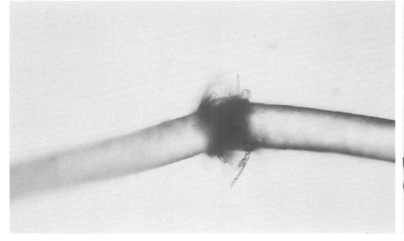

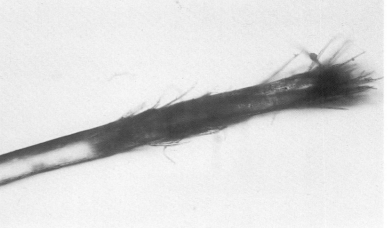

Fig. 22.40   Trichorrhexis nodosa. Small grey-white nodules occur. They are partial fractures of the hair shaft. Trauma is the cause in most cases. By courtesy of Dr. R.P.R. Dawber, Oxford.

Trichostasis Spinulosa

This is a relatively common condition of young adults and the abnormality appears to be the production of multiple vellus unmedullated hairs from a single hair follicle which at the surface of the skin is surrounded by a keratinous sheath (Figs. 22.41 and 22.42). The condition is seen predominantly on the shoulders, back, arms, front of the chest and abdomen. Depilatory waxes may be of benefit.

Fig. 22.41 Trichostasis spinulosa. Multiple vellus unmedullated hairs arise from a single hair follicle, which is surrounded by a keratinized sheath at the surface giving a pigmented appearance. The skin feels rough.

Fig. 22.42 Trichostasis spinulosa. This is a closer view of the patient in Fig. 22.41.

23 Disorders of Pigmentation

Production of Melanin

Phenylalanine

⬇

Tyrosine

⬇

Dihydroxyphenylalanine (DOPA)

⬇

Dopaquinone ➡ Cysteinyldopa

⬇ ⬇

Melanin **Phaeomelanin**

Fig. 23.1 Table illustrating the stages in the production of melanin.

PIGMENTARY DISORDERS RELATED TO MELANIN

Melanocytes are normally found in the epidermis around the basal cell layer in an approximate proportion of 1:5 basal cells. Melanocytes are seen as clear cells in routine sections of the skin because they do not stain with haematoxylin and eosin. They are derived from the neural crest and have a dendritic form. They inject neighbouring keratinocytes with melanosomes, which contain melanin. Each melanocyte serves several keratinocytes. There are the same numbers of melanocytes to be found in both negroid and Caucasian skin. The difference in pigmentation is accounted for by the number, size and distribution of the melanosomes present in any one melanocyte. The function of melanocytes is to produce melanin which acts as a protection against ultra-violet light irradiation. Any individual has a basic constitutional degree of pigmentation with a facultative response largely to ultra-violet light but also to MSH (melanocyte stimulating hormone) and ACTH (adrenocorticotrophic hormone).

Melanin is derived from phenylalanine via intermediates, a reaction which is under the control of the enzyme tyrosinase (Fig. 23.1). If the reaction is continued and melanin is oxidized, a colourless compound results. This is how hydrogen peroxide or intense ultra-violet light irradiation bleach the hair. The colour of red hair is due to phaeomelanin which is formed from dopaquinone via a reaction with cystein.

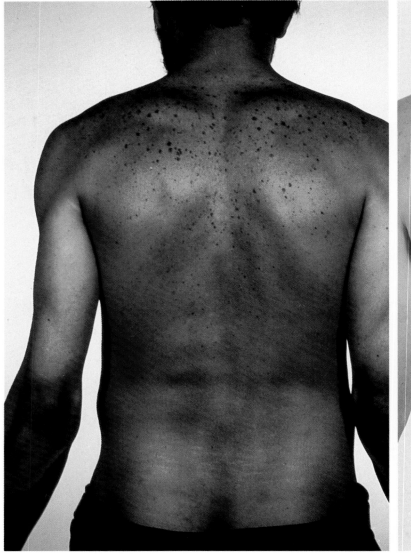
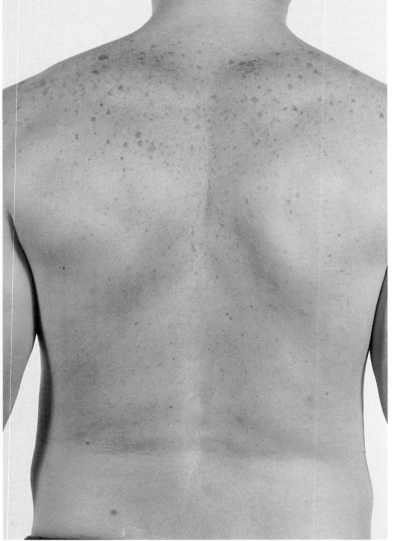

Fig. 23.2 Addison's disease. There is a generalized increase in pigmentation (left), which is particularly striking when compared with the normal skin colour after treatment (right). By courtesy of Dr. T. Cundy, King's College Hospital.

Examination of pigmentary disorders under the Wood's light, which is an artificial ultra-violet light source of a wavelength of approximately 365 nanometres, reveals the localization of the disorder. Epidermal pigmentary abnormalities are detected under the light whereas dermal disorders are not. Thus pityriasis versicolor and freckles which are epidermal disorders of pigmentation are accentuated under the Wood's light.

Normal skin colour is made up of four pigments, haemoglobin, oxyhaemoglobin, melanin and carotene. The pink skin of a Caucasian individual is due to the visibility of the red pigment oxyhaemoglobin in the superficial blood vessels. The pallor of anaemia and the blue or purple of cyanosis are functions of diminished amounts of haemoglobin in the first instance and of reduced (deoxygenated) haemoglobin in the second. Carotene is a yellow substance found in the subcutaneous fat.

Disorders of Hyperpigmentation
Generalized, Diffuse Hyperpigmentation
Apart from the genetic and sun-induced causes of hyperpigmentation there are several important pathological causes.

HORMONAL CAUSES OF HYPERPIGMENTATION. The first presenting feature of Addison's disease is a gradual increase in pigmentation of the skin generally (Fig. 23.2). This is particularly obvious in the skin creases of the palms (Fig. 23.3) and soles, in the flexures, in scars (Fig. 23.4), along the nails and on the buccal mucous membranes (Fig. 23.5) and gums. The patient may also note a failure to lose a summer tan in the winter months. The condition is caused by increased production of MSH and ACTH in response to hypoadrenalism. A similar hyperpigmentation occurs in Cushing's syndrome due to a basophil adenoma of the pituitary, or an ectopic source. A very striking hyperpigmentation occurs in Nelson's syndrome which arises after bilateral adrenalectomy for adrenal hyperplasia, when pituitary peptide production from a functioning chromophobe tumour is completely unopposed. Hyperpigmentation is also seen in chronic renal failure secondary to increased circulating levels of MSH which is normally degraded by the kidney. Oestrogens also appear to have some effect on melanogenesis and in pregnancy generalized hyperpigmentation is often noticed, particularly of the nipples, linea alba, axillae and genitalia.

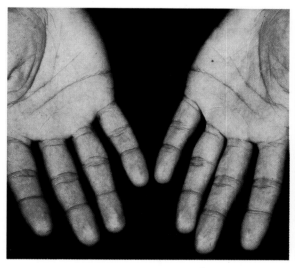 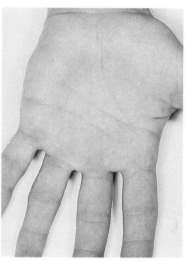 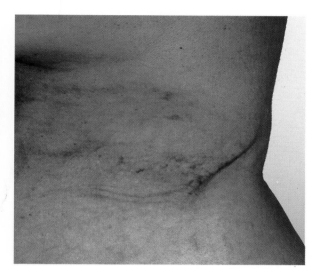

Fig. 23.3 Addison's disease. The palmar skin creases are hyperpigmented (left). This disappears with treatment (right). By courtesy of Dr. T. Cundy, King's College Hospital.

Fig. 23.4 Pigmented adrenalectomy scar. In Nelson's syndrome, the unopposed functioning pituitary tumour produces the same pigmentary anomalies as in Addison's disease. By courtesy of Dr. T. Cundy, King's College Hospital.

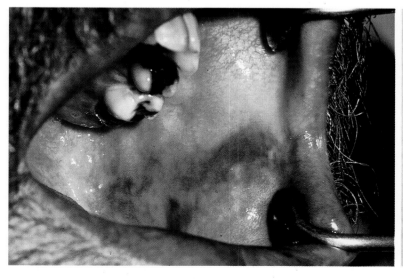 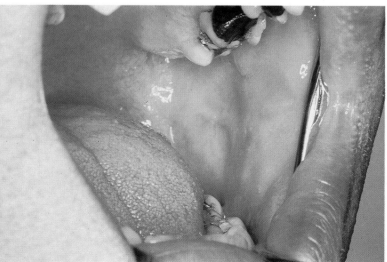

Fig. 23.5 Addison's disease. Pigmentation occurs on the buccal mucous membranes (left). This disappears with treatment (right). By courtesy of Dr. T. Cundy, King's College Hospital.

METABOLIC DISEASE. Hyperpigmentation is seen in any patient with wasting or cachexia, for example due to overwhelming tuberculosis, carcinomatosis or malabsorption. Nutritional disorders, and in particular vitamin B12 deficiency, can produce hyperpigmentation. Hyperpigmentation particularly in sun-exposed areas occurs in primary biliary cirrhosis and porphyria cutanea tarda (Fig. 23.6). In haemochromatosis a striking pigmentation occurs in the vast majority of cases. The pigmentation may be brown-black, bronze or blue-grey and the distribution is similar to that in Addison's disease with accentuation in the sun-exposed areas. The different shades are due to a combination of melanin deposition and haemosiderin. Haemochromatosis is a disorder of iron metabolism which leads to cirrhosis and diabetes mellitus, but frequently hyperpigmentation precedes overt manifestations of the other symptoms.

DRUG CAUSES. A number of drugs have been recorded as producing pigmentation of the skin. The better known of these is chloropromazine, which may cause a slate-grey discoloration, probably due to a metabolite which binds to melanin, although more commonly it produces hyperpigmentation secondary to its phototoxic effects. A number of drugs act in this way (Fig. 23.7). Busulphan produces a similar pigmentation to that seen in Addison's disease. Arsenic produces a raindrop pigment-

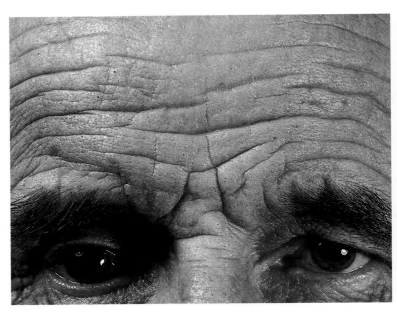

Fig. 23.6 Porphyria cutanea tarda. Hyperpigmentation may occur in solar exposed areas. Considerable solar elastosis has also resulted in furrowing of the skin.

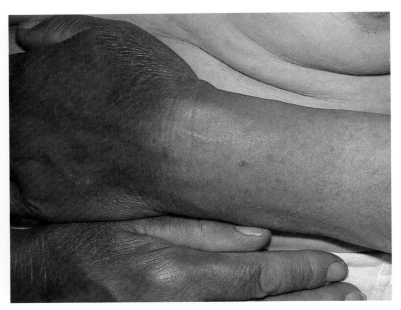

Fig. 23.7 Hyperpigmentation resulting from drugs. Moduretic may produce a phototoxic eruption. Erythema is present on the wrists and secondary hyperpigmentation on the hands.

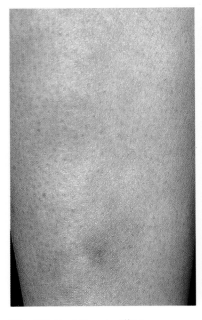

Fig. 23.8 Minocycline pigmentation. A focal blue discoloration may occur. By courtesy of St. John's Hospital for Diseases of the Skin.

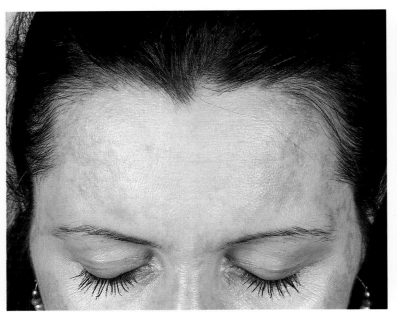

Fig. 23.9 Melasma. The forehead is a common site. This patient had received treatment for six years without success.

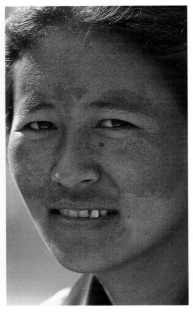

Fig. 23.10 Melasma. This is common in coloured skin. Ultra-violet light is the most common cause.

ation. Minocycline can produce a striking focal blue discoloration in the skin (Fig. 23.8). Topical nitrogen mustard produces hyperpigmentation. Argyria secondary to chronic ingestion of silver produces a blue-grey discoloration of the skin particularly in sun-exposed areas due to the deposition of silver.

Localized Hyperpigmentation

MELASMA. This is a common condition resulting from melanin deposition in the skin of the face. Various degrees and shades of patchy pigmentation occur on the forehead (Fig. 23.9), cheeks, upper lip, nose and chin. The condition is more common in women and certainly pregnancy and the oral contraceptive pill are factors in its aetiology. Once pigmentation has occurred it may or may not disappear with parturition or discontinuing the contraceptive. Although oestrogens are thought to be partly responsible, the condition does occur in men, particularly those with darker skins who live in sunny climates.

All patients note that the disease becomes worse in the sun (Fig. 23.10). Treatment is unsatisfactory but hinges on fastidious use of sun screens and physical avoidance of ultra-violet light irradiation with the concomitant use of hypopigmenting creams containing hydroquinone. Even with these measures the condition may persist indefinitely.

Post-Inflammatory Hyperpigmentation

This is probably the most common cause of increased pigmentation locally in the skin. It is much more common in dark skins and constitutes a problem because it can be many years before the hyperpigmentation fades, if at all. Any inflammatory disease is capable of producing pigmentary disorders including *acne*, *eczema* and *psoriasis*. The cause of the hyperpigmentation may be difficult to detect. The description of the preceding eruption, the distribution and morphology of the pigmentation are all of the utmost importance. *Lichen planus* in particular almost always produces hyperpigmentation in whatever race. It is quite striking and may be persistent. The diagnosis can be suspected because the patient may admit to a preceding pruritic eruption and the pigmentation is found in the sites usually affected by lichen planus (Fig. 23.11).

FIXED DRUG ERUPTION. The patient may admit to episodic inflammation in the site of the pigmentation (Fig. 23.12).

PITYRIASIS ROSEA. The pigmentation is predominantly of the trunk (Fig. 23.13) and the site of the herald patch may be discernible.

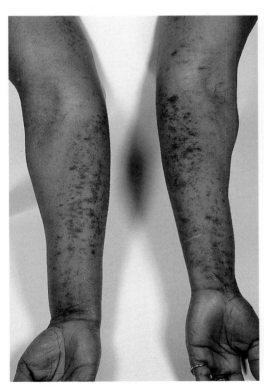

Fig. 23.11 Post-inflammatory hyperpigmentation (lichen planus). The pigmented lesions are symmetrical and occur in the same distribution as lichen planus. The flexor surface of the arms and wrists is a common site.

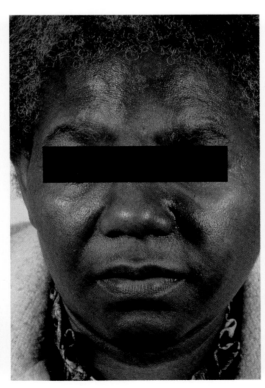

Fig. 23.12 Fixed drug eruption. This patient has been taking laxatives containing phenolphthalein. A persistent hyperpigmentation on the face followed recurrent attacks of erythema and oedema.

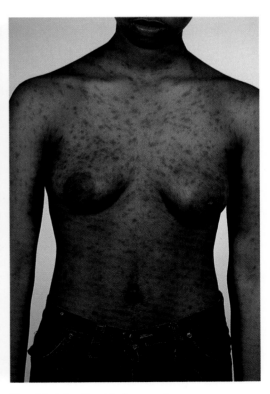

Fig. 23.13 Post-inflammatory pigmentation (pityriasis rosea). The eruption was confined to the trunk and upper arms. The lesions are oval and pityriasis rosea was the most likely cause.

PHYTOPHOTODERMATITIS. Pigmentation (Fig. 23.14) follows the inflammatory reaction between ultra-violet light and psoralen producing plants. The patient may not appreciate the connection.

ERYTHEMA DYSCHROMICUM PERSTANS (ASHY DERMATITIS). This is an unusual but striking, presumably post-inflammatory, hyper-pigmentation of the skin. The eruption consists of symmetrically placed, often figurate ashen-coloured patches varying from a few millimetres to a number of centimetres in diameter (Fig. 23.15). It occurs particularly over the trunk and is seen in patients with coloured skins. It tends to be persistent. The cause is unknown. The diagnosis is suspected after known causes of post-inflammatory pigmentation have been excluded.

POIKILODERMA OF CIVATTE. This is a common condition particularly of adult women. There is a mottled pigmentation sometimes with atrophy and telangiectasia of the sides of the neck (Fig. 23.16). It is thought to be due to a combined effect of ultra-violet light irradiation and photosensitizing chemicals present in perfumes which have been applied to the skin. It occasionally occurs on the face. There is no specific treatment but avoidance of perfumes and photo-protection are advocated.

Disorders of Hypopigmentation
Generalized Hypopigmentation

HYPOPITUITARISM. Deficiency of pituitary trophic hormones results in gonadal failure followed by hypothyroidism and eventually by adrenal insufficiency. The effects on the skin are seen as sparseness of body hair and males will note that the need to shave becomes much reduced. The skin is soft, wrinkled and pale. The colour is due in part to hypopigmentation secondary to MSH deficiency and partly to the anaemia which accompanies the disease.

ALBINISM. There are various types of this disorder which are inherited on an autosomal recessive basis and are due to a failure of melanocytes (which are present) to produce melanin. It is a disorder of non-functioning or absent tyrosinase. This effects the skin, hair (Fig. 23.17) and eyes. In complete types of failure the skin is milk white, the hair is pale blonde and the iris is translucent. Such individuals burn in the sun and are at risk from the development of squamous cell carcinoma of the skin. The disease is thus a disaster in coloured races in non-temperate climates. The eyes are pale pink due to the translucent iris and patients suffer from photophobia, nystagmus and poor vision. Photo-protection, regular surveillance of the skin for malignant change and ophthalmic care are necessary. The *Chediak-Higashi syndrome* is a variety of oculocutaneous albinism often found in cases of consanguinity. It is associated with recurrent staphylococcal and streptococcal infections and neurological and haemotological complications such as anaemia, neutropenia and thrombocytopenia. It commences in childhood and is ultimately fatal. Lymphoma may develop.

Phenylketonuria

This is an autosomal recessive disorder of metabolism due to a deficiency of phenylalanine hydroxylase which is responsible for the conversion of phenylalanine to tyrosine. This results in an accumulation of phenylketones which are toxic to cerebral neurones and cause mental retardation and neurological abnormalities if untreated. The disorder is diagnosed by routine testing of the urine of all neonates. The condition is treated by restricting the dietary intake of phenylalanine. The cutaneous changes are of pigmentary dilution of the skin, hair and eyes.

23.6

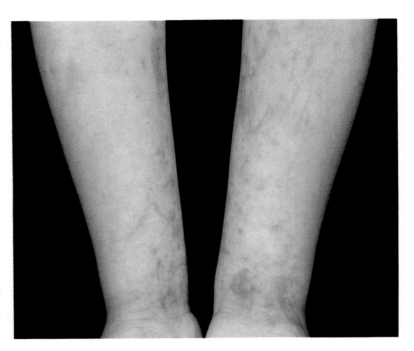

Fig. 23.14   Phytophotodermatitis. Interaction between ultra-violet light and psoralen producing plants causes streaky hyperpigmentation. By courtesy of St. John's Hospital for Diseases of the Skin.

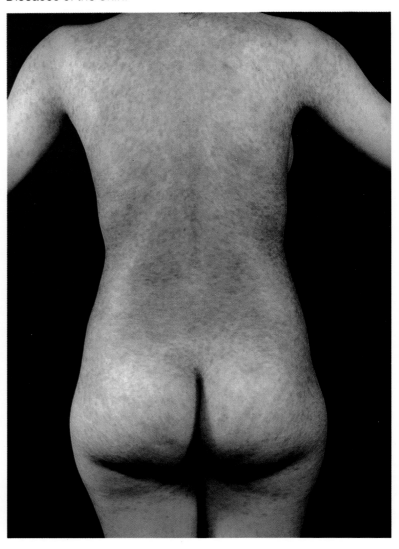

Fig. 23.15   Ashy dermatitis. The patches are ash grey in colour and may become confluent. The trunk is especially affected. Ashy dermatitis is more common in pigmented individuals. The cause is unknown. By courtesy of Professor E. Wilson-Jones, The Institute of Dermatology.

The affected individuals are therefore fair, have blonde hair and blue eyes, although there are exceptions to this. The affected individuals have poor tolerance of sunshine as a result of the failure to be able to produce melanin. The consequences of this inborn error of metabolism are entirely preventable.

Piebaldism

This is an autosomal dominant inherited condition resulting from a failure of the migration of melanoblasts to the skin from the neural crest or a failure of proper differentiation of melanocytes from melanoblasts. The condition results in vitiligo-like hypomelanotic macules with hypermelanotic macules within them, occurring in a certain distribution associated with a white forelock of hair known as poliosis. The hypomelanotic macules occur in a characteristic distribution and are thus seen on the mid-upper arms to the wrists, mid-thighs to the mid-calves (Fig. 23.18) and back. The condition is present at birth. The patients are usually otherwise perfectly healthy.

Localized Disorders of Hypopigmentation
Vitiligo

This is a common disorder which can be of devastating social significance particularly in coloured peoples. It is an acquired loss of melanocytes which are absent histologically. It can occur at any age (Fig. 23.19). Occasionally there is a family history of the disorder. There is an association with organ specific auto-immune disorders such as thyroiditis and Addisonian adrenal insufficiency and it is therefore thought to be due to an auto-immune destruction of melanocytes.

The condition is usually but not always symmetrical. Patches are sharply demarcated with irregular borders (Fig. 23.20) and the margins are sometimes hyperpigmented. The lesions are depigmented and therefore have a chalk-white coloration. The condition particularly affects the flexures, the backs of the hands, face, around orifices (Fig. 23.21) and over bony prominences. The condition can vary from mild to extensive or even universal involvement. The skin itself feels and appears normal,

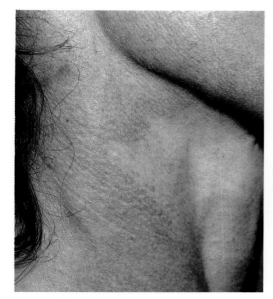

Fig. 23.16 Poikiloderma of Civatte. A reticulate pigmentation, atrophy and telangiectasia occurs most commonly in women on the side of the neck. The condition is thought to result from an interaction between photosensitizers in cosmetics and ultra-violet light.

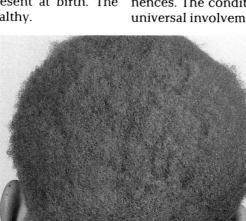

Fig. 23.17 Albinism. The skin is almost white and the hair is flaxen yellow due to absent or non-functioning tyrosinase.

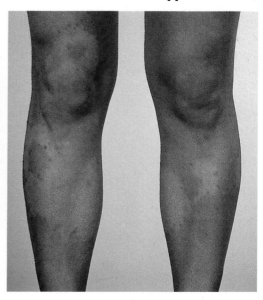

Fig. 23.18 Piebaldism. Hypermelanotic macules occur within hypomelanotic patches on the upper regions of the shins.

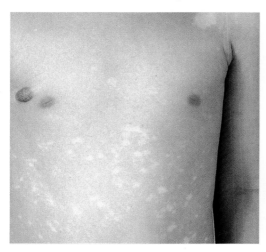

Fig. 23.19 Vitiligo. This condition may commence at any age. It is less noticeable on pale skins.

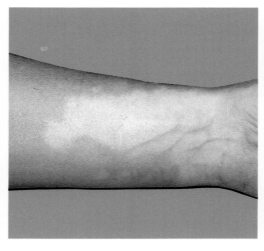

Fig. 23.20 Vitiligo. The lesions are sharply demarcated with irregular borders and have a chalk white coloration.

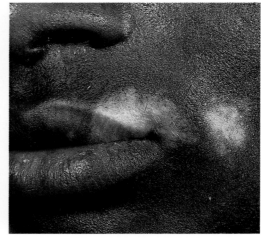

Fig. 23.21 Vitiligo. The condition can be disfiguring.

other than the loss of pigment. Spontaneous repigmentation does occur, particularly in a patchy manner and especially in coloured races (Fig. 23.22). The repigmentation is derived from melanocytes which migrate from the hair follicles. Clinically this produces a stippled appearance and the pigmentation can be seen surrounding hair follicles. Hair in vitiliginous areas of skin grows white (Fig. 23.23). Vitiligo may be associated with alopecia areata (Fig. 23.24). Burning of the vitiliginous patches (Fig. 23.25) will occur in the sun but the incidence of malignant change is surprisingly low.

A variant of this disorder is the so-called halo naevus (see Fig. 5.63) as described by Sutton. This is vitiligo occurring around a junctional naevus and will result in complete removal of the naevus followed by repigmentation. It is of interest that antibodies to melanocytes can be demonstrated in such patients.

Treatments of vitiligo are unsatisfactory. The stigma associated with the condition in many societies produces demand for advice. Spontaneous repigmentation does occasionally occur in pigmented races. Topical steroids are sometimes effective. Photosensitizing agents such as trimethylpsoralens taken orally or topically followed by exposure to ultra-violet irradiation may be of benefit. Natural sunlight is more effective than artificial long wave light sources. Vitiligo of the mucous membranes or extremities does not respond well to this treatment. Dihydroxyacetone can be used as a dye to stain the skin and thus disguise the white patches, but this does not have a very high patient acceptance. Patients can be taught how to camouflage the skin with Covermark cosmetics. Prevention of tanning of the surrounding skin by the use of sun screens and the avoidance of exposure to ultra-violet sunlight is helpful in the Caucasian, since it is more noticeable in the tanned individual and less so in the natural state. Very occasionally, if vitiligo is extensive, depigmentation of the remaining normal skin may be tried with twenty percent hydroquinone.

Post-inflammatory Hypopigmentation

Post-inflammatory hypopigmentation of the skin is an end-result and if there are no active lesions present it is a question of deducing what condition gave rise to the hypopigmentation. A description of the eruption from the patient and the distribution of the eruption on examination may aid diagnosis. Hypopigmentation of the skin, whilst occurring in Caucasians, is a much more common problem in pigmented races.

PITYRIASIS ALBA. Pale, but not white, patches occur solely on the faces of children (Fig. 23.26) and young adolescents. It is extremely common in coloured races.

PITYRIASIS VERSICOLOR. This is regularly confused with vitiligo. However, the condition is largely seen on the trunk (Fig. 23.27), the lesions are asymmetrical and of various shapes and sizes, and not chalk-white as in vitiligo (Fig. 23.28). The condition occurs in both white and black skins and is due to a temporary paralysis of melanocyte function due to a product of the fungus *Malassezia furfur*.

HYPOPIGMENTED ECZEMA. Discoid eczema in young people may be confused with pityriasis versicolor, but hypopigmentation is usually seen on the limbs (Fig. 23.29) and frequently active areas of eczema are also present. Scrapings from these areas will be negative for fungus unlike pityriasis versicolor.

DISCOID LUPUS ERYTHEMATOSUS. This may produce hypopigmentation in the skin often with concomitant scarring (see Fig. 18.9). This eruption is particularly seen on light-exposed areas and in particular on the face.

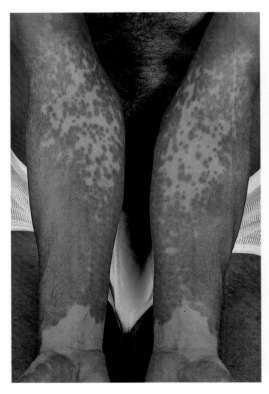

Fig. 23.22 Vitiligo. Repigmentation may occur in coloured races, but is not usually complete. Vitiligo is usually symmetrical.

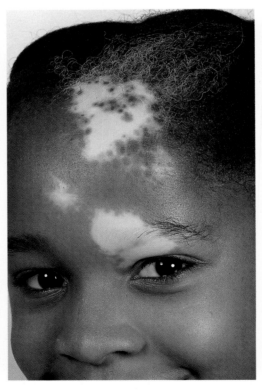

Fig. 23.23 Vitiligo. The hair in affected areas is white.

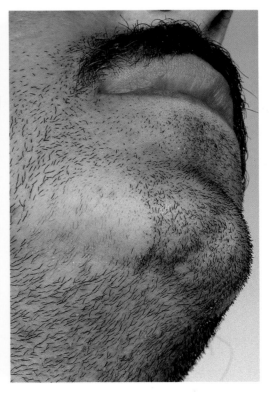

Fig. 23.24 Vitiligo and alopecia areata. The skin is white in the patch of alopecia. Both disorders are thought to have auto-immune involvement.

IDIOPATHIC GUTTATE HYPOMELANOSIS. This is a common condition consisting of well-circumscribed, small white macules on the skin of sun-exposed areas other than the face (Fig. 23.30). It is usually seen in sun-damaged Caucasians but it does also occur in pigmented races. The lesions are frequently seen on the anterior surfaces of lower legs and also on the arms and occasionally the abdomen. Although common, they are seldom of concern to the patient, but they are an indication of solar damage.

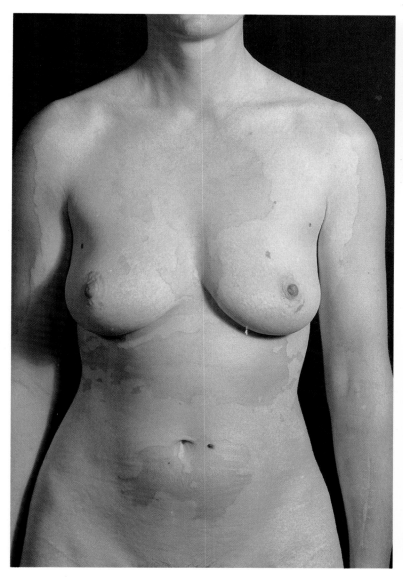

Fig. 23.25   Vitiligo. As a result of the lack of melanocytes, the patient will burn readily in the sun. This patient was undergoing treatment with psoralens and ultra-violet light. By courtesy of St. Mary's Hospital.

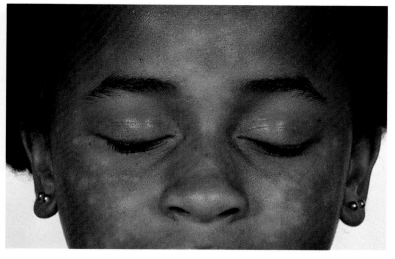

Fig. 23.26   Pityriasis alba. Scattered hypopigmented but not depigmented patches occur on the faces of young children or adolescents. The condition ultimately resolves.

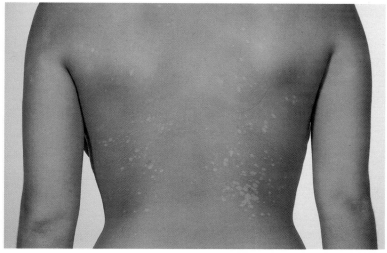

Fig. 23.27   Pityriasis versicolor. Scattered hypopigmented macules of various shapes and sizes occur asymmetrically on the trunk.

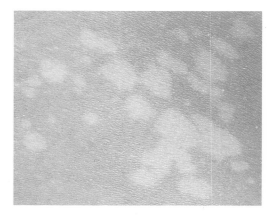

Fig. 23.28   Pityriasis versicolor. This is a close-up of Fig. 23.27. The lesions are hypopigmented (off-white) not depigmented (white), as in vitiligo.

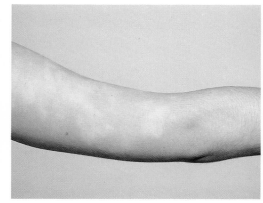

Fig. 23.29   Hypopigmented eczema. Discoid eczema in young adults may leave post-inflammatory hypopigmentation. The limbs are commonly affected.

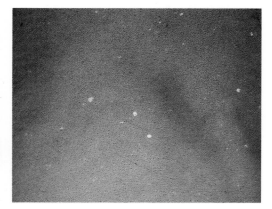

Fig. 23.30   Idiopathic guttate hypomelanosis. Well-circumscribed white macules occur particularly on the lower legs. They may be induced by too much solar exposure.

NON-MELANIN PIGMENTARY DISORDERS OF THE SKIN

Jaundice is the most common non-melanin pigmentation of the skin and is caused by the deposition of bile pigments in the skin and sclerae. The pigmentation of haemochromatosis is partly due to melanin but also to iron deposition in the skin. Localized deposition of iron is common as a result of stasis eczema and ulceration of the lower legs and is due to haemosiderin deposition following extravasation of red blood cells. Haemosiderin is also deposited in the skin of the lower limbs in various conditions due to capillaritis.

Carotenaemia

Carotene is a naturally occurring pigment of the skin which can produce a disproportionate orange discoloration of keratin in individuals who eat a large number of carrots or oranges. The yellow pigmentation is particularly obvious in the palms (Fig. 23.31) and soles. A similar discoloration occurs in patients receiving oral carotene in the treatment of erythropoietic protoporphyria. The skin also appears yellow in hypothyroidism, nephritis and diabetes.

Ochronosis (Alkaptonuria)

This is a rare recessive inborn error of metabolism. The patients lack homogentisic acid oxidase so that a polymer of this acid accumulates as a dark pigment in the urine and connective tissue. The pigmentation is a blue or blue-grey colour and is most visible when the skin overlying cartilage or tendons is thin. Thus it is noticeable over the pinnae (Fig. 23.32), tip of the nose, costochondral junctions and extensor tendons of the hands. Since the pigment is excreted in sweat, those areas well supplied with sweat glands, such as the axillae and genital areas, may be pigmented and the underclothing may be stained. The most important consequence of this disease is the development of a disabling arthritis. Treatment at the present time is unsatisfactory.

Ochronosis occurs in coloured people who use high concentrations of hydroquinone to lighten their skin. An arthropathy does not occur.

Exogenous Causes

Mepacrine, an anti-malarial drug, causes yellow discoloration of the skin. Silver, usually ingested only in those working with the metal, may be deposited in the skin producing a slate-blue discoloration; this is particularly accentuated in sun-exposed areas. Gold very rarely produces a blue-grey discoloration when given parenterally. Exogenous pigments (Fig. 23.33) may become imbedded in the skin during tattooing or as coal dust in miners. Various chemicals stain the skin temporarily, e.g. iodine, dihydroxyacetone, dithranol and potassium permanganate.

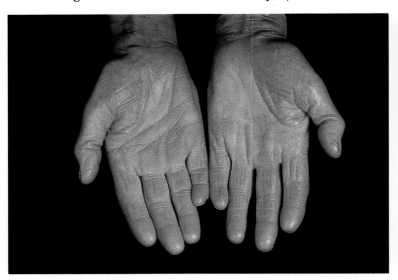

Fig. 23.31 Carotenaemia. A yellow discoloration of the skin occurs. The palms are particularly affected. By courtesy of St. John's Hospital for Diseases of the Skin.

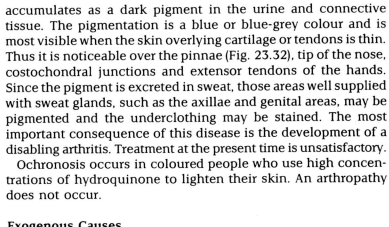

Fig. 23.32 Ochronosis. Blue-grey pigmentation is visible over the pinna. By courtesy of St. Mary's Hospital.

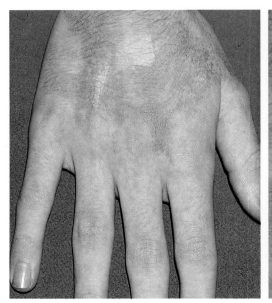
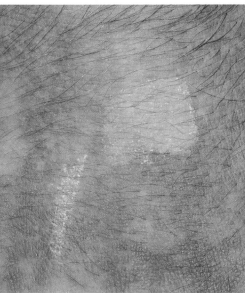

Fig. 23.33 Exogenous pigment. This adolescent complained of pigmentation on the hand (left). The dirt was easily scraped away to reveal normal skin underneath (right).

24 Psychological Disorders
of the Skin

Most skin disorders cause some psychological suffering to the patient, largely because they are so clearly visible. Some patients feel that they may be ostracized, particularly those with psoriasis. Others feel embarrassed, for example those with too much or too little hair. To the doctor accustomed to more serious complaints, these imperfections may seem trifling and may be dismissed as cosmetic, but the patient's anguish persists. The degree of involvement of the skin is no guide to the degree of unhappiness. Mild acne vulgaris or psoriasis may be devastating to one patient, whereas severe disease may apparently be well tolerated by another. Undoubtedly the symptoms of the skin disease, particularly pruritus, may be extremely disturbing emotionally to the patient. Anyone who has questioned a patient who is suffering from scabies will know the profound effect the irritation may have on their tranquility.

Although some authorities seek to deny it, significant life events probably do influence the development or exacerbation of skin disease in many cases. All dermatologists are familiar with compelling histories which are difficult to discount and

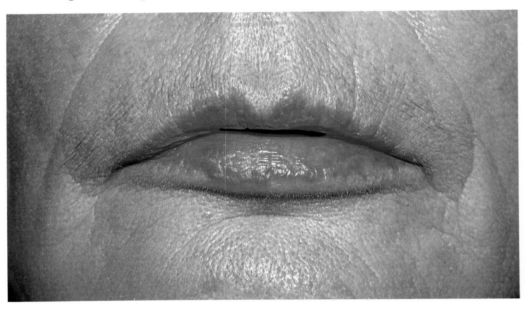

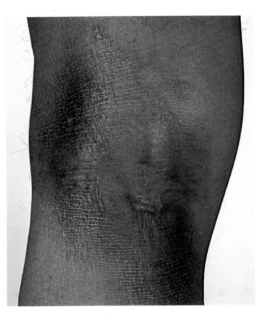

Fig. 24.1 Dermatological non-disease. This lady complained bitterly about her sore lips and mouth but there were never any abnormal physical signs on examination. She was depressed and her symptoms resolved within a few weeks of therapy.

Fig. 24.2 Lichen simplex. The skin creases are very prominent from continual rubbing. The plaque is well-defined.

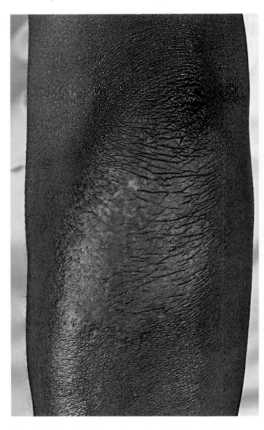

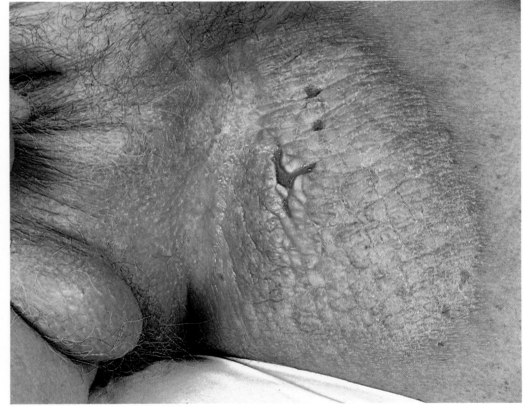

Fig. 24.3 Lichen simplex. Lichenification of the extensor surface of the forearm below the elbow is a common site.

Fig. 24.4 Lichen simplex. Lichenification (thickening of the skin and prominent skin creases) is present on the inner upper thigh.

certainly patients are not sceptical about their influence. In particular, alopecia areata, atopic eczema, pompholyx, psoriasis and herpes simplex may be exacerbated by stress. On the other hand, these disorders do not respond to psychiatric drugs or psychological techniques other than those of a basic supportive nature and active dermatological therapy is singularly more impressive in most cases.

Perhaps the greatest advantage the dermatologist has over colleagues in other specialities is that the skin is readily accessible for examination. If a patient makes a complaint referring to the skin and no abnormality is found, it is likely that the symptom has a psychological origin. The most common complaints are itchy eyelids, sore mouth (Fig. 24.1) and symptoms involving the genitalia. Patients with itchy eyelids are usually women. They have often consulted several doctors including ophthalmologists and are told that there is nothing wrong but they are usually given a cream. Examination is totally unrevealing but specific enquiry reveals anxiety or depression. Similarly, patients complain of a sore mouth and often tingling or burning of the tip of the tongue. They consult dentists and general physicians and often have extensive investigations but there are no abnormal physical signs on examination and the patient is usually depressed. Anti-depressants may be very effective.

In men, soreness and redness of the penis is a common complaint. Examination may reveal minimal erythema but nothing else. The condition often indicates marital disharmony or sexual guilt and counselling is required. In a similar manner, skin cancerophobia and venereophobia can be readily recognized without extensive investigation because of the lack of physical signs and the underlying depression can be diagnosed and treated.

LICHEN SIMPLEX (Localized Neurodermatitis)

This is a common, extremely itchy condition which is readily recognizable and in the main amenable to therapy, although chronic cases undoubtedly occur. The eruption consists of a well-defined lichenified plaque, usually on one side of the body corresponding to the handedness of the patient. Lichenification is a response of the skin to continuous rubbing or scratching. It is seen classically in atopic eczema, which is a pruritic skin disorder but can be induced in any skin by constant friction. The skin is thickened and the skin creases are very prominent (Fig. 24.2). These well-defined patches are seen particularly on the nape of the neck, the eyelid, just below the elbow (Fig. 24.3), on the extensor surface of the forearm, on the back of the hand, on the upper inner thigh (Fig. 24.4), on the outer aspect of the ankle or calf, around the natal cleft, and on the labium majorum (Fig. 24.5) or scrotum (Fig. 24.6). The unilateral nature of the eruption should arouse suspicion of the diagnosis. In a minority of patients, widespread patches of lichen simplex can occur. On the lower legs (Fig. 24.7) these may be difficult to distinguish from hypertrophic lichen planus and a biopsy may be necessary. These lesions tend to be persistent and the condition is then known as *lichen simplex chronicus*.

The lesion is not a sign of deep psychological disturbance but often is initiated during a period of stress. It persists, however, even though the stress has been removed, because the lichenified skin is intensely pruritic in its own right. Treating the skin with a powerful corticosteroid such as clobetasol propionate ointment with exhortations not to scratch the area coupled with oral antihistamines will affect a cure in the majority of patients. Counselling is necessary if the cause is still present. Lichen simplex chronicus responds poorly to treatment, however, since it is a result of chronic neurosis.

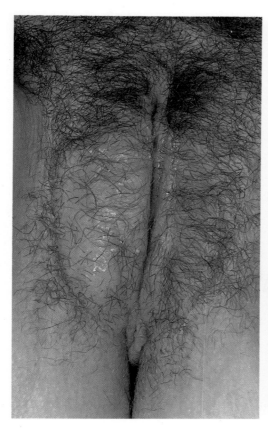

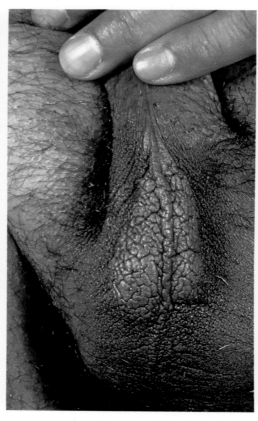

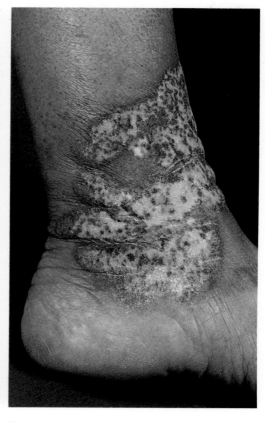

Fig. 24.5   Lichen simplex. The eruption is well-defined, unilateral and lichenified on the labium majorum.

Fig. 24.6   Lichen simplex. Continual rubbing of the skin results in lichenification. The lesion is well-defined. The skin is thickened and the skin creases are accentuated.

Fig. 24.7   Lichen simplex chronicus. Lichen simplex responds to powerful topical steroids, especially under occlusion but in some patients the condition tends to relapse and is chronic.

PRURIGO

This is a chronic disorder of the skin, characterized by generalized pruritus and widespread excoriation, largely on the limbs and upper back. The small of the back is spared because most patients are unable to reach it successfully to scratch. Excoriations (Figs. 24.8 and 24.9) with minor degrees of fresh haemorrhage in recent lesions, or surrounded by hyperpigmentation in long-standing lesions, are characteristic of this condition. In some patients, actual nodules (Fig. 24.10) develop as a result of the chronic scratching (nodular prurigo).

The diagnosis is one of exclusion, for it is extremely important that all the causes of generalized pruritus are searched for and eliminated. The patients admit that they scratch the skin, but the condition does not respond to psychotherapy or psychotropic drugs and it may yet be that a specific cause will be found. Treatment of this condition is extremely difficult, although topical steroids under occlusive bandages are of temporary benefit, particularly in hospital. Injection of the nodules with steroids can also be of benefit.

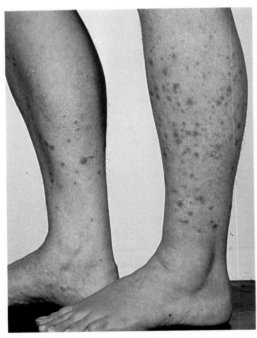

Fig. 24.8 Prurigo. Widespread excoriations occur in the absence of any cutaneous or systemic explanation.

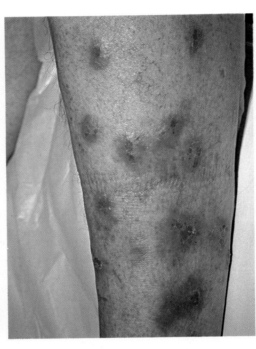

Fig. 24.9 Prurigo. In long-standing cases the skin becomes thickened as well as excoriated.

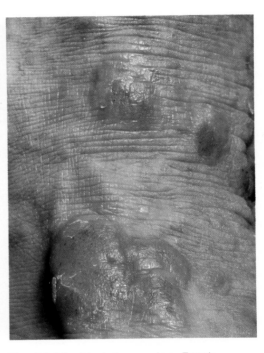

Fig. 24.10 Nodular prurigo. Frank nodules may result from chronic scratching of the skin.

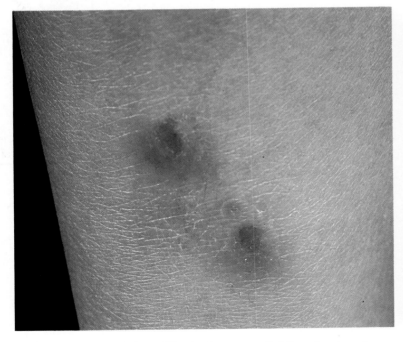

Fig. 24.11 Excoriations. The lesions are slightly raised and fresh haemorrhage is visible on the surface. By courtesy of St. John's Hospital for Diseases of the Skin.

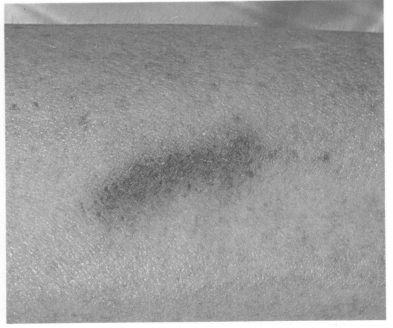

Fig. 24.12 Neurotic excoriation. This lady developed one or two linear excoriations on her arm over a few months. She had insight into the cause of her anxieties and the lesions resolved with simple psychotherapy.

NEUROTIC EXCORIATIONS

This condition is of a more acute nature and is short-lived once the precipitating cause has been identified and rectified. The patient complains of generalized itching and fresh excoriations (Figs. 24.11–13) are found on the limbs and upper back. It is clearly important to exclude a pruritic skin disorder or a systemic reason for itching. The condition is usually a reaction to unsatisfactory circumstances either at home or at work. Occlusive bandages are helpful.

ACNE EXCORIEE DES JEUNES FILLES

This is a common disorder confined to women. It commences

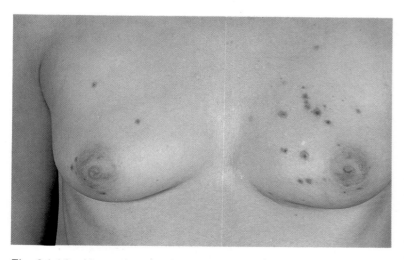

Fig. 24.13 Neurotic excoriations. In this case scratch marks were limited to the breasts. The patient accepted psychiatric help and her anxieties were successfully treated. By courtesy of St. Mary's Hospital.

during early adult life on the face. Some authorities doubt whether acne is present at all, but the patients believe that they can see spots and deal with them by mechanically interfering with them, usually by squeezing or picking. The physical signs therefore are of excoriations on the face which tend to leave post-inflammatory pigmentation and scarring (Fig. 24.14). Although the patients freely admit that they do pick at their skin, it is extremely difficult to convince them that this is detrimental to their skin and to break the habit. The psychological disturbance is not gross but the neurosis is chronic and may represent an immature personality with the lesions becoming a protective excuse for the inadequacies of their lives. This condition is chronic and does not respond to psychological help. Treatment with oral antibiotics as for acne vulgaris is not very helpful.

PRURITUS ANI AND VULVAE

Both these localized forms of itching are common. The diagnosis is made on examination by the absence of physical signs. The condition tends to wax and wane in intensity. The patients with pruritus ani are often introspective, obsessional and mildly hypochondriacal. Women with pruritus vulvae may have marital problems. Pruritus ani is chronic and does not respond well to any treatment. By the time the patient is referred to the specialist, he or she will have compiled a sizeable list of unsuccessful topical remedies. Sometimes patients become sensitized to one of the topical medications they have been using and a dermatitis (Fig. 24.15) results (*dermatitis medicamentosa*). Frequent causes of sensitization are preparations containing topical anaesthetics and antibiotics. The condition responds to identification of the allergens by patch testing and topical steroids.

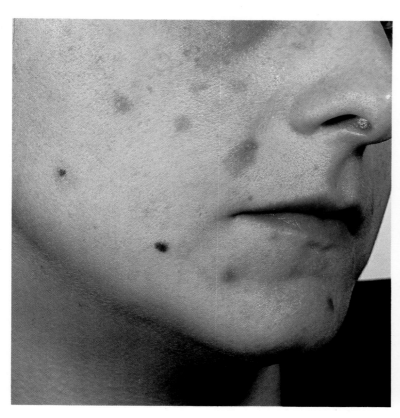

Fig. 24.14 Acne excoriée des jeunes filles. This woman picks at her skin and produces excoriations which result in unsightly post-inflammatory pigmentation.

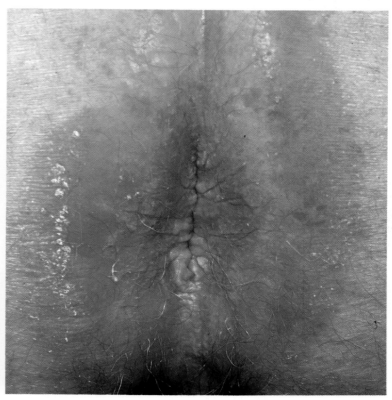

Fig. 24.15 Dermatitis medicamentosa. There are no abnormal physical signs in pruritus ani but a dermatitis may result from sensitization to a topical medicament such as a local anaesthetic or antibiotic. By courtesy of St. John's Hospital for Diseases of the Skin.

TRICHOTILLOMANIA

This is a disorder of young children and presents as a loss of hair, resulting from a habit of twisting or pulling the hairs of the scalp. It may be likened to nail biting and is a form of habit tic. There is usually an asymmetrical patch of partial hair loss (Fig. 24.16) corresponding to the handedness of the patient and the hairs are broken off at different levels (see Fig. 22.29). It is not of deep psychological significance, and in the majority of patients the condition resolves with time. However, occasionally the disorder is seen in the mentally disturbed (Fig. 24.17) and then the prognosis is poor. It is important to exclude the common disorders of hair loss in children which are alopecia areata and tinea capitis. In the former, there is complete loss of hair in the patch involved and the scalp looks completely normal. In the latter, there are inflammatory changes to be seen on the scalp in addition to the loss of hair.

DELUSIONAL PARASITOPHOBIA

This is a condition almost solely of middle-aged or elderly women. The patients are truly deluded in that they tenaciously hold the belief that they are infested and they remain unconvinced even though medical examination of their clothing and skin refutes the point. By the time they reach the specialist, they have been told by one or several doctors that they are not infested and they have usually changed doctors as a result. They often have called in the public health authorities to fumigate their lodgings and they will bring specimens to the consultation to prove the infestation. These specimens are usually scales of skin not parasites. The parasitophobia is usually the only delusion and management centres around colluding with the patient whilst urging them to take oral medication to eliminate the 'parasites' from within. The psychotropic drug pimozide can be extremely helpful in this respect. In a significant number of patients the delusion will pass, but other patients are singularly difficult to help. The suggestion of referral to the department of psychological medicine is usually greeted with antagonism.

DERMATITIS ARTEFACTA

This is rare and indicates deep psychological disturbance. The patient totally denies that he or she is responsible for the destructive lesions of the skin (Fig. 24.18) and indeed confrontation to this effect results in the patient seeking help elsewhere. The diagnosis is suggested because the cutaneous physical signs do not conform to those of a recognized skin disease. The face (Fig. 24.19) and hands (exposed sites) are usually affected. In particular the lesions tend to be of bizarre shapes, for example linear or rectangular (Fig. 24.20).

Various methods are used to produce the lesions from the application of caustics (if these are used inexpertly signs of trickling of the fluid may be seen) to some form of instrumentation (Fig. 24.21). Elucidation of the reasons for the artefact may be possible in some cases and then the prognosis for recovery is quite good (Figs. 24.22 and 24.23), but in the majority this is a disastrous condition to manage. It does not respond to psychotropic drugs or to psychiatric referral. Indeed the patient will reject the latter. If the manifestation is on a part of the body which can be occluded, for example with plaster of Paris, the skin will rapidly heal but inevitably break down when the patient is able to interfere with it once more. However, this manoeuvre will help to confirm the diagnosis. The condition is largely confined to females and the nursing profession has a higher incidence. The patients show an indifference to the unsightliness of the damage to the skin and some have other hysterical symptoms, whereas others have more deep, psychological disturbances.

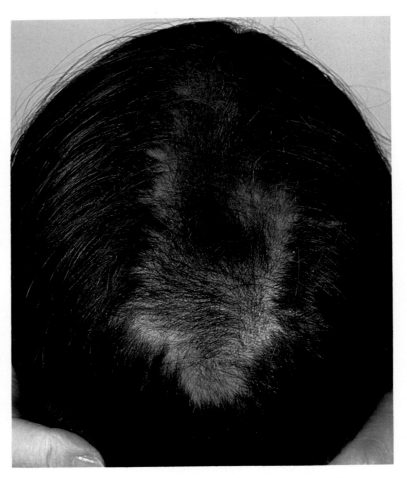

Fig. 24.16 Trichotillomania. The loss of hair is partial and is usually linear to the side of the scalp.

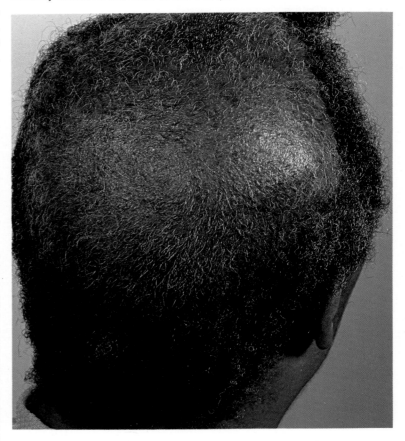

Fig. 24.17 Trichotillomania. This disturbed lady had broken off most of the hairs on the back and the top of the scalp. The hair on the front of the scalp is intact.

24.6

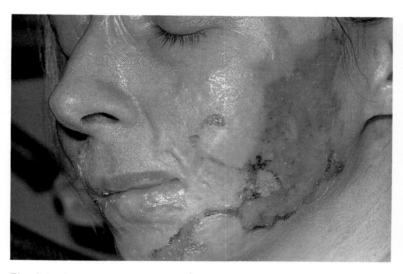

Fig. 24.18 Dermatitis artefacta. There is a bizarre-shaped area of ulceration of the face with scarring from previous lesions. This degree of self-mutilation has a poor prognosis. The patient had already seen four dermatologists and a psychiatrist and subsequently visited several more.

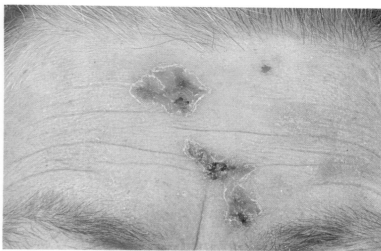

Fig. 24.19 Dermatitis artefacta. The excoriations are of various shapes and do not conform to a recognized intrinsic skin disorder.

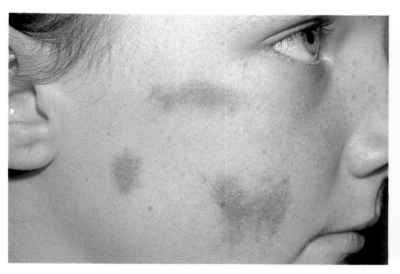

Fig. 24.20 Dermatitis artefacta. Linear excoriations present a bizarre rectangular pattern.

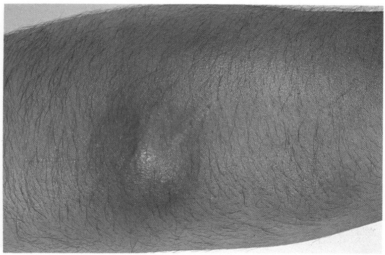

Fig. 24.21 Dermatitis artefacta. This woman developed many lesions simulating boils, but swabs were negative for bacterial infection. The lesions were secondary to injections of an unidentified foreign material.

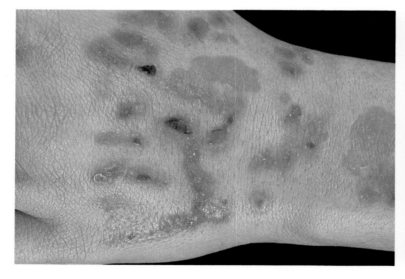

Fig. 24.22 Dermatitis artefacta. Linear excoriations were present on the back of this hand only, with no cutaneous abnormalities elsewhere. This girl did recover after her troubles with her boyfriend had been resolved. By courtesy of St. John's Hospital for Diseases of the Skin.

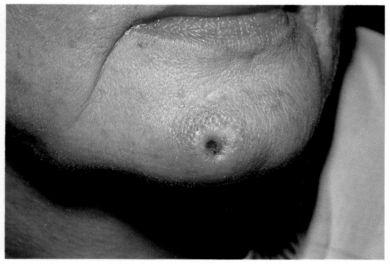

Fig. 24.23 Dermatitis artefacta. This ulcer was eventually believed to be self-induced. Biopsies and X-ray of the jaw were negative. It healed when the cause of the patient's anxiety was discovered. She had a carcinoma of the bowel, the symptoms of which she suspected but had been afraid to reveal.

Index